The Economics of Health and Medical Care

OTHER INTERNATIONAL ECONOMIC ASSOCIATION PUBLICATIONS

The Economics of Health and Medical Care)

Proceedings of a Conference held by the
International Economic Association at
Tokyo

EDITED BY
MARK PERLMAN

A HALSTED PRESS BOOK

JOHN WILEY & SONS
New York – Toronto

First published in the United Kingdom 1974 by
THE MACMILLAN PRESS LTD

*Published in the U.S.A. and
Canada by Halsted Press, a
Division of John Wiley & Sons, Inc.,
New York*

Library of Congress Cataloging in Publication Data

Conference on Economics of Health and Medical Care,
 Tokyo, 1973.
The economics of health and medical care.

"A Halsted Press book."
 1. Medical economics—Congresses. I. Perlman,
Mark, ed. II. International Economic Association.
III. Title. [DNLM: 1. Economics, Medical—Congresses.
2. Public health administration—Congresses. WA540
E19 1973]
RA410.A1C6 1973   338.4'7'3621   73–20107
ISBN 0–470–68051–2

Printed in Great Britain

Contents

Acknowledgments

There are many to be thanked.

The Program Committee, which in the I.E.A. tradition is the intellectually critical one, had five active members: Professor Martin Feldstein (Harvard University, U.S.A.), Mr Michael Kaser (Oxford University, U.K.), Professor Shigeto Tsuru (Hitotsubashi University, Japan), Professor Hirofumi Uzawa (Tokyo University, Japan), and the undersigned (University of Pittsburgh, U.S.A.), who with Professor Tsuru served as co-chairman.

Professor Tsuru had a superb Conference Secretariat. It was headed by Mr Denzo Izumi, who was assisted by Mrs Teruko Morikawa, Mr Kenji Miyamoto and others.

There was generous financial support from several Tokyo businessmen and newspapers, thus enabling the International Economic Association to cover most of the travel expenses of non-Japanese participants.

The copy-editing was done by Dr Ruth Bilgrey Waxman. The checking of all mathematical equations was the work of Professor Asatoshi Maeshiro of the University of Pittsburgh.

Professors Fritz Machlup, Luc Fauvel and Austin Robinson (respectively President, Secretary and Series Editor) and Miss Mary Crook, all of the International Economic Association, were present at the Conference and played key roles in expediting the publication of the book.

MARK PERLMAN

Pittsburgh, Pennsylvania, U.S.A.
July 1973

List of Participants

Professor A. B. Atkinson, University of Essex, Colchester, U.K.

Dr D. Bell, Brooking Institution, Washington, D.C., U.S.A.

Professor M. Bronfenbrenner, Duke University, Durham, North Carolina, U.S.A.

Dr U. Christiansen, Danish Building Research Institute, Copenhagen, Denmark

Mr M. H. Cooper, University of Exeter, Exeter, U.K.

Mr A. J. Culyer, Institute of Social and Economic Research, University of York, York, U.K.

Dr K. Davis, Brookings Institution, Washington, D.C., U.S.A.

M. J.-P. Dupuy, Centre de Recherche sur le Bien-être (CEREBE), Paris, France

Mr T. Ema, Social Security Agency, Tokyo, Japan

Professor K. Emi, Hitotsubashi University, Tokyo, Japan

Professor R. G. Evans, University of British Columbia, Vancouver, Canada

Professor L. Fauvel, International Economic Association, Paris, France

Professor M. S. Feldstein, Harvard University, Cambridge, Massachusetts, U.S.A.*

M. A. Foulon, Centre de Recherches et de Documentation sur la Consommation (CREDOC), Paris, France

Dr B. Friedman, Brown University, Providence, Rhode Island, U.S.A.

Professor V. R. Fuchs, Center for Advanced Study in the Behavioral Sciences, Palo Alto, California, and New York University, New York City, U.S.A.

Dr M. Grossman, National Bureau of Economic Research (N.B.E.R.), New York City, U.S.A.

Dr R. M. Hartwell, Nuffield College, Oxford, U.K.

Professor K. Imai, Hitotsubashi University, Tokyo, Japan

Professor M. Intriligator, University of Southern California, Los Angeles, California, U.S.A.

Mr S. Jinushi, Social Development Research Institute, Tokyo, Japan

Mr M. Kaser, St Antony's College, Oxford, U.K.

Dr T. Kawakami, Suginami Kumiai Hospital, Tokyo, Japan

Dr B. H. Kehrer, American Medical Association, Chicago, Illinois, U.S.A.

Dr E. Kleiman, Hebrew University of Jerusalem, Jerusalem, Israel

Professor J. Lave, Carnegie-Mellon University, Pittsburgh, Pennsylvania, U.S.A.

Professor L. Lave, Carnegie-Mellon University, Pittsburgh, Pennyslvania, U.S.A.

Professor S. Leinhardt, Carnegie-Mellon University, Pittsburgh, Pennsylvania, U.S.A.

Professor E. Lévy, Université de Paris–IX Dauphine, Paris, France

Professor E. Liefmann-Keil, University of Saarland, Saarbrucken, West Germany

Professor F. Machlup, Princeton University, Princeton, New Jersey, U.S.A.

Professor C. Moriguchi, Kyoto University, Kyoto, Japan

Professor M. Perlman, University of Pittsburgh, Pittsburgh, Pennsylvania, U.S.A.

Dr C. E. Phelps, RAND Corporation, Santa Monica, California, U.S.A.

Mr J. D. Pole, Department of Health and Social Security, London, U.K.

Professor E. A. G. Robinson, Marshall Library, Cambridge, U.K.

* Professor Feldstein, who served on the Program Committee and who prepared a paper, was actually absent from the Comference because of illness.

Introduction

Mark Perlman

A conference? To hold it or not to hold it? Several factors seem to make a conference on health and medical care timely. First, few economic topics are more pressing; the rate at which the share of medical expenditures in the national product accounts of most industrialized nations is rising suggests, even shouts for, the need for great priority in analyzing causes and consequences. Second, there has been almost a century's experience since Bismarck first introduced the thought that industrialized society was responsible for medical care for the self-supporting citizen; moreover, within the past three decades country after country has moved to experiment in its own way with creating the institutions necessary to satisfy the health expectations of its own people. Thus, a variety of national experiences exists, and comparisons of these experiences are generally useful. Third, economists have been intermittently considering the cost of health care and the value of health care ever since the time of the Political Arithmeticians – specifically since Sir William Petty (one-time Professor of Surgery at Oxford and all-time economic genius) introduced the topic of the economic value of a preserved life to scholars working in the economics tradition.

Yet in spite of these reasons for holding a conference, the operative question remained whether those working in the field of economics of health had enough solid achievement as well as common inter-nation bases to justify an expensive international conference. One way around this hurdle was to insist that health care, not just medical care, be considered.

A second preliminary decision was to confine the papers to work done in industrialized nations; this step made investigation of the feasibility of a conference easier, because in industrialized nations there is a convergence of demographic considerations. (It is not that there are necessarily more data or better analysts working on industrialized countries than elsewhere.) Most preliminary work has revealed the critical importance of the age, educational and distribution-of-wealth composition of countries in the social handling of what might be termed the health industry.

The next query was whether there were sufficient institutional similarities between the various industrialized countries' medical care systems to make worthwhile comparisons of results, methods or even objectives. Preliminary examination suggested that the answer to this question was complex. Most industrialized nations have markedly increased inputs into their respective health sectors; indeed, they have done so almost willy-nilly. Yet in these countries there are few, if any, reliable (even relevant) measures of health output. Without output measures, comparisons lose most meaning. Here divergence of view among the program planners emerged. The one which ultimately dominated was that lack of good systematic output data was even more a reason for having an international meeting than for not having it. Getting analysts to work together for as little as a week could focus pressure for solution of the provision of output data. Such a thrust might well prove to be one of the more important long-run empirical contributions that the International Economic Association could make to the subject. At the same time, comparisons of analytical method and input considerations would be intellectually beneficial.

Table 1 shows the organization of the Conference, held in Tokyo at the Tokyo Prince Hotel from 2 April through midday of 7 April 1973.

The Principal Findings

Part I. The two initial papers were selected to put the health and medical care problems into an appropriate perspective. Both authors noted that historically it has not been the contributions of technologically sophisticated medical care which account for improved health in the urban areas of industrialized nations; rather it has been the rise of average nutritional levels and the application of sanitary reform with respect to both pure water distribution and centralized sewage-pumping systems.

Another point raised in these historical overviews was the need to get some stable measurements of health, and that improvements in life expectancy were very crude proxies for studying the output of various kinds of health and medical care programs.

The tone of both papers was essentially optimistic, with both authors concluding that the economists' usual analytical techniques, when applied to sophisticated data, would yield a satisfactory social return on the necessary intellectual investment.

Part II. The nine papers in this part were initially conceived as dealing with problems of the national supply and demand for health and medical services. As they turned out, however, there were several denominators – which were by no means common.

Two papers dealt with international comparisons. Dr Kleiman studied the public/private split in responsibility for the provision of medical care. His model has a beguiling neatness; his conclusion is a disturbing realization that privately financed care and socially financed care are not, in practice, easy substitutes. Professor Fuchs's paper had an even more disturbing tone. He found that the conventional wisdom (rising national per capita income was positively associated with increasing average longevity) was no longer 'true'; instead, life-style (with affluence in many instances destroying longevity) plays an important role. Fuchs did grant, however, that the form national medical delivery systems took did still affect, albeit in limited degree, life expectancy.

Professor Evans (Canada) sounded clearly what became a terribly loud theme. The economist's favorite constructs, supply and demand schedules, were largely confusing in the health area because the supplier (generally a physician) told the demander (generally a medically unsophisticated patient) what the latter needed and wanted.

Mr Cooper's paper on the British National Health Service (N.H.S.) expanded this same theme, even if Cooper's paper actually precedes Evans's.

Professor Liefmann-Keil's paper on the West German pharmaceutical supply code (prescriptions by physician) spelled out in no small detail how the market system has been bent to serve the physicians' and the pharmaceutical manufacturers' interests. Again, it is the supplier who tells the demander what the latter needs, wants and will pay for.

The Culyer and Cullis paper, also on the British N.H.S., studied the alleged inefficiencies grafted on the N.H.S. by allowing private patients in N.H.S. hospitals. Their conclusion was that the present mixture was not going to be made significantly more efficient if private patients were driven to completely private hospitals.

Professor Rosett's paper (actually given before the Culyer and Cullis one) added a most interesting analytical point, but this time in the context of the American institutional scene. In comparing non-profit to proprietary hospitals, he concluded that the former offered greater net efficiencies to the decision-making physician. Thus, the income-maximizing decision-maker preferred to maximize his interests by forgoing money profits (as found in proprietary hospitals) in favor of the service facilities for him associated with non-profit institutions.

The Kawakami paper offers further thought on this theme of the contradictions between facile market models and the hospital and similar medical care institutions, as they have developed. Kawakami's paper deals with the current Japanese medical care delivery system.

The Newhouse and Phelps paper dealt with 1963 American data on the demand for medical care. Price elasticities were found to be small, which seems logical if one realizes the importance most buyers

TABLE 1

CONFERENCE ON ECONOMICS OF HEALTH AND MEDICAL CARE

Session	Topic	Chairman	Papers*	Discussants
I	Economic History of Health and Medical Care	S. Tsuru	M. Perlman, U.S.A., University of Pittsburgh R. M. Hartwell, U.K., Nuffield College, Oxford	M. Kaser, U.K., St Antony's College, Oxford R. N. Rosett, U.S.A., University of Rochester
II	Health Care Systems I	F. Machlup	T. Kawakami, Japan R. N. Rosett, U.S.A., University of Rochester E. Kleiman, Israel, Hebrew University	K. Emi, Japan, Hitotsubashi University T. Ema, Japan, Social Security Agency M. Shinohara, Japan, Seikei University
III	Health Care Systems II	E. A. G. Robinson	M. H. Cooper, U.K., University of Exeter A. J. Culyer, U.K., University of York E. Liefmann-Keil, West Germany, University of Saarland	A. B. Atkinson, U.K., Essex University R. G. Evans, Canada, University of British Columbia S. Jinushi, Japan, Social Development Research Institute
IV	Demand-Associated Problems I	L. Fauvel	C. E. Phelps, U.S.A., RAND Corporation R. G. Evans, Canada, University of British Columbia V. R. Fuchs, U.S.A., Stanford University	M. Grossman, U.S.A., National Bureau of Economic Research B. H. Kehrer, U.S.A., American Medical Association L. Lave, U.S.A., Carnegie-Mellon University

attach to medical care purchases. Wage income elasticities similarly confirmed expectations and were found to be positive. Other non-wage income and third-party insurance considerations confirmed expectations.

Part III. Here are three papers on the handling of the impact certain specific demands on the provision of medical care. The Grossman and Benham paper analyzes the impact of health in American labor market performance. Not only does it ask whether improved health adds measurably to production, but it also asks whether improved income adds to improved health and the allied aspects of household management. Dr Friedman's paper considers the impact that the American Medicare system (designed for the elderly) has had on the general allocation of resources for one type of medical care service (breast cancer management) not usually associated with the Medicare receivers; he finds that in absolute terms the treatment breast cancer patients receive has increased (reflecting technological advance) since Medicare was instituted. In sum, the whole medical system has expanded to absorb both the augumented Medicare demand and the technologically induced demand of breast cancer victims. Finally, Dr Christiansen's paper reports in detail on a method for analyzing the impact of demand for accident services in Copenhagen.

Part IV. The nine papers in this part reflect research on rather specific health care problems. Dr Davis analyzes the reasons for the expansion of American hospital costs, estimating *ad seriatim* the various causes. Professor Sloan's paper estimates how responsive American physicians are in terms of hours worked to changes in weekly and hourly earnings. The Lave-Lave-Leinhardt paper proposes and examines by simulation a model considering the impact of counseling, clinic and hospital options on patient choice of service; not unexpectedly, the nature of the illness (not the patient care options) is the principal determinant, but the options do play roles of some significance – particularly critical in a system used to over-capacity.

The Williams paper, written within the context of the British National Health Service, directs attention to what he (Williams) thinks a planning error: possible supply is estimated and then allocated (probably imperfectly) among competing claims. He thinks more work should now be done on estimating the aggregate demand for service, rather than starting from the supply side alone.

The Atkinson paper, also conceived from within the British institutional context, focused on the wisdom of the government affecting the demand side by prophylaxis (in this case anti-smoking) regulation.

The Intriligator–Kehrer paper deals with the trade-offs between physicians and other professional and paraprofessional medical care personnel. It estimates these trade-offs in terms of hours, comparative (direct and interactive) wage effects and the role of worker-supplied investment or capital.

The Yett–Drabek–Intriligator–Kimbell paper is an attempt to develop a macro-model of the American medical system. It relies upon no fewer than 37 behavioral and identity equations and attempts to predict utilization rates and prices.

Two of the papers deal with the rather profound measurement of output problems. Professor Feldstein's paper introduced and tested some ideas pertaining to linear measurement of the quality of hospital care. Professor Lévy, by way of contrast, rejected linear scales for measuring general health quality and suggested something in the way of a profile system for estimating the individual's health status; presumably these profiles could in some way be aggregated to yield estimates of the 'health of nations'.

Part V. The two concluding papers, like the opening two, were intended to provide perspective. M. Dupuy's paper considered the problem of whose rationalty was being used as the logical basis for medical care systems. He was particularly concerned that economists not force their *Weltanschauung* on the examination of the physician–patient relationship; the medical efficiency topic is too critical to be left either to the experts on efficiency (the economists) or the experts on medicine (the physicians). In truth, the topic requires a much broader base, if useful insights are to be produced and implemented. Mr Kaser's paper, which closed the Conference, again stressed the load or responsibility which society tends to force on the physician: he must act as seller and adviser to the buyer; he must cooperate with, yet fight off, public administrators' interventions on the costs and administration sides.

One of the great values of the Conference is its indication, to scholars working in the field, of the unevenness of the 'line of intellectual settlement,' some particularly neglected subject lacunae, and the need for improved data and semantic discipline to sharpen the focus of questions being asked. In sum, this Conference volume reflects the wide variety of research activities, each geared to the problem as perceived within a particular nation's institutional setting.

Some Concluding Observations

The price of any *ex ante* program estimate is only too clearly seen in the *ex post* product. I, as editor, have maintained (with one very minor adjustment) the sequential order of the program by interposing the summary records of the discussion and the debate in the sequence in which they occurred. Yet it is apparent from the way I have divided the volume into parts (it is not even necessary to admit this point by bald statement) that the contracted-for papers in many instances did not fit the original matrix. Parts I and IV would have fitted together nicely; the fact is, however, that the philosophic emphasis found in Part IV – possibly one of the more useful parts – had not been foreseen. Moreover, Parts II and III overlapped and were intentionally non-homogeneous.

In a few instances the authors revised the papers as originally given. In each such instance, notice has been taken in this volume to indicate that what we are printing is a revised version; one limitation on the revision of papers was to preclude any author (or authors) choosing to use the opportunity to revise the paper to make redundant (or even silly) specific criticisms, comments or discussion as summarized by Professor Martin Bronfenbrenner, our very active rapporteur.

Great effort has been made to process this volume quickly. Inevitably there is a trade-off of quality for speed. I hope that our trade-off provides interested scholars a comfortable saddle on which to sally forth.

Part One

Economic History and the Economics of Health and Medical Care

1   The Economic History of Medical Care

R. M. Hartwell

NUFFIELD COLLEGE, OXFORD

The history of medical care divides into two periods, separated by the Industrial Revolution. If the history of mankind can be described as 'the history of poverty, dirt and disease', these three major obstacles to wealth, health and population growth have been overcome only in the advanced economies of the last two centuries. Nevertheless, the inheritance of the pre-industrial age was (a) a great deal of medical knowledge which was ineffective operationally and (b) ideas of social control (of doctors) and prevention (e.g. of leprosy, plague, etc.). The Industrial Revolution (including an agricultural revolution and, therefore, a nutritional revolution) was followed by a public health revolution (mid-nineteenth century) and a medical revolution (only in the twentieth century). For most of history, medical care has been irrelevant in the determination of aggregate social indices whatever comfort it may have brought to particular individuals.

I

'The history of mankind is the history of its diseases.' This firm statement by a Swedish medical historian is a rare admission about the historical role of disease. Folke Henschen goes on to argue that

It is understandable that historians usually do not think medically. Their interest is first captured by the repeated growth of states in the course of history, their rise and fall, their religions and ideologies, their leaders, mild elders, noble tyrants or inhuman despots. For historians such themes as justice, the demand for freedom, the destructive instinct, productivity, social and economic conditions and the general development of civilization have been of paramount importance. But powerful historical factors (and grim rulers) like crop failure, famine and in particular the great epidemics have in general hardly attracted interest to the degree they deserve. Infectious diseases . . . have probably been the most dangerous enemies of mankind, much more so than war and mass murder. When one studies the constant epidemics of the past and the deficiency diseases on land and at sea, one realizes that the whole of civilization could have succumbed, and one is constantly surprised that mankind has survived.

As an economic historian, however, I would amend Henschen's generalizations to: '*The history of mankind is the history of poverty, dirt and disease.*' Life for most men for most of history has been a constant struggle for survival, in an insanitary environment, against poverty and disease; for much of mankind today it is still so. Constant shortage of food and malnutrition, with recurring crop failures and famines, and constant exposure under living conditions which ignored the basic elements of public health, to infectious diseases, with recurring onslaughts of great epidemics, were the essential characteristics of human societies up to the eighteenth century. This vicious cycle of poverty, dirt and disease was broken, first, by the Industrial Revolution, beginning in England in the eighteenth century, which dramatically increased man's capacity to produce goods and services, and thus enabled economic growth and a long-term, sustained increase in living standards and population; second, by a public health movement, which invested heavily in environmental improvements and which gradually enforced standards of hygiene in increasingly concentrated urban communities; and third, by the medical conquest of infectious diseases, the result of considerable investment in medical research, which reinforced the ability to survive already boosted by the decline of universal chronic malnutrition and by the making of a healthier environment. Only in the twentieth century, however, and only in the advanced economies, has there been a convincing solution to the old historical problems of under-nourishment, lack of hygiene and endemic and epidemic disease.

It is not surprising, therefore, that all past societies have had theories of disease and forms of medical care. As anthropologists demonstrate, 'In all human groups, no matter how small or technologically primitive, there exists a body of belief about the nature of disease, its causation and cure, and its relation to other aspects of life, ([19] p. 88). All societies have a knowledge of medicine, often remarkably effective, and attempt to identify and classify diseases, and to prescribe specific remedial treatment. All societies have individuals and/or institutions concerned with the identification and remedy of disease. All societies have devoted resources to medical care. The historians' records, also, clearly prove the past universality of the cultural response to disease and, from the beginnings of the written word, chronicle accounts of disease, epidemics and medical care. Hippocrates' extant writings on medicine date from *c.* 425 B.C., but there are other records – Egyptian papyri, and Indian and Chinese writings, for example – which are older. And as the survival of surgical instruments and other medical artefacts proves, there was also systematic treatment of disease in ancient societies whose written records are otherwise uninformative.[1] The first great advances in medicine and medical care were made in Greece and Rome. The Greek contribution to medicine was to free it from magic and to make it scientific, to give the doctor something like his modern professional status, and to define an ethic for the relationship between doctor and patient (the Hippocratic oath, 'the nucleus of all medical ethics'). The origins of medical care had been, undoubtedly, in magic and religion on the one hand, and in empiricism on the other; and magic and empiricism still dominate primitive medicine. The Greeks, however, developed 'the art of healing', consisting 'in acting with some degree of scientifically exact knowledge of *what* was being done and *why*' ([8], p. 15). The Greeks made medicine and medical care secular and rational; they also firmly enunciated the principle of providing free medical care to the sick poor, a principle of social action which survived the hazards of a changing European civilization through to the twentieth century. Thus, some form of the public provision of medical care for the sick poor has existed in Western society since the Greeks. Rome added to this principle an institution, the hospital, a by-product of an extensive empire and efficient military system, and of 'the Roman genius for organization.' Greek doctors had had their surgeries, but the Romans developed hospitals for soldiers and the sick poor, institutions which were both publicly and privately endowed ([31], pp. 56–9, 84–7). These Roman *valetudinaria*, with their essential character as public and charitable institutions, were the direct forerunners of the modern hospital.

Greece and Rome were relatively advanced societies, socially stratified, with a wealthy class prepared to pay for medical services, and with accepted social obligations towards the sick poor; but the fall of Rome was followed, in Europe, by a long-term decline in medical knowledge and medical care [31, 28, 25]. The medicine of Greece and Rome, however, was conserved and advanced by the Arabs, so that with the remarkable revival of European civilization in the twelfth century and beyond, medieval medicine was able, through the Arabs, to draw directly on the knowledge and experience of the ancient world. Post-Roman medicine was Christian in inspiration and practice; it became an essential part of the life of the monasteries where it was 'the Christian office of healing'. The basic motivation was charity, but diagnosis and care were based on such

---

[1] For example, no surgical texts have survived from Assyria and Babylonia, but surgical instruments have ([31], pp. 14–15).

ancient therapeutic knowledge as had survived, on empiricism, on some increases in knowledge, and on a belief in miracles (and hence on the use of Christian ritual and holy relics for therapy). Monastic medicine and the doctor-priest, with services dispensed freely, dominated Europe until about the twelfth century. Thereafter, however, increasing wealth, the foundation of universities with medical faculties, the advance of medical knowledge on a wide front and the revival of Greek–Arab medical texts led to the emergence and rapid dominance of the secular medical practitioner and to the establishment of public hospitals. The expansion of medical care facilities was mainly the result of an increasing demand, but advances in medicine were the outcome, also, of the new knowledge, not autonomous but much sustained by the Renaissance quest for understanding man. With the 'rebirth of science' there was an awakening interest in anatomy, the establishment of modern descriptive anatomy and, aided by the continuous practical experience of war, improvements in surgery. At the same time there were advances, not so marked, in the understanding of disease, and the beginnings of internal medicine with increasing understanding of physiology. Perhaps the most significant development in medical care, however, was the idea of disease prevention. In particular, the widespread incidence of leprosy and the periodic visitations of the plague led to explicit theories of contagion and infection, and to a policy of preventive action in the form of quarantine. The secularization of doctors came quickly, of hospitals more slowly, and both were subjected to increasing public control. Even though medieval society interpreted the doctor's duty to his patient in terms of Christian principles, the contractual nature of the relationship was also recognized and, at the same time, there was recognition of the social importance of disease and attempts at control.

The social control of doctors, which varied considerably from country to country, took the form of regulation of professional conduct. As P. L. Entralgo points out, with the particular example of medieval Spain: 'The civil authorities of the Middle Ages framed rules that regulated many of a doctor's activities: medico-legal provisos, rules concerning hygiene, medical responsibility, fees, the preparation and price of medicine, and so forth ([8], p. 100).[1] Not only were doctors subjected to a wide variety of legally enforced regulations, they were expected, as a matter of civil prudence and Christian duty, to give free treatment to the sick poor. And for this purpose also, civil authorities, along with the Church, provided hospitals where such poor could be treated. The most decisive social action and

---

[1] For the regulation of doctors in London in the middle ages, see Clark [6], chap. 1.

public expenditure against disease, however, was the attempt to control the spread of infectious disease, especially the plague and leprosy. The earliest anti-plague regulations that have survived were made at Reggio (Italy) in 1374; Venice pioneered maritime quarantine in 1403; cities like London gradually evolved elaborate administrative machinery for the enforcement of plague regulations which survived into the nineteenth century ([17], pp. 405–8). Leprosy, more continuously dreaded even than the plague, inspired policies of rigorous isolation: there were reckoned to be some 19,000 leprosaria in Christendom in 1200, the first having been established in the sixth century.[1] Neither quarantine nor leprosaria were effective as preventive devices. The plague declined dramatically in Europe in the eighteenth century for reasons which are still debated; leprosy began to decline in the same century, again for reasons which are not clear.[2] The coincidence of the decline of both diseases, and of smallpox, with the beginnings of the period of modern economic growth and the 'population explosion', however, suggest the therapeutic importance of better nutrition and improving hygiene rather than of specific medical advances in the classic period of the Industrial Revolution.

What, then, was the 'state of play' on the eve of the Industrial Revolution? Firstly, there had been, between the twelfth and eighteenth centuries, remarkable advances in science, including medicine. Advances in physical and biological sciences had led directly to the formulation of medical theories to explain the working of the human body as well as to analyse the nature of disease. Advances in physiology and the rise of clinical teaching improved the doctor's power of diagnosis and put the theory of disease on a more scientific basis. Improving knowledge of anatomy had further aided the surgeon and obstetrician. If the main impulse to medicine before the eighteenth century had been in the understanding of the working of the human body, that of the eighteenth century was increasingly in the systematic clinical analysis of disease. Secondly, there had been the proliferation of hospitals in the form of charitable institutions; thus, Britain in the reign of Henry VII had 200 lazar houses and 500 hospitals ([7], appendix B). Numbers multiplied noticeably in the eighteenth century, before the Industrial Revolution. In London, for example, there were two medieval foundations in existence in 1700, which were supplemented, before 1780, by five other general hospitals founded in 1719, 1721, 1733, 1740 and 1745 ([2], p. 4). Thirdly, there had been the secularization and

---

[1] The exact figure can be doubted, but the importance of leprosy in the medieval world can be seen in its influence on art ([15], pp. 107–18).

[2] On the decline of the plague, see Hirst [17], Shrewsbury [26] and Helleiner [147]. On leprosy, see Henschen [15].

professionalization of the doctors. From the twelfth century, several Councils of the Church had forbidden priests to practise medicine outside of the monasteries, and from the same date there was the increasing appearance of the secular doctor, stemming originally from the famous medical school of Salerno ([8], pp. 62, 64, 74). Numbers of doctors, however, remained small, even in large cities; for example, Paris in 1500 was reckoned to have had only twenty-one *médecins*. A noticeable growth in numbers occurred only in the seventeenth and eighteenth centuries. The first steps towards professionalization came from the universities, which clearly established standards of professional knowledge, and which exercised considerable authority over practitioners. But the division of the profession between the professionally trained and the untrained, the latter often including the surgeons and apothecaries, made control difficult; thus, untrained and unlicensed 'doctors' were to be found in every town. From the fifteenth century professional organizations, like the Royal College of Physicians of London, exercised increasing control over professional standards and practice ([6], chap. 4). Fourthly, there had been varying degrees of public control and public provision of medical care. On the one hand there were the leprosaria, quarantine houses and public hospitals, and the preventive regulations that went with them; on the other, there was the regulation of doctors and the appointment of public officials for medical care. There were in France, in the fifteenth century, *médecins fonctionnaires* with duties not unlike a modern medical officer of health, and *médecins ordinaires* whose job it was to deal with the plague and sanitation. In the eighteenth and early nineteenth centuries the common law courts of England decided that the overseers of parishes should provide medical care for the poor, so that by 1834 about half of England's parishes already had a medical officer ([18], p. 680). In Castile [after 1422] there was a state and municipal institution called the *protomedicat* with disciplinary powers over the physicians and surgeons and with a tribunal of judges (*alcades*) and examiners to test the competence of aspirants ([6], pp. 34–5). The degree and effectiveness of control varied from country to country, and over time, and control generally was less effective by the early eighteenth century than it had been in the early sixteenth and, for example, was always less effective in England than it was in Spain. Nevertheless, doctors were never quite free from control and, in varying degrees, from public scrutiny and accounting. By the beginning of the nineteenth century, however, the doctor in France, England, Germany or the United States 'exercised his profession largely unhampered by regulations' [21, 11].

The results? What effects did medical care have on societies before the Industrial Revolution, say up to 1800? What determined the volume, organization and effectiveness of medical care? Briefly, the answers to these questions are: Medical care had little or no effect on the incidence or cure of disease, or on mortality rates, at any time before the nineteenth century. The volume of medical care was always small, with numbers of 'qualified' doctors small in relation to total population, and hospitals in such small supply that their baneful character as 'gateways to death' [14, 23] was unimportant in determining mortality trends. Effective medical knowledge was limited. Most medical care was provided in the home, using a combination of home remedies, magic, folklore, religion and patent medicines (which were in widespread use in the eighteenth century), and when outside advice was sought, it was often provided by cheap and unqualified practitioners ([35], pp. 234–51). The organization of medical care was, in general, in the hands of independent doctors, often unsystematically trained, only partly organized into professional associations, only partly controlled by public authorities; doctors dealt mainly with private, well-to-do, fee-paying patients but also provided some free service to the sick. Public expenditure on medical care was minimal, with some expenditure on hospitals, some employment of medical officials and some expenditure on 'public health' (for example, scavenging); there was, however, clear recognition of the need to control some diseases (like the plague) and patchy recognition of the desirability of ensuring standards of professional competence. As regards the public or private control of disease, only vaccination (at the end of the period) was effective in remedying a mass killer, and the dramatic decline of the plague in Europe, the most important medical event in the history of disease before the Industrial Revolution, seems unconnected with medical improvements. About the plague in Britain, for example, Shrewsbury writes that 'There is no evidence that the peoples of these islands had any inkling of the decisive part played by the house-haunting rat in the genesis and maintenance of epidemics of plague' ([26], p. 6). The beginnings of the decline of ancient killers such as leprosy and malaria, similarly, are largely inexplicable, except in terms of increasing standards of living. Practically no progress had been made in public health, expecially in the growing towns and cities which were already 'gateways to death'. But population was increasing *before* the Industrial Revolution, along with the decline of some diseases. The result of a decisive improvement in nutrition? McKeown, Brown and Record have argued, for example, that 'The reduction of mortality and the rise of population in the late eighteenth and early nineteenth century were probably due to a significant increase in food supplies, which spread throughout Europe from the seventeenth century' ([24],

p. 382). The causes of the advances in health and longevity before the Industrial Revolution are thus to be sought in agricultural rather than in medical improvements, to increasing investment in food production rather than to increasing investment in medical care. It is important to remember, however, that public concern about, and the public control and provision of, medical care goes back at least to the Greeks. It is a mistake, therefore, to attribute the present-day, universal demand for public responsibility in medical care either to recently formulated economic theories about public goods, or to recently acquired social ideologies of interventionism. From the Greek concept of *philia*, through the Christian concept of charity, to the modern concept of *social cost*, there is a continuing theme of social obligation and a continuing policy implication of intervention. The egalitarianism of the treatment of acute illness among the free-men of Plato's Athens, and the egalitarianism of the treatment of all illness for the whole population of the nationalized health services of modern Britain, have much in common, even if the effectiveness of the treatment afforded to the Greeks differed markedly from that now given to the British.

II

The long-run effects of the Industrial Revolution on health, and on the provision of medical care, were extremely favourable, but in the shorter run, up to and beyond the mid-nineteenth century, the effects were also harmful. This harmful impact of industrialization on health can be attributed to the facts that the Industrial Revolution *preceded* the modern revolution in medical knowledge which finally ensured the effective control of infectious diseases, while at the same time it created new health hazards which were solved only by advances in medical knowledge and by massive investments in public health. The Industrial Revolution marked 'the great divide' in the rate of production of goods and in the rate of growth of population: before it, output, population and real income per capita were rising slowly or not at all; after it, there was much faster economic growth, with population rising at an almost frightening rate, and with sustained increases in the rate of growth of output and real income per capita [13]. The dramatic breakthrough in the production of food enhanced the power to survive and brought down death rates, especially infantile mortality rates [9]. Agricultural output in Europe increased massively over the eighteenth and nineteenth centuries, more than keeping pace with the rate of growth of population, and output was supplemented increasingly in the nineteenth century from non-European sources. The nutritional decline in the death rate, however, was temporarily halted in the mid-nineteenth century as the health hazards of industrialization and urbanization increased, before remedies were sought, found and paid for. In Britain, for example, the death rate declined from the beginnings of the Industrial Revolution up to 1831, was almost stable until 1871, and declined continuously thereafter until 1921. Industrialization had immensely increased health problems by concentrating population *before* solving the problems of urban sanitation and infectious disease. The population of nineteenth-century Britain, for example, was increasing at a rate which doubled it in just over fifty years, and most of the increase went into towns and cities which were not public health equipped. In Britain, as elsewhere in Europe, there was little regulation of building, inefficient garbage and sewage services, and inadequate and insanitary water supplies. In particular, the substitution of the water-closet for the privy, an undoubted advance in individual comfort and hygiene, created a serious and increasing social problem. 'What was now to happen to this new and rapidly swelling flood of liquid sewage?' ([12], p. 8).

The problems of urban health were threefold: first, *technical*, involving civil engineering problems on the one hand, and medical problems, especially the theory of disease and contagion, on the other;[1] second, *administrative*, involving questions of control (central versus local, voluntary versus official, amateur versus professional, etc.); third, *economic*, involving the important questions of who should pay and how. Questions of control and payment were intermingled: individual action was expensive and almost useless; collective action by agreement was almost impossible because of conflicting economic interests and high transaction costs. The only solution lay in government action, especially as health hazards multiplied. 'Conscious design could hardly have produced conditions more agreeable to the spread of infectious diseases and the cost of living amid such filth was a sickly and uncertain existence' ([16], p. 37). Endemic disease was supplemented, terrifyingly, by a new epidemic disease which regularly devastated Europe – cholera. The career of 'King Cholera' [22] was short and deadly, from the 1830s to the end of the century, and its periodic and lethal visitations did much to stimulate public action for improved sanitation and water supplies. Generally, public health legislation was everywhere opposed on the grounds of its cost (and, sometimes, because of its centralizing, anti-liberal character), and everywhere was delayed by those who were protecting vested

[1] For examples, see the amusing, if serious, debate in Britain about the appropriate shape (egg-shaped?) of the sewer-drain [30]. The accepted mid-century theory of contagion was the 'miasmic', which argued that disease came from breathing air contaminated by miasma arising from decomposing animal and vegetable matter.

interests or who were opposed to increasing taxation. Nevertheless, there was increasing recognition of the public-good character of health and the need, in consequence, for public investment in health. 'Public health is public wealth', wrote the English barrister, Edward Jenkins.

> Every person laid aside by ill health is so much subtracted from the power and capacity of the state; and more than this, every person so laid aside is a drain upon the resources of the state. It takes more money to keep him than if he were well; one or more other persons in health are withdrawn from productive operations to expend their strength and time upon his recovery. If one-third of a town, or city, or state, is suffering from disease, there is cast upon the other two-thirds a proportionately greater amount of exertion than would otherwise be required of them, and there is extracted from them a proportionately greater contribution to the general expenditure, while there is less capacity both of work and contribution in the whole community [20].

The increasing acceptance of such cogent argument, common sense, cholera, humanitarianism, medical research and civic pride were among the varied motives which produced the 'sanitary idea'. Certainly, after mid-century there was recognition of the harmful externalities associated with poverty, dangerous occupations, unhygienic environments and infectious and epidemic disease; there was recognition of the link between poverty and disease, occupation and disease [33], and environment and disease; there was recognition that health could be protected and improved, at a cost, and with compulsory controls. Thus, there was increasing public expenditure for adequate garbage collection, sewage disposal and clean water provision, in addition to medical services. Dirt was no longer tolerable since it affected not only the poor and dirty but also the rich and clean. As an English lawyer, H. E. Pember, argued about Parliament's indecisiveness on this matter: 'A great mistake was made when Parliament receded [after 1848] from the general principle . . . that people should have no prescriptive right to remain dirty' ([10], Q. 4788). (The British Sanitary Act of 1869 remedied that mistake by giving local authorities compulsory powers over hygiene.) Everywhere in Europe legislation multiplied and expenditure increased. In Britain, for example, a series of Acts after 1846 gave central and local authorities by 1870 comprehensive control over the environment and, in an age of *laissez-faire*, a truly remarkable range of powers.[1]

[1] See Appendix (pp. 17–18) for an account of British legislation and its effects between 1846 and 1866.

Similarly in the United States, where, for example, the urban dweller drinking filtered water increased from 30,000 in 1880 to over 20 million by 1920 ([16], p. 38). The big gains in health in most countries came towards the end of the nineteenth century, when more efficient medical care supplemented the gains already achieved by improved nutrition and better public health, but death rates had turned down before this. In England and France, for example, mortality rates came down after 1871, the result mainly of civic efforts which reduced metropolitan disease ([4], chap. 10). Dirt, as a killer, was already on the way out.

The next great steps in the conquest of disease were medical. Increasing wealth led to an increasing demand for medical care as a consumer good. At the same time the professionalization of doctors, with carefully defined standards of training, ensured the increasing competence of the medical profession [5, 11, 21]. The training of doctors centred on the hospitals which multiplied and became institutions, not only of medical care, but also of teaching and research. Thus was established a mutually reinforcing process of medical training and research in universities and hospitals, a process of increasing investment in the human capital of doctors, in hospitals and in medical research. Doctors were prominent in the public health movement, which eliminated or reduced some of the causes of preventable mortality; biologists and doctors as researchers, aided by other scientists, were also able to identify the causes of infectious disease. Identification and cure of infection, however, was achieved only with public assistance for research, for the compulsory notification of disease and for the free provision of isolated hospital accommodation for communicable diseases. As with public health, the essential move was from the care of individual patients to the medical control of populations with correspondingly expensive public investment. With the biological identification of great infectious killers of the nineteenth century – cholera, tuberculosis, typhoid, etc. – 'death control' on a large and effective basis became technologically possible. In the context of increasing wealth, the increasing private demand for medicine, and the increasing willingness of governments and communities to invest in health, made 'death control' economically possible. Thus, the old infectious and epidemic diseases retreated, and two other groups of diseases (cardio-vascular diseases and tumours, diseases connected with increasing expectation of life) became more prominent. As Henschen points out: 'Many infectious diseases are by nature originally cosmopolitan, but now confined to backward parts of Europe and the rest of the world, especially the great tropical and sub-tropical countries where over-population, illiteracy, malnutrition, poverty and wretched hygiene make their continued existence possible' ([15], p. 33).

In most societies patients have been treated in the home, and only modern 'Western' society has produced large numbers of hospitals as important centres of medical care. As was pointed out above, the hospital is of ancient origin but in its immediately pre-modern form it was a custodial institution for the sick poor; for centuries it had a role of 'passive caretaking' rather than of positive remedial treatment; it was voluntary and charitable, and had the primary aims of caring for the helpless and of protecting society from dangerous infection. The period of the Industrial Revolution, up to and beyond 1900, however, was a period of great expansion of hospitals, and of their changing character. Many of the great European hospitals were founded or rebuilt in the eighteenth century; more were added in the nineteenth. This 'hospital and dispensary movement', for example, added 154 such institutions in the British Isles between 1700 and 1825; even so, there were only about 3,000 patients in hospitals in 1800, and even in 1851 there were only 7,619 ([31], p. 194). At the beginning of the nineteenth century, moreover, one of the pioneers of public health declared that medical knowledge in hospitals consisted of 'nurses' gossip, and sick men's fancies, and the crude compilations of blundering empiricism' ([29], p. 21). Hospitals were for the poor, not for respectable artisans or the well-to-do; hospitals were dangerous institutions for the inmates, not just because of the relative inefficiency of surgery and medicine, but mainly because of the danger of infection. As two medical historians have argued persuasively, for the period before the discovery of antiseptics, the patient who entered a hospital without a fatal disease could easily succumb to a fatal disease which he contracted there by infection ([23], p. 125). The outstanding change in the role of the hospital, achieved only after 1900, was the shift from the home to the hospital, for all classes of society, for the major phases of individual medical care. This occurred only after an expansion and improvement in hospital services, a development which depended on the willingness and ability to support increasing expenditure on hospitals, either voluntarily or through taxation, on medical improvements which lessened the chances of infection, and on an increasing provision of skilled personnel, especially doctors and nurses [1]. The long-standing voluntary character of hospitals made them relatively open to social pressures, and, for example, increasing awareness of the dangers of infection both loosened private purses and made for more decisive action by local and central governments. Hospitals were created, not only for categories of sick who had special claims on society (like soldiers) or posed special threats (like those suffering from infectious disease), but also as social investment in the maintenance of a healthy population. By 1909 there were 2,412 hospitals in the United Kingdom, 2,024 in Germany and 1,524 in France [34], pp. 297–8). These were of two main types – those owned by independent charitable foundations and those owned by public authorities – and the balance of expenditure and authority was swinging towards the public authorities. In Britain, for example, the majority of the sick in institutional care by the end of the nineteenth century were in publicly owned institutions. Payment for hospital care, likewise, was already being catered for by insurance, and the development of hospital insurance schemes had been part of the movement for self-help and mutual aid which characterized the nineteenth-century working class. Indeed, B. Abel-Smith has argued that 'patients' direct payments, unaided by insurance, have never contributed much to the running costs of European hospitals' ([3], p. 221). The hospital, also, was the base of the publicly employed doctor, and gave him the opportunity for specialization. Elsewhere, in rural areas for example, and especially in the poorer parts of Europe, doctors were employed by civic authorities to supervise public health provisions and regulations, and to cater for the medical needs of the poor, using as their base the dispensary or polyclinic.

What, then, was the state of play in 1900? What effect did medical care have on societies during the Industrial Revolution? What determined the volume, organization and effectiveness of medical care during this period? Briefly, the answer to these questions are: Medical care services still had little effect on the incidence or cure of disease, or on mortality rates, before the second half of the nineteenth century; thereafter, however, meaical care became increasingly effective, although nutrition and public health continued to dominate mortality trends. The volume of medical care expanded continuously from the beginning of the Industrial Revolution, the result of increasing demand from rising real incones; the numbers of qualified doctors increased, as did also the numbers of hospitals, dispensaries and clinics, and the numbers of supporting services (for example, dentists and nurses); more medical care was catered for institutionally, and at the public expense. The doctors generally remained an independent, fee-earning profession, but one which had expert training and which was organized into professional associations, much dependent on public hospitals for specialist experience, and including a large number of publicly paid, official doctors catering for the poor. Medicine became more effective than it had ever been: on the one hand, when antiseptics made infection easy to control in institutions and the biological identification of diseases made cures easier to discover; and on the other, when improving living standards (the result of economic growth) and improving living conditions (the result of expenditure on public health) made the individual healthier and more robust and, hence, more able to withstand diseases, especially those which thrived on malnutrition (for example, turberculosis) and lack of hygiene (for example, cholera). The reduction in the nineteenth-century death rate can be accounted for almost entirely by a decline in the deaths from infectious disease,[1] the result mainly, before the last years of the century, of improved nutrition (privately paid for) and improved public health (publicly financed). In the nomenclature of our age, the industrial and agricultural revolutions resulted in a nutritional revolution, followed by a public health revolution, and only finally by a medical revolution. The public health revolution was induced by the obvious public bads of growing urban concentrations, the medical revolution by the increasing demand for medical care (mainly as a consumer good) from increasingly wealthy societies. The most important change over the period before industrialization was in the recognition of, and in the strenuous efforts to propagate and finance, preventive social action against disease. On the finance of medical care, apart from the willingness to invest publicly in health, the important change was the development of various schemes of health insurance, with as yet voluntarism as the basis of contributions. Voluntary insurance schemes, not surprisingly, were pioneered by the working classes, and were the direct forerunners of compulsory health insurance. The transition from a private and voluntary to a public and compulsory system of health insurance occurred after this period, but arguments for compulsion and public responsibility were already being loudly voiced, and listened to. Again, the idea of public responsibility for the sick poor was being generalized into the idea of public responsibility for the sick. The debate about medical care was about to change from discussion about responsibility to discussion about efficiency. 'Once one accepts the citizen's right to receive medical care as a broad philosophy underlying a century or more of European history', B. Abel-Smith writes, 'the considerable difference in financing systems between countries become matters primarily of detail'. ([3], p. 231) I would say, rather, 'matters primarily of efficiency'.

The lesson of history? For most of history medical care was largely ineffective or even harmful, and whatever comfort it gave to individuals, and whatever its role in promoting increasing medical knowledge, it was irrelevant in the determination of social aggregates.

---

[1] The 'infectious diseases' included 'the infectious fevers (such as measles, scarlet fever, whooping cough, smallpox and diphtheria), and tuberculosis, typhoid, paratyphoid, dysentery, influenza and syphilis'.

Medical care was important socially and intellectually, relatively unimportant economically, and unimportant for vital statistics.

APPENDIX
BRITISH PUBLIC HEALTH LEGISLATION, 1846–1866
(from Stewart [32] pp. 6–7)

'Then followed, in rapid succession, the Acts for Promoting the Establishment of Baths and Washhouses, both in Great Britain and Ireland, in 1846; the Towns' Improvement Act in 1847; the Public Health, the Nuisances' Removal, and the City of London Sewers' Acts in 1848; the Metropolitan Interments Act in 1850, followed in 1853 by a similar Act for the whole of England, the Act to Encourage the Establishment of Lodging houses for the Labouring Classes, and the Common Lodging Houses' Act in 1851; the Metropolitan Water Act in 1852; the Smoke Nuisance Abatement (Metropolis) Act, and the Act to Extend and make Compulsory the Practice of Vaccination, in 1853; the Merchant Shipping Act, with its stringent provisions for the preservation of the health of our merchant seamen, in 1854; the Diseases Prevention, the Metropolis Local Management, the Metropolitan Buildings, and the Nuisances' Removal Amendment Acts, in 1855; and the Public Health Act, 1858, which abolished the General Board of Health, and vested its powers in the Privy Council. Since then there have been added to the statute book the Acts for the purification of the Thames in 1858 and 1866; the Nuisances' Removal Amendment Act in 1860; the Act for preventing the Adulteration of Articles of Food and Drink in the same year; the Acts (passed in 1860, 1861, and 1864) which included under the provisions of the Factory Acts women and children employed in bleaching and dyeing works, in lace factories, and in the manufacture of earthenware, of lucifer matches, of percussion caps and cartridges, of paper staining and of fustian-cutting; the Vaccination Amendment Act in 1861; the Act for the Seizure of Diseased and Unwholesome Meat, and the Alkali Works Act, in 1863; the Sewage Utilization Act in 1865; the Labouring Classes' Dwelling Houses Act, and the Sanitary Act, in 1866.

'Let us attempt to condense into a few sentences the great principles embodied in this vast mass of legislation. They are as follows:– That the employment of women and children in laborious occupations for which they are physically unfit, is physiologically as well as politically and morally wrong; that the sanitary state of our large towns, and the condition, physical as well as moral, of our labouring population, are matters of imperial interest, which we cannot with impunity neglect; that various diseases, which prevail among us, either epidemically or endemically, and are attended with a high mortality, depend wholly or in part on neglect of the laws of health and disregard of the common decencies of life, and are in great measure preventible by a few simple precautionary measures; that a sufficient supply of pure air and water is essential to health, and therefore, that the overcrowding of workshops, dwellings, and schools, the contamination of the air by smoke or other irritating foreign particles, by noxious gases, the product of organic decomposition, and by chemical fumes, and the pollution of water by sewage and other refuse should, as fruitful sources of disease, be prevented; that the establishment of baths and washhouses, and the erection of suitable dwellings for the labouring classes should be encouraged; that efficient drainage should everywhere be promoted, but that the conversion of streams and rivers into common sewers is a monstrous perversion of the gifts of Providence and a great, public wrong; that the practices of conveying persons smitten with contagious or infectious disorders in hackney carriages, and of retaining the decomposing remains of the dead in the crowded abodes of the living, are full of peril, and therefore to be discouraged; that with the view of discovering and removing such evils as affect directly or indirectly the health of the community, medical officers of health and inspectors of nuisances are needed, the latter not to wink at the continuance of nuisances, but to ferret them out and drag them to the daylight, the former to report from time to time the results of inspection and inquiry to the proper authorities, with such suggestions as may seem to him best fitted to remedy existing abuses; that it is the duty of local authorities to take cognizance of and remove all nuisances and impediments to the public health, and to promote such measures as may be conducive thereto; that, in the event of the local authority declining to act, any inhabitant of any parish or place may complain to a magistrate, who shall proceed as if he were the local authority, with a view to the abatement of the nuisance complained of; and finally, that, in the event of a local authority making default in providing its district with sufficient sewers or water supply, complaint may be made to a Secretary of State, who shall inquire and proceed in the matter as he may see fit; in other words, that every facility shall be given to the inhabitants for compelling the local authority to perform its duty. Let us note in addition, that since 1858, we have had in the Privy Council a Public Health Department, which presents us annually with a volume full of interesting and important material, and exercises a summary jurisdiction in times of epidemic visitation.'

REFERENCES

[1] Abel-Smith, B., *A History of the Nursing Profession* (London: Heinemann, 1960).
[2] ——, *The Hospitals, 1800–1948* (London: Heinemann, 1964).
[3] ——, 'The History of Medical Care', in E. W. Martin (ed.), *Comparative Development in Social Welfare* (London: Allen & Unwin, 1972).
[4] Ayers, G. M., *England's First State Hospitals, 1867–1930* (London: Wellcome Institute of the History of Medicine, 1971).
[5] Carr-Saunders, A. M., and Wilson, P. A., *The Professions* (Oxford: Clarendon Press, 1933).

[6] Clark, G., *A History of the Royal College of Physicians of London* (Oxford: Clarendon Press, 1964).

[7] Clay, R. M., *The Mediaeval Hospitals of the British Isles* (London: Methuen, 1909).

[8] Entralgo, P. L., *Doctor and Patient*, trans. F. Partridge (London: World University Library, Weidenfeld & Nicolson, 1969).

[9] Eversley, D. E. C., and Glass, D., *Population in History* (London: Edward Arnold, 1965).

[10] *First Report of Royal Sanitary Commission*, Parliamentary Papers (1868–9) xxxii.

[11] Fishbein, M., *A History of the American Medical Association, 1847 to 1947* (Philadelphia: American Medical Association, 1947).

[12] Flinn, M. W., Introduction to A. P. Stewart and E. Jenkins, *The Medical and Legal Aspects of Sanitary Reform* (Leicester Univ. Press, 1969).

[13] Hartwell, R. M., *The Industrial Revolution and Economic Growth* (London: Methuen, 1971).

[14] Helleiner, K. F., ' The Vital Revolution Reconsidered', *Canadian Journal of Economic and Political Science*, xxiii (Feb. 1957).

[15] Henschen, F., *The History of Diseases*, trans. J. Tate (London: Longmans, 1966).

[16] Higgs, R., *The Transformation of the American Economy, 1865–1914* (New York: Wiley, 1971).

[17] Hirst, L. F., *The Conquest of Plague* (Oxford: Clarendon Press, 1953).

[18] Hodgkinson, R. G., *The Origins of the National Health Service* (London: Wellcome Historical Medical Library, 1967).

[19] Hughes, C. C., 'Ethnomedicine', in *International Encyclopedia of the Social Sciences* (New York: Macmillan–Free Press, 1968) vol. x.

[20] Jenkins, E., *The Legal Aspects of Sanitary Reform* (London: Robert Hardwicke, 1867).

[21] Little, E. M., *History of the British Medical Association, 1832–1932* (London: British Medical Association, 1933).

[22] Longmate, N., *King Cholera: The Biography of a Disease* (London: Hamish Hamilton, 1966).

[23] McKeown, T., and Brown, R. G., 'Medical Evidence Related to English Population Change in the Eighteenth Century', *Population Studies*, ix (Nov. 1955).

[24] ——, —— and Record, R. G., 'An Interpretation of the Modern Rise of Population in Europe', *Population Studies*, xxvii (Nov. 1972).

[25] Major, R. H., *A History of Medicine* (Oxford: Blackwell Scientific Publications, 1955).

[26] Shrewsbury, J. F. D., *A History of the Bubonic Plague in the British Isles* (Cambridge Univ. Press, 1970).

[27] Sigerist, H. E., *Medicine and Human Welfare* (New Haven: Yale Univ. Press, 1941).

[28] ——, *A History of Medicine*, vol. i (New York: Oxford Univ. Press, 1951),

[29] Simon, J., *On the Aims and Philosophic Method of Pathological Research* (London, 1847).

[30] ——, *English Sanitary Institutions* (London: Cassell, 1897).

[31] Singer, C., and Underwood, E. A., *A Short History of Medicine* (Oxford: Clarendon Press, 1962).

[32] Stewart, A. P., *The Medical Aspects of Sanitary Reform* (London: Robert Hardwicke, 1867).

[33] Thackrah, C. T., *The Effects of Arts, Trades and Professions, and of Civic*

States and Habits of Living, on Health and Longevity: with Suggestions for the Removal of Many of the Agents which Produce Disease, and Shorten the Duration of Life (Leeds: Baines & Newsome, 1832).

[34] Webb, A. D., *The New Dictionary of Statistics* (London: Routledge, 1911).

[35] Withers, C., 'The Folklore of a Small Town', *Transactions of the New York Academy of Sciences*, VIII (May 1946).

2 Economic History and Health Care in Industrialized Nations

Mark Perlman
UNIVERSITY OF PITTSBURGH

The focus is on three points:
Medical care delivery is only a subset of health protection systems. Indeed, from a historical standpoint, nutritional improvement, establishment of sanitary control and the spread of educational achievement in industrialized nations have been clearly more significant for improving the health of nations (particularly in the reduction or postponement of mortality) than medical delivery has been.

Second, our imperfect mortality data (which are about all we presently have) must be supplemented by a sophisticated collection of morbidity data so that we can compare output to the variety of inputs we are so frantically collecting. The design for such data collection must basically be the responsibility of epidemiologists and biostatisticians; only after they have completed their tasks can the analytical contributions of economists ring true.

Finally, the two methods upon which economists have relied, investment in human capital (essentially an aspect of benefit–cost studies) and production function analysis (leading to an examination of substitutabilities), have inherent logical inadequacies. None the less, the product has served to improve our understanding of the problems and probably thereby to improve the quality of the health institutions serving our various communities.

It is reasonable to expect that these techniques, coupled with better data and refined perceptions of the priority of problems, will serve us even better in the future.

There are several good reasons why a session on the economic history of health care should not only be included in this meeting, but should actually come at its outset. The major reason is that research, like many activities, is subject to fashion enthusiasms or fads. To prevent such excessive enthusiasm, it is always desirable to strive for perspective. The economic historian's contribution is not only to add time-dimension to the data included, but, even more important, to provide caution about, as well as insight into, the processes of defining problem boundaries (cf. [1]). Thus, the major purpose of this paper is to draw attention, from the very outset of these meetings, to the various perceptions of the topic to show how the parts fit together and perhaps to indicate lacunae which should be filled in.

I. SOME LIMITATIONS OF THE HISTORICAL LITERATURE

There was early identification between disease and organized social activity. In the Bible there appear a welter of references to epidemics thwarting governmental policies and consequently disrupting civilian as well as military pursuits. When one turns to modern history, the impact of plague and other diseases and their effects on population levels are well chronicled. Indeed, whatever may be meant by the 'economic take-off' seems to have waited for the elimination of plague as a principal cause of population stagnation. Helleiner of Toronto has developed a most interesting thesis on just this point [19], and his study is typical of a desirable kind of historical work.

Notwithstanding the Helleiner example, until relatively recently health was treated, if at all, as a private good, and its manipulation was relegated to a not very benevolent Divine Providence, influenced by personal prayer as occasionally reinforced by pious microeconomic works. In so far as social action was concerned, it seems to have been principally limited to the isolation of lepers (from the standpoint of contagion – an act now considered all but unnecessary) and to the enlargement of private prayer through the building of public monuments like churches after Divine intercession, in response to prayer, had proved its worth by stopping epidemics in their course.

It was in the nineteenth century when health became, in part at least, redefined as a public or social good. There are those who attribute this changed approach to the impact of the smallpox vaccination program. On this topic there is already a fascinating and growing literature [29]. Another explanation ties the new interest to some radical philosophers, to the members of the London Political Economy Club, to the facts of several cholera epidemics in London, and to the peculiar personalities of Edwin (later Sir Edwin) Chadwick the irredoubtable Miss Nightingale and Sir John Simon. Other names like William Farr and Dr Southward Smith should also be added, but as the focus of this paper is not on individuals' contributions, discussion here is inappropriate.[1] My own view is that the English sanitary movement was motivated more by a desire for the efficiencies of a centralized technocratic civil service than by a desire for improving the productivity or the happiness of the populace. This judgment will have to be explained elsewhere; yet, it is consistent with findings by Finer [17] and Lambert [23], to mention but two (however, cf. [13]).

On the whole, historians have focused most on great men, great ideas, and on certain clearly specified professions. Dubos's study [12] of the French genius, Louis Pasteur, is a marvelous study of the heroic figure – an example of Carlyle's view that history is the deeds of great men. Brian Abel-Smith [2, 3] and Rosemary Stevens [31] are two social scientists who have written important comparative and longitudinal histories of such key institutions as hospitals and nursing.

But virtually no one has speculated about the impact of the institutions which shape the health of the great numbers of people before they are ill or before they are conscious of the infirmities of chronic disease and old age. There is still to be made a critical analysis of the School of Public Health movement initiated around the First World War by Professor William Henry Welch and the Rockefeller Foundation. The Johns Hopkins School of Hygiene was the first effort; it brought together, in the name of preventive medicine, the disciplines of epidemology, biostatistics and sanitary engineering; not unexpectedly, it left out economics, an omission explicitly corrected in the last decade. This ignoring of economics has been more than matched by the more recent parochialism of economists whose interest in health policy still all too frequently proceeds with scant, if any, reference to contributions by the disciplines established in medical and public health schools.

My point is that this ignoring of the multidisciplinary dependence is a vital gap; in the absence of its being filled, we economists often look at the wrong immediate causes where we should be thinking about earlier or even prime causes. The historical literature has not helped us, and this is not only a pity, but a need worthy of immediate remedy.

[1] The eschewing of this line of investigation should in no sense suggest that I think it of minimal current relevance. In the history of health care great names and great theories are many. Hippocrates, practicing in Epidaurus four centuries before the Christian era, set forth the rules for the ethics of medical care; they are still dominant. Galen, preaching two hundred years later in Pergamon, had important ideas about medical care delivery; he set up a health care facility which clearly involved multi-phasic diagnosis and treatment. As we come closer to the present, examples proliferate.

II. WHAT ARE HEALTH SERVICES?

The economics of health involves considerably more than the supply of, or demand for, hospital space, physician or nursing time, or even what the gross national product accounts describe as 'medical care' (cf. [1], [4], [5]). Even the study of the spectrum of prices, however they are determined and administered, and the development of attendant cost–benefit ratios are also only a small part of the topic.

(1) The Supply Side

If we turn first to the supply side, we find that, among economists, almost everyone defines the topic in terms of medical care delivery. And although there is enough in this functional definition to justify several sessions at this Conference, my opinion is that there has been, and is still today, far more to the study of improving health care delivery than the study of the role of physicians, other medically trained personnel, or clinics and hospitals. Improving health is accomplished both in treatment and prevention; not only by curing the ill but, even more, by improving the environment of the workplace, the home, and even the urban/regional setting. These latter changes, more often than not, are principally non-medical in perception and execution. Historically, improved nutrition, centralized high-pressure water service, sewage service and improved housing have had a greater impact in lowering infant mortality rates and improving life expectancy than any improvements in medical care delivery. This view, derived from mortality data and from a careful perusal of the literature on medical technology, is now generally accepted [25, 26, 27]. So much for my preliminary remarks on the need for broadening the study of the supply side.

(2) The Demand Side

Studies of the demand for health services have been few in number. We have included in this Conference several papers which estimate usage (effective demand). Work done by Timothy D. Baker, M.D., and by me in 1962 in Taiwan produced several interesting insights [8], some of which have been partly confirmed by others. Professor Ronald Andersen's group, including specifically Professor Odin Anderson, using a National Opinion Research Center (American) sample [6], has made important contributions and has gone on to compare the American effective utilization pattern with the Swedish in a study in which he collaborated with Dr Bjorn Smedby, a physician and faculty member of Uppsala University. These studies all suggest that effective utilization of medical care services is determined by chance (a somewhat stochastic incidence of disease by age group), wealth (often measured by family income level) and social class. Baker's and my Taiwan study surprised us by indicating that urban/rural location was not a significant factor in explaining who saw physicians; rather, wealth was a significant indicator: the rich in the country got as much as the rich in the urban area – it was just that the proportions of the poor in rural areas (as adjusted for age) are relatively higher [8]. A second Johns Hopkins study in Turkey inferred the same situation prevailing [32]. But Grossman's excellent recent book finds otherwise anent American data [18]. I hasten to add, however, that the demand for expenditure of funds for prevention of food pollution, prevention of environmental pollution and other kinds of epidemiological effort should share this *a priori* reason for recognition. *Reculons pour mieux sauter.*

(3) *Other Approaches*
For our purposes it is also useful to organize thinking about health services in other ways. First, there is the division between clinical (generally curative) services and preventive (prophylaxis) services. This distinction is more real than is often apparent; confusion stems from the fact that immunology (a major element in preventive medicine) is clearly physicians' job-territory while much, if not most, of the rest of preventive medicine is handled by non-physicians. Confusion is further exacerbated because a great deal of the work done under the rubric of clinical or curative medicine draws little on the scientific skill of the physician, but heavily on his patience, understanding and a willingness to listen non-normatively to individuals weighed down by the burdens of conscience and/or alienation. In all events, the important point here is simply to note that the historical record clearly shows that emphasis only on clinical and/or physician care or labor substitutes for such care reveals a critical naïveté.

Another approach is to look at the whole health field by drawing a distinction between efforts made to augment health in order to encourage production, and efforts made to augment health in order to improve consumption. The former stresses health as an 'intermediate product', the latter as a 'final product'. Much of the recent work on health care has been identified with the assumption that 'investment in health' reduced private and social costs and, consequently, paid for itself. Employers, for example, quickly learned the lesson that if industrial accidents were prevented, industrial accident insurance premiums could be reduced, and private costs to the firm and/or industry would consequently be less and profits or wages consequently more. The irrefutable neatness of this logic has at times spilled over to a further assertion that if illness could also be prevented, regular workers would be present in the optimum numbers, and productivity would increase with earnings rising. For many reasons, the implied assumption should be fully specified to make this argument – that worker health is almost everything – completely tenable.[1] In any case, while the cost to firms of industrial accidents is clearly measurable in the form of increased insurance premiums, the element of loss because of the absence of the regular (usual) employee is less perceptible. Yet one has to have far better data and a better understanding of the assumption (more complete information) to draw useful generalizations.[2]

Consideration of health as a consumer good involves reconsideration of the whole set of accustomed analytical apparatus. This approach stresses that the individual and/or the community spends on health because he wants to be healthy in order to improve the quality of life. He does not justify this expenditure on the basis of a change in his anticipated income flow. Quite the contrary, he may justify this expenditure by its making it possible for him to get along with less income (not having to pay for medical care) and consequently making it possible for him to enjoy more leisure or to enjoy more profoundly what leisure he already has. Expenditure on medical care in this event lends itself only tangentially to the use of the human capital approach. A recent most interesting National Bureau of Economic Research monograph, mentioned in another context below, does touch, but only tangentially, on this point: '. . . healthy time has a negative income elasticity. If the consumption aspects of health were at all relevant, then a literal interpretation of the observed income effect would suggest that health is an inferior commodity; however, this is not the only possible interpretation of the results' [18].

Many nations, ranging from the right-wing nineteenth-century Bismarckian autocracy to twentieth-century centrally planned

---

[1] I think the case can often be made that the interruptions in workers' job attendance are not as important as the quality of management.

[2] Yet to drop the matter on this basis is a major error, because there is another important element to this question. In developed countries, particularly because of a preference for social welfarism and a decision to pay for it by income and payroll taxes, there has been, in part at least, an increasing substitution of physical capital goods for labor. With the advent of job-guaranteeing provisions, labor in manufacturing is no longer the variable cost it once was, and machines are no longer the fixed costs they once were. Thus, where there might have been an argument once that a 'healthy worker' was the obvious key to competitive success, there is now increasing economic reason for preventive maintenance on machines. I do not aver that all workers are 'outmoded'; indeed, had I the time I would probably argue that there is an empirical case for showing that increased investment in physical capital correlates very well with increased reliance upon professional and less specialized white-collar (rather than manual) labor. Consequently, whatever was once true about the health of the manual worker is probably as true, or more so, now in the case of the professional and white-collar laborers. But that is another essay.

socialist economies, have used an *a priori* perception of their citizens' desire for health services as a major element in their political programs. If we lack hard data confirming the details of these decisions, there is, at least, considerable prima-facie evidence suggesting that these choices have been made; countries relying less on central planning, in so far as they have moved towards providing state welfare services, have increasingly replaced market allocation of health care services with some form of bureaucratic allocative power. What I have in mind here is the kind of health service provided by the various Scandinavian countries, the British National Health Service, the American Medicare/Medicaid Program and, finally, such intriguing mechanisms for decreasing (at least at first thought) health care by making certain forms of prepaid health programs fully tax-deductible.

There are, of course, other ways to approach the topic from the economists' tradition. But these three, (1) the clinical as contrasted with the preventive. (2) the focus on substitutabilities in shaping supply and/or the focus on the determinants of demand, and (3) the approach of investment in health for production purposes compared to expenditure on health for improved consumption, all seem to me to make sense.

III. HEALTH DATA

What we know about a community's health has historically been inferred from certain vital statistics data which are, to say the least, poor proxies for what we would like to know. The United Nations Secretariat, to cite one of the better examples, uses infant mortality data to infer population growth rates [34]. Of necessity, demographers and economists have to use death certificates; although they are better sources than anything else generally available, they remain poor sources. Such certificates are invariably prepared by personnel who are given information by mortally ill individuals or by their relatives and friends. Thus, the basic demographic data (age, occupational experience and educational level) are poor. The health information is, in all probability, equally poor because 'cause of death' is usually impressionistic (not confirmed by a pathologist's post-mortem study) and usually describes only one cause when more than one is likely to be the case. Yet what is the most serious gap is that mortal illness, although an important element of the disease picture, provides only a small portion of disease data. Disease, whether chronic or episodic, can result in only one death certificate per individual; the important element in terms of pain and interruption of production and/or consumer activity in most instances will not result in such a certificate.

Of recent years attempts have been made to register (ultimately to measure) the incidence of disease. Initially, these attempts were inspired by the desire to contain contagious disease (epidemics). Smallpox and cholera, to mention two out of a much longer list, inspired sufficient fear so that reasonably accurate counts were made. But the perception of the presence of the disease was unsystematic. Recent research suggests that only one in three of those who had significantly reproducing cholera organisms in their gastrointestinal tracts is aware of his classic cholera symptoms; another one in three is aware only of the discomforts of 'accustomed' diarrhea; while the third is unaware of any deviant symptoms, but is a carrier none the less. Clearly, patient perception is not a very reliable measure of disease symptoms; as such, then, patients may not be a very good source of disease incidence data.

Clinical observations by trained medical personnel are better. Yet these are very expensive processes. Of recent years, some countries have used a multi-phasic process to find out about disease incidence. More such research is probably needed. And if the cost is high, consider how much is spent in the health sector without any systematic measure of product and of objectives; the image of needless groping for a pin in the dark come to mind. We do have, however, sophisticated non-quantitative evidence on disease experience. Pathology, one of the most intellectual and scientific areas of medical practice, has records for over a century on many disease patterns – including incidence *sequelae;* the histories of epidemics, as perceived by trained eyes, give us information from which stable inferences can be drawn. These inferences relate not only to the incidence of disease, but also to changes in symptoms and lasting effects. Difficulty arises when medically untrained research scholars (including, specifically, economists) start making inferences about incidence of disease from unreviewed observations; that is, where economists have depended upon data unexamined or 'uncertified' by competent pathologists or epidemiologists. These data lacunae should be filled and there are prima-facie reasons for doing it soon. Unfortunately, economists must wait until others have done that work; only then will economists have the data necessary for their own work. Or, to put the matter bluntly, as perception of the importance of health care grows, it is mandatory that economists recognize that their tools can be used only on adequately understood data.

Aside from these biologically scientific sources of health data, there are other useful sources. Among these are records of civil contracts found in health insurance relationships. Insurance carrier experience with income assurance policies, written as annuities, yields considerable information about health in certain labor-force sectors.

Although, it is true, most of this information applies to the wealthy part of the population, nonetheless inferences can be drawn. Civil litigation records, particularly in accident cases involving loss of earning capacity or even chronic pain conditions, are other rather well-balanced sources for learning something about trends in health expectation.

The point of all of the foregoing is that economists, working in the health area, have to use both caution and ingenuity in obtaining their data because systematic, stable data have yet to be collected. As elsewhere, collection of the data and their analysis requires sophistication.

IV. SOME CURRENT APPROACHES

In the recent period, economists, perhaps manifesting some atavistic classicalism, have tended to approach their studies of the economics of health care from the standpoint of the complexities of production. Two perceptions seem dominant. One stresses that the costs of disease and illness are paid either by the worker or by the consumer; consequently it is possible, indeed likely, that the cost of avoiding such disease or illness pays of itself by increased income flow or the lowered cost of goods and services. This approach is professionally identified as the 'investment in human capital' approach.

The other, production-centered, orientation attempts to improve the efficiency of health care delivery systems. This improvement can be accomplished on the microeconomic level – the physician's office, the hospital or even the administration of a particular health care insurance system. It can also be accomplished on macroeconomic levels involving choices within the financing of, and, particularly, operational specialization within, national health schemes. This approach is basically oriented to the ultimate construction of appropriate production functions and stresses the determination of viable trade-offs (substitutabilities) of the various inputs into the production process.

There are other approaches as well; but although I discuss them at the end, they have not, as yet, attracted as much research effort.

(1) *The Investment in Human Capital Approach*
Particularly when expenditure on health is viewed as an intermediate product and is used to lower prices by reducing factor costs, there are advantages to capitalizing the incremental factor income flow associated with good health. The idea for this is undoubtedly old: contemporary literature really starts with Louis Dublin's and Alfred J. Lotka's 1946 work [11]. More recently, several authors have studied losses of earnings associated with specific diseases. Names

like Weisbrod [37], Fein [14], Klarman [20, 21, 22] and Rice [30, 35, 36] come to mind. Their method is somewhat over-generously called the 'benefit–cost' approach to studies of particular diseases. In fact, what they are, are studies of the capitalized values associated with alleged net benefits if the disease had not occurred or had been cured at known costs. None of these studies estimates the indirect costs of specific disease eradication programs. Moreover, in most instances the alleged benefits of the elimination of the disease preclude all probabilities of the 'patients' having other debilitating diseases. Moreover, the assumptions relating to earnings (essential to estimating the costs of the disease or of the potential benefits of health) center on averages, the revelance (to say nothing about the reliability) of which is shaky. My point is simply that these studies are very general approximations, perhaps intended to show the potential usefulness of a method rather than to show why one health preventive or cura-tive policy is superior (of a higher social or personal priority) over another. This level of analysis has been micro-analytically focused; its obvious primary purpose is to identify what disease conditions cause the greatest social and/or private loss. Ultimately, given the estimates of what prophylaxis or cure can do and what they should cost, the path to inference about policy choices should be straight and well illuminated. From the analytical standpoint, Feldstein's 1967 paper suggests ways to deepen such policy choices ([16], but cf. also [14], [15]).

(2) *The Production Function Approach*
The production function approach covers a wide sweep. Histories of hospital cost experience [2, 3], the historical costs of training various types of professionals, and ways to determine from an accounting standpoint the cost-effectiveness of combining under the aegis of one institution or group of institutions ultimately lead to knowledge which can be fitted into the mold of a production function. Bits and pieces of particular experiences can be fitted together to give under-standing of technologically possible trade-offs and the costs of savings associated therewith. What is intriguing is the variety of levels of aggregation which can be employed to formulate these production functions. And again, once they have been identified, the inference is clear; policy or empirical validation follows.

The production function technique applies not only to the costs of training para-professionals and professionals and to the running of hospital departments and hospitals; it also, ultimately, extends to studying the operation of whole health care systems. There is a burgeoning literature on the topic; nonetheless, it still suffers from a 'bits and pieces' orientation. To this particular point I shall refer at this paper's end. Here I want simply to note that the topic, narrowly perceived, is technically difficult, with at least two considerations serving to muddy its clarity.

First, there is the need to understand that efficiency has to be qualified by considering the need to maintain some degree of standby capacity. Unfortunately, disease incidence is, in the aggregate, not stably stochastic [9, 28]; instead, disease surges in waves, and whatever value there is to the criterion of production efficiency has to be much modified if a modicum of compassion is to be allowed. But there is another complication as well.

There is a question of many kinds of barriers. Some are technical: physicians require expensive training, the sheer enormousness of the cost of which serves to limit the size of the corps. This technical constraint is reinforced by what Sidney and Beatrice Webb called the 'device of restriction of numbers', or self-interest phenomena. Yet there are other factors which restrain the substitutabilities options. Social insistence upon very high-quality training for all personnel has often been used to thwart attempts to provide some medical care for those who presently can expect to receive none. Also, legal regulations, probably more wise than stupid, restrict choices of alternatives and serve to prevent para-professionals from filling in where the supplies of professionals are so small as to push prices skyward.

V. CONCLUDING OBSERVATIONS

Perhaps the most neglected area of study is the one tying environmental and nutritional influences to health care efforts. It is hard, these days, to escape hearing about awful environment and the need to incorporate the cost of pollution into our systems of national accounts and our perceptions of production costs. Yet it is in precisely this area that the economic historian's word is so needed.

For the flies of a horse-powered transporation system are remembered by few in the industrialized world, except the historian. The great cities of the industrialized world existed before they had intricate sewage and drainage systems. And there was a time, less than five generations ago, when the British Parliament had to suspend debate because of the stench from the river Thames. Pollution eradication is becoming the intellectual passion, the *idée fixe*, of our generation; it is wise to recall that the evil is not new, and its eradication will do what it has done in the past: shift health concern from an overburdened medical care delivery system to an area where we hope it can be handled more efficiently – preventive health problem services (but cf. [24]).

No less significant is the need to focus on the economic consequences of nutrition reform [10]. It may well be that this area, so
little understood by physicians, by development economists ([33]
and, particularly, [38]) or, for that matter, by anyone else, will
become the great research mother-lode. In any event, little has thus
far been done.

REFERENCES

[1] Abel-Smith, Brian, 'Health Priorities in Developing Countries: The
Economist's Contribution', *Health Services*, II (1972) 5–12.
[2] ——, *A History of the Nursing Profession* (London: Heinemann, 1960).
[3] ——, *The Hospitals, 1800–1948* (Cambridge, Mass.: Harvard Univ. Press,
1963).
[4] ——, 'The Major Pattern of Financing and Organization of Medical
Services that have Emerged in Other Countries', *Medical Care*, III (Jan–Mar
1965) 33–40.
[5] ——, *Paying for Health Services: A Study of the Costs and Sources of
Finance in Six Countries*, Public Health Papers No. 32 (Geneva: World
Health Organization, 1967).
[6] Andersen, Ronald, and Anderson, Odin W., *A Decade of Health Services:
Social Survey Trends in Use and Expenditures* (Chicago and London: Univ.
of Chicago Press, 1967).
[7] ——, Smedby, Bjorn, and Andersen, Odin W., *Medical Care Use in Sweden
and United States: A Comparative Analysis of Systems and Behavior*, Center
for Health and Administrations Study No. 27 (Univ. of Chicago, 1970).
[8] Baker, Timothy D., and Perlman, Mark, *Health Manpower in a Developing
Economy. Taiwan: A Case Study in Planning* (Baltimore: John Hopkins
Press, 1967).
[9] Barlow, R., *Economic Effects of Malaria Eradication*, Bureau of Public
Health Economics Research Series No. 15 (Ann Arbor: Univ. of Michigan,
1968); also in *American Economic Review, Papers and Proceedings*, LVII
(May 1967) 130–48.
[10] Drummond, J. C., and Wilbraham, A., *The Englishman's Food*, rev. ed.
(London: Cape, 1958).
[11] Dublin, Louis I., and Lotka, Alfred J., *The Money Value of a Man* (New
York: Ronald Press, 1946).
[12] Dubos, Réne J., *Louis Pasteur: Free Lance of Science* (Boston: Little Brown,
1950).
[13] Eversley, D. E. C., 'The Home Market and Economic Growth in England,
1750–80', in E. L. Jones and G. E. Mingay (eds.), *Land, Labor and Population in the Industrial Revolution*. (London: Edward Arnold, 1967).
[14] Fein, Rashi, *Economics of Mental Illness*, Joint Commission on Mental
Illness and Health Monograph No. 2 (New York: Basic Books, 1958).
[15] Feldstein, Martin S., *Economic Analysis for Health Service Efficiency*,
Economic Analysis No. 51 (Chicago: Markham, 1968).
[16] ——, 'Measuring the Costs and Benefits of Health Services', in *The Efficiency
of Medical Care* (Copenhagen: World Health Organization, 1967).
[17] Finer, S. E., *The Life and Times of Sir Edwin Chadwick* (London: Methuen,
1951).
[18] Grossman, Michael, *The Demand for Health: A Theoretical and Empirical*

Investigation, National Bureau of Economic Research Occasional Paper No. 119 (New York: Columbia Univ. Press, for N.B.E.R., 1972).

[19] Helleiner, K. F., 'The Vital Revolution Reconsidered', *Canadian Journal of Economic and Political Science*, XXIII (1957) 1–9.

[20] Klarman, Herbert E., 'Present Status of Cost–Benefit Analysis in the Health Field', *American Journal of Public Health*, LVII, 11, (Nov 1967) 1948–52.

[21] ——, 'Socioeconomic Impact of Heart Disease', in *The Heart and Circulation*, 2nd National Conference on Cardiovascular Disease (Washington, D.C.: Federation of American Societies for Experimental Biology, 1965).

[22] ——, 'Syphilis Control Programs', in R. Dorfman (ed.), *Measuring Benefits of Government Investments* (Washington, D.C.: Brookings Institution, 1965).

[23] Lambert, Royston, *Sir John Simon, 1816–1904, and English Social Administration* (London: MacGibbon & Kee, 1963).

[24] Lave, L. B., and Seskin, E. P., 'Air Pollution and Human Health: The Quantitative Effect, with an Estimate of the Dollar Benefit of Pollution Abatement, is Considered', *Science*, CLXIX (1970) 723–33.

[25] McKeown, Thomas, Brown, R. G., and Record, R. G., 'An Interpretation of the Modern Rise of Population in Europe', *Population Studies*, XXVI, 3 (1971) 345–82.

[26] ——, and Brown, R. G. 'Medical Evidence Related to English Population Changes in the Eighteenth Century', *Population Studies*, IX (1955) 119–41.

[27] ——, and Record, R. G., 'Reasons for the Decline of Mortality in England and Wales during the Nineteenth Century', *Population Studies*, XVI (1961) 94–122.

[28] Newman, Peter, *Malaria Eradication and Population Growth with Special Reference to Ceylon and British Guiana* (Ann Arbor: Bureau of Public Health Economics, Univ. of Michigan, 1965).

[29] Razzell, P. E., 'Population Change in Eighteenth Century England: A Reinterpretation', *Economic History Review*, XVIII (1965) 312–32.

[30] Rice, D. P., 'Measurement and Application of Illness Costs', *Public Health Reports*, LXXXIV (Feb 1969) 95–101.

[31] Stevens, Rosemary, *American Medicine and the Public Interest* (New Haven: Yale Univ. Press, 1971).

[32] Taylor, Carl E., Dirican, Rahmi, and Deuschle, Kurt W., *Health Manpower Planning in Turkey* (Baltimore: Johns Hopkins Press, 1968).

[33] ——, and Hall, M. F., 'Health Population and Economic Development', *Science*, CLVII (1967) 651–7.

[34] United Nations, *Age and Sex Patterns of Mortality: Model Life-Tables for Underdeveloped Countries*, Population Studies No. 22 (New York, 1955).

[35] United States Public Health Service, *Economic Costs of Cardiovascular Disease and Cancer, 1962*, Health Economics Series No. 5, Publication No. 947–5 (Washington, D.C.: Government Printing Office, 1965).

[36] ——, (Rice, Dorothy P.), *Estimating the Cost of Illness*, Health Economics Series No. 6, Publication No. 947–6 (Washington, D.C.: Government Printing Office, 1966).

[37] Weisbrod, Burton A., *Economics of Public Health: Measuring the Economic Impact of Diseases* (Philadelphia: Univ. of Pennsylvania Press, 1961).

[38] ——, Andreano, R. L., Baldwin, R. E., Epstein, E. H., and Kelley, A. C., 'Disease and Economic Development: The Impact of Parasitic Diseases in St Lucia (Madison: Univ. of Wisconsin, Feb 1971; unpublished).

Summary Record of Discussion

Following the initial formalities of opening and organizing the Conference, discussion began on the historical papers by Dr Hartwell and Professor Perlman.

Although *Mr Kaser* was the scheduled discussant of Professor Perlman's paper, he identified himself more with the long continuity of medical-economic history demonstrated by Dr Hartwell and embodied in his phrase 'All societies have devoted resources to medical care'. Perlman's was by contrast focused on a nineteenth-century revolution, when health care gained its present dimension of social provision (and that, Perlman claimed, due to bureaucratic ambition rather than embrace of a social objective). Mr Kaser contested Perlman's interpretation of the medieval Christian as led by his Church exclusively to personal salvation. Monastic hospitals were clear evidence of a social concern, even though today's inverse correlation of ill-health and welfare was often transformed into a direct one (as, for example, in mortification of the flesh or the 'offering up' of infirmity). The visitor to Magdalen College, Oxford, could see the embodiment of the Church's dual policy in the open-air pulpit from which a monk preached pious fortitude to the sick being cared for in the quadrangle below. Perlman was of course right in implying that it was not until the nineteenth century that professional medicine was able significantly to reduce mortality; previous improvements were largely effected by nutrition, environmental and public health measures, three areas on the present efficiency of which Perlman rightly invited the health economist to give more priority.

Professor Rosett was the scheduled discussant of the Hartwell paper. He immediately struck a note which was to pervade discussion in later sessions, by querying the common view that doctors had killed as many people as they cured until the nineteenth century, and therefore had done society no good. They had accomplished a great deal, in Professor Rosett's view, by reducing discomfort, providing symptomatic relief, and thereby improving the quality of life. (Illustrations were the reduction of the number of the seriously crippled, and the relief to sufferers from hare-lip and cleft palate.) It is important that these effects be remembered. If medical care becomes largely a public responsibility, improvement of the quality of lives may be as significant as saving them. In fact, according to Professor Rosett, quality-of-life aspects of medicine seem to be downgraded in existing public medical systems, which stress care for major ailments and subject patients with less serious ills to rationing and waiting. Somewhat paradoxically, quality-of-life medicine is provided better by the free market, and the comparative advantage of public systems lies in dealing with catastrophic medicine.

The floor was opened to interpellations after Professor Rosett's discussion. The first speaker, *Dr Phelps*, felt that the physician's major task is usually the provision of information of a diagnostic or prognostic sort, except perhaps in the two extreme cases of hypochondria and terminal illness. *Professor Rosett* accepted this addition to his own case, stressing also *preparation* for invalidism and/or mortality. He felt that the continuity of care associated with the private system's doctor–patient relationship was important in this connection.

Dr Christiansen defended public medicine against these criticisms. In Scandinavia at least, discomfort is not neglected, especially not in orthopedic surgery. He particularly opposed any 'division of labor' proposals which would limit the public system to extreme cases of illness, which of course would make the system look bad because of high mortality rate.

Professor Fuchs made three points, not in conflict with the two papers. (1) Early medicine seems to have done more harm than good. (2) The social-psychological role of the physician in 'legitimizing the sick man's social role' can likewise be performed by faith-healers and witch-doctors. (3) The demand for medical services may be either exogenous to the medical system or created endogenously by that system. Thus, even with the same sort of medical system, demand varies from one culture to another.

Professor L. Lave formalized certain views presented earlier by presenting medical care as a matrix, with consumption and investment as 'benefit' or 'demand' vectors, and with public and private systems as 'supply' vectors. (Until medical efficacy reached a certain level, only the consumption aspect was important, and medicine contributed little 'human capital investment'.) Professor Lave saw symptomatic relief as the historical role of private medicine, and the provision of special facilities like pest-houses and leprosaria as the historical roles of public medicine. Efficacy, however, brought with it 'public good' aspects, and demands that these be made available more widely. Professor Lave concluded that even today a case could be made for limiting the public interest in medicine to 'investment' and 'human capital' aspects, with consumption left largely to the private sector. *Professor Rosett* in reply, felt that the consumption–investment distinction is more valid in theory than in practice, especially when account is taken of short-period investment.

Professor Williams feared that the historical approach might be misleading, in neglecting the long-period cumulation of small real improvements, both as regards medicine proper and as regards other approaches to health. In nutrition, he cited the treatment of obesity, alcohol and tobacco. In public health and hygiene, he feared that the marginal productivity might be negative in the long term, through lowering the population's level of natural immunity. One should also consider the increased pressure on the medical system from rising population density generally, as well as such specific problems as industrial and traffic accidents. In short, Professor Williams felt that the papers had understressed the case for medicine.

Professor Robinson introduced a Malthusian note, feeling that distinctions are necessary between benefits to individuals (patients) and to society as a whole. He wondered, for example, what the actual effects of the eradication of malaria have been in both regards. Passing specifically to development problems, Professor Robinson cited Bangladesh (where approximately two-thirds of increased income goes to support increasing population) as an example of environmental controllers threatening civilization, via population explosion, on a scale comparable with the nuclear-bomb threat from physics. He saw the Japanese record as due largely to greater success in controlling population growth, although perhaps at the cost of another form of social disarray (pollution). Was not the Black Death basically a good thing, inasmuch as the British record dates progress from this event? In summary, Professor Robinson questioned the convention of judging the social contribution of medicine by its effects on mortality and life expectancy.

Returning to the quality-of-life discussion, *Professor Leinhardt*, himself a sociologist, suggested the explicit introduction of sociology into the discussion, and with it the importance of non-quantitative variables. The term 'quality-of-life', he felt, is itself a vector, depending upon history and culture. People in different cultures express their demands for health differently, seeking different sources, and dealing with these sources differently. Part of our problem may be that medical systems are monolithic, and take insufficient account of these differences.

Professor Liefmann-Keil stressed the interdependence of medical history and the history of economic thought. Individual doctors have been interested in economic problems, François Quesnay being an obvious case in point. Others, particularly in Germany, have attempted to compute the value of human life, the costs of specific illnesses and the economic benefits obtainable by reductions in mortality rates. She hoped that the present Conference might lead to more interdisciplinary contact between medicine and economics.

Dr Christiansen's second interpellation was anti-Malthusian. He felt that the growth of cities in advanced countries had been due more to internal migration than to population growth, and that the need for public investment there was due primarily to cultural lags in adjusting our habits to technological change, especially motorization. He also objected to economists' stress on human capital citing, E. J. Mishan as urging the complete abandonment of this particular concept.

Dr Kleiman felt that individual welfare contributes to that of the nation when the length of individual productive life is increased and the capital–labor ratio is changed accordingly. These gains, he felt, were amenable to individual computations of the indifference curve variety in framing demands for health.

Health care was regarded as a public good, Dr Kleiman continued, in ancient legal systems. He cited the laws of Hammurabi, Moses and Imperial Rome. In more recent times, increased national income and social equality have increased the stress on public health. These effects are all increased by rising expectations in every country, inspired by reports of progress elsewhere.

Professor J. Lave undertook the defence of economists against charges of being too narrow and of asking the wrong questions. She admitted, however, a certain occupational bias for looking at inputs as surrogates for outputs, because health inputs are more easily measured than health outputs. She also raised the question of the allocation of health inputs at the two extremes of terminal and preventive medicine, and wondered how such decisions would or could be made rationally, either in a public system by health authorities or in a private system by individuals.

Mr Pole and *Mr Kaser*, in different contexts, stressed problems of data unreliability. Mr Pole was concerned with morbidity and 'cause of death' data within the United Kingdom, whereas Mr Kaser felt that international comparisons and classifications at any given time were just as non-comparable as intra-national ones at different points in history.

The writers of the two papers had the closing words.

Professor Perlman, as co-chairman, had tried to organize his paper in a form reflecting what had been perceived from the early abstracts of the accepted papers as the frame of the Conference as a whole. His first point had been to consider the limitations of historical literature, stressing that medical care is one entity and other forms of health were others. Second, he had tried to break down 'the health of the nations' into its supply and demand aspects. On the supply side, he felt Galen and Hippocrates had been virtually as good as anything generally available before 1900. On the demand side, we really have no historical measures, especially if we recognize the distinction between preventive and curative medicine and consider the para-medical contributions of nutrition, sanitation and education. Third, he (Professor Perlman) had tried to improve the 'data' discussion by stressing the distinctions between health, mortality and life expectancy. (He believes the relation between mortality and morbidity to be highly unstable.) Fourth, he proposed to criticize most economists for staying too closely within standard economics and, more recently, for stressing analytical techniques designed to estimate the capitalized value of investment in human capital over the value of consumption activity as seen in the quality-of-life. (Centrally planned economies, Professor Perlman felt, make better decisions here.) On production functions, Professor Perlman accepted their use but feared they might be misleading, unless they included such other variables as sanitary engineering along with medical care as causative variables. At the same time, he defended some health benefit–cost analysis on the principle that a partly bad statement may be preferable to none at all, and that, by analogy, many national income data are little or no better than those of health economics. And as a final note (in answer to Dr Klieman) he expressed the view that modern epidemiology represents a major advance over the religious and quasi-religious laws of the ancients, because modern studies are based upon science rather than upon revelation.

Dr Hartwell began his own summary by defending the historical approach, on the ground that contemporary concerns may decline in importance later on, and vice versa. He repeated his conclusion that lack of medical care has been less important (as compared with disease, malnutrition and unsanitary conditions) than is believed in standard demography. The main factors in later improvements have been, he felt, in public health, nutrition and sanitation, rather than in medical care (or, for that matter, the Industrial Revolution). For some reason not yet fully understood, a number of 'great killers' all declined in the eighteenth century – plague, smallpox, malaria and leprosy. Only in the case of smallpox was there much 'medical input'. Another reason why medicine could not have done either much good or much harm before approximately 1900 was that there was so little of it that earlier improvements (or errors) had affected only the few. And even in the present century, Dr Hartwell believed increasing medical care less important than, for example, education in affecting the general population.

As four major elements of continuity in the historical record, Dr Hartwell cited (1) preventive medicine and public health, (2) the regulation of the medical profession itself, and its responsibility for the sick poor, (3) the increasing importance of sanitation, and enforcement of minimum standards of cleanliness, and (4) the rise of social insurance, orignally on a voluntary basis.

Replying to one or two points brought out in the discussion, Dr Hartwell felt that the demand for medical care as a public good was related less to increasing medical efficacy than to increasing national income and wealth. He also said that the marginal efficacy of non-medical factors remains positive for the developing countries despite 'population explosion' factors, and doubted the seriousness of overpopulation problems in the developing economies with which the Conference primarily deals.

Part Two

Problems of the Demand for and Supply of Health Services, and the Relation of Mortality to Economic Activity

3 The System of Medical Care in Japan and its Problems

Takeshi Kawakami

SUGINAMI KUMIAI HOSPITAL, TOKYO

This paper describes the evolution of medical care in Japan with considerable analytical attention to the emergence of several economic system 'contradictions'. These contradictions include the profitable operation of hospital units and widespread location of these units, scholarly merit of students and ability of families to pay full tuition costs, and the market ethos and the humanitarian instinct. The nature of disease problems has, of recent years, changed. The paper concludes by turning to the problem of improving the health care delivery system within the framework of the kind of market economy Japan presently has.

I. GENERAL PICTURE OF MEDICAL CARE IN JAPAN

It is indeed true that, despite some deepening contradictions, medical care in Japan, during one hundred years of her modernization, has made considerable progress in response to the developmental process of capitalism. Although it is a matter of great importance which index of progress to choose for assessment in making socio-economic analysis of medical care, here at the outset I should like to refer to some statistical figures in order to clarify both the changes in the last hundred years and the present status of medical care in Japan.

Table 3.1 demonstrates how a series of technical innovations in medical care and the expansion of the social security system have caused substantial changes in the life expectancy, the mortality rate and the order of causes of death in Japan. It also indicates the prevalence of abortion, which is peculiar to post-war Japan, and the increasing coverage of the medical insurance system.[1]

Table 3.2 shows the numbers of doctors, of medical colleges and of hospitals. Attention should be paid to the high percentage of the private colleges and hospitals.

[1] The population covered by the medical insurance system in 1970 appears to be too large, but this is due to some overlapping in the process of statistical compilation.

TABLE 3.1

VITAL STATISTICS 1970, JAPAN: LIFE EXPECTANCY, MORTALITY RATE, ORDER OF DEATH CAUSES, INFANT MORTALITY RATE, ABORTION AND THE COVERAGE OF MEDICAL INSURANCE

Stages	Life expectancy Male	Life expectancy Female	Mortality rate (per 1000 persons)	Order of causes of death (1)	(2)	(3)	(4)	(5)	Infant mortality rate (per 1000 live births)	Abortion[g]	Population ('000)	No. of persons covered by medical insurance ('000)
From Meiji Restoration to the golden age of the practitioner system (1868–1900) 1876	42·8[a]	44·3[a]	20·8[c]	Pneumonia Bronchitis	Tuberculosis	Apoplexy	Gastro-enteritis	Senility[d]	155·0[f]	—	43,847[i]	—
Socialization of medical care (1900–36)	44·8[b]	46·5[b]	22·2	Pneumonia Bronchitis	Gastro-enteritis	Tuberculosis	Apoplexy	Senility[e]	173·2	—	69,590	1,941[j]
1917 to immediately after the war (1945–)	50·1	54·0	14·6	Tuberculosis	Pneumonia Bronchitis	Gastro-enteritis	Apoplexy	Senility	76·7	246,104[h]	78,101	37,129
1947 up to the present	65·3	70·2	7·6	Apoplexy	Cancer	Heart Disease	Senility	Pneumonia Bronchitis	30·7	1,063,256	93,419	93,079[k]
1960 1970	69·3	74·7	6·9	Apoplexy	Cancer	Heart disease	Accidents	Senility	13·1	7,320,033	102,738	103,943

[a] 1891-8. [b] 1926-30. [c] 1900. [d] 1900. [e] 1920. [f] 1900. [i] 1900. [j] 1900. [h] 1949. [k] 1961. [g] Reported by the Eugenic Protection Law.

Source: The 12th Life Tables; Abridged Life Tables (1970), prepared by the Insurance Bureau, Ministry of Health and Welfare.

TABLE 3.2

SURVEY OF MEDICAL INSTITUTIONS; SURVEY OF PHYSICIANS, DENTISTS AND PHARMACISTS

Stages	No. of doctors[a]	No. of medical colleges			Annual graduates	No. of hospitals			No. of beds
		Total	Public	Private		Total	Public	Private	
From Meiji Restoration to the golden age of the practitioner system (1868–1900) 1879	33,503[b] (96·0)	34	16	18	0	159	124	35	··
Socialization of medical care (1900–36)	46,060 (83·0)	16	12	4	1,393	2,904	1,749	1,055	39,574
1917 to immediately after the war (1945–)	70,620 (90·4)	74[c] 64[d]	52[c] 47[d]	22[c] 17[d]	2,424[c] 4,353[d]	4,412	880	3,532	276,811[g]
1947 up to the present	103,131 (110.4)	46	33	13	about 3,400[e]	6,094	1,894	4,200	686,743
1960 to 1970	118,990 (114.7)	59	35	24	5,535[f]	7,974	1,832	6,142	1,062,553

[a] Figures in brackets are per 100,000 population. [b] Among these, 1,817 obtained a license by examination. [c] 1946. [d] 1947. [e] 1954. After the defeat in the war, sweeping integration and abolition of medical colleges took place. With the establishment of the new college system, they were reconstituted into 46 colleges. For a fairly long time after that, no new medical college was set up. (Yet increases in student numbers were seen.) [f] The fixed number in April 1972. With the opening of the medicine faculty in Akita University as a breakthrough, many medical colleges were newly established. Except for Jichi Medical College (which was attached to the Ministry of Local Autonomous Bodies), all were private. [g] 1949.

Source: *The History of Eighty Years in Japanese Medical Care System.*

TABLE 3.3

CHANGES IN THE NUMBER OF HOSPITALS BY SCALE

	1951	1960	1970
Total	3,796	6,094	7,974
20–29 beds	1,627	1,454	1,214
30–39	446	717	803
40–49	235	439	740
50–99	673	1,373	1,828
100–149	305	708	1,078
150–199	142	436	616
200 and over	368	1,067	1,695

Source: Survey of Medical Institutions, 1951, 1960, 1970.

Table 3.3 gives the changing composition of hospitals by size (in terms of the number of beds); it should be pointed out that the fact that more than 50 per cent of small hospitals with fewer than 100 beds are private is indicative of the peculiarity of Japanese medical care.

Table 3.4 shows the number of radiograph and electrocardiograph appliances possessed by clinics in three benchmark years. Although it is not necessarily appropriate, in view of the nature of medical technique, to infer the technical level of medical practitioners only by the number of such appliances in their possession, this table gives us at least some indication of that level so far attained by Japanese doctors. Unless we pay more attention to this aspect of medical care, the 'socialization of medical care', which has thus far been limited to the sphere of medical care payment, cannot be extended to encompass the medical care system as a whole.

TABLE 3.4

NUMBER OF GENERAL CLINICS IN POSSESSION OF RADIOGRAPH APPLIANCES AND ELECTROCARDIOGRAPH APPLIANCES

		Clinics[b]	
		With beds (%)	Without beds (%)
1951	Radiograph	7,109 (53·8)	9,995 (31·5)
	Equipment for laboratory examination[a]	8,001 (57·5)	13,023 (31·9)
1960	Radiograph	15,541 (65·5)	17,534 (50·7)
	Electrocardiograph	5,569 (23·4)	7,583 (21·5)
1969	Radiograph	22,314 (75·1)	22,812 (59·1)
	Electrocardiograph	17,204 (57·0)	20,884 (51·5)

[a] In 1951 electrocardiograph appliances were not yet in wide use.
[b] Figures in brackets show the percentage rate of clinics which were equipped.
Source: Survey of Medical Institution, 1951, 1960, 1969.

TABLE 3.5

GROSS NATIONAL MEDICAL CARE EXPENSES
(estimated)

	Gross medical expenses (in 100 million yen)	Annual rate of increase (%)	Percentage to national income
1949	1,133	—	4·1
1950	1,154	1·9	3·4
1951	1,163	0·8	2·6
1952	1,540	32·3	2·9
1953	2,070	34·4	3·5
1954	2,436	17·7	3·7
1955	2,715	11·5	3·7
1956	2,915	7·4	3·6
1957	3,243	11·3	3·5
1958	3,531	8·9	3·7
1959	3,899	10·4	3·5
1960	4,426	13·5	3·3
1961	5,462	23·4	3·5
1962	6,511	19·2	3·7
1963	7,966	22·3	3·9
1964	9,895	24·2	4·2
1965	11,737	18·6	4·5
1966	13,522	15·2	4·5
1967	15,643	15·7	4·8
1968	18,419	17·7	4·4
1969	21,519	16·8	4·4
1970	25,534	18·7	4·3

Source: Prepared by the Department of Health and Welfare Statistics, Ministry of Health and Welfare.

Table 3.5 gives the estimated gross value of national medical care expenses since 1949. As the figures in this table do not include the extra bed charge and attendance service fees, it cannot be denied that they underestimate the actual amount.

Tables 3.6 and 3.7 offer the growth in the output of medical supplies and the percentage occupied by the charge for drugs in the total medical care charges. These two tables together imply that medical care in Japan has increased its dependence upon drugs under the high economic growth.

II. ACCUMULATING CONTRADICTIONS IN JAPANESE MEDICAL CARE

It is true that the system of medical care in Japan has made great progress during its transition from 'modernization' to 'socialization',

TABLE 3.6

OUTPUT OF DRUG SUPPLIES

	Output (in million yen)	Annual rate of increase (%)
1950	31,916	2·9
1953	75,647	29·1
1954	78,468	3·7
1955	89,539	14·1
1956	103,767	15·9
1957	125,147	20·6
1958	130,712	4·4
1959	150,000	15·0
1960	176,012	17·9
1961	218,075	23·9
1962	265,596	21·8
1963	341,141	28·4
1964	423,225	24·1
1965	457,639	8·1
1966	507,108	10·8
1967	563,257	11·1
1968	688,953	22·3
1969	842,514	22·3
1970	1,025,319	21·7

Source: Prepared by the Pharmaceutical Affairs Bureau, Ministry of Health and Welfare.

TABLE 3.7

DRUG CHARGES (involving injections)
AS PERCENTAGE OF
MEDICAL CARE EXPENSES[a]

1960	21·5
1961	25·1
1962	28·7
1963	31·8
1964	36·8
1965	38·2
1966	38·9
1967	42·2
1968	39·6
1969	41·9
1970	43·2

[a] Calculated from charge point statistics in the government-managed health insurance in the month of May each year.

Source: Prepared by the Insurance Bureau, Ministry of Health and Welfare, Social Medical Care Survey.

supported by the expansion of social security in the course of the democratization process and also by a series of modernizations in medical technology. But at the same time it has encountered some serious problems in the course of the reconstruction and development of Japanese capitalism during the twenty-seven-year post-war period. These problems derive their essential nature from the very structure of the social system in Japan, although the inherent defects in the medical care system itself can hardly be discounted. As there is no space available for the detailed analysis of the specific problems confronting Japanese medical care, we shall have to be satisfied with a brief survey focusing mainly on the problem areas where the solution is urgently called for.

(1) *The Medical Care System*

Since the war, the law provides that hospitals should have 20 beds or more. In 1971, 57·3 per cent of the hospitals had 100 beds or fewer. With this number of beds it is difficult to sustain hospital finance. Thus, inevitably, such hospitals place an emphasis on out-patients, and the competition with clinics cannot be avoided. This results in an anarchic flow of patients, disrupting the systematic and qualitative differentiation of hospitals as against clinics. Middle-sized and even large hospitals, which cannot secure enough income within the limit of the medical care insurance system, survive only with the introduction of extra-charge beds. Thus, only the people with large incomes can hope to receive long-term treatments in the hospitals today.

While some urban hospitals are on their way to expansion and mechanical modernization on the financial basis of extra-charge beds, the number of doctorless districts is increasing year by year. Even in the cities, deficiencies in the emergency medical care system make some districts doctorless at night and on holidays, thus inviting discontent among the citizens concerned.

As to the functional differentiation in medical care between treatment and pharmacy, there has been much talk in support of such differentiation in principle ever since the Meiji Restoration. But in practice there has been little progress in this regard up to this day.

As to health centers, which constitute the primary institution for preventive medicine, they have suffered from the lack of resident doctors, with a post-occupancy rate of less than 50 per cent for more than ten years now. Such a situation causes 'hemiplegia', as it were, of these centers.

As for the rehabilitation and intermediary facilities, they are still in the stage where their importance has only begun to be recognized.

(2) *Medical Education*

Today, many hospitals in Japan suffer from a chronic lack of sufficient manpower, often causing serious functional impairment. The shortage of doctors, the central agents in medical care, was first felt in the clinics of remote corners of the country and also in the smaller local hospitals, but today it is felt in large urban hospitals as well. The employment of part-time doctors, originally intended as a temporary makeshift, is now a universal practice. The existence of a large number of part-timers among doctors is a reflection of the inadequacy of the salary system of the doctors in hospitals within the framework of the medical care system in Japan. On the surface, the shortage of doctors comes from the absolute limitation in the number of doctors in the face of the increased demand in medical care, and also from the unbalanced concentration of doctors in the cities. But the question is how and why such a situation has come about.

When the war was over, the Public Welfare Ministry was optimistic about the problem of the number of doctors; rather it was concerned with a possible surplus of them. Later it gradually turned out that doctors were in short supply, but the Ministry took no definite action for increasing their number, apparently under pressure from the Medical Association which was concerned with its vested interest. However, mounting discontent among the people, arising from the shortage of doctors, the need for bringing up successors to the members of the Medical Association, and the crippled condition of public hospitals and health centers, were all factors that cooperated in making the Public Welfare Ministry change its policy towards finally approving new medical colleges, which had long been held down, in the general tide of the 'Build More Colleges' boom.

Even then, however, the original plan was to approve mainly *private* medical colleges; but, under the pressure of public opinion, the government was finally compelled to open more *public* medical colleges as well, resulting, for the first time after the war, in a rush to medical colleges in 1971.

In Japan today, one can enter public medical colleges only under severest competition, while private medical schools are generally said to collect 10–20 million yen per aspirant as the entrance fee. Here it is clearly shown that the very training of medical doctors has an aspect which smacks of lucrative business.

The training of nurses who, together with doctors, constitute the cardinal part of the medical team, has been undertaken, with a few exceptions, mainly by practicing medical institutions themselves. The poor quality of the working conditions for nurses (severe and low-paid midnight duties, etc.), labor intensification and meager wages are the factors which aggravate the shortage of nurses further. It has been pointed out that only a half of the 500,000 qualified women are actually working as nurses.

As to the post-graduate training of doctors, the intern system, introduced after the war under the direction of the occupation authorities, turned out to be only nominal and lacking in substance and, in reality served as the source of unpaid labor. The system was abolished in 1967 under opposition from medical students and young doctors. In the course of this movement against the intern system, there arose struggles in medical colleges to break up the so-called *ikyoku*[1] system, which had been the symbol of the feudalistic element in Japanese medicine ever since the Meiji Restoration. This struggle actually ignited the campus turbulence of the late 1960s. In the wake of this conflict, the authorities came up with a proposal for the specialized doctor system in place of the existing degree system, which had long kept young doctors unpaid and tied for nearly ten years to the college hospitals or large hospitals. There have been opposition movements against this proposal in some of the medical societies. The controversy stands in a stalemate at present, and the solution is still being sought.

(3) *Medical Security*

The greatest problem besetting Japan's medical security today is a huge deficit in the social insurance account (especially in the government-managed health insurance). As the reconstruction from the ruins of the war progressed and the scope of coverage by the social security in medical care expanded, the problem of deficit in the social insurance account gradually arose and the deficit in the health insurance managed by the government attained a serious proportion for the first time in the fiscal year 1954. The direct cause of the deficit was, no doubt, an increase in the demand for medical care and the soaring cost of tuberculosis treatment. But it should not be forgotten that the basic problem behind it was the low income of the insurance subscribers.

During the following two decades, many problems in medical care came to be discussed, but they can be summarized, essentially, as the problem of medical charges. The policies in the hands of the government were two-sided: namely, to collect more insurance fees and/or to cut down the expenses in the payment for the medical treatment. It can be said that which policy was actually taken depended upon the balance of power between the paying side (i.e. the Health Insurance Societies Association and the government) and the receiving side

[1] Literally, it means a 'medical office unit'. But it used to be almost a guild-type organization with hierarchical structure.

(i.e. the Medical Association). Thus, the general public has a strong impression that the problem of medical care boils down to the history of the struggle between these two sides. It is to be regretted that such an impression obscures the essential nature of the Japanese medical security system.

At the beginning, there were several categories of social insurance schemes embodying differences in the payment rate, which reflected the view of private enterprises and the government that social security was a mutual aid system of the employees and that it could be utilized as an arm of labor management policy.

But as the strains of the policy of rapid economic growth became intensified, the category of social insurance covering low-income subscribers could no longer be taken care of by the principle of mutual aid as is characteristically shown in the government-managed health insurance which now has an accumulated deficit of 300 billion yen, with a monthly increase in the deficit of 10 billion yen. With the rise in the power of employees, the deficit eventually came to be covered by the national treasury. On the other hand, the accounts of health insurance societies of large enterprises with higher-income subscribers have been in the black all this time.

Thus, it has been the constant proposal of the government in recent years to merge the accounts of both classes of insurance, thereby reducing the burden upon the national treasury. This is the so-called 'overall adjustment of social insurance finance', aiming at the transition from the existing system of mutual aid inside the enterprises to that of nationwide mutual aid. Such a transition, however, is not easy inasmuch as there arises an inevitable conflict between the stand which the society *in toto* can take and the stand which an individual capitalist member is constrained to take.

(4) *The Structure of Diseases and the Structure of Medical Technology*

Owing to a series of post-war technological innovations, infectious diseases have receded, and instead, diseases of adulthood and of old age (as represented in malignant tumors, apoplexy, heart disease, etc.) and mental disorders have come to the front. Although basic medical researches on these diseases are by no means adequate enough, competent technology has been developed to cope with them which, together with the long-term treatment generally required for such diseases, necessitates the rising cost of medical care.

Further, as a result of the strains in the rapid economic growth policy, *kogai* (environmental pollution) diseases, occupational diseases and labor accidents have gained pominence over infectious diseases. Concerning such *kogai* diseases as Minamata disease (methyl-mercury poisoning), Itai-itai disease (cadmium poisoning) and Yokka-ichi asthma, lawsuits over their compensations have been in progress. Besides these diseases there continue to arise, one after another, new types of problems such as photochemical smogs, exhaust-gas lead poisoning, dangerous and contaminated foods, and so forth.

As to occupational diseases, by contrast with their pre-war localization in mines and plants with inferior conditions, today they haunt anywhere, as shown by the key-puncher's disease in modern offices of large cities.

Labor accidents, too, are becoming larger in scale and more frequent in occurrence, as seen in the great explosion (1963) in the Mi-ike coal mine which, in addition to the dead, left a large number of patients suffering from carbon monoxide poisoning.

Kogai, labor accidents and occupational diseases are essentially external diseconomies resulting from the 'rationalization' of industry at the sacrifice of the very human beings; and their solution is what modern capitalism is pressed for.

Further in this connection, a class of diseases originating from some medical treatment or drugs themselves has to be pointed out as an important problem in medical care today. The traditional inclination towards the use of drugs in the technical structure of Japanese medical care (the drug consumption per capita is said to be twice that of foreign countries), the relative neglect of safety, coupled with the rapid growth of the drug industry, have collaborated in producing numerous medicogenic diseases, unparalleled in other countries. Typical examples are the thalidomide deformity and the Smon[1] disease. Preventive inoculations are compulsory in Japan today, and the ill-effects arising from them have just entered the arena of public debate.

III. LIMITATIONS TO 'SOCIALIZATION OF MEDICAL CARE' IN JAPAN

The greatest contradiction besetting the system of medical care in Japan lies in the fact that, while the medical care charge payment system (medical care insurance) has been completely socialized, medical care is still provided through the private practitioner system, the same system that has obtained ever since the Meiji Restoration. In other words, it is the inevitable result of the 'socialization of medical care' within the limitation of a capitalistic form of medical care. However, in attempting to solve this contradiction, the government tends to try to put the medical care system under its

[1] Subacute myelo-optico-neuropathy.

control. Therefore, there is a possibility of its colliding with the practitioners on much more fundamental issues than the setting of medical care charges as such.

The true problem actually lies back of this; it lies in the Japanese peculiarity that the 'socialization of medical care' has been expanded to its maximum while limiting its scope only to the charge payment system. It is dangerous to discuss mechanically the socialization of medical care without examining this problem. If left as it is, the 'socialization' of medical care will turn out, in reality, to be bureaucratization, and there is a good possibility of its going against the true requirements of medical care.

Thus, it is now necessary to reconsider the implications of 'socialization' in the sphere of medical care in order to find the way out of the contradictions confronting medical care in Japan. If one is to cope with the problem of the socialization of medical care in its true sense, one will have to take into consideration the following four aspects of the problem:

(*a*) medical charge payment system (medical care insurance);
(*b*) the system and institutions of medical care;
(*c*) medical education;
(*d*) drug and medical industries.

All these for aspects are involved in the provision of medical care in our society; and in contrast to other commodities and services, it is too complex to be treated mechanically in terms of simple demand and supply. Among the above four factors, (*a*) reflects simply the functional side (as a service) of medical care, and is essentially reducible to the matter of pure monetary exchange, even though the valuation may differ between the doctor and the patient or the diagnosis and treatment may involve drugs and medical instruments. (*b*), (*c*) and (*d*), on the other hand, strongly reflect structural characteristics of the medical system, requiring large capital investment and involving the principle of private property. The capital invested in land and medical equipment per individual practitioner might be small, but the sum for all practitioners of the country would be enormous. The same situation applies to hospitals, medical colleges, the drug industry and the medical instrument industry.

The socialization of aspect (*a*) is theoretically possible within the framework of the capitalist system, although there may be technical problems concerning apportionment of the cost and the means of payment in the social insurance system, and also there may be opposition from the practitioners who have been accustomed to the principle of free practice.

By contrast, the socialization of aspects (*b*), (*c*) and (*d*) runs into a basic question of the capitalist system, namely, interference with the principle of private property. To circumvent such a conflict would require a tremendous amount of investment in bringing all the facilities under public administration.

Thus, the policy adopted in Japan has been to socialize, with a certain degree of success, only aspect (*a*) with limitations in payment rates, based on the principle of mutual aid.

On the other hand, no attempt has been made concerning aspects (*b*), (*c*) and (*d*), which have been, in fact, deliberately left untouched. Even what could be properly taken care of with public investment by the government has been left to private profit considerations. One example is the entrance charge collected by private medical colleges. It is only natural that a medical student who enters a medical college and pays an entrance fee of something like 10 million yen will be induced, when he begins practicing ten years later, to try to recover his early investment even while working within the security system which is completely socialized in principle so far as its payment aspect is concerned.

There is also a contradiction in that the payments to doctors are under the regulation of the social insurance scheme while the drugs used in the treatment are produced under the free enterprise system. Similar incongruities are numerous, and it is exactly the attempt to patch up these inconsistencies that has given rise to the various knotty problems confronting medical care in Japan.

From these discussions it is clear that the situation in Japan is worthy of a thorough study as an example of the complete socialization of the aspect of the medical charge payment system without touching upon other aspects such as medical education, the drug and medical industries, etc. Here there is also a challenge for the economics of medical care under modern capitalism.

Such 'socialization of medical care' as attempted in Japan is the consequence of the long-standing policy of the government, since the Meiji era, of shifting to the practicing doctors and to the people the cost of what is essentially in the nature of public investment in the sphere of medical care. The neglect in this sphere is nothing but the other aspect of the pre-war policy epitomized in 'Industry and Commerce First' and 'Rich Nation and Strong Soldiers', as well as the post-war policy of rapid economic growth. If we focus upon the restricted 'socialization of medical care' in Japan which touches only upon the medical care charge payment system, we cannot but recognize both the merits and demerits which arise from the combination of the free-of-charge service to patients and the reward in proportion to performance to doctors. Omitting a detailed analysis here, one may say, in summary, that the merit lies in bringing into the open the latent demand for medical treatment, while the demerit lies in the tendency of medical costs to soar thus magnifying the deficit problem of medical insurance.

Concerning the analysis of the present deficit problem, the paying side (the government and the Health Insurance Societies Association) and the receiving side (the Medical Association) hold totally different views. The former maintains that it results from the time-economizing on service by doctors for the purpose of increasing the number of cases treated and from the occasional overcharging, both of which ensue from the very system of the free-of-charge service and the reward in proportion to the services rendered. In this respect, there does exist a system of checking operated out of a fund from the medical charges that examines in detail all the bills handed in by doctors; and the above contention may be too one-sided. Although, at any rate, this problem does not pertain to the essential nature of the matter, it remains, in reality, as one of the shadowy aspects of medical care in Japan.

On the other hand, the Medical Association points out that causes soaring medical charges are the increase in demand for medical treatment, the change in quality of the treatment and the innovations in medical technology.

All of these factors as pointed out by both sides, are not completely without grounds, if seen from the actual experience of medical care. Since judgment on the relative importance of various factors as a cause of the deficit problem affects the choice of countermeasures to be adopted, it is necessary, when there exist conflicting opinions, somehow to resolve the differences, in itself not a simple task.

Lastly, it should not be forgotten that the drug and medical industries are reaping profit while the paying side (the government and the H.I.S.A.) and the receiving side (the Medical Association) keep on contesting over the details of the health insurance scheme. The road to 'insurance for every citizen' ('the socialization of medical care') has actually been an important factor in the rapid growth of the drug and medical industries and also in the promotion of labor–capital cooperation in large enterprises. No thorough investigation of the deficit problem of medical care insurance is possible without studying this part of the picture.

IV. THE PROSPECT OF MEDICAL CARE IN JAPAN

The system of medical care in Japan, like that in other advanced capitalist countries, has acquired a number of contradictions that have become grave social problems urgently in need of solution. Without a doubt, the 'socialization of medical care' is quite relevant here as an important clue to their solution. The future of Japanese medical care will depend on the manner in which we succeed in bringing about this 'socialization'.

The 'socialization of medical care' in Japan has been pushed forward only in the limited sphere of the medical care charge payment system. And even at present, this policy is difficult to change, and it attempts to solve all the problems within this payment system. The system and institutions of medical care, medical education and the medical supplies industry, too, remain as major issues which Japanese capitalism will have to face in the near future. Nevertheless, they have not been faced squarely thus far. If such an attitude continues, the system of medical care in Japan will continue to pile up further contradictions.

Even if attempts were made to meet this dilemma through encompassing the entire nation in a single mutual aid system, a question which, in itself, has become a momentous political issue, it will not solve various contradictions which have been discussed in this paper. In order to find a rational way to the solution of such contradictions, it is essential to convert the present policy into a new one predicated on the condition that the government assumes the ultimate responsibility in public investment which, in the past, has been the burden borne by the medical practitioners and, consequently by the patients. Further, in view of the new situation where the informational revolution is making inroads in the field of medical care, the plan for systematizing medical care should be worked out, and then further efforts must be exerted to realize that plan.

There is a tendency now for the 'systematization of medical care', instead of the 'socialization of medical care', to begin to take the lead in the field of medical care. This trend is not wholly welcome since, in Japan, the 'socialization of medical care' was pursued only in a limited sphere and the new slogan of the 'systematization' is being brought forth apparently to divert public attention from the task of fulfilling the agenda of the 'socialization of medical care', Actually, as a prerequisite to carrying out the 'systematization of medical care', the 'socialization of medical care' should be accomplished on a full scale. Until then, the system of medical care will not benefit either the people or those engaged in its practice. The time is really opportune for us to make a thorough inquiry into the system of medical care in Japan from the viewpoint of combining the 'systematization of medical care' as well as its 'socialization'.

At the same time, a new concept of regional health service is being brought forward as a solution to the accumulated contradictions which Japanese medical care now faces. Although the term is interpreted in different ways among its advocates, it is at least certain that here is a key towards linking the 'socialization' and the 'systematiza-tion' in the sphere of medical care because a practical problem such as this cannot avoid resolution.

In Japan, the future system of medical care depends largely on how it treats the first-line medical practitioners. It is true that Japanese medical practitioners at present are distrusted by the people and the mass media. However, it is dangerous to rely on 'bureaucratic control', under the name of the 'socialization of medical care', in view of the fact that there are merits in the medical practitioners' system such as the large number, relatively high medical standard and better service than is available in public medical care institution. Disputes over these problems will continue for some time between the Japan Medical Association and the government.

In this connection, there would be a possibility of much distortion of the medical care system if the technological aspect of medical care were planned with a focus only upon the medical specialist. Medical care for the people will best be accomplished through seeking to raise the standard of medical technology and enabling general medical practitioners to collaborate, and then making efforts to help hospitals where the medical specialist can work. This is also true in any other sub-fields of medical care.

If this point is left vague, partitioning medical care into small compartments, there will be a danger that any specific (economic, for example) analysis may make the mistake of 'looking at the trees and not at the forest'. In this regard, the history of medical care in Japan clearly shows that technological analysis must, by all means, precede the socio-economic one.

4 Proprietary Hospitals in the United States

Richard N. Rosett
UNIVERSITY OF ROCHESTER, N.Y.

It has been traditionally argued that short-term private hospitals in the United States are predominantly non-profit voluntary institutions because they owe their origins to the charitable hospital of the nineteenth century, because they enjoy tax and other advantages over profit-making hospitals, and because Americans abhor the idea of profiting at the expense of the sick.

Though all three arguments contribute to an explanation, they are incomplete. The charitable tradition and the abhorrence of profit-making explain why non-profit hospitals have been granted tax exemption and other legal advantages. But what incentive is there to accept these advantages if the condition attached to them is that profit, including the profit flowing from the advantages, must be forgone? It is argued that the profits of a physician-owner come partly in the form of service provided by the hospital, and that the proportion of profit taken in this form grows as the size of the hospital and its medical staff grow. Thus, the non-profit hospital is preferred to the profit-making hospital because, paradoxically, it is the more profitable form.

Since the modern hospital owes its origin to a charitable tradition, it seems hardly surprising that proprietary hospitals provide so few of the beds in which Americans are cared for. Yet if one compares the services provided by the charitable hospital of the eighteenth and early nineteenth centuries with those provided now, and if one considers the change in the sort of patient cared for, a puzzle does appear that needs explanation.

The early charitable hospital was an institution established for the care of the sick poor who could not be cared for at home. Frequently it was adjoined to an almshouse. Too often it was little more than a place in which to die. The development of anesthesia, modern surgical techniques and sophisticated medical treatment have converted the hospital into a source of highly effective treatment that is unobtainable elsewhere. In the modern hospital, the sick poor are still the beneficiaries of charity. They are treated at public expense or through philanthropy. But the same voluntary non-profit institutions that provide these services for the poor sell them to those who can afford to pay for them, and the question is why?

Again the answer seems simpler than it really is. Voluntary hospitals enjoy advantages in their competition with proprietary hospitals. They are tax-exempt, can raise interest-free capital, and have been – though this advantage has largely disappeared – exempt from certain kinds of legal liability for damages, so that those who can afford to buy hospitalization appropriate to themselves some of the charity intended by society to benefit the poor.

This answer is incomplete because it overlooks the role of the physician who admits his patient to the hospital and who is responsible for the care the patient receives there. In an important sense, the physician is the natural proprietor of the hospital to which he admits his patient. While the physician is responsible for prescribing treatment, the hospital assumes responsibility for supervision of the patient in the physicians' absence, including immediate response to emergencies. To a large degree, this places the use of hospital resources under the control of the physician. His availability, the frequency of his visits and the amount of time he spends with the patient determine the amount of supervision the hospital must provide and the frequency with which it will need to deal with emergencies. In principle, of course, it would be possible to account for hospital inputs and to charge the individual patient or his doctor for them, but practical considerations, like the cost of keeping such accounts and the advantages of risk-sharing, seem to rule this out. Since, therefore, the physician is free to choose that mixture of his own inputs and the hospital's inputs that will go to produce a given level of care for his patient, he will make the choice on the basis of the relative costs to himself of inputs. If he is the sole owner of the hospital, the cost to him of the hospital's inputs is their market value. If he is not, the cost to him is inevitably less. Thus there is a profit to be realized through the physician's ownership of a hospital that cannot be otherwise realized. If this argument is correct, it is not the paying patient who appropriates charitable benefits in the form of hospital care, but rather it is the physician who realizes the benefits by substituting hospital inputs for his own in caring for the patient.

A physician who establishes a small hospital for the care of his own patients must decide whether he wants to organize it as a proprietary hospital from which he can profit directly, or whether he wants to organize it as a non-profit hospital and convert its tax-exemption, its interest-free capital and its other advantages into payments in kind by relieving himself of some of the leisure-time interruptions usually taken to be an inevitable part of the physician's life. Apparently neither form of organization overwhelmingly dominates the other since, of hospitals with fewer than 25 beds surveyed by the American Hospital Association in 1969, half were proprietary and half were voluntary with the fraction falling as the size of the hospital grows. This relationship is shown in Table 4.1.

TABLE 4.1

GENERAL MEDICAL AND SURGICAL
HOSPITALS SURVEYED BY THE
AMERICAN HOSPITAL ASSOCIATION, 1969

Number of beds	Number of hospitals		Percentage of hospitals	
	Non-profit	Proprietary	Non-profit	Proprietary
Under 25	117	122	49	51
25–49	540	254	68	32
50–99	741	225	77	23
100–199	827	122	87	13
200–299	462	20	96	4
300–399	287	5	98	2
400–499	160	0	100	0
500 and over	146	0	100	0

Explanations for the predominance of voluntary hospitals like those advanced by Arrow (1963) and by Steinwald and Neuhauser (1970), are appealing, but do not explain the strong correlation between size and non-profit status. Arrow hypothesizes that subsidies are passed on to the patient, and that patients and physicians are antagonistic to the idea of profiting from the care of the sick. Steinwald and Neuhauser accept the idea that tax-exemption and charity give the non-profit institution a competitive advantage, and they then attribute the persistence of the proprietary hospital to its superior adaptability under new and changing circumstances. But Arrow must explain why we do not abhor profit-making in small hospitals or in the sale of life-saving drugs, or in medical practice itself, but not in hospitals. And he must explain why profit-making becomes more and more abhorrent as the size of the hospital grows.

Similarly, Steinwald and Neuhauser, who offer convincing evidence that small proprietary hospitals evolve into large voluntary hospitals, must explain what induces a proprietor to abandon his profit and adopt the voluntary non-profit form of organization as his hospital grows larger.

One plausible explanation for the latter is that larger hospitals are more likely to occur in densely populated areas where competition from voluntary hospitals forces the proprietor to choose between adopting the non-profit form or going out of business. Unfortunately, this speculation will not stand the empirical test. For a given size, a hospital is more likely to be proprietary the larger the metropolitan area in which it is located. In 1969, for example, in rural areas in the United States, there were 606 general short-term hospitals with 50–99 beds. Of these, only 13 per cent were proprietary. Of the 135 such hospitals in Standard Metropolitan Statistical Areas (S.M.S.A.s) with populations greater that 2·5 million, half were proprietary. For hospitals with 100–199 beds, the comparable proportions are 6 per cent and 24 per cent. This relationship, which is remarkable for its uniformity across all hospital and S.M.S.A. sizes, suggests that competition from voluntary hospitals *per se* is not sufficient explanation for the shift from the proprietary to the voluntary form as hospitals grow. Actually, this observed effect of S.M.S.A. size requires an explanation. Speculating, I offer the suggestion that the proprietary hospital is viable if it can specialize.

Still we are left with the question of why hospitals are more and more likely to become voluntary as they grow. The answer seems to lie in the theory of the collective good. As the hospitals grow in size, as more and more physicians share the use of its resources, the incentive to economize becomes weaker and weaker for each individual, even if they share the ownership of the hospital. The sole proprietor of a 20-bed hospital can increase his own profit by one dollar for every dollar he spares in the use of hospital resources, but each of the 10 physician-owners of a 200-bed hospital can increase his profit by only ten cents. Of course, there are social pressures that operate in a small group to impose non-monetary costs on the individual, but as the group grows in size, this is less and less effective. Thus, as the hospital grows in size, the advantages of the proprietary form diminish relative to those of the voluntary non-profit form. Since the owners of the large hospital are taking their income in the form of services anyway, why not enjoy tax-exemption and other benefits of non-profit organization?[1]

Unfortunately, direct evidence for this explanation of the shift from the proprietary to the voluntary non-profit form of organization is difficult to obtain. The very factors that are responsible for a hospital's growth tend to obscure the evidence, if it indeed exists, that

[1] Nursing homes enjoy the same advantages as hospitals when they adopt the non-profit form of organization. They stem from the same charitable traditions. Yet they are predominantly profit-making with 85 per cent of the non-government beds under control of proprietary institutions. The difference between these and hospital beds is that admitting physicians can profit from the services hospitals provide to their patients, but that no one can profit from the services provided to a nursing home patient except the proprietor.

physicians who practice in large hospitals substitute hospital resources for their own time in caring for their patients. The uncertain nature of demand for medical care and the law of large numbers combine to make large hospitals more efficient than small ones. If a hospital wants to avoid the risk of being unable to meet emergency demands for its services, the optimal occupancy rate is an increasing function of its size. Hospitals with fewer than 25 beds operate at an average occupancy rate of under 0·6. Hospitals with more than 200 beds operate at a rate above 0·8. Were this the only advantage of large size, it would be relatively easy to test a hypothesis about the relation between cost and hospital size. Indeed, it is tempting to interpret the strong positive correlation between size of hospital and expense per patient-day or number of personnel per patient-day as evidence to support the hypothesis. But large hospitals offer sophisticated forms of treatment that are expensive, that require large labor inputs and that can operate efficiently only on a large scale or in a large market. It is difficult to disentangle the effect of these services from the hypothesized effect of size on the physician's use of hospital resources. In fact, it may even be impossible. Though patients undoubtedly benefit from intensive care, even those benefits may be shared with the physician who can, because of them, safely be spared from the bedside of a critically ill patient.

Analysis of hospital accounts is now under way, and may eventually yield evidence relevant to the hypothesis, but so far the results are ambiguous. It is possible, however, to offer direct evidence on the value which physicians attach to the services provided by hospitals.

Assume that physicians, choosing a city in which to practice, take account of the profitability of practice and the quality of life they will lead. Profitability will be determined by the demand for services, the amount of competition and the availability of cooperating factors of production. The quality of life will depend on location, climate, recreational resources and many other factors that are difficult to quantify. In a given city, the physician can trade quality of life for profit at a rate given by the prevailing fee structure. If $\pi =$ profit and Q is quality of life, the physician maximizes

$$U = U(\pi, Q) \qquad (1)$$

subject to a budget constraint relating π and Q.

Measurements of π are available for 27 S.M.S.A.s in the form of profit of solo practitioners in 1967 as reported to the Internal Revenue Service. As a measure of hospital resources that benefit the office-based physician, I have taken hospital-based physicians ($HBMD$) per thousand population. Per capita income (Y) is taken as an important factor influencing the level of demand for physicians'

TABLE 4.2

SELECTED CHARACTERISTICS OF 27 S.M.A.s

	Average profit solo practice $	General practitioners per 1000	Medical specialists per 1000	Surgical specialists per 1000	Other specialists per 1000	Per capita income $	Hospital based physicians per 1000	Hospital beds per 1000	Dentists per 1000
San Bernardino-Riverside-Ontario, Calif.	35,636	0·2160	0·1829	0·2606	0·1691	2,910	0·2256	3·6141	0·5491
St Louis, Mo.-Ill.	34,947	0·1439	0·2377	0·2921	0·1552	3,299	0·4607	4·9077	0·5360
Dallas, Tex.	34,639	0·1903	0·2500	0·3673	0·2089	3,469	0·3766	3·5747	0·5882
Anaheim-Santa Ana-Garden Grove, Calif.	33,607	0·3375	0·2313	0·3724	0·2378	3,515	0·1717	2·6738	0·6430
Detroit, Mich.	32,875	0·1473	0·2049	0·2716	0·1658	3,624	0·4331	3·3819	0·5642
Paterson-Clifton-Passaic, N.J.	32,849	0·2055	0·2910	0·3183	0·1976	3,838	0·2896	3·2859	0·7264
Los Angeles-Long Beach, Calif.	32,144	0·3399	0·3390	0·4087	0·2975	3,879	0·3421	3·6722	0·6573
Buffalo, N.Y.	31,938	0·1925	0·2607	0·3371	0·1640	3,199	0·5595	4·9899	0·7011
Atlanta, Ga.	30,236	0·1371	0·3253	0·4112	0·2008	3,476	0·3475	3·3059	0·5349
Newark, N.J.	28,869	0·2329	0·3444	0·3807	0·2106	4,181	0·4108	4·2077	0·7599
San Francisco-Oakland, Calif.	28,806	0·2912	0·4832	0·5006	0·3932	3,798	0·4996	4·4450	0·8999
Baltimore, Md.	28,110	0·1884	0·2537	0·3471	0·2190	3,327	0·8747	3·8667	0·4826
Houston, Tex.	27,981	0·2419	0·2430	0·3334	0·2251	3,224	0·3413	4·5225	0·5475
Washington, D.C.-Md.-Va.	27,217	0·1827	0·3413	0·3980	0·2802	3,813	0·4841	3·1026	0·6717
Cincinnati, Ohio-Ind.-Ky.	27,021	0·2513	0·2534	0·2663	0·1599	3,239	0·4397	3·6650	0·4269
Minneapolis-St Paul, Minn.	27,019	0·2712	0·2322	0·3242	0·2281	3,683	0·4452	5·7761	0·8398
San Diego, Calif.	26,826	0·3478	0·2401	0·3867	0·2618	3,166	0·2476	2·7087	0·6972
Chicago, Ill.	26,690	0·2453	0·2351	0·2868	0·1917	3,964	0·4877	4·3672	0·6745
Denver, Colo.	26,409	0·2478	0·3593	0·4639	0·3061	3,446	0·6585	4·7149	0·7288
Pittsburgh, Pa.	25,975	0·2230	0·2042	0·2953	0·1529	3,138	0·4060	4·9549	0·6223
Milwaukee, Wis.	25,677	0·2008	0·2289	0·3066	0·2166	3,520	0·3505	4·4897	0·7183
Seattle, Wash.	25,445	0·3267	0·2863	0·3840	0·3113	3,826	0·4427	3·3267	0·8840
Portland, Oreg.-Wash.	21,926	0·2517	0·3215	0·4236	0·2204	3,388	0·3882	4·2362	0·9544
Philadelphia, Pa.-N.J.	21,646	0·2328	0·2689	0·3115	0·2183	3,343	0·6098	4·3240	0·6124
New York, N.Y.	20,408	0·2603	0·4156	0·3830	0·3177	3,813	0·9291	4·5288	0·9397
Cleveland, Ohio	20,222	0·1777	0·2943	0·3431	0·2123	3,705	0·6910	4·0926	0·6545

services, and the number of hospital beds per thousand population (*BEDS*) is a measure of hospital capacity. These all come from the 1970 survey of physicians conducted by the American Medical Association. As a proxy measure for the quality of life, I have taken the number of dentists per thousand population. Dentists are similar in education and income to physicians. Though their tastes may not be identical to physicians', to the extent that they are similar the number of dentists per thousand population may be taken as a measure of those qualities that make a city an attractive place to live in. Dentists rarely admit patients to the hospital and so this ratio may be assumed to be unaffected by *HBMD* or *BEDS*.

For the 27 S.M.S.A.s in the sample, Table 4.2 gives these data as well as the number of physicians per thousand population. These are office-based practitioners in private practice. Four categories are distinguished: general practitioners, medical specialists, surgical specialists and other specialists. Data pertaining to physicians, hospital beds, per capita income and dentists are all from 1970.

Each of the four variables, *Y*, *HBMD*, *D* and *BEDS*, can be thought of as operating on the budget constraint. An increase in *Y* increases the demand for services without increasing the supply of cooperating factors of production, and without changing the resources that affect the quality of life. The disequilibrium will be corrected by an increase in the number of physicians, but since this will dilute the fixed supply of cooperating factors, the flow will stop short of reestablishing the old level of π. The first row of Table 4.3

TABLE 4.3

PARTIAL CORRELATION COEFFICIENTS

Coefficient of	*General practitioners per 1000*	*Medical specialists per 1000*	and *Surgical specialists per 1000*	*Other specialists per 1000*	π
Y/HBMD, D, BEDS	−0·12	0·30	0·01	0·09	0·16
HBMD/Y, D, BEDS	−0·22	0·41	0·20	0·35	−0·58
D/Y, HBMD, BEDS	0·52	0·45	0·54	0·61	−0·46
BEDS/Y, HBMD, D	−0·25	−0·22	−0·33	−0·40	0·07

Coefficients greater than 0·3 are significant at the 5 per cent level in a one-tailed test.

gives partial correlation coefficients between *Y* and the numbers of physicians in each category. The coefficients for general practitioners and medical specialists are consistent with the observation that internists and pediatricians replace the general practitioners as income rises. Independent evidence (based on analysis of 300 S.M.S.A.s) supports the low elasticity of the number of surgeons with respect to income. The coefficient for π is as expected.

An increase in *HBMD* shifts the budget constraint in the sense that it reduces the physician's own input to a unit of his service without cost to him. But an increase in *HBMD* also represents a source of competition with the private practitioner in the form of clinics and emergency services. This competition affects the general practitioners most heavily. The net effect of *HBMD* depends on the relative importance of these two opposite forces. Ignoring the competitive threat of *HBMD*, an increase would lead, in the absence of mobility, to lower fees and increases in both π and Q. Entry of physicians, however, would lead ultimately to lower π and higher Q. This can readily be seen if we consider that fees will certainly be lower if both the number of physicians and *HBMD* are raised while demand is unchanged. The effects of *HBMD* are shown in row 2 of Table 4.3. The competitive effect dominates in the case of G.P.s, but the effect on the number of specialists is positive and the effect on π is negative as expected.

The effects of *D*, given in row 3, are unambiguous; increasing *D* increases the numbers of all physicians and decreases π.

It is the effect of *BEDS* that is most interesting and that provides the strongest support offered here for the hypothesis that for a physician there is a trade-off between profit and the services provided him by the hospital. An increase in *BEDS* might be thought attractive to physicians, but all four partial correlation coefficients are negative and the π coefficient is positive, though small. But if *HBMD* is, as hypothesized, a collective good, its dilution through an increase in *BEDS* while *HBMD* is held constant would lead to a decrease in the number of physicians, an increase in fees and an increase in π.

While a strong case has been made that physicians value the services of hospital-based physicians, it does not necessarily follow from this alone that physicians choose between admitting their patients to proprietary hospitals from which they can profit and admitting them to voluntary hospitals from which they receive payment in kind. It is possible to account for 70 per cent of all hospital-based physicians. They are interns and residents and fewer than 1 per cent of them are employed in proprietary hospitals. The other 30 per cent, the full-time staff physicians, are not easily accounted for, If it could be shown that proprietary hospitals employ fewer physicians per bed, including interns, residents and full-time staff physicians, the case would be considerably strengthened. As things stand now, however, we must be content with evidence that the services of these hospital-based physicians are valued by private practitioners and that they are treated as a collective good.

REFERENCES

Arrow, Kenneth, 'Uncertainty and the Welfare Economics of Medical Care', *American Economic Review* (1963).
Steinwald, Bruce, and Neuhauser, Duncan, 'The Role of the Proprietary Hospital', *Law and Contemporary Problems* (1970).

DATA SOURCES

American Dental Association, *Distributions of Dentists in the United States by State, Region, District, and County* (Chicago, 1972).
American Hospitals Association, *Journal of the American Hospital Association*, various issues.
American Medical Association, *Distribution of Physicians in the United States*, 1970 (Chicago, 1971).
U.S. Department of Health, Education and Welfare, *Income of Physicians, Osteopaths, and Dentists from Professional Practice, 1965–69* (Washington, D.C., 1972).

5 The Determinants of National Outlay on Health[1]

Ephraim Kleiman

HEBREW UNIVERSITY OF JERUSALEM

This paper investigates international differences in per capita levels of health outlay and in their division between private and public components. The findings support the hypothesis that households, having decided on their desired level of outlays in view of their health conditions and their income, then adjust to allow for the provision of health services by the public sector. Similarly, it holds that the public sector behaves in a parallel manner, adjusting its level of outlays on health services to allow for qualities acquired privately by households. However, from the standpoint of each of the two sectors, the services provided by the other one are imperfect substitutes for those provided by itself.

I. INTRODUCTION

The purpose of this study is to identify the factors determining the level of the national expenditure on health and, in particular, its distribution between the public and the private sectors of the economy. Pryor has argued that as the share of public expenditure on health in G.N.P. varies considerably among nations while that of the total national expenditure does not, public and private health expenditures must be good substitutes for each other.[2] I shall attempt here to test this contention, as well as the one that a country's economic system has no effect on the public expenditure on health.

II. THE DATA

The statistical results presented here are those of an international cross-section analysis. The data were taken from the U.N. *Yearbook of National Accounts Statistics, 1970*, the U.N. *Demographic* and

[1] I am grateful to Mrs Z. Galyam, a graduate student in the Department of Economics, for assistance with the calculations; and to the research committee of the Eliezer Kaplan School of Economics and Social Sciences for financial support.

[2] F. L. Pryor, *Public Expenditures in Communist and Capitalist Countries* (London: Allen & Unwin, 1968) p. 171.

Statistical Yearbooks and the I.L.O.'s *Yearbook of Labour Statistics, 1971.* At this stage of the investigation, size of sample was sacrificed to comparability of data. Consequently, the sample is much smaller than originally planned. It consists of sixteen countries or territories, which do, however, represent various stages of economic development. In six of them per capita national product (at factor costs) amounted in 1968–9 to less than U.S.$350, in three it exceeded $2,000, falling in the $650–1,500 range in the remaining seven.[1] Where absolute values, rather than relatives, are used, they were transformed into U.S. dollars through the exchange rates quoted in the U.N. *Statistical Yearbook.*

III. THE INDEPENDENT VARIABLES

Allocations of expenditure are made in the face of budget constraints. They may be expected, therefore, to vary with income. However, health services are not purchased for their own sake but rather as intermediate inputs in the production of health levels. This production will be cheaper the larger the stock of health inherited from the past: with the breeding-grounds of the *Anopheles* drained, the current costs of malaria prevention are considerably reduced. It may also be affected by expenditure on items other than health services: better diet raises disease resistance; lower housing density reduces the chances of contamination.[2] Both the size of the inherited stock and the volume of health-augmenting consumption are, ultimately, associated positively with income. The substitution and income effects which increases in them generate might thus be expected to strengthen the tendency of the health levels 'consumed' to increase with income. On the other hand, the decline in the marginal cost of health levels in terms of health service inputs means that, valued at the margin, the rise in the total volume of income forgone in exchange for health will be slower than that in the latter; and it may therefore rise more slowly than income, or even decline with it.[3] Thus, the net

[1] Included in the sample are, in ascending order of per capita income: Thailand, Korea, Southern Rhodesia, Malaysia, Taiwan, Fiji, Singapore, Jamaica, Austria, Italy, Israel, Finland, United Kingdom, Australia, Sweden, United States. The data are for the years 1968 or 1969, except for Malaysia, the data for which refer to 1967. Estimates of public health outlays for Israel were received from the Israel Central Bureau of Statistics. For data appendix, see pp. 80–1.

[2] On the complementarity between income and health, see Pryor, op. cit., pp. 153 ff. For the treatment of health as a stock, see M. Grossman, 'On the Concept of Health and the Demand for Health', *Journal of Political Economy* LXXX (Mar–Apr 1972) 223–55.

[3] Changes in the relative cost of health services, as distinguished from health levels, operate presumably in the opposite direction; because of the high labour intensity of these services, their cost may be expected to rise with income.

effect of income on outlays for health services is far from being
a priori clear.

Three alternative measures of income were used:

NNP   net national product per capita, at factor prices, in U.S.
      dollars;
CP   private consumption per capita, in U.S. dollars, an approx-
      imation of the disposable income of households.

In international comparisons, both measures raise an index-number
problem, aggravated by the arbitrariness of some of the rates of
exchange used. We therefore also experimented with a pure-number
measure:

CP/F the inverse of the share of expenditure on food in private
      consumption.

While the private component of health expenditure is constrained
by income, the public one may be expected to be affected by government's attitude regarding its role as supplier of services in general.
As alternative measures of this attitude we used:

CG/CP   the ratio of public, non-military consumption to
        private consumption;
CG/GDP the share of public, non-military consumption in the
        gross domestic product (at market prices).

As has been pointed out by Tobin, the degree of inequality which
society may be ready to tolerate in the distribution of goods such as
health is often lower than that it finds tolerable in the distribution of
income.[1] Consequently, the greater the income inequality, the more
health services have to be supplied by the public sector, to bring the
health distribution to the desired degree of equality. As for private
health outlays, they will be invariant to income inequality only if,
within each country, the marginal propensity to consume them is
constant. For lack of a better comparable measure we approximated
the degree of inequality by:

W   the share of labour in national income.

As has been pointed out above, the expenditure necessary to
produce a given health level may vary with the characteristics of the
population concerned. The most obvious of these, the state of health
as measured by morbidity, is in itself a function of current health
expenditure. But other traits are affected by such expenditures only in
the long run. We tried to introduce the following variables:

[1] J. Tobin, 'On Limiting the Domain of Inequality', *Journal of Law and
Economics*, XIII (Oct 1970) 263–77.

D15   the percentage of population less than 15 years old;
D60   the percentage of population aged 60 or over.

These two groups are popularly regarded as requiring more health care than the working-age population.

B   the crude birth rate, which may be expected to raise the costs of maintaining a given health level;
U   the share of population living in localities of 100,000 or more inhabitants;
L   the life expectancy of birth (simple average for both sexes), as a summary measure of the prevailing health level.

IV. THE NATIONAL OUTLAY ON HEALTH

We first tested the dependence on the independent variables of the per capita national outlay on health, H. This consists of: the expenditures of households on medicinal and pharmaceutical products, services of physicians, hospital fees, etc., and their net payments to private accident and health insurance companies; the expenditures of non-profit institutions on the services they provide; and the expenditures of all levels of government on the provision of health services (exclusive of transfers to non-profit institutions and to households). Of the three income measures, both net national product and private consumption per capita provided equally good explanations of health expenditures, but the former did it in a linear and the latter in an exponential relationship. In addition, both the relative size of the public sector's consumption and labour's share of income exert some influence on the level of health expenditures:[1]

$$H = 0.73 + 0.079 \ NNP + 1.800 \ CG/CP - 0.874 \ W \quad \bar{R}^2 = 0.967. \quad (1)$$
$$(0.03) \ (14.92) \qquad (2.43) \qquad (1.79)$$

The positive influence of CG/CP suggests that as government increases its role in the provision of services in general, it also sets itself higher targets with respect to the health services it provides.[2] Note, however, that this explanation is acceptable only on the

---

[1] Figures in parentheses show ratios of coefficients to their standard errors. As we hypothesize not only the existence but also the sign of the independent variables' effects, their significance should be evaluated in a one-tailed test. With 13 degrees of freedom, the probability of the ratio observed for the negative coefficient for W in equation (1) is less than 5 per cent; of the positive one for CG/CP, just above 1 per cent. The logarithmic relationship with CP, which is as good as the linear one with NNP, is not improved, however, by the introduction of the other two variables.

[2] Both here and elsewhere in this study, the explanation provided by the alternative measure of governmental attitude, CG/GDP, was much weaker than that provided by CG/CP.

assumption that households do not regard health services provided publicly to be perfect substitutes for those acquired privately.

As for the labour share, its being only a rough approximation for the degree of income equality, the interpretation of its negative effect is somewhat risky. Because of its positive association with per capita income it could be argued to represent a correction for a linear estimation of what may actually be a curvilinear relationship, i.e. for *H* increasing with *NNP* at a decreasing rate. However, of the four forms tested, the semi-logarithmic one – which represents such a relationship – provided the poorest fit.[1] We may conclude that phenomena associated either with equality of with the labour share itself tend to depress the national outlay on health. Estimates derived from cross-section studies of household budgets show private health expenditure to be income-elastic – indicating the marginal propensity to consume health services to increase with income within individual countries.[2] This would cause the *average* expenditure to be larger, given average income, the greater the inequality in the distribution of incomes. As mentioned earlier, equity considerations may be expected also to cause both the non-profit institution's and governments' health outlays to be larger the greater the income inequality. Furthermore, inequality is presumably positively associated with the relative remuneration of professionals, including medical personnel. This would again serve to raise outlays on health services with inequality.

With the exception of *U*, the demographic variables tested are significantly correlated with both income and health expenditures.[3] Once the variability due to income has been removed, the correlation of most of them with *H* is almost eliminated, while that of *U* now becomes significant.[4]

$$H = 25{\cdot}05 + 0{\cdot}074 \; NNP - 0{\cdot}316 \; U - 0{\cdot}717 \; D15 \quad \bar{R}^2 = 0\,964. \qquad (2)$$
$$\quad (0{\cdot}86) \quad (12{\cdot}65) \qquad (1{\cdot}86) \qquad (1{\cdot}10)$$

The higher population density in large urban centres is supposed to assist the spread of contagious diseases which, together with

---

[1] The corresponding values of $\bar{R}^2$ for the association on *NNP* above were: 0·960 in a linear relationship; 0·953 in a double-logarithmic one; 0·811 in a semi-logarithmic one; ·811 in an inverse-logarithmic one. Natural logarithms were used.

[2] Thus, for example, in Israel the income elasticity of the health expenditure of households was found to be 1·3. See N. Liviatan, *Consumption Patterns in Israel* (Jerusalem: Falk Project for Economic Research in Israel, 1964) Table 28.

[3] At the 1 per cent significance level. Highest association obtained with logarithms of the economic variables, i.e. the demographic variables rise or decline with income at a diminishing rate.

[4] The value of the correlation coefficient changes from 0·063 to − 0·454, which is just below the 5 per cent significance level.

industrial pollution, may be expected to raise the amount of health services required to attain a given health level. Can the fact that, with income accounted for, the effect of urbanization is to *reduce H* be interpreted as indicating the salubrious effect of country life to be largely a romantic myth? The benefits of the latter may well be offset by economies of scale made possible by the higher population density of cities, and by higher levels of outlays on health-augmenting commodities, such as housing.[1] Further investigation of this effect should therefore also cover the expenditure on such health-affecting services as water supply and sewage which are not presently included in health expenditure data.[2]

The physical quantities of goods required to satisfy given needs are, generally speaking, smaller for children than for adults. Per capita income figures, unadjusted for age structure, underestimate the satisfaction levels more, the younger a country's population is.[3] The effect of $D15$ on any expenditure which rises with income should therefore have been positive. Its negative coefficient in equation (2) is thus of some interest, despite its low significance, It negates the popular image of the young and the elderly being the main consumers of health services. The great multiplicity of medical treatments supplied to the young, and the high frequency with which they are supplied, seem to be more than offset by the relatively low per-unit cost of some of them, such as vaccinations. Calculating H on the alternative assumptions that $D15 = 0$ and $D15 = 100$, we estimate the health expenditure per adult and per child, respectively. For the mean values of the other variables the latter amounts to 29 per cent of the expenditure per adult.[4] However, $D15$ is negatively associated with $D60$. If the elderly consume more health services than do working-age adults, our calculations underestimate the health

[1] Even in the plumbing-conscious United States, 72 per cent of all rural farm dwellings lacked flush toilets in 1950, as against 24 per cent only of the urban ones, and 55 per cent of the former had no piped running water, as against less than 2 per cent of the latter. See *Statistical Abstract of the United States, 1958*, p. 765.

[2] See United Nations, *A Manual for Economic and Functional Classification of Government Transactions* (New York, 1958). Attention should also be paid to the fact that in the case of some items it is the capital outlay which is recorded, not the annual cost.

[3] See M. K. Bennett, 'International Disparities in Consumption Levels', *American Economic Review*, XLI (Sep 1951) 632–49; E. Kleiman, 'Age Composition, Size of Households, and the Interpretation of Per Capital Income', *Economic Development and Cultural Change*, XV (Oct 1966) 37–58.

[4] Derived from a linear relationship such as that of equation (2), this estimate has the drawback that it varies considerably with the level of income for which it is calculated. Postulating a logarithmic relationship, the relative expenditure per child was estimated at only 7 per cent of that of an adult, irrespective of the values of the other independent variables.

expenditures on a child relative to an adult. But even then, they do suggest the former to be smaller than the latter: the expenditure on the elderly would have to be almost three times that on working-age adults for the latter expenditure to be exceeded by that on children.[1]

The demographic variables of equation (2), when introduced in addition to income, provide an explanation of H which, in terms of R^2, is practically as good as that provided by the economic or institutional ones of equation (1). But they fail to add any extra explanation. This need not necessarily mean that we are faced with two alternative causal explanations of H: both CG/CP and W might, in their own turn, be affected by demographic conditions. We may, perhaps, obtain some clarification of this point by considering separately the private and public components of health expenditure.

V. PRIVATE AND PUBLIC COMPONENTS

The national outlay on health is the outcome of decisions made by units with distinctly different rules of behaviour. While services provided by non-profit institutions and by various level of government may be good substitutes for those purchased by households, the factors determining the volume provided by each of them need not be identical. Unfortunately, internationally comparable data do not provide separate estimates for non-profit institutions. These will be treated here as part of the household sector.

(1) *Private Outlays*
We tried to explain the per capita level of private health outlays, HP, by those variables which, in the previous section, were interpreted as operating through the decisions of households, and by HG, the per

---

[1] In the present sample, the relationship between the two age groups is $D60 = 0.316 - 0.604\ D15$. Thus, with $D15 = 0$, 32% of the population will be 60 or more, while with $D60 = 0$, 52% will be under 15. Denoting the expenditures per child, adult and the elderly by HY, HA and HE respectively, we have:

$$H_{(D15=0)} = 0.68\ HA + 0.32\ HE$$
$$H_{(D60=0)} = 0.48\ HA + 0.52\ HY$$

so that

$$\frac{HY}{HA} = \frac{H_{(D60=0)}}{H_{(D15=0)}} \frac{0.68}{(0.52} + \frac{0.32}{0.52} \frac{HE}{HA}) - \frac{0.48}{0.52}.$$

Calculated from equation (2) for the mean values of the other variables, this is, equal to:

$$\frac{HY}{HA} = 0.384\ \frac{HE}{HA} - 0.107.$$

capita level of public outlays. By far the best results were obtained using a linear relationship:

$$HP = 32 \cdot 15 + 0 \cdot 076 \, NNP - 0 \cdot 839 \, W - 0 \cdot 240 \, U - 0 \cdot 632 \, HG \quad \bar{R}^2 = 0 \cdot 946$$
$$(1 \cdot 52) \, (14 \cdot 22) \qquad (1 \cdot 98) \qquad (1 \cdot 64) \qquad (4 \cdot 48) \qquad\qquad (3)$$

The most interesting result here is the appearance, with a negative sign, of HG.[1] This may be interpreted as indicating that the units of the private sector, having decided on the amount of services they wish to consume, adjust their actual purchases to allow for the free provision of similar services by government. However, they seem not to regard such services as perfect substitutes for those acquired privately.

The association between HP and the demographic variables tested is much weaker than for H. It rises once income has been accounted for, but, with the exception of U, decreases again after the inclusion of HG. In particular, the correlation with the age structure is virtually reduced to zero.[2] This suggests that considerations associated with these variables do not affect the decisions of households explicitly, but only through their effect on the level of public outlays on substitutable services.

(2) *Public Outlays*

The investigation of the rules determining per capita public health outlays raises the question of the budget constraints under which government operates. In other words, what is the magnitude to which public outlay on health may be expected to be systematically related: is it the national income (or product) as a whole, or is it some share of it which, for political or economic reasons, constitutes the effective limit on public spending? Lacking any other evidence on the existence of such a limit,[3] we represented the notion of it by CG/CP – the ratio of public, non-military consumption to the private one. On the assumption that equity considerations affect governmental decisions, the labour share, W, has also been included, as well as the per capita level of private outlays. The dependence of HG on NNP

[1] In a simple correlation the association between HG and HP is positive.

[2] The introduction of income alone not only strengthens the associations between the remaining variance in HP and $D15$ and $D60$, but also changes their signs – the former's to negative, the latter's to positive. In view of the negative effect of $D15$ on H, it is tempting to interpret this as indicating that the burden of providing health care for children falls on households, while that of providing for the elderly is carried by government. However, the explanation provided by NNP and $D60$ ($\bar{R}^2 = 0 \cdot 866$) is weaker than that provided by NNP and HG alone ($\bar{R}^2 = 0 \cdot 926$), or by equation (3) – $\bar{R}^2 = 0 \cdot 946$.

[3] See, e.g., R. Musgrave, *Fiscal Systems* (New Haven: Yale Univ. Press, 1969).

itself, is clearly of the exponential (double-logarithmic) form.[1] When all other variables have been introduced, we have:[2]

$$\ln HG = -10 \cdot 09 + 1 \cdot 474 \ln NNP + 0 \cdot 052 \; CG/CP + 0 \cdot 037 \; W - \quad (4)$$
$$\quad (6 \cdot 18) \quad (3 \cdot 58) \qquad\qquad (1 \cdot 45) \qquad\qquad (1 \cdot 37)$$
$$0 \cdot 009 \; HP \quad \bar{R}^2 = 0 \cdot 877.$$
$$(1 \cdot 80)$$

Other things being equal, HG will rise more than proportionately with per capita product. If we disregard the low statistical significance with which CG/CP enters equation (4), its effect can be said to be in the direction hypothesized. Not so that of the labour share, W. This, however, may well be only a correction for the form of the relationship used: in a pure linear relationship, the effect of W is negative. In both, however, it is of low significance.

The negative effect of HP in equation (4) indicates that, in a symmetry to the behaviour of household, government also sets itself some desired level of health services, adjusting its expenditure to allow for their private acquisition. Because of the interdependence of equation (3) and equation (4), and of the peculiar form of the latter, discussion of the substitution relationship implied here is deferred to the next section.

To judge by their simple correlation coefficients, the demographic variables, in particular the age structure, are strongly associated with public health outlays. This, however, turns out to be only a reflection for the dependence of HG on income, with which the demographic variables are associated. With income accounted for, all traces of these correlations practically vanish.[3]

VI. THE SUBSTITUTABILITY OF PRIVATE AND PUBLIC OUTLAYS

The interdependence of HP and HG means that the estimates of their regression coefficients in equations (3) and (4) may be biased. We

---

[1] The value of $\bar{R}^2$ for the double-logarithmic form (with NNP as the only independent variable) is $0 \cdot 800$, while for the linear, semi-log and log-inverse relationship it falls between $0 \cdot 523$ and $0 \cdot 559$.

[2] For the linear version of e.g., (4), $\bar{R}^2 = 0 \cdot 852$. However, this is due to the effect of HP; when this variable is left out, the linear form yields $\bar{R}^2 = 0 \cdot 647$ compared to $\bar{R}^2 = 0 \cdot 853$ for the exponential one. The use of $\ln HP$ instead of HP resulted in poorer results than those of, e.g., (4) – $\bar{R}^2 = 0 \cdot 855$.

[3] e.g. the correlation between $\ln HG$ and $D15$ is reduced from $-0 \cdot 850$ to $-0 \cdot 016$ once $\ln NNP$ has been included.

therefore experimented with a number of two-stage least-squares estimates. The best, consistent results were provided by:[1]

$$HP = 60 \cdot 25 + 0 \cdot 073 \ NNP - 1 \cdot 630 \ W - 0 \cdot 204 \ HG \quad \bar{R}^2 = 0 \cdot 876. \qquad (5a)$$
$$\quad (2 \cdot 07) \ (7 \cdot 41) \qquad (2 \cdot 83) \qquad (1 \cdot 29)$$

$$\ln HG = -11 \cdot 48 + 2 \cdot 006 \ \ln NNP + 0 \cdot 066 \ CG/CP - 0 \cdot 014 \ HP \quad R^2 = 0873.$$
$$\quad (6 \cdot 25) \ (5 \cdot 78) \qquad\qquad (1 \cdot 91) \qquad\qquad (2 \cdot 31)$$

$$(5b)$$

The relationship described by the second equation is, approximately:

$$HG = 10^{-5} \ NNP^2 \ 1 \cdot 068^{CG/CP} \ 1 \cdot 014^{-HP}. \qquad (6)$$

This form makes the elasticity of substitution of private for public outlays increase with the level of the latter. Halving HP with respect to its mean value increases HG by 33 per cent; doubling HP decreases HG by 42 per cent.[2] While such a relationship cannot be ruled out on theoretical grounds, it cannot be easily defended either. The increase of the elasticity with the value of HP suggests that the true relationship (ignoring other variables) may be a combination of a constant income elasticity and a constant marginal rate of substitution:

$$HG = NNP^\alpha - \beta HP.$$

As α and β cannot be estimated simultaneously, we adopted an iterative procedure, estimating β given alternative values of α. Using values of HP calculated from a regression on the exogenous variables, the highest value of $\bar{R}^2$ was obtained for $\alpha = 1 \ 25$:[3]

[1] The corresponding first-stage estimates were:

$$HP = 64 \cdot 18 + 0 \cdot 064 \ NNP - 1 \cdot 658 \ W \quad \bar{R}^2 = 0 \cdot 870$$
$$\quad (2 \cdot 16) \quad (8 \cdot 80) \qquad (2 \cdot 80)$$
$$\ln HG = -8 \cdot 24 + 1 \cdot 379 \ \ln NNP + 0 \cdot 084 \ CG/CP \quad \bar{R}^2 = 0 \cdot 830.$$
$$\quad (6 \cdot 04) \quad (5.54) \qquad\quad (2 \cdot 18)$$

For the last estimate, somewhat better results were obtained when $\ln CG/CP$ was used. See, however, footnote 3, below.

[2] The last element in equation (6) gives the proportion to which HG will be reduced compared to its value when $HP = 0$. For the mean value of the latter, \$40·56, this amounts to 0·57, as compared with 0·76 for $HP = 20$ and 0·33 for $HP = 80$.

[3] CG/CP may be expected to have an equiproportionate rather than equal absolute effect on HG. The alternative procedure would therefore be to estimate the coefficients of $\ln (HG + \beta HP) = a + \alpha \ln NNP + \delta \ln CG/CP$, for various values of β. However, some of the calculated values of HP were negative enough to rule out this method.

Postscript: I am no longer sure that $\alpha = 1 \cdot 25$ is, indeed, the best result. The higher the value assumed for α, the lower is the regression coefficient of NNP^α in equation (7), various combinations of two yielding results of fairly equal statistical significance.

$$HG = -39.04 + 0.004\,NNP^{1.25} + 2.878\,CG/CP - 0.217\,HP \quad \bar{R}^2 = 0.620 \quad (7)$$
$$\quad (2.04)\,(1.02) \qquad\qquad (2.55) \qquad\qquad (0.42)$$

Equations (5) and (7) show public health outlays to be poor substitutes for private ones from the point of view of households, and vice versa from that of governments. A number of explanations may be proffered: (a) Low efficiency of the public sector in producing health services, so that even if the services themselves are perfect substitutes, the outlays on them are not. However, were this the only explanation, the marginal rate of substitution of HP for HG should have been higher than 1. (b) Non-identity of public and private preferences, so that the marginal utility to households of a dollar's worth of services of the type provided by government is smaller than that of a dollar's worth of services purchased privately. Households may even regard public services to be utility-decreasing, as exemplified by the bonus paid by the Indian government to males undergoing free-of-cost vasectomies. Similarly, an increase in private expenditure on, say, face-lifting surgery would not be considered by most of today's government as justifying a cut-down in their outlays on health services. Many of the services provided by the two sectors may therefore be non-competing, and even complementary from the point of view of both – an increase in the quantity acquired of the one raising demand for the other. (c) Divergence of the 'distributional weights' which government attaches to services enjoyed by different groups in the community, from those of the actual income distribution.[1] In particular, if government wishes to provide low-income groups with more services than they would have consumed otherwise, the resultant decline in private outlays cannot offset the increase in public ones.

The allocation of health expenditures between the two sectors is illustrated in Fig. 5.1 below. For a given level of income and of the other variables, the GG' line shows the various combinations of private and public outlays regarded as equivalent by government; PP' shows the same – from the point of view of households. It can be easily seen that unless the two lines intersect there will be only public or only private, services, as the case may be. (With GG' lying throughout above PP', the outlay which government regards as desired in the absence of private outlays exceeds that with which households are satisfied, even if public services only are to be available.) Furthermore, E will determine a stable allocation only if the slope of PP' with respect to the HP axis exceeds that of GG'. Otherwise the allocation will be unstable, fluctuating between private

---

[1] See Tobin, op. cit.; also Pryor, op. cit., *passim*.

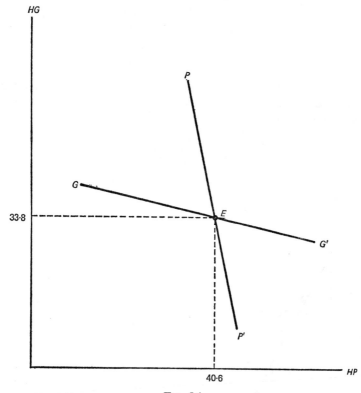

FIG. 5.1

outlays only and public ones only, or (slopes identical) it will be indeterminate.

How does the allocation react to changes in income? Ignoring the other variables (or, rather, their association with income), we have:

$$dHP = \frac{\partial HP}{\partial Y}dY + \frac{\partial HP}{\partial HG}dHG \qquad (8a)$$

$$dHG = \frac{\partial HG}{\partial Y}dY = \frac{\partial HG}{\partial HP}dHP \qquad (8b)$$

For the equilibrium allocations this yields:

$$\frac{dHP}{dY} = \frac{\dfrac{\partial HP}{\partial Y} + \dfrac{\partial HP}{\partial HG}\dfrac{\partial HG}{\partial Y}}{1 - \dfrac{\partial HG}{\partial HP}\dfrac{\partial HP}{\partial HG}} \qquad (9a)$$

$$\frac{dHG}{dY} = \frac{\dfrac{\partial HG}{\partial Y} + \dfrac{\partial HG}{\partial HP}\dfrac{\partial HP}{\partial Y}}{1 - \dfrac{\partial HG}{\partial HP}\dfrac{\partial HP}{\partial HG}}. \tag{9b}$$

With public outlays being imperfect substitutes for private ones and vice versa, the denominator in equations (9) is always positive, and their signs depend only on those of the numerator:

$$\frac{dHP}{dY} > 0 \text{ if } \frac{\partial HP}{\partial Y}\bigg/\frac{\partial HG}{\partial Y} > -\frac{\partial HP}{\partial HG}$$

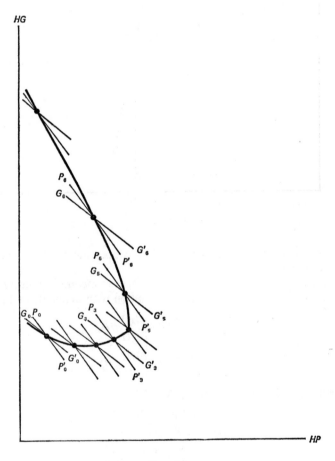

Fig. 5.2

$$\frac{dHG}{dY} > 0 \text{ if } \frac{\partial HP}{\partial Y} \bigg/ \frac{\partial HG}{\partial Y} < -\frac{1}{\dfrac{\partial HG}{\partial HP}}$$

With $(\partial HP/\partial Y)/(\partial HG/\partial Y)$ constant, the sign and size of $(dHP/dY)/$ (dHG/dY) will also be constant, and will depend on the magnitude of the former ratio relative to the marginal rates of substitution of private for public outlays in the two sectors. We have seen, however, that the dependence of the two sectors' health outlays on income do not follow the same rules: while the marginal propensity of the private sector to spend on health is constant, that of the public one increases with income. Therefore, $(\partial HP/\partial Y)/(\partial HG/\partial Y)$ will decrease as income rises, and the development path of allocation will not follow a straight line.

As has been pointed out before, for the allocation to be stable:

$$-\frac{1}{\dfrac{\partial HG}{\partial HP}} > -\frac{\partial HP}{\partial HG}$$

Therefore, as illustrated in Fig. 5.2, very low income levels may satisfy simultaneously the conditions for $(dHG/dY) < 0 < (dHP/dY)$. As income rises, and $\partial HG/\partial Y$ increases ($\partial HP/\partial Y$ remaining constant), a point will be reached at which dHG/dY becomes positive: increases in income will now result in increases in both the private and the public components of health outlays. Finally, from some level of income onwards, dHP/dY will be negative: any further increases in income will cause the public component to increase by more than the total national health outlay.

APPENDIX

	HP $ (1)	HG $ (2)	H $ (3)	NNP $ (4)	CP $ (5)	CP/F (6)	CG/CP % (7)	CP/GDP % (8)	W % (9)	D15 % (10)	D60 % (11)	U % (12)	B % (13)	L (years) (14)
Australia	69 110·8	38·0	148·8	2,134	1,606	4·92	15·5	9·1	67	29	12	67·3	20·5	71·0
Austria	68 30·0	60·0	90·0	1,188	938	3·63	22·7	13·4	66	24	20	31·7	15·1	69·9
Fiji	68 5·5	0·7	6·2	308	241	3·49	18·2	11·6	63	45	4	–	35·4	68·1
Finland	69 29·8	70·7ᵃ	100·5	1,523	1,056	3·23	27·1	14·6	63	25	13	17·7	13·7	68·5
Israel	69 64·6	22·7ᵃ	87·3	1,311	1,075	3·84	28·7	19·0	59ᵇ	33	10	34·0	27·0	71·0
Italy	69 63·4	18·1	81·5	1,253	981	2·72	17·7	11·3	56	32	15	28·1	16·8	69·8
Jamaica	68 7·4	25·0	32·4	829	703	2·93	17·9	10·9	63	46	7	23·6	32·9	64·6
Korea	69 5·0	0·1	5·1	182	155	2·10	9·6	6·7	39	41	6	29·0	35·6	52·4
Malaysia	67 3·9	3·9	7·8	248	199	2·16	21·7	13·7	50	44	6	10·8	35·2	64·6
Singapore	69 11·1	11·7	22·8	767	519	3·46	9·6	6·5	50ᶜ	41	5	100·0	23·3	68·2
Southern Rhodesia	69 2·0	3·5	5·5	242	158	4·85	17·8	10·5	57	47	3	26·5	48·4	51·4
Sweden	68 85·4	144·0	229·4	2,582	1,791	3·93	32·6	17·8	74	21	19	18·3	13·6	74·2
Taiwan	69 11·7	1·3	13·0	269	199	2·39	12·2	7·0	51	43	5	34·1	28·1	68·1
Thailand	69 6·9	0·7	7·6	131	122	2·03	10·6	7·1	30	43	5	7·1	42·8	56·2
United Kingdom	69 1·9	75·6	77·5	1,530	1,225	4·24	20·7	13·1	78	24	19	40·5	16·2	74·8
United States	69 209·6	58·6	268·2	3,816	2,854	6·35	20·1	12·3	73	29	14	28·4	18·2	70·3

ᵃ Received directly from Israel Central Bureau of Statistics.
ᵇ Exclusive of the remuneration of members of cooperatives and collectives.
ᶜ No data available – Malaysia's figure arbitrarily ascribed.

Col. (1): Total private medical care and health expenses – from (1a); divided by population – from (2a); multiplied by exchange rate for U.S.$ – from (3).

Col. (2): Government health expenditure – from (1b); divided by population – from (2a); multiplied by exchange rate – from (3).

Col. (3): Col. (1)+Col. (2).

Col. (4): Net national product at factor prices = national income at market prices *minus* indirect taxes net of subsidies – from (1c). divided by population – from (2a).

from (1a).

Col. (7): Government final consumption *minus* defence expenditure – from (1b); divided by total private consumption expenditure – from (1a).

Col. (8): Government final consumption *minus* defence expenditure – from (1b); divided by gross domestic product at purchasers' values – from (1c).

Col. (9): Compensation of employees – from (1d); divided by national income at market prices *minus* indirect taxes net of subsidies – from (1c).

Col. (10): Percentage of population under 15 years of age – from (2b).

Col. (11): Percentage of population aged 60 or over – from (2b).

Col. (12): Percentage of population living in localities of 100,000 and more – from (2c).

Col. (13): Crude birth rate per thousand – from (2d).

Col. (14): Unweighted average of male and female expectation of life at birth – from (2e).

Sources:

(1a)   U.N. *Yearbook of National Accounts Statistics, 1970*, vol. I, Private Final Consumption Expenditure by Object (number of table varies).

(1b)   Ibid., Government Final Consumption Expenditure According to Purpose (number of table varies).

(1c)   Ibid., vol. II, Table 10.

(1d)   Ibid., vol. I, National Income and National Disposable Income (number of table varies).

(2a)   U.N. *Demographic Yearbook, 1970*, Table 4.

(2b)   Ibid., Table 6.

(2c)   Ibid., Table 9.

(2d)   Ibid., Table 3.

(2e)   Ibid., Table 20.

(3)   U.N. *Statistical Yearbook, 1970*, Table 186.

Summary Record of Discussion

This session took up three disparate papers, by Dr Kawakami on the Japanese health care system, by Professor Rosett on American private hospitals, and by Dr Kleiman on the determinants of private and public expenditure on health. Because of their disparate character, these papers were discussed separately.

A. *Dr Kawakami's paper*

The formal discussant, *Professor Emi*, made four primary critical observations:

1. At least one more basic table is necessary, to summarize the complex Japanese health insurance system for the benefit of non-Japanese readers.

2. Dr Kawakami, finds a conflict or, in Marxian terms, a 'contradiction' between what he calls 'socialization' and 'systematization' in the Japanese health care system. His suggestions for its solution are, however, inadequate. He is clearly on the side of further socialization, but should be more specific: where should the system go from where it is now, and by what steps? Also, what precisely is to be socialized further: the drug industry? the incomes of medical practitioners?

3. Dr Kawakami has discussed systematization as designed to delay socialization by drawing attention away from it. On the other hand, Professor Emi wondered whether systematization might not be a step towards socialization.

4. Is there any way of combining private enterprise with socialization of medical care? Admitting the primary importance of medical science and medical technology to the health care system, we should not forget the importance of proper resource allocation, as provided by a market system.

In replying to Professor Emi, *Dr Kawakami* was joined by *Professor Uzawa*. The main purpose of the paper, according to Dr Kawakami and Professor Uzawa was to stress the need for socialization rather than to provide a complete consensus as to the meaning of the term. To them, however, socialization includes (1) a guarantee of equal access of all persons to medical services, together with (2) public control over the cost of these services.

Evaluating the Japanese system in terms of progress toward these goals, it appears that after the Meiji Restoration of 1868 the market system has in fact dominated. As socialization has proceeded after the Second World War, contradictions have developed between the payment system (which has indeed been largely socialized) and the institutions providing medical care, medical education and medical goods (which remain largely private). The resulting difficulties are described in Dr Kawakami's paper.

Socialization need not mean complete nationalization, but it does require a planned program of devoting public resources to construct and maintain the physical and human resources of the medical care system.

Systematization and socialization need not conflict, but the relations between the two have not been made clear in the present Japanese system. Advocates of systematization advocate computerizing and automation as methods of cutting the costs of medical care, to the neglect of the non-mechanical aspects of medical problems.

The present system provides medical services in kind, together with public payment of doctors' fees. This system provides wrong incentives for both patient and doctor behavior. Patients use medical services too often for minor ailments, while doctors try to maximize 'secondary receipts' from the sale of medicines, tests and examinations under an elaborate 'point system'. In addition to being an unwise resource evaluation, this system erodes the professional ethics of the Japanese physician.

Discussion from the floor was largely statistical and institutional. *Professor Evans* and *Mme Sandier* expressed surprise that health care in Japan seemed to consume only a nearly constant proportion of the Japanese G.N.P., and that (since the share of drugs in medical care expenditure was rising) the non-drug share of health care in G.N.P. appeared to be falling. This is most unusual, and so is the rising share of drugs; in many other countries the share of hospitals has risen faster. *Mr Cooper* wondered whether the figures in Dr Kawakami's tables included private as well as public expenditures for medical care. *Professor Robinson* suggested that differential price movements might be involved and proposed that Dr Kawakami's tables be put in constant prices. *Professor Tsuru* believed that the appropriate specific deflators might not be available, but might be approximated. *Professor Evans* wondered about the reliability of such Japanese sectoral deflators as existed, and was assured by *Professor Shinohara* that the sectoral price indices of the Japanese Economic Planning Agency were comparable in reliability to those of the United Kingdom.

Professors Bronfenbrenner and *Moriguchi* offered institutional interpellations. Professor Bronfenbrenner's feeling was that the paper was somewhat too abstract in neglecting two particular aspects of the Japanese health care system under heated discussion in the current press. These are (1) the size of the system's budgetary deficit, and (2) the conflict between quantity and quality in Japanese medical education, which has recently resulted in a proliferation of lowgrade private medical colleges supported by exorbitant student fees. Professor Moriguchi mentioned the endemic conflict between physicians and pharmacists. The pharmacists complain that physicians sell their own prescription drugs; the physicians complain that too many drugs are available without prescription from pharmacists, and that pharmacists feel too free in offering medical advice.

Closing the discussion of the Kawakami paper, Dr Kawakami and Professor Uzawa expressed the view that the Japanese statistics reflected genuine anomalies as compared with similar figures from other countries, and that these were due largely to the charge payment system. Doctors are paid, they pointed out once more, on a point system which gives too high weights to medication and examinations. At the same time, the statistics exclude some of the expenses not covered by medical insurance and therefore less adequately reported, particularly nursing care and 'extra-charge' hospital beds.[1] While the published statistics do not suggest that the medical profession is highly profitable, the fees of private medical schools indicate the contrary. Of course, doctors may not be completely rational in desiring their sons to inherit their medical practices and private hospitals, and in paying the high fees of private medical colleges. This same desire to pass on one's practice and income to one's son, regardless of the son's aptitude and ability, is a main factor in the current erosion of Japanese medical ethics. Furthermore, other sorts of medical care personnel, particularly nurses, remain badly underpaid in Japan.

B. *Professor Rosett's paper*

Mr Ema, the scheduled discussant for Professor Rosett's paper, was unable to attend this session, and was replaced by his colleague, Dr Kiikuni. Their discussion is a joint product, as the two men had collaborated in preparing it.

Dr Kiikuni began his discussion with diffidence. It is difficult for a Japanese to understand the American proprietary hospital system on the basis of the Japanese system, because the two are so different. Professor Rosett's main point was the shift from the proprietary to the voluntary hospital as the size of the hospital increases. The physician expects more income from a proprietary hospital, but at the cost of less leisure and of more services than he would contribute to a voluntary hospital of the same size. In addition, voluntary or non-profit hospitals have advantages in tax exemption, capital formation and limited liability. Since costs seem to rise more than proportionately to hospital size, Dr Kiikuni thought this factor largely responsible for the Rosett phenomenon, and wished to ask three questions: (1) Is the private proprietary hospital dying out in the United States? (2) How can one explain the concentration of proprietary hospitals in particular areas, such as Texas and Southern California? (3) What will be the effect of multi-hospital holding companies?

Professor Rosett argued that, as a given proprietary hospital increases in size, more physicians admit patients, and the degree to which any particular physician can profit will decline more than proportionately to any increase in leisure. This, rather than increasing cost, may be the key reason why proprietary hospitals are predominantly small. He had no explanation for the special phenomenon of Southern California and Texas. Hospital chains and holding companies, he felt, were new phenomena on which it was too early to comment. He recognized, however, the possibility that they might offer 'housekeeping' advantages by centralization.

Mr Culyer opened discussion from the floor by wondering why *corporate* hospitals do not develop, instead of *voluntary* ones, to meet the problems of increasing size.

Professor Perlman expressed the view that large hospitals were so different from small ones that no simple rational model like the Rosett one could take adequate account of the difference between them. They differ, for example, in the demographic characteristics of their patients, in their

---

[1] Some details regarding the coverage of Japanese medical statistics were provided at this point by *Dr Kiikuni*.

need to maintain standby capacity and (in many cases) in their teaching responsibilities.

Professor Sloan and *Dr Davis* raised statistical questions relative to the Rosett model. Professor Sloan made five principal suggestions: (1) Explicit allowance for case-mix differences between hospitals. (2) Inclusion of a separate hospital profit variable. (3) Expansion of the number of Standard Metropolitan Statistical Areas (S.M.S.A.s) covered, since Rosett's Table 4.3 shows anomalous negative partial correlation coefficients between the number of beds and other variables; these may be due to simple bias. (4) Consideration of the number of hospital-based physicians as being jointly determined with the dependent variable (physicians' income) rather than as an independent variable. (5) Consideration of some variable other than the number of dentists in an area as a surrogate for a 'quality of life' variable.

Dr Davis's criticism was more sweeping. She proposed expansion of the model to include specification of the demand as well as the supply side, and feared that Rosett might be limiting himself to a single equation of a simultaneous equation system. In addition to agreeing with Professor Sloan's point (5) above, Dr Davis believed physicians' fees not independent of hospital charges, and suggested that the number of hospital-based physicians in each area be respecified as a proportion of the total number of physicians in the area.

Professor Rosett rose to answer these and allied questions about his study. Answering Mr Culyer, he said that in explaining why voluntary hospitals replace proprietary hospitals, it is not sufficient to cite advantages of the voluntary such as tax-exemption. One must also explain what incentive the proprietor has to abandon his profit. He had also been asked about the replication of small proprietary hospitals fulfilling the functions of fewer larger ones, but he doubted this, since a larger number of admitting physicians would still be required. As for case-mix differences mentioned by so many of his critics, he felt the difference was largely a matter of size in hospital.[1]

C. *Dr Kleiman's paper*

Introducing this paper, *Professor Shinohara* expressed the view that, public and private health expenditures were good, if not perfect substitutes for each other, and that this result stands up when other variables are added to estimating equations. The point is important when one seeks to forecast total health care expenditures on the basis of planned or projected public ones.

With specific regard to the paper by Dr Kleiman, Professor Shinohara made a number of technical suggestions:

1. Relative prices should also be considered in estimating the elasticity of substitution between the two types of medical care.

---

[1] *Professor Sloan* suggested at this point that causation might operate in the direction opposite to that presumed in the Rosett model. Proprietary hospitals, being equipped to handle only a relatively small range of illnesses, perforce remain small, regardless of the preferences of the proprietors.

2. There is a much stronger cross-sectional association between total health expenditures and *NNP* than between public health expenditures and *NNP*. In 11 of 16 countries in the Kleiman sample, health expenditures are more than 70 per cent public, but the others are outliers.[1]

3. Dr Kleiman uses the labor share as a proxy for the level of income inequality in his equation, but it is a poor proxy, especially in countries where agricultural production is important.

4. The relation of household consumption expenditures for health care with public expenditures for the same purpose shows a high degree of substitution.

5. In summary, he (Professor Shinohara) saw no great difference between Dr Kleiman's work and that of Pryor, whom Dr Kleiman criticized.

Dr Kleiman began his reply by the assertion that what his papers really needed was a 'health' variable, inasmuch as purchases of health care are not measures of either health output or health utility in different countries. He was using a definition of substitution involving two quantities and one price, as in estimating the cross-elasticity of demand. Contrary to Professor Shinohara, he believed his own estimate of 0·6 for this elasticity to be significantly lower than Pryor's earlier assumption of 1·0. With regard to his measure of inequality, however, he accepted Professor Shinohara's criticism, not only relative to the agricultural share but also relative to the distribution of labor income itself, which varies in equality from one country to another. He admitted also an element of statistical bias in his results, in that his figures for non-military government expenditures included those on health care. Despite this bias he believed he had shown that the imperfect substitutability of public for private outlays may result in Wagner's Law – the proportion of total public expenditures increases with the national income – applying likewise to public health care expenditures specifically.

M. Foulon raised several additional statistical points, his basic conclusion being that Dr Kleiman's results were not very reliable because of the non-comparability of his observations, and that for many purposes a three-vector breakdown of private, public and semi-public health care services might help. M. Foulon's more specific points were:

1. The definition of 'private' and 'public' sectors varies from one country to another. For example, a greater proportion of hospital expenditures are included in the public sector in Britain and Scandinavia than in France and Italy, with Japan in an intermediate position. The distinction is administrative, not economic.

2. Dr Kleiman's independent variables are not really independent. For example, the labor share is not independent of the degree of urbanization, and the ratio of public to private consumption of health is not independent of demographic and particularly age variables.

---

[1] Dr Kleiman dissents from Professor Shinohara's view; Kleiman urges inspection of columns (1) and (3) of his appendix.

3. With reference to age variables, the proportion of young children under 3 years of age may be more important than the proportion under 15.

4. Is Dr Kleiman's labor share an approximation to gross or net inequality (gross or net of income taxes and transfers)? In the U.S.S.R. the labor share is approximately 98 per cent, but the degree of inequality is larger than in Sweden or Israel. Dr. Kleiman and Mr Kaser disagreed with M. Foulon as regards the Soviet situation: the former insisted that the 98 per cent figure is much too high, when allowance is made for capital allotments and indirect taxes; the latter's point was that approximately 30 per cent of Soviet consumption is free and, therefore, equal.)

Dr Christiansen expressed the opinion that the sample sizes relied upon by both Professor Rosett (27) and Dr Kleiman (16) were too small to warrant the sweeping conclusions of both these papers.

Dr Kleiman, in closing the discussion, insisted on the importance of the substitution relation between private and public health care in predicting future growth of public expenditure on health. He felt that the three-sector division suggested by M. Foulon was even more subject to cross-country incomparabilities than his own conventional two-sector one. He did not feel that the grossness or netness of the inequality measure made a great difference. Accepting Dr Christiansen's point in principle, he explained that he had started his study with observations on 44 countries, but had reduced his sample size to 16 because of assorted data problems in the other 28.

A few minutes were left before the close of this session, and were used for general comments upon the three papers. *Mr Cooper* began this period by saying that Japan's problems seemed to him fairly typical. For example, there are 'shortages' of doctors everywhere, and similarly 'excess demands' for medical care. He believed these terms lack empirical content in the health case. As for the Japanese budget deficit, he wondered whether this could be in large measure the result of prolonged bed rest and expensive drugs in tuberculosis cases. *Dr Kawakami* and *Professor Uzawa* denied this. With the introduction of antibiotics and new location of hospitals, tuberculosis-related expenditures have been falling since the mid-1950s.

Professor Intriligator would have liked to see more discussion of particular 'scarcity areas', primarily rural, in the Kawakami paper. The *Kawakami – Uzawa* reply was that the problem of health in rural Japan is part of the larger problem of Japan's sacrifices in achieving growth, in that the Japanese government has neglected all sorts of rural public services. In medicine, experiments are now under way to increase the role of TV in both diagnosis and treatment. *Professor Moriguchi* added that the problem was not primarily one of urbanization, because the shift of doctors to the cities has been less than the parallel shift of the population as a whole. The 'real' rural area, however, remains in shortage.

Dr Kehrer raised three questions on the Rosett paper: (1) Does not a higher-income area attract increased supplies of cooperant factors of production as well as of physicians themselves? (2) Why, if profit is found objectionable in large hospitals, is it not equally objectionable in the provision of drugs and other services? (3) Proprietors can sell hospitals to communities at rates allowing for future earnings; should not this point be considered in the paper?[1] *Professor Rosett* claimed that (1) was covered by his partial correlation analysis, while (2) was ancillary to the point of his paper and he had not realized (3) might be of importance.

[1] *Dr Phelps* added that the transfer process sometimes works in reverse with, proprietary chains and holding companies buying small community and other voluntary hospitals.

6 Economics of Need: The Experience of the British Health Service

Michael Cooper
UNIVERSITY OF EXETER

Twenty-five years of employing 'need' as the main allocative device within the Health Service has demonstrated that 'need' is capable of almost infinite interpretation. In a zero-price market no level of provision exists to eliminate excess demand and remove the necessity for rationing. This rationing function has never been explicitly recognized, but has fallen by default upon the medical profession as the main decision-makers of the Service. Doctors, however, have claimed the complete clinical freedom to act solely in the interests of each individual patient while being accountable only to their own personal consciences. As a consequence, rationing has taken place only implicitly, resulting in inconsistencies of medical practice and in inequalities of provision. Further, need being limitless, the Service has found it easier to claim shortages of resources than to examine critically their current deployment. A better understanding of the process by which the need for medical care is determined and a re-examination of the rationality of clinical freedom is attempted.

I. INTRODUCTION

Over 20 per cent of the British national income consists of goods and services supplied by the state at zero prices. In turn, some 25 per cent of this provision is accounted for by the National Health Service. This paper examines some of the problems which the Health Service has encountered in the last quarter-century as a consequence of charging zero prices and using 'need' as the main allocative device.

II. THE ORIGINAL ASSUMPTIONS

The intention of the Health Service Act, 1946, was to establish access to health care resources, as a 'human right', to all those shown to be in need. Nationalization was to ensure that sufficient of the country's resources were diverted from other ends to meet fully all genuine health needs, while provision at zero prices at the time of consumption was to ensure that no one in need was deterred from demanding.

Health care was to be no longer rationed amongst competing claims by the willingness and ability to pay a market clearing price. Instead, the state accepted responsibility for ensuring that sufficient resources were made available to meet society's needs as defined and assessed by the medical and allied professions. The professions, in turn, were guaranteed complete clinical freedom to decide what was in the best medical interests of patients and, in effect, to allocate resources as they alone saw fit.

The underlying assumptions were, firstly, that 'need' is finite, and secondly, that once defined, the nation could afford to divert sufficient resources to meet it fully. At zero price, rational individuals would attempt to consume *OW* resources in Figure 6.1. This would exceed

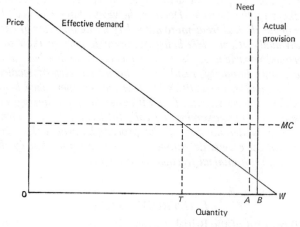

FIG. 6.1

the professions' assessment of need by some amount (*AW*), owing to the existence of hypochondria and various forms of abuse. The profession was charged with seeing that any such cases progressed no further than the initial visit to a general practitioner's surgery. Further, as 'needs' would be equal to, or slightly less than, the actual level of provision, the profession was assured complete and unconstrained clinical freedom to pursue the best interests of their patients, while being accountable to no one but their consciences. It was also thought almost self-evident that nationalization would result in more health resources (*OB* as against *OT*), as well as in those resources being more equitably distributed.

III. THE NEED TO RATION

In practice, need has proved to be a relative, not an absolute, concept. There was, and is, no finite allocation of resources that could eliminate all health care needs. Even in the relatively rare instances in which professions have formed consensus views as to adequacy, such levels of provision have proved in practice to be inconsistent with competing claims upon national resources. Exercises reported elsewhere have shown that the total cost of achieving even the main goals of different social agencies can amount to many times a country's total national income.[1]

The processes by which the demand for, and the supply of, health care resources are matched are illustrated in Fig. 6.2. The demand process begins with an individual's own assessment of his health state. If his assessment is positive, he then has to decide whether to convert his 'want' for better health into a 'demand' upon health care resources by presenting himself to some medical agency for care and/ or advice. Demands are therefore simply 'expressed wants'. Needs, on the other hand, are those demands deemed to require attention by a medical expert. That is to say, they are someone else's view of our health state. The Health Service differs from the normal market in that the individual does not have to convert his wants into effective demand and is therefore not constrained from visiting the doctor by his ability, or otherwise, to pay.

On the supply side, the quantity of resources devoted to health care is administratively determined. Nationalisation does not lead to abundance. Clearly, the resources available are constrained by the competing claims of other social agencies, by other demands on public resources and by society's reluctance to sacrifice private goods and services.

In practice, the scope for an individual to regard himself as in 'want' of health care is virtually unlimited. Wadsworth *et al.*, for example, recently found that 95 per cent of Bermondsey considered themselves unwell during the fourteen days prior to questioning.[2] Roghmann and Haggerty, in Rochester, N.Y., found that during a 28-day survey period adults claimed to be suffering from at least one

[1] Y. Dror, *Publicity Policy Making Re-examined* (San Francisco: Chandler, 1968) p. 165.
[2] M. E. J. Wadsworth, R. Blaney and W. J. H. Butterfield, *Health and Sickness: The Choice of Treatment* (London: Tavistock Press, 1971).

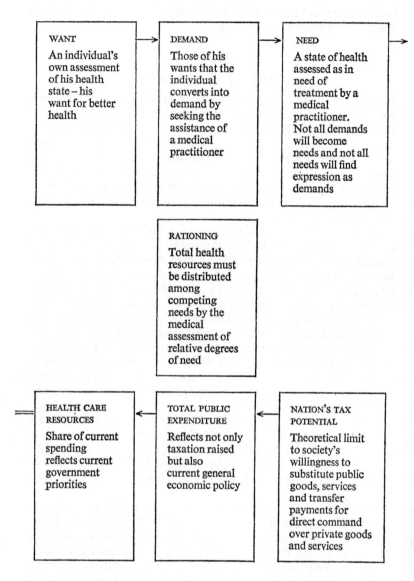

FIG. 6.2 The accommodation of want to supply

Source: Taken from M. H. Cooper, 'Rationing and Financing Health Care Resources', in N. Hunt and W. D. Reekie (eds.), *Management and the Social Services* (London: Tavistock Press, 1973).

disorder on over 20 per cent of the days in question.[1] Further, 46 per cent of the United States draft are reported to be rejected on 'genuine' medical grounds.[2] Clearly, to feel unwell is normal.

Fortunately for the Health Service, not all health wants find expression in demands, while some 30 per cent of those that do, by-pass the doctor and go directly to the chemist in search of 'over the counter' remedies. Whether these are the more trivial disorders, however, remains an open question.

The factors which determine whether an individual consults a doctor or not are highly complex and far from fully understood. Kessel and Shepherd have rather disturbingly found little obvious medical difference between patients who, over a ten-year period, never saw their doctor and those with the average number of atten-dances.[3] Job satisfaction personality and the stability of the family background have all been found materially to alter consultation rates.[4] There are also real costs involved in converting wants into demand. Deterrents include the necessary expenditure of time and energy plus for example, such factors as concern not to overwork the doctor. Further, the sheer availability of manpower and resources will profoundly influence demand. The knowledge that there are queues will obviously deter many would-be patients from demanding care. Indeed, in the long run, demand will tend to gravitate towards whatever level of provision there happens to be.

Once the patient is in contact with the doctor, the doctor is faced with the choice of treating, referring to a specialist or doing nothing. Again the decision-making process is complex and far from fully understood. No doubt, however, in addition to the patient's physical and mental well-being, class, education, manners and degree of persistence will all play a significant part. The dice are heavily loaded against the doctor deciding to do nothing. If a patient expresses a want it is difficult to show him he is mistaken, still more to expose him as a malingerer.

Need is, in any case, a medical opinion, not a medical fact. It is one of many possible points along a continuum. What levels, for example, of blood sugar or emotional stress are abnormal are not matters

[1] K. J. Roghmann and R. J. Haggerty, 'The Diary as a Research Instrument in the Study of Health and Sickness Behaviour', *Medical Care*, x (1972) 142.

[2] Reported in *Prospects for Health* (Office of Health Economics, 1971) p. 15.

[3] N. Kesse and M. Shepherd, 'The Health Attitudes of People who Seldom Consult a Doctor', *Medical Care*, iii (1965) 6.

[4] See, for example, P. J. Taylor, 'Personality Factors Associated with Sick-ness Absence', *British Journal of Industrial Medicine*, (1968) 105, and J. T. Shuval, 'The Sick Role in a Setting of Comprehensive Care', *Medical Care*, x (1972) 50. These factors are further discussed in *Medicine and Society* (Office of Health Economics, 1972).

which readily attract medical unanimity. It is likely to be only those conditions at the extreme end of the continuum, where life is immediately threatened by inaction, that will be universally considered as need.

The scope for individual medical interpretation of need is well illustrated by the facility with which numbers of British dockers, until recently considered fit, have managed to find doctors who genuinely consider them unfit and therefore eligible for redundancy from the docks and for the consequential 'golden handshake'. Similarly, a leading professional footballer was recently found, upon attempting to change clubs, to be suffering from a 'serious' congenital heart disorder. He continues to play football for his old club, unimpaired by his new-found health state. Again, Rosenham at Stanford has managed to plant eight normal people into mental hospitals where they remained undetected for as long as they could endure it. Further, within a mental hospital warned of impending planted 'normal' patients, one consultant detected 41 and another 23 out of a population of 193 entirely genuine patients.[1] Perhaps, however, the most striking example which can be cited is the fact that hospital surgeons in the United States manage to find twice as many patients per capita in need of surgery as do their British counterparts. This contrast is made all the more surprising when allowance is made for the existence of a large medically deprived population in the United States due to the price barrier.[2]

Collectively the profession appears to reassess its conception of need in line with actual levels of provision. Feldstein, for example, pointed out in 1967 that any attempt to allocate funds to hospital beds based upon medical assessment of the need for them as reflected in admissions and waiting lists was likely, in practice, to have little or no meaning.[3] Need seemingly tends to grow in line with provision, as doctors react to any expansion in supply by realigning their conception of need further along the possible continuum. In his study of 177 large acute hospitals, Feldstein found that both admissions and length of stay increased with bed availability and could discover no indication of a level of bed provision which would have fully satiated doctors' demands. Thus, like an iceberg, the more resources devoted to melting it, the more need seems to float to the surface.

As medical science enjoys roughly the same degree of exactitude as

---

[1] D. L. Rosenham, *Science*, 20 Jan 1973.

[2] Scope for medical abuse exists in both countries. Fee per item of service might tempt some consultants to perform 'unnecessary' operations, while the salary system might tempt some not to perform 'necessary' operations.

[3] M. S. Feldstein, *Economic Analysis for Health Service Efficiency* (Amsterdam: North-Holland, 1967).

economics (and scarcely more unanimity of opinion), the patient who is insistent is bound to use up considerable quantities of scarce resources. The doctor makes his need decisions in face-to-face confrontations with patients anxious to be helped, and he is, in turn, anxious not to appear helpless.

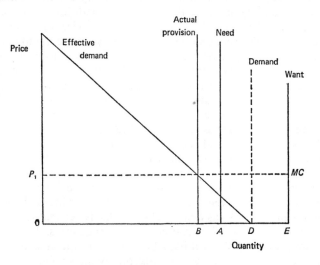

FIG. 6.3

Fig. 6.3 illustrates the probable outcome of the Health Service's inception upon supply and demand. Demand (*OD*) is shown to exceed actual provision (*OB*) by a wide margin. Demand will, in fact, tend to coincide with effective demand at zero price. To the extent, however, that individuals link the consumption of health care to the payment of tax prices, demand will fall short of *OD*.

On the other hand, wants which have little to do with health care as such may find expression as demands on the Health Service simply because the Service is there and free of charge. The lonely, for example, may go to the doctor in default of any other social welfare agency to turn to. Further, the state calls upon doctors in Britain to act as general social policy agents. Individuals are expected to consult a doctor, not only for medical treatment, but also to legitimize absence from school or work, to obtain state sickness benefit certificates, to gain arbitration on the need for an abortion, or even simply to get the back of a passport photograph signed. Therefore it is feasible, if somewhat unlikely, that demand might even exceed strictly health wants (*OE*).

Again, although one would normally expect need (OA) to fall some way short of demand, as doctors discouraged 'unnecessary' calls upon their time, it might conceivably exceed it. This result would follow if the so-called 'iceberg of sickness' could be somehow made explicit. Considerable evidence exists of health states that would be clearly defined as 'in need' if they ever found expression in demand.[1] Individuals may be unaware that they have conditions which would be technically defined as 'sick' if they sought advice, or, again, may be well aware of the condition but consciously choose not to demand any help. This might be out of fear of discovering an appalling disease, or because they are convinced that little could, in any case, be done to relieve their condition. Quite serious disorders can be 'lived with' by a combination of self-treatment and a change of life-style. In the event, research has shown that many conditions not reaching the doctor are as serious if not more so than, those that do.

Clearly, want, demand, need and the level of provision are all interrelated in a complex and, as yet, little understood pattern. Medical assessment of need is a function of actual provision, demand, medical progress and factors individual to each doctor. Gaps will inevitably exist between what is technically feasible and what is operationally possible, as well as between what is demanded and what is supplied. The line of causation will run both ways. The level of provision, for example, will itself be a function (albeit sometimes a weak one) of the level of need as assessed by the profession.

What emerges as certain from this section is that there will always be excess demand for resources and a problem of rationing demands amongst OB resources. In the market-place this would be achieved by a price rise to P_1. In the Health Service, the problem of rationing has fallen to the medical and allied professions.[2]

IV. RATIONING BY NEED

The main decision-makers in the Health Service are doctors, but they have not seen their role as being one of rationing at all. Rather, they have insisted upon complete clinical freedom. They have remained 'accountable only to the patients whom they serve and to their own conscience'.[3] If need had proved, in fact, to be an absolute and the

[1] See S. Israel and G. Teeling-Smith, 'The Submerged Iceberg of Sickness in Society', *Social and Economic Administration*, I, 1 (1967).

[2] It can also be seen from Fig. 6.3 that whether or not the market solution would result in more or fewer resources depends upon the position that is assumed for the best curve.

[3] D. R. Cook, 'The Reorganisation of the N.H.S.: Viewpoint of the G.P.', *Journal of the Royal Society of Health*, XCII, 1 (1972).

nation could, in theory, have afforded to allocate the appropriate level of resources, then it would have been possible (but not necessarily desirable) to grant the profession immunity from normal market forces. In other professions, freedom is constrained by the client's willingness and ability to pay: in the case of health, the constraint is ultimately the state's willingness and ability to pay.

The misconception as to the nature of need, combined with the insistence (however imaginary it may have been in practice) upon complete clinical freedom, have meant that rationing has taken place in a largely unplanned and uncoordinated manner. This has inevitably resulted in misallocations of existing resources, plus an insatiable thirst for more.

Inconsistencies in medical practice are to be found at all points in the rationing process (illustrated in Fig. 6.4). The decision as to whether to refer a patient to a specialist, whether to hospitalize, and how long to retain him in a hospital bed, all show inexplicable variations between doctors, hospitals and regions. Further, there is a rapidly growing literature indicating the existence of much current medical treatment which, if not actually detrimental to the patient's health, certainly has no positive material effect upon it.

The general practitioner is clearly critical to the whole rationing process. It is to he who decides whether any given demand should proceed any further than his consulting room. General practitioners, however, have displayed no consistency in the number of episodes of sickness which they deem as worthy of the attention of a specialist. Scott and Gilmore, for example, found a variation in the proportion of patients referred to hospital during a year, between practices in Edinburgh, of from 0·6 per cent to 25·8 per cent.[1]

Although it has been shown that as high as 83 per cent of referrals to consultant surgeons go no further than the initial interview and without any pathological or X-ray investigation, Ashford and Pearson have shown, in Exeter, that general practitioners with high referral rates also prove to have high hospital admission rates.[2]

It has been estimated, by Crombie and Cross, that 25 per cent of the patients in hospital in Birmingham had no therapeutic or diagnostic need to be there.[3] The obvious subjectivity of such

[1] R. Scott and M. Gilmore, 'The Edinburgh Hospitals', in G. McLauchlan (ed.), *Problems and Progress in Medical Care* (London: Oxford Univ. Press, 1966).

[2] G. Forsyth and R. F. L. Logan, *Gateway or Dividing Line* (Nuffield Provincial Hospitals Trust, 1968), and J. Ashford and N. G. Pearson, 'Who Uses Health Services and Why?', *Journal of the Royal Statistical Society*, series A, CXXXIII, 3 (1970).

[3] D. L. Crombie and K. W. Cross, *The Medical Press* (London: Routledge, 1959) pp. 242, 316, 340.

Patient's own assessment	Action taken	G.P.'s assessment	Action taken	Specialist's assessment	Medical action taken	Effect
1. In want	1. Sees doctor	1. In need	1. Refers	1. In need	1. Treatment (a) Proven (b) Unproven (c) Unsound (d) Inappropriate (e) Alleviate (f) Comforting 2. No treatment (a) None technically possible (b) None available (c) Low priority 3. Second-best treatment	1. No effect 2. Cure 3. Survival 4. Death 5. Reassurance
				2. Not in need	1. Referred back 2. Self-medication	As above
		2. Not in need	2. Treated	None	As with specialist	As above
			None	None	1. Second opinion 2. Self-medication	As above
	2. Sees pharmacist	None	None	None	1. Self-medication 2. Advised to see doctor	As above
	3. None	None	None	None	None	1. Survival 2. Death
2. Not in want	None	None	None	None	None	As above

Fig. 6.4   The National Health Service rationing process

judgments is revealed, however, by the fact that Mackintosh *et al.* arrived at a figure of 4 per cent for the same area. After re-analysis for comparability between the studies, a figure of 13 per cent was arrived at, but with the rider that non-medical needs had been such that only 4 per cent could, in practice, have been denied admission.[1]

Once admitted to hospital, the length of stay for any given condition varies manyfold between hospitals, even after standardization for age and sex, and after rejecting extreme values which show high fluctuations from year to year. The variation between lengths of stay following treatment for hernia is fivefold, for appendicitis sixfold, and for bronchitis and pneumonia ninefold.

Little or no evidence exists to support the contention that those consultants who habitually insist upon using more resources are, in reality, materially altering the condition of their patients. In the case of hernia, Morris *et al.* established, in 1968, that discharge from hospital after one day had no observable effect upon the patient, as compared with discharge after one week.[2] The current national average stay for this condition, however, remains 11 days, while some hospitals average 21 days.

Clearly, different doctors are taking different actions when confronted with similar health states. This is not, of course, to argue that either human beings or their ailments are all exactly similar. Clearly, patients cannot all be discharged after the minimum length of stay irrespective of their actual medical condition. What is being suggested however, is that patients should be discharged after the minimum acceptable period in the clear absence of any good reason to the contrary. There should always be explicit and positive reasons for variations from the scientifically established practice.

While it is true that doctors have to adjust their aggregate demands so that they are consistent with available resources, clinical freedom means that they are individually neither adjusting from, nor to, a common base line or conception of need. What one general practitioner sees as meriting a referral will still differ radically from that of another even if all general practitioners are forced to adjust to changed supply circumstances.

Clinical freedom is also, of course, the freedom to be wrong. There is a growing body of evidence that much medical practice is, if not unsound, then at least unproven.[3] Large-scale cancer surgery, insulin treatment for mature diabetes, tonsillectomy, and bed rest

---

[1] J. M. Mackintosh, T. McKeown and F. N. Garratt, *Lancet* (1961) p. 815.

[2] D. Morris, A Ward and A. J. Hendyside, *Lancet* (1968) p. 681.

[3] A. L. Cochrane, *Effectiveness and Efficiency: Random Reflections in the Health Services* (Nuffield Provincial Hospitals Trust, 1972).

for both coronary heart disease and tuberculosis are some examples which have been widely examined and found wanting.

Surgery for small-cell cancer of the bronchus, for example, has been shown, by controlled trials, to lessen rather than lengthen a patient's life expectancy when compared with treatment by radiotherapy alone.[1] Again, in the case of tuberculosis, the World Health Organization has shown that even in the poorest areas of Madras treatment at home was no less effective than that in hospital.[2] Yet in Britain the average length of stay in hospital remains at 70 days.

Perhaps even more serious is the literature pointing to the rise of iatrogenic diseases or DOMP (diseases of medical practice). Malleson quotes the story of Solomon at Harvard who added to his medical reputation by curing his over 50-year-old patients of being confused and forgetful by denying them their usual supply of prescribed barbiturates.[3] A dramatic example of global DOMP was revealed by a study conducted in Hanover, which suggested that the main reason why the German mortality rate from appendicitis was three times higher than any other country's was that appendectomy was performed there three times as often. A follow-up of 959 cases revealed that only one in four patients had actually been suffering from acute appendicitis. The appendix was healthy but the patient was dead.[4] In the United States, a decline in the appendectomy rate has been accompanied by a parallel fall in the mortality rate.

It is certain that much medical treatment is inappropriate, unproven or even unsound, but will authorities ever be united in deciding which? Indeed, even if there were unanimity as to which treatments did no positive good, does it follow that they would be universally discontinued as unnecessary? Such treatment, it could be claimed, provides hope and temporary reassurance to many otherwise hopeless cases. Few doctors are prepared to tell a patient that the hope of effective treatment is so low that he should go home and, unaided, wait to recover or die. The question is, however, what level of resources can the country afford to allocate to such ends, however desirable, and, again, after the decision, ought there not to be some uniformity of practice between doctors and hospitals?

Very little current medical practice has ever been subjected to the same rigorous testing to which, say, all new pharmaceuticals are

[1] Medical Research Council, *Lancet*, II (1966) 997.

[2] Quoted by A. L. Cochrane in W. A. Laing (ed.), *Evaluation in the Health Services* (Office of Health Economics, 1971) p. 20.

[3] A. Malleson, *Need Your Doctor Be So Useless?* (London: Allen & Unwin, 1973).

[4] S. Lichtner and M. Pflanz, 'Appendectomy in the Federal Republic of Germany: Epidemiology and Medical Care Patterns', *Medical Care* (Ann Arbor), IX (1971) 311.

subjected. The objection to the evaluation of medical and surgical practices seems to centre upon the ethics of denying a control group of patients a possibly helpful treatment, purely as a consequence of a random numbers table. There seems, however, to be little justification to this objection in those cases where the treatment is already widely considered suspect. Bed rest, for example, appears to be an admirable candidate for evaluation. It is expensive in resources, and practice already varies widely throughout the country.

There is, however, little point in evaluation if clinical freedom is to continue to mean freedom to be eccentric and to ignore scientific evidence without any attempt to refute it.

V. PLANNING BY NEED

The misunderstanding as to the nature and extent of need has resulted in little or no effective planning and control. Research into various aspects of need has been sparse and uncoordinated. The result has been the persistence of the very inequalities between regions, hospitals and specialities that the Health Service was, in part, formed to remove.

Further, the fact that need is a relative concept has meant that the scope to claim a shortage has been almost infinite. Demands for more resources and manpower have always been simpler than critical self-appraisal of current practices. Scope for economies persists even in the strictly non-medical aspects of the Health Service's administration.

The central machinery for assessing the purpose, direction and priorities of the Health Service has always existed. The original intention of the 1946 Act was that the Regional Hospital Boards should be the agents of the Central Department. In practice the regions have enjoyed considerable autonomy, with circulars passing down the system with little more status than suggestions.

Clear-cut, obtainable, national standards have never existed. The system has worked upon the basis of maximum downward delegation with minimal upward accountability. Even the shaping of long-term plans has emerged as the sum of individual authorities' aspirations or as extrapolated trends of usage, rather than as the consequence of any research into the probable dimensions of future need. Planning has amounted to, in the words of one of the Service's Chief Medical Officers, 'the use of last year's budget with a bit added here and a bit taken off there'. 'We never ask ourselves the big questions', he continued.[1]

[1] J. H. F. Brotherston, in W. Latham and A. Newberry (eds.), *Community Medicine in Teaching, Research and Health Care* (London: Butterworths, 1970) p. 131.

The initial allocation of resources in 1948 exactly reflected the pre-1948 imbalances. Further, subsequent distributions of manpower and finance have largely preserved them intact. By 1969, according to the then Minister in charge, geographical inequalities remained the 'single most difficult problem' to be faced.[1] The author and A. J. Culyer have pointed out elsewhere that there are two-fold variations between Regional Boards in the number of consultants and general practitioners per capita, and in expenditure upon both medical and surgical supplies.[2] Sheffield, for example, is less well endowed than Oxford on over thirty indices of provision. What is not clear, however, is whether it is Oxford, Sheffield or neither that is efficient. Certainly, there are no obvious signs that morbidity is lower in Sheffield, or any signs that its citizens are suffering from any deprivation. Such differences in provision rates certainly require more careful scrutiny and justification than they have received to date. Why, for example, do the children of the Oxford region require twice as many tonsillectomies as those in Sheffield?

Until 1971, no explicit effort was made to allocate resources to Regional Hospital Boards on the basis of a need formula. According to the current Under-Secretary of State for Health, 'We had not developed any acceptable system of measuring the relative needs of regions'.[3] Even in the absence of such indicators, however, equality of provision per capita would seem a more rational objective than two-fold variations. The current formula, although crudely based upon population weighted by age and sex, cases treated and the current supply of beds, is nevertheless an important step forward.[4]

Attempts to rationalize the distribution of general practitioners by

[1] Richard Crossman, reported in the *Guardian*, 27 Nov 1969.

[2] M. H. Cooper and A. J. Culyer, 'Equality and the N.H.S.: Intentions, Performance and Problems in Evaluation', in M. Hauser (ed.), *The Economics of Medical Care* (London: Allen & Unwin, 1972).

[3] Michael Alison, personal communication, 27 July 1972.

[4] Each of the factors is used to determine theoretical allocations for the individual regions:

(a) Population: the national total revenue moneys are divided in direct proportion to the weighted populations served in each region.

(b) Beds grouped under specialities are multiplied by annual costs of providing hospital services based on national average costs per inpatient week (similarly for outpatient attendances).

(c) Cases (inpatients and outpatients) by specialities are multiplied by the appropriate national average costs of treating a case.

A combined theoretical allocation is then derived by adding one-half of the population-based allocation and one-quarter of each of the other two calculated figures and making a few adjustments for such factors as higher rates of pay in the London area. The formula excludes teaching hospitals. Equality under the formula is to take place gradually over the next ten years.

a system of negative direction involving the closing of adequately doctored areas to newcomers met with some success as long as the supply of newcomers continued to expand. With the decline in numbers, however, the more unfashionable and already under-doctored areas suffered most. The percentage of population living in areas officially designated as under-doctored fell from 52 per cent in 1952 to 17 per cent in 1961. Between 1963 and 1967, however, with the decline in general practitioner numbers, this percentage rose to 38 per cent, but it is now dropping again and is currently standing at 29 per cent.

Similar discrepancies also exist between different categories of patients and hospitals. Bed-week costs, for example, vary from £23·29 for the mentally handicapped (slightly less than the cost of keeping a man in prison) to £76·56 for acute hospitals and £112·25 for London teaching hospitals. These differences are reflected in even the non-medical costs. Catering costs vary from £3·15 a week for the mentally handicapped to £7·39 in acute hospitals and £11·60 in London teaching hospitals. Such differences obviously cannot be explained by variations in medical dietary needs.[1]

The insatiability of need has led to continuous demands for additional health resources. Medical manpower is a case in point. Between 1949 and 1969, hospital doctors increased by 90 per cent, while the total British work-force increased by only 10·5 per cent. Last year a record number of new doctors were added to the register, and medical school places will have doubled by 1979 compared with the situation ten years ago. Nevertheless, it is possible to make a case for still more. Over 50 per cent of junior hospital doctors, 15 per cent of general practitioners and 15 per cent of nurses were born overseas. A world trade in doctors which involves Britain in importing some 700 a year from countries like India and Nigeria, with doctor/population ratios of 0·7 and 0·02 per 1,000 respectively, while simultaneously exporting 400 a year to the United States and Canada with ratios of 1·60, hardly seems a firm foundation for the Health Service.

Shortage, within the context of an administered market, can mean only a shortfall from some technically defined ideal. It may well be that such an ideal is itself a constant function of actual provision and is unobtainable. Certainly, any claim for more manpower must be seen in the light of competing claims upon scarce skilled resources. A well-founded case is necessary, but not sufficient grounds, for obtaining more. Further, such a case must follow, and not precede, a careful scrutiny of current practices and the conventional deployment of manpower.

[1] *Hospital Costing Returns for Year Ending March 1972* (London: H.M.S.O., 1973).

VI. MANAGEMENT AND NEED

Although there now exists a clear management hierarchy within the nursing profession,[1] consultants and general practitioners remain independent and unaccountable. Clinical freedom has prevented the role of general manager from evolving and has made consensus government through committees the only viable alternative.

The lack of normal chains of management has resulted in the kinds of misallocation of resources within hospitals reported by Logan *et al*. This team found, for example, that the allocation of beds between consultants was seriously out of line with their respective requirements.[2] Even in strictly non-medical areas, the Health Service's efficiency has been seriously questioned. The service is, in effect, Britain's largest hotel and laundry chain. One-quarter of the total hospital budget goes upon supplies and equipment, mostly in common use. Suppliers complain of irregular and unplanned purchases, duplicated orders, and having to deal with several departments within one management committee area.[3] The Public Accounts Committee complains of failures to select the cheapest gas and electricity tariffs and of small-scale purchases of even the more common user goods.[4]

The scope for management in the medical side has been severely limited, while on the other, incentives have been largely lacking. The current government is pledged to the administrative reform of the system.[5] There is to be a two-tier structure with 14 Regional Boards overseeing 92 Area Boards. Basically, 6,000 Regional, Hospital Management and Executive Council committee members are to be replaced with 1,600 in a more unified system. The whole structure is to be compatible with the geographical boundaries envisaged for the new local authorities which come into being in 1974. Within each Area Board there are to be Community Health Councils for each district. Their task will be to feed back local opinion and to act as 'visitors' to the health amenities in their locality. These councils are to have tongues but not teeth. They are to have the power merely to report their views to the Area Board but not to take any action.

Great hopes for the new structure have been expressed in terms of

---

[1] *Report of the Committee on Senior Nursing Staff Structure* (Salmon Report) (London: H.M.S.O., 1966).

[2] R. F. Logan *et al.*, *Dynamics of Medical Care* (1973).

[3] See *Hospital Purchasing* (Office of Health Economics, 1972).

[4] *2nd Report of the Committee of Public Accounts* (London: H.M.S.O., 1972).

[5] *The Future Structure of the National Health Service* (London: H.M.S.O., 1970); *N.H.S. Reorganisation: Consultative Document* (London: H.M.S.O., 1971); *National Health Service Reorganisation: England*, Cmnd. 5055 (London: H.M.S.O., 1972).

the introduction of modern management techniques. Formidable barriers exist, however, in the form of tradition, emotion and professional self-interest, and it is these which will finally determine how the legislature's intent is translated into practice. In the event, the reorganization may prove to be little more than the illusion of change.

Even if faithfully translated, the plan does not hold out great promise of radical change. Although the general practitioner service is now to be under the same umbrella as the rest of the Service, it nevertheless retains its own committees and old terms of practice. Within the hospital system the concept of a chief executive continues to be rejected, if anything, with more force than before. Management teams at each level are to be 'groups of equals, no member being the managerial superior of another'.

The strictly hierarchical nursing profession will continue to be 'coordinated' with the representatives of the other professions. The role of the committee doctors, for example, will be to represent the consensus view of their colleagues; or 'to express views when they have, or that it is reasonably likely that they will be able to obtain, the support of their colleagues'. At the district level (i.e. the level concerned with the actual delivery of care), the management team 'will act as a consensus forming group, i.e. no decision will be taken that overrides the opposition of a team member'.[1]

A structure which depends to this extent upon consensus government is unlikely to encourage any new managerial virtues. Further, it seems unlikely that the medical profession will suddenly discover a capacity for unanimity. Indeed, the plan seems unlikely to satisfy either those demanding more rational and explicit line management or those hoping for greater decentralization and democratization.

VII. CONCLUSIONS

The Health Service was founded upon a basic misconception of the nature of the need for health care resources. The conception of sickness as an unambiguous and absolute state led to the false hope that unmet need could be abolished. In practice, sickness has been found to be a relative, state capable of almost infinite interpretation by both potential patients and the medical profession. There has proved to be no allocation of national resources which would eliminate the necessity for the Health Service to ration its services among excess competing claims upon them.

[1] *Management Arrangements for the Reorganised National Health Service* (London: H.M.S.O., 1972).

The process by which final demands upon the Service are determined is complex and certainly involves many non-medical considerations which remain only poorly understood. What emerges as certain is that demand tends to outstrip supply. Rationing, however, has never been explicitly organized, but has hidden behind each doctor's clinical freedom to act solely in the interests of his patient. Any conflict of interest between patients has been implicitly resolved by the doctor's judgments as to their relative need for care and attention. The clinical freedom to differ widely as to their conception of need has led to inconsistencies of treatment between patients, and to the allocation, without challenge, of scarce resources to medical practices of no proven value.

A study of the processes by which treatments – formerly accepted as standard, but revealed by scientific inquiry or clinical trial as wanting – are finally rejected by the entire profession, would prove illuminating. Judging, for example, by the survival of the leech bottle until after the First World War, the process is, to say the least, ponderous.

Clinical freedom has enjoyed a rationality under the traditional conception of need that is severely undermined with its better understanding. It survives, partly at least, as a consequence of the widespread view that sickness is an unambiguous state which, following diagnosis, suggests a standard and self-evident treatment which would attract universal agreement from a profession composed of individuals of high, but largely homogeneous, talent. The truth is that consultants and general practitioners vary in ability and intellect as much as do any other group of graduates. The competent but undistinguished may benefit from the guidance, encouragement and shared responsibility which comes with more hierarchical professional structures. The incompetent and indolent need the exposure and accountability of line management. All would probably profit from the incentive offered by the prospect of further advancement above the rank of consultant.

The medical profession, however, claims that management is inconsistent with good medicine. Undoubtedly, the present system is perfectly consistent with bad medicine. The profession dominates current management while at the same time rejecting it. Consensus government has led to compromise and inefficiency.

For their part, the Central Department has been content to delegate responsibility downwards so that even long-term plans have reflected the sum of regional hopes and aspirations. The lack of research into indicators of need has enabled gross inequalities of provision to persist on the grounds that, in the absence of any evidence to the contrary, they might in fact, however accidentally, reflect needs.

Further, the nature of need has enabled the Service continuously to claim shortages of manpower and other resources. It has remained easier to demand more of the taxpayer than critically to re-examine current practices and to prune out waste.

The most apparent need in the Health Service is for more information of all kinds, at all levels. Regular flows of tailored data are required, for example, on resources available by locality and specialty, usage patterns and the variables that determine them, unmet demands, the evaluation of treatment, and so on. Doctors need to know if they differ from their colleagues; the Service needs to know why. Statistics gathered to make up tables in the *Annual Report* are not enough.

Few would deny that the Health Service was an enormous step forward in British social policy, but several steps remain to be taken. This paper has tried to pose the question as to whether, with a better understanding of need and in the absence of complete clinical freedom, unavoidable rationing would not take place more rationally, consistently and efficiently, to the mutual benefit of taxpayer and patient.

7 Private Patients in N.H.S. Hospitals: Waiting Lists and Subsidies[1]

Anthony J. Culyer and J. G. Cullis

INSTITUTE OF SOCIAL AND ECONOMIC RESEARCH,
UNIVERSITY OF YORK

Private practice by National Health Service (N.H.S.) consultants in its hospitals is alleged both to inflate the lists of those (N.H.S. patients) waiting for admission as inpatients and to involve substantial transfers that internalize no externality and that are, moreover, regressive. This paper shows that, on certain assumptions, the short-term effects of removing private practice in N.H.S. hospitals include only minor (positive or negative) effects on waiting lists. In the longer run, if private hospitals can provide sufficient substitute care and of other inputs (such as consultant time in the N.H.S.) do not fall and inpatient referrals do not rise faster than the trend, then substantial reductions may be gained. The paper also shows that the present structure of charges does not cover the full costs of care and that net transfers to private patients may take place, even allowing for the tax price paid by such patients.

I. INTRODUCTION

Ever since Aneurin Bevan conceded the continuation of private practice in Britain's health system during the protracted medical politics preceding the inception of the N.H.S., it has remained the subject of – sometimes quite bitter – controversy. At least a part of this controversy has been ideological, but with this we shall not be concerned here. The continued existence of private practice has also presented difficulties for those seeking to derive formal rationalizations of the N.H.S. in terms of manageably simple welfare functions [1,8]. In this paper we examine a small part of the total set of analytical problems posed by the existence of private practice in N.H.S. hospitals – the impact upon the lists of non-paying patients

[1] Acknowledgment is made to the Department of Health and Social Security for a grant to the Department of Economics and Related Studies and the Institute of Social and Economic Research at the University of York for research in the economics of hospital waiting lists. We are also grateful to members of the Health Economics Research Programme at York for discussion of these and related issues.

waiting for admission to hospital and the method of charging used
for use of N.H.S. facilities. These two problems, between them, have
proved an embarrassment to responsible officials in the management
of the N.H.S., partly because there have been some well-publicized
cases of abuse but, more importantly in our view, also because
officials and other experts appear not to have had any ready answers
to charges that (*a*) private practice causes waiting lists and waiting
times for N.H.S. patients to be longer than they need be, and that
(*b*) the system of charges is such that private patients (on the whole,
relatively wealthy citizens) are subsidized by the N.H.S.[1] It is, of
course, a basic part of the 'constitution' of the N.H.S. that treatment
of private patients using its facilities should not prejudice the treatment of non-paying patients.

II. WAITING LISTS

Hospital waiting lists in the N.H.S. are of three types: (*a*) the outpatients with appointments waiting to see consultants (or the average
time between an appointment and being seen by the consultant); (*b*)
the patients waiting for a first appointment as an outpatient (or the
length of time between referral to a consultant and being seen by
him); (*c*) the numbers waiting for admission as an inpatient (the
aveɪage time between being put on the inpatient waiting list and
being admitted). The major public concern, and ours, is with (*c*),
defined officially as a 'record of patients who, though needing hospital
treatment, must wait because there is no appropriate bed available' [9].

In 1971 there were 5,289,000 deaths and discharges in N.H.S.
hospitals in England and Wales (excluding psychiatric cases) of
whom 114,856 were paying inpatients, or 2·17 per cent.[2] The waiting
list for all N.H.S. hospitals (excluding psychiatry again) stood at
520,048 at 31 December 1971. Of these, about 10 per cent are admitted within a month, another 15 per cent are admitted within one
to three months; another 15 per cent are admitted within three to six
months of being put on the list and 20 per cent within six to twelve
months. About 40 per cent have to wait from one to five years or even
longer (3½ per cent wait over five years).[3] The thɪee most popular

---

[1] See, for relatively sober discussions on waiting lists [4] paras, 967–90,
2121–9; on charges, *ibid.*, paras. 828–77, 2055–91.

[2] Some inpatients may have been readmitted and discharged a second time
or died during the second stay. Deaths and discharges thus tend to overstate
the number of inpatients treated since they are a record of inpatient *spells*.

[3] Waiting list data are far from accurate. One study [7] indicated that principal
sources of waiting list inflation are (*a*) about 15 per cent due to patients already
treated or who have died, and (*b*) another 15 per cent who no longer wish to be
admitted.

specialities for private practice in hospital were general surgery, gynaecology and traumatic and orthopaedic surgery – the three specialities with the longest N.H.S. waiting lists. Surgery and gynaecology accounted for 97 per cent of the numbers waiting for non-psychiatric care (also exclusive of geriatrics and chronic sick).

The arithmetic in this paper is conducted on the basic assumption that seems to have been shared by discussants of problems of private patients and hospital waiting lists, namely that paying patients and N.H.S. patients are competing essentially for *beds*. An implication of this assumption is that beds are the only effective constraint on hospital throughput, which we do not think realistic. The kinds of modification required to the basic argument in recognition of a more realistic hospital service supply function are briefly touched upon later. Meanwhile, we follow tradition in supposing the naïve view to be true.

If private practice were to be removed from N.H.S. hospitals,[1] the impact on waiting lists for N.H.S. patients would depend principally upon:

(*a*) relative occupancy rates for what used to be private and N.H.S. beds;

(*b*) relative durations of stay for private and N.H.S. patients;

(*c*) the extent to which private patients could be absorbed into the private-sector institutions;

(*d*) the length of private patient waiting lists.

On the assumption of full absorption of private patients into private institutions, we estimate that N.H.S. hospital waiting lists could fall by as much as 15·9 per cent[2] if the higher occupancy of N.H.S. beds (79·7 per cent) were to apply to the released pay-beds (whose occupancy by *all* patients was 72·0 per cent[3]) and if patients treated in

---

[1] If private practice *per se* is not to be abolished, the (official) case for permitting its existence in N.H.S. hospitals, rather than relegating it entirely to private-sector institutions, is basically threefold: (*a*) N.H.S. hospitals are, on the whole, better equipped than private-sector hospitals and nursing homes and it has been considered unjust to deny superior publicly owned facilities to any set of patients whether paying or not paying; (*b*) N.H.S. hospital private practice reduces the necessity of having part-time consultants moving excessively between different institutions; (*c*) the more time consultants spend in N.H.S. hospitals, the more time they are likely to have available for treating N.H.S. patients in excess of their contractually obligatory number of 'sessions'.

[2] Using 1968 data. Since the 1968 Health Services and Public Health Act, pay-beds are no longer separately designated or set aside in N.H.S. hospitals. Only the total number of private paying patients being treated at any one time in a particular hospital is subject to control, not the beds they use.

[3] Pay-beds are not reserved for the *exclusive* use of private patients. In 1968, private occupancy of pay-beds was 61 per cent and N.H.S. patient occupancy

them had the same length of stay as N.H.S. patients (15·35 days) rather than the average length of stay of private patients (9·44 days).[1] The gain would be larger than 15·9 per cent of course, if the patients taken off the waiting list – who would tend to be non-priority patients – had a shorter length of stay in hospital.

On the alternative polar assumption that erstwhile private patients in N.H.S. hospitals all join the N.H.S. queue, the waiting list would *increase* by at least 3·8 per cent[2] if the former private patients are treated at the *N.H.S.* average duration of stay. If the N.H.S. can treat the former private patients with the average duration of stay associated with private practice, there would be a *decrease* in the waiting list of between 1·5 per cent and 2·5 per cent, depending on whether additional patients admitted from the waiting list as a result of the increased occupancy rate take up bed-days according to the N.H.S. or the private patient average.

None of these calculations allows for the existence of private patient waiting lists. In December 1968, however, these amounted to only just under 2,000 patients, and would have relatively small impact on the N.H.S. inpatient waiting list.

Since 1968, pay-beds are no longer designated in N.H.S. hospitals. As a consequence, it would seem that the advantage to be had from an increase in overall occupancy rates, if it were ever real (see footnote 3 on p. 110), has disappeared.

Thus, if we suppose that in the short term the throughput of patients in private-sector hospitals is a given rate, the most optimistic estimate of the impact of removing private practice from N.H.S. hospitals would be of the order of a 1 or 2 per cent reduction. The impact on waiting times would depend, of course, upon the management of the waiting list. Changes in private practice are not, *ceteris paribus*, likely to have much effect on either the average wait or the

---

11 per cent. N.H.S. bed capacity utilisation included the utilization of 'amenity' beds, which are available to N.H.S. patients desiring privacy not required on medical grounds, for a fee, under section 4 of the 1946 National Health Service Act and the 1968 Health Services and Public Health Act. However, the differential in occupancy of private and N.H.S. beds may well have been due as much to recording failures by hospital staff as to any real factor. It seems that non-paying patients in pay-beds are sometimes not counted. If N.H.S. patients in pay-beds are consequently attributed to N.H.S. beds, the pay-bed occupancy rate should be adjusted upwards and the N.H.S. bed occupancy rate adjusted downwards.

[1] This differential, arises we believe, from the case-mix of private surgical practice, rather than from any other factors. Unfortunately, we have no data on private patients by speciality.

[2] 'At least' if it is the case that longer waits are associated (for clinical reasons) with shorter stays in hospital.

variance of wating times.[1] Most commentators would agree, we think, that there exist a number of far more promising methods of tackling the waiting list problem than the abolition of private practice. We conclude, therefore, that the costs of private practice in terms of increased waiting lists are not as large as has frequently been supposed.[2]

The preceding arithmetic and, indeed, much of the conventional discussion of waiting lists takes an implicitly fixed-proportions production function for hospitals. Quite clearly, however, a shift in the balance of private care as between public and private institutions will affect the supply of other factors to hospitals – in particular, the supply of consultant time. In addition, even the total abolition of all private practice (supposing 'black markets' in medical services to be effectively suppressed) would have an effect, it is alleged, on the emigration of young doctors in that it affects the future pecuniary returns to being a consultant in some important specialties.[3]

The response of waiting lists to changes in bed capacity is far from clearly understood. For one thing, the stock of available hospital beds has been steadily reduced in recent years as a matter of Health Service policy (though patient throughput capacity[4] has increased at the same time), implying, superficially, that beds are in excess supply rather than excess demand. More important, however, has been the observed relationship between bed stock and inpatient waiting lists. For several years it was thought that waiting lists could be used as an indicator of the excess demand for inpatient beds and that increases in the stock could reduce waiting lists. Feldstein, however, in a series of applied studies, made the disconcerting discovery that hospital bed supplies appeared to *create their own demand* [5, 6].

While there are a number of theoretical explanations based upon

---

[1] The classification schemes of patients according to priority currently used and the efficient management of waiting lists are currently under consideration by the Department of Health and Social Security.

[2] 'If you look at the total waiting list in the Department's annual report and look at the total number of empty beds available in the country at any given moment and the number of consultants who are working less than whole-time it is very simple arithmetic to show what the consultants could do in the other two-elevenths of the time using these beds to the full advantage. They could wipe out the waiting list in a very short time.' Dr D. Stark-Murray in evidence to the Expenditure Committee [4] para. 2121).

[3] We doubt whether any *current* difficulties in obtaining private practice affect many doctors' decisions to emigrate, but it would be exceedingly rash to suppose that the entire abolition, or severe curtailment, of private practice would not have a serious affect. Men may not become doctors *solely* for pecuniary reasons, but they would not be men if their incomes were unimportant to them.

[4] Throughput capacity $= \dfrac{\text{No. of available beds} \times \text{occupancy rate} \times 365}{\text{Average duration of stay}}$.

the behaviour of doctors and patients, each of which would be consistent with this finding (for example, that G.P.s refer more patients to consultants when bed capacity rises and consultants recommend more patients for admission as inpatients[1]), there is a great lack of information about how individual actors in the system actually do react. There is also evidence that when genuine through-put capacity increases, the waiting list actually does fall [3]. One's intuitive response that rejects the 'supply creates its own demand' view of hospital activity is strengthened by such evidence. The key, however, lies in the adjectival qualifications *genuine* throughput capacity. Clearly, a hospital's ability to manage any throughput of patients depends not only upon the available stock of beds and the ways in which it is managed, but also upon other cooperating factors of production and the way they are managed. If, for example, beds were not the effective constraint on greater throughput, but some other factor – such as operating theatres or surgeon availability – one would no longer expect any negative correlation between bed supply and inpatient demand. If bed throughput capacity increased, other factors constant, capacity utilization would be expected to fall. Even if other factors can be adjusted, as they can within limits, it would be unusual (given conventional forms of the production function) to expect utilization to increase in the same proportion as the bed capacity factor.

If increases in bed capacity are accompanied by smaller propor-tionate increases in other factors, it is clearly possible for capacity utilization to fall (or to remain more or less constant), for throughput to rise and for (possibly more) consultants to place more cases – especially the non-urgent ones – on the waiting list. But it would be misleading to describe this phenomenon (if it is one!) as 'supply creating its own demand'.

In short, the relationship between bed capacity and waiting lists is unlikely to be a simple one. We are at present exploring some of these relationships – including the relationships between waiting lists for inpatient admission and waiting lists for first appointments – in order to clarify the complex and important functional interdependences that may exist. Unfortunately, it is too early as yet to report any results.[2]

---

[1] Explicit consideration of these possibilities in simple models does not, how-ever, yield very plausible first-shot results (see [2]).

[2] A substantial amount of operational research is being and has been undertaken in the matter of optimizing the management of waiting lists. While not regretting these efforts it is, however, our view that the difficulties inherent in obtaining major changes in managerial practice in British hospitals are very substantial unless there are also substantial changes in incentive and control structures. At present, we believe that understanding the underlying functional relationships –

III. SUBSIDIES

The 'who subsidizes whom' argument is double-edged. On the one hand, it is argued that private patients subsidize N.H.S. patients because (*a*) they pay both the small earmarked health tax (the 'contribution') and the implicit tax price of N.H.S. care without receiving benefits as N.H.S. patients, and (*b*) because any progressivity in the tax structure implies that private patients (being, on the whole, wealthier than other patients) pay higher implicit tax prices. On the other hand, it is argued that N.H.S. patients subsidize private patients, since charges for the use of N.H.S. staff and facilities are not 'properly' based (the consultant's fee for his own personal service is, of course, a matter between him and the private patient). In our opinion, there can be little doubt that the imperfections, if any, in the N.H.S. charges for private patients could not be so gross as to outweigh the tax prices implicitly paid by private patients.[1]

The analytically more interesting question relates, however, to the obligation of the N.H.S. to recoup, so far as it is possible, the total cost of providing services for private resident patients. Some allowance may also be made for capital costs in so far as these appear to be 'proper and reasonable' to the Secretary of State.

The injunction of the N.H.S. does not correspond with the marginal cost pricing rule(s!) that have figured so prominently in the pricing policies of public enterprise, for these are supposed – in principle – to ensure optimal (in a partial equilibrium sense) consumption rates of publicly provided goods and services. The N.H.S. charges, by contrast, are supposed, we presume, to exclude any element of subsidy to N.H.S. patients. They are supposed, between them, to pay the full cost of the N.H.S. resources they use up. Moreover, we infer that this average cost that the charges are to cover is not the average *social* cost but the average *fiscal* cost. The

---

with given management procedures – promises to be more helpful in solving the waiting list problem. The parameters are certainly more in the control of central administration.

[1] In 1969–70 there were an estimated 18·36 million taxpayers in England and Wales and the cost met from all sources of finance by the national health and welfare services net of charges to persons using the services at the central government level amounted to £1,441 million implying an average tax price of £78·49. If the 109,144 private patients in England and Wales in 1969 paid this tax price (a minimum estimate), the average direct charges paid by these people of £80·63, calculated on the basis of the £8·8 million estimated receipts from pay-beds in 1970–1, would have to be short of the correct amount by not less – and probably more – than the implicit tax price, £78·49, for private patients to be subsidized by the rest of the community.

charge, in short, is equity-based rather than efficiency-based, where the equity principle is referring to shares in public expenditure, their share of which private patients should repay to the fiscal authorities in full.

The matter thus reduces to a reasonably straightforward accounting procedure, and practice has been to base charges upon the average inpatient costs of the type of hospital in which a private patient is receiving treatment.[1] A question of controversy arises, however, in the matter of accounting for capital and depreciation costs, for it has been widely claimed that it is in respect chiefly of these costs that the subsidy to private patients is given.[2]

Were it an efficiency question, analysis suggests that capital costs incurred in the past are irrelevant in pricing decisions. The only relevant capital costs would be the depreciation implicit in retaining some (non-designated) hospital capacity for private use over the forthcoming planning period of a year. As it is an equity question, however, the costs to be recouped from private patients must presumably be the capital costs incurred in the base year, suitably deflated for changes in the price level, averaged out over the expected life of the capital equipment and with the resulting annual sum (adjusted for N.H.S. patient usage) divided between the expected number of private patients in the next accounting period.

Taking the average capital cost of a new hospital bed at current prices to be about £20,000, assuming the expected life of the asset to be fifty years, a 61/72 share in the bed of private patients and an average length of stay of private patients of 9·44 days, this implies a charge of about £6·50 per week or £8·77 per private patient spell in hospital.

It is not clear whether equity also requires implicit interest to be paid for the creation of private patient capacity in N.H.S. hospitals, though it would appear consistent with what we take to be the objective of private patient charges that deferred payments for the use of previously created capacity should include interest. If this is correct, then, at 10 per cent, an addition of £26·22 per week must be made to the £6·50, making a total capital charge of £32·72.

The figure of £32·72 is very much higher than the £1 per week capital charge retrieved by the N.H.S. in 1972 and is not very far

---

[1] The five types are Regional Hospital Board long-stay hospitals; R.H.B. psychiatric hospitals; R.H.B. acute and other hospitals (in which most private patients are found); London teaching hospitals; and provincial teaching and R.H.B. university teaching hospitals.

[2] Strictly speaking, the capital cost should be the marginal capital expenditure on the extra capacity implicitly built for private patients, averaged over the number of private 'beds' thus provided, not the average of the total capital cost.

short of the sum suggested by Meacher as being the appropriate one.[1]
The derivation of the £1 charge is not clear, though it appears to be
related to the 1963 rating valuation for hospitals ([4] para. 875).
Rating valuations are, of course, irrelevant to this charge if our
equity interpretation is correct,[2] though the charges should be adjusted
annually to maintain the real value of the capital cost repayment.

IV. CONCLUSIONS

We make three brief conclusions from this discussion:

  (i) The evidence does not suggest that private practice has any
      serious effect on the length of N.H.S. inpatient waiting lists.
 (ii) The evidence does suggest that, on equity grounds, private
      patients pay too little of the capital expenditure incurred on
      their behalf.
(iii) The central case against private hospital practice, that it is
      unfair because it enables 'queue-jumping', is independent of
      and intrinsically different from the objections discussed in
      this paper. It is a moral argument not dependent on, or
      strengthened by, the basically factual matters discussed here.

REFERENCES

[1] Culyer, A. J., 'Medical Care and the Economics of Sharing', *Economica*
    (1969).
[2] —— and Cullis, J. G., 'Economics of Hospital Waiting Lists', unpublished
    paper (Univ. of York).
[3] Dodson, R. M., 'Planning for Out-patient Surgery', Ph.D. dissertation
    (Univ. of Lancaster, 1971).
[4] Expenditure Committee, 4th Report, *National Health Service Facilities for
    Private Patients* (London: H.M.S.O., 1972).
[5] Feldstein, M. S., 'Hospital Bed Scarcity: An Analysis of the Effects of
    Inter-Regional Differences', *Economica* (1965).
[6] ——, 'Hospital Planning and the Demand for Care', *Bulletin of the Oxford
    University Institute of Economics and Statistics* (1964).
[7] Grundy, F., Hitchens, R. A. N., and Lewis-Faning, E. (Welsh National
    School of Medicine), 'A Study of Hospital Waiting Lists in Cardiff (1953–
    1954): A Report Prepared for the Board of Governors of the United Cardiff
    Hospitals'.
[8] Lindsay, C. M., 'Medical Care and the Economics of Giving', *Economica*
    (1971).
[9] Ministry Circular H.M.(62)45.

[1] Michael Meacher suggested that £45 per week might be appoximately right
on the basis of a capital cost of £18,000 per bed ([4] para. 873). The apparent
lowness of the capital charge currently imposed suggests that other charges for
the use of N.H.S. services, such as pathological laboratories, may be too low as well.
    [2] They are, moreover, also irrelevant on efficiency grounds.

8 Consumer Protection, Incentives and Externalities in the Drug Market

Elisabeth Liefmann-Keil

UNIVERSITY OF SAARLAND

The purpose of this paper is to analyse the influence of the requirements of prescription for ethical drugs on the position of the different participants in the drug market (D.M.). The consequences, intended and expected, of enforcing regulation introduced to protect the ignorant consumer, namely prescription requirements for a growing share of drugs, are – as the paper demonstrates – not achieved. It is well known that the ignorance of the consumer is of special importance for the structure of the D.M. It is also well known that the pharmaceutical industry has an exceptionally strong position in the D.M. When examined, the protection of the consumer proves to be, first of all, not a protection of the demand (the consumer or patient) but a special legal framework for protecting the physician and the pharmaceutical industry. The incentives for the physician and the pharmaceutical industry to monopolize information and knowledge in respect to ethical drugs are strengthened. The additional introduction of a social sickness insurance scheme or a national health service turns out to fortify the monopolistic positions of the physician and the pharmaceutical industry, induced by present consumer protection. The position of the consumer is thus further weakened. The guarantees of quality and safety are imperfect, the economic interests of the consumer disregarded. The intention to achieve a reduction in social costs results in additional social costs.

I. INTRODUCTION

The purpose of this paper is to deal with a rather neglected subject in the field of health economics, the development of the market for (prescription) drugs (D.M.). This market for an essential input in health services is characterized as well by the importance of its product as by its institutional capacity to impede potential externalities. Two additional peculiarities have, in many countries resulted in regulations to protect the consumer from misusing or abusing drugs and to avoid the possibilities of externalities (that is,

involving impacts on persons whose consent is not necessary for the
decision): the existence side by side of complex beneficial curative
effects and dangerous side-effects[1] and an insufficiency of information among the consumers of drugs.

There are two well-established theories of government regulation.
The one says: 'Protection may be intended primarily for the
protection and benefit of the public.' The other says: 'Such regulation
may serve as a façade for the protection of certain elements in the
regulated industry.' The regulatory process may encourage special
incentives to strengthen the position of groups of sellers participating
in the market.[2] As R. N. McKean recently assumed: 'Even government regulation of itself or of the private sector, though often
intended to do something about externalities, will typically generate
other externalities.'[3]

I intend in this paper to investigate such effects and, particularly,
the incentives and costs caused by the legalized protection of the
consumer in the D.M.: *the prescription.*

The consideration of the situation in the D.M. is based on the
following assumptions:

(a) A regulation favouring the consumer, such as in most highly
industrialized countries, as, e.g., in the Federal Republic of
Germany (F.R.G.), i.e. a prescription by a physician necessary
for the purchase of selected drugs.

(b) No insurance or public service schemes (this assumption does
does not apply to sections IV and V).

(c) The behaviour examined is the behaviour of groups, not of a
single individual.

(d) There is almost no competition between physicians.

In submitting the paper I agree with Alchian and Allen that 'it
may be captious to emphasize that such constraints (as protections)
have their "costs", but these kinds of costs are often overlooked or
ignored by proponents of restrictive or protective legislation'.[4] The

[1] They comprise curative poison (digitalis), substitutes of food (vitamins) and
indispensable medicines (insulin), as well as special kinds of amenities (analgesics)
or something like luxury goods (like, sometimes, tranquillizers).

[2] R. Urban and R. Manke, 'Federal Regulations of Whiskey Labelling: From
the Repeal of Prohibition to the Present', *Journal of Law and Economics*, XV, 2
(1972) 423.

[3] R. N. McKean, 'Property Rights, Appropriability and Externalities in
Government', in G. Wunderlich and W. L. Gibson, Jr (eds), *Perspectives of
Property Rights* (University Park. Pennsylvania State Univ. Press, 1972) p. 52.

[4] A. Alchian and W. R. Allen, *Production and Exchange* (Belmont, Calif.:
Wadsworth, 1969) p. 418.

costs for one group may be the benefits cultivated for other groups. The groups participating in the D.M. are: the consumer, the physician, the pharmacist and the pharmaceutical industry. What are the characteristics of these groups caused by consumer protection?

II. THE GROUPS PARTICIPATING IN THE DRUG MARKET

(1) *The Consumer*

Following the new approach in the theory of demand by Lancaster and Becker, consumer demand is characterized by two choices that are to be distinguished:[1]

- (a) The choice of an *output*; that is, the ascertaining of preferences and of the bundle of characteristics desired for the satisfaction of the consumer.
- (b) The choice of an *input*; that is, the goods possessing the characteristics wanted. Such choice presupposes some knowledge about the 'consumption technology'.

In the D.M. the consumer ought to know, on the one hand, the diagnosis and the suitable treatment (the characteristics) and, on the other hand, the pharmaceuticals appropriate for the treatment. In reality, however, the consumer's knowledge of both these aspects is – as mentioned before – generally inadequate.[2] It is currently felt that customer liability would lead to transaction costs being relatively high. These high transaction costs are a special reason for supporting a protection of the consumer.[3]

Similar information situations for the consumer exist today also in other markets. They are not exceptional, especially in highly industrialized countries. In the D.M., however, it is a traditionally acknowledged and carefully cultivated state of affairs which requires a special solution. The function of control is transferred, therefore, from the principals to the agents who have to be experts. This is a procedure which is also evident, e.g., in the relationship between the stockholder and banks. In the D.M. it is confirmed by an institution enforcing the consumer to abandon some of his property rights. As Abba Lerner has recently shown, being able to make choices requires

[1] K. J. Lancaster, *Consumer Demand: A New Approach* (New York: Columbia Univ. Press, 1972) pp. 15 ff.

[2] Only the moment of visiting the physician is sometimes left as a matter of the consumer's decision. Up to today the patient generally performs the first diagnosis.

[3] R. N. McKean, 'Products Liability: Implications of Some Changing Property Rights', *Quarterly Journal of Economics*, LXXXIV (1970) 617 ff.

the ability to exercise property rights.[1] Such an exercise is questionable if information and knowledge are unsatisfactory, as is the case in the D.M. Exercising property rights signifies, normally, a twofold process. It is divided, on the one hand, into decision-making and control and, on the other hand, the actual exercising of ownership rights. The prescription compels the consumer, as owner of his income and/or wealth, to transfer some of the first-mentioned rights to the physician. The latter is assumed to act as a substitute, leaving to the consumer in this area only his ownership rights. The prescription enforces, in this way, a separation of ownership rights from the rights to control. Accordingly, the consumer is left in a situation where he is induced to neglect benefits, the value of which he cannot appreciate because monitoring the physician's behaviour would be extremely expensive.

(2) *The Physicians – the Mediators*
Four peculiarities characterize the mediators and their behaviour in the D.M.:

   (*a*) Medical education enables the physician only to inform the consumer about the necessary output (the diagnosis and some treatment).
   (*b*) The physician faces the possibility of becoming liable for a treatment. He is usually insured against liability.
   (*c*) The physician's education with respect to the 'consumption technology' i.e. the input, the goods possessing the characteristics desired, is rather modest. Moreover, the physician has continuously to renew his knowledge of this technology. Today he relies for this information primarily on the services offered by the pharmaceutical industry.
   (*d*) The physicians, as a group, have the monopoly to prescribe. They recommend and order the drugs to be used by their patients.
   (*e*) These decisions are mainly technological decisions. The physician controls the demand, but he does not control the costs. He exerts almost no economic control. As the late Senator Kefauver said: 'The man who orders does not buy, and the man who buys does not order.'[2]

The physician as the principal decision-maker dominates the demand for drugs. As a technician, therefore, he has to consider a kind of supplier liability. In this respect, he depends chiefly on the services of the pharmaceutical industry. Surprisingly, he does not depend on the services of the pharmacist.

[1] A. Lerner, 'The Economics and Politics of Consumer Sovereignty', *American Economic Review, Papers and Proceedings*, LXII (1972) 258.
[2] E. Kefauver, *In a Few Hands: Monopoly Power in America* (Harmondsworth: Penguin Books, 1965) p. 8.

(3) *The Pharmacist*

The functions of the pharmacist are decreasing. Nevertheless, the distribution costs are relatively high. They raise the expenditures for drugs in most highly industrialized countries to about 70–90 per cent above the producer's price.[1] The pharmacist still retains his special knowledge of the consumption technology. He still belongs to a licensed group of experts. The pharmacist's position in the D.M., however, is limited to that of being more or less a retailer or store-keeper and (in a very reduced area) an adviser. In some countries the physicians retain the right to dispense drugs; in other countries the physician may be the owner of a chemist's shop.

Today, in some countries, as in the F.R.G., the pharmacist enjoys a special kind of protection in the form of a legalized retail-price maintenance. Therefore, he is very much interested in retaining his privileges. The reduced functions permit us, in this paper, to ignore the present limited influence of this group.

(4) *The Pharmaceutical Industry*

As mentioned before, this industry operates in a special legal frame-work. It is characterized by protection intended to favour both the consumer and the producer. The first kind of protection imposes laws on the industry requiring special care in the production of drugs and laws restricting the practice of advertising. The second kind of protection results from the advantages connected with patents, trademarks, etc. Therefore, there is not free access to certain parts of the market for producers, and a rather expensive access to others. As a seller of drugs the industry does not depend greatly on the demand of the retailing pharmacist or of the consumer. It depends, basically, on the demand created by the physician. The customer to be protected and managed is the physician. With the transfer of the consumer liability to the producer and physician, this relationship has been particularly strengthened.

III. THE PROTECTION IN THE DRUG MARKET

Protection is the protection of somebody and/or something. The proponents usually suppose that it is possible to isolate the effects of protective measures, that their influence may be limited to the effects intended. They overlook what McKean calls 'intervention costs'.

---

[1] T. D. Rucker, 'Economic Problems in the Drug Distribution', paper presented at the Annual Meeting of the Pharmaceutical Wholesalers Association, 8 Mar 1972 (mimeographed), and E. Liefmann-Keil, 'Überlegungen zur Verbesserung der Position der gesetzlichen Krankenversicherung auf dem Arzneimittelmarkt', *Pharmazeutische Zeitung*, XI, 41 (1972) 1483 ff.

They neglect such originally not intended costs, as 'protective effects' or 'shadow costs' which affect other groups or cause feedbacks to the protected.[1]

Until now the studies made of the D.M. have for the most part concentrated on the supply side. It has been demonstrated, that 'the misallocation of resources has been made possible by the existence and abuse of the patent privilege for ethical drug products and processes by a number of measures which the industry has taken'.[2]

This kind of institutional framework certainly supplements the protection introduced in favour of the consumer. Nevertheless, the special protection of the demand side has its own impact on the situation in the D.M. It results in special incentives influencing the supply of medical services.

The instruments chosen by governments in the interest of the consumer are:

(a) The description of drugs at a registry office with the declaration of the content, etc.
(b) The obligation of the consumer to obtain a prescription before being able to purchase 'ethical drugs'.

The purpose of both instruments is to enforce the realization of special obligations, be it for the producer or consumer, be it for a demand to be restricted or for a careful use. The prescription may be regarded as the official acknowledgment of the ignorance of the consumer with regard to the purchase and use of drugs. The prescription means transferring a demand for medical services, the liability for a special kind of product, to the physicians, who at the same time act as suppliers in the field of diagnosis and treatment. These preventive interventions vary from country to country. There are drugs which have to be prescribed in one country but not in another. The proportion of ethical drugs supplied and used in relation to all drugs supplied varies from country to country. The share of ethical drugs in the total number of drugs in the F.R.G. is estimated by the pharmacists to be 27–28 per cent. The share in the total sale of drugs by the public pharmacies is estimated to be about 53 per cent in the F.R.G., For the United States and for Sweden the figure is about 60–70 per cent.

The constraints characterizing the D.M. are intended to control the demand and to restrict the supply, etc. They have, however, a kind of expansion effect, favouring the protection of other groups. Such

[1] For the concepts mentioned, see McKean, 'Property Rights', p. 36, and Alchian and Allen, op cit., p. 422.
[2] H. Steele, 'Monopoly and Competition in the Ethical Drug Market', *Journal of Law and Economics*, v (1962) 132.

effects are reflected in the corresponding constraints imposed on the consumer making choices.[1] As choice, by definition, involves the consideration of costs, limiting choices means restricting the calculation of costs. Substituting the decision of a representative for a consumer's decision means, beyond that, adding the competitive interests of the substitute. The restrictions permit other groups to appropriate the corresponding benefits. In supplying their medical services these groups are permitted to impose an all too selfish a use on the consumer.

Regarding the different groups participating in the D.M. and, chiefly, in the ethical drug market, there is no group left without some protection. The consumer has his protection, there are the protections derived from the consumer protection favouring the groups supplying medical services, there are the special protections added favouring the producers of drugs. All these protections are more or less assumed to be justified by the need to protect the consumer without considering the costs for the consumer and potential externalities.

(1) *The Protection of the Consumer*

This reveals itself as a deceptive substitute for the individual search by the consumer for information and knowledge. The price the consumer has to pay for these substitutes consists in the separation of the rights of ownership and control, and in the substitution of his liability by a physician's and a producer's liability. It is assumed that the consumer does nothing but profit from using the physician's knowledge of the consumption technology and the suitable output for the treatment of the patient, as perfect or imperfect as it may be. Four disadvantages are generally overlooked:

(*a*) With the physician's conscious or unconscious concentration on the consumption technology, economic control is more or less set aside.

(*b*) With the selection of special products, with the smaller range of choices, the consumer has (for a relatively large part) only an option to buy higher-priced products as a consequence of the different restrictions[2] which are sometimes, more or less irrationally priced,[3] plus the costs of the physician's information and insurance and the producer's insurance.

---

[1] A. A. Scitovsky, 'Changes in the Costs of Treatment of Selected Illnesses, 1951–1965', *American Economic Review*, LVII (1967) 1194.

[2] For an example of such consequences see W. Benham, 'The Effect of Advertising on the Price of Eyeglasses', *Journal of Law and Economics*, XV, 2 (1972) 337 ff.

[3] Rucker, op. cit., pp. 7–8.

(c) The opportunities lost by the purchaser who has other preferences. He may like, e.g., to retain his own liability, to depend
less on the physician or to accept a lower level of quality.

(d) The splitting of ownership and control. There will remain the
risks of obtaining an inappropriate prescription, of an inferior
recovery, the danger of overmedication and of additional expenditures to compensate for allergies, etc.[1]

The consumer suffers from the weakening of his incentives to
exercise his property rights, to inform himself, or to control the
economic as well as the technological decisions and performances.
His behaviour in respect to illness and recovery is shaped by the
physician. He is left with the presumption or fact that some services
are improperly priced, that there are still externalities.

(2) *The Adjustments of the Physicians*

What are the incentives to the physician resulting from the consumer
protection? The enforcement of the prescription and the connected
shift of the decision-making to the physician rest on the assumption
that 'the social demand for a guaranteed quality can be met this
way'.[2] The only relevant counterpart to quality is special knowledge,
an ability to control the quality, an accomplishment only in the
interest of the consumer. The performance of such a guarantee
proves, however, to be imperfect and accidental. What. therefore, is
the result of the enforcement of the legal prescription to the physician?

(a) He is not only granted a special monopoly but also the right to
appropriate many of the rewards connected with the guarantee
of the quality of the drugs.

(b) He enjoys the right to prescribe, that is, to handle a special
'necessary' exclusion principle, supplementing the usual exclusion principle, the price (without, generally, having the
right to sell the drugs).

(c) He is guaranteed a certain demand for his services. As the
consumer is obliged to ask for a prescription, the physician
is subsidized in a special way.

(d) The probability of complaints by the patients is not too great
because such a procedure would mostly be without prospects.
The consumer knows that to sue means a kind of gamble. In
any case, also, the physician is interested in risk reduction.[3]

[1] For the United States, these costs, in hospitals only, have been estimated to
be about $3 billion. (*Neue Züricher Zeitung*, 18 July 1972.)

[2] K. J. Arrow, 'Uncertainty and the Welfare Economics of Medical Care',
American Economic Review, LIII (1963) 996.

[3] R. A. Bauer, 'Risk Handling in Drug Adoption: the Role of Company
Preference', *Public Opinion Quarterly*, XXV (1961) 559.

These circumstances comprise, for the physician, new complementing incentives. The complement the restricted access to the physician's market results from the duty to possess a licence or a certificate. For a long time the physicians insisted on restricted entry to their own market. This has changed in the last few years. The physician is now interested in ensuring a growing demand for his own services. Such a tendency matches very well the incentives arising out of the right to prescribe. It intensifies the incentives to enlarge the kind of services supplied as well as the number of ethical drugs.

With the prescription, governments have strengthened the position of the physician as a mediator and a channel of information to the consumer. Although the physician is appointed to be a protector, he is at the same time granted his own protection. Moreover, the physician is also induced to use the incentives resulting from the assumptions of the ignorant consumer. Prescriptions signify, for the consumer, a guarantee of quality and of better treatment, like a high price or a trademark. This is an additional incentive to increase the number of drugs available only on prescription. It may, e.g., also stimulate overmedication.[1]

(3) *The Adjustments of the Pharmaceutical Industry*

The adjustment of the physician is followed by adjustments in the pharmaceutical industry. The industry profits from the special position of the physician. He is, for the industry, a powerful controller of the demand for drugs. The failure of an effective control by the consumer favours the seller and price-searcher. For the single drug, the industry is confronted with a rather low price elasticity (supported by the protective practices) and a relatively higher substitution elasticity. As competition and, especially, advertising for the consumer are prohibited, the struggle for the customer concentrates on the physician. The pharmaceutical industry has, in this situation, two special incentives:

(*a*) To make good use of its position as a price-setter. The consequences are relatively high profits, plus a tendency to concentrate, control and maintain prices.

(*b*) To exploit the physician's dependence on the industry with regard to information.

The producers are interested in cementing their relations to the protective mediators by different forms of promotion. For the United States, 85 per cent of the expenditures for these purposes have

[1] Ch. Müller, 'The Overmedicated Society: Forces in the Marketplace for Medical Care', *Science*, CLXXVI, 4034, 5 May 1972, p. 488.

been classified by an expert as 'an economic waste ... designed to fortify producer sovereignty.[1] The protectors who are assumed to protect the consumer are, in reality, protecting only themselves and also the industry. 'Overall remarkably little of the available evidence suggests that consumers are protected by [such] regulations.[2]

IV. THE ADDITIONAL INFLUENCE OF SOCIAL INSURANCE AND/OR PUBLIC SERVICE SCHEMES

The introduction of social insurance or public services in the field of health has two implications:

(a) The consequences of financing by contributions or by a system of general taxation.

(b) The consequences of zero-pricing for most of the medical services.

They strengthen the position of the supply, i.e. of the physician as well as of the pharmaceutical industry. They complement the monopolistic positions already existing by the introduction of authorities who have their own special interests in the performance of zero-pricing and indirect financing. They also bring about a change regarding exclusion principles. Demand has to face a substitute for price, another exclusion principle, waiting. The usual exclusion principle, the price, is explicitly removed by the introduction of special financing schemes. Both the retained principles (prescriptions and waiting) are handled by the physician. He, therefore, also dominates the consequences of zero-pricing. In this respect, both principles have almost a doubling effect. They intensify the reduction of the consumer control. These kinds of consequences have been characterized by Arrow in this way: 'In general any system which, in effect, insures against adverse final outcomes automatically reduces the incentives to good decision-making'.[1] The private transaction and information costs are internalized. The financing systems combine the technical protection with an additional kind of economic protection. The latter turns out to be practically a kind of disguised income redistribution. Thus, economic controls are left to official authorities. In addition to the consequences already

[1] Rucker, op. cit., p. 4.

[2] W. A. Jordan, 'Producer Protection, Prior Market Structure and the Effects of Government Regulations', *Journal of Law and Economics*, xv, 1 (1972) 175.

[3] K. J. Arrow, 'The Organization of Economic Activity: Issues pertinent to the Choice of Market versus Non-market Allocation', in *The Analysis and Evaluation of Public Expenditures: The P.P.B. System*, vol. i, submitted to the Joint Economic Committee (Washington, D.C.: U.S. Government Printing Office, 1969) p. 55.

mentioned, this internalization produces a new problem, demonstrated by multinational firms, the possibility of externalities in the world economy.

V. CONCLUSIONS

What are the costs of the efforts to protect the consumer? What are the unintended externalities generated by the regulations to reduce the externalities expected?

Perhaps the best way to handle these questions would be to use the new approach in the theory of demand mentioned before. The comparison of the results with the goals may be accomplished by defining the output as the goals and the input as the characteristics wanted.

(1) *The Output*

Do the goods, i.e. the protective measures, possess the characteristics needed?

   (*a*) The enforcement of the substitution mentioned before may often suffer from the fact 'that people who make decisions to [use] certain items do not necessarily have the same preferences as those for whom they are sought'.[1] The consumer has less incentive and chance to reveal his preferences and to improve his information. The consumer is consciously kept in a weak position. Protection is not meant to change this fact. On the contrary, the presupposed assumption of a basic ignorance of the consumer is apt to fortify this situation.[1]

   (*b*) Regarding his preferences and needs, the consumer is interested in having alternatives. He needs conditions which enable him to control the activities of the supply, be it the supply of actual services or the number of producers. In a market, supply is usually intended to communicate to the consumer a variety of choices based on its ability to create new possibilities. But the more the available choices are restricted by artificial means, as in the case of pharmaceuticals, the greater is the distortion that may exist between the pattern revealed by the exchange process and the product–price relation. To the degree that the products and the demand are directly or indirectly regulated and standardized, each act of purchasing conveys less information from the consumer to the producer. Communication between

---

[1] Alchian and Allen, op. cit., p. 418.
[2] K. Gronhaug, 'Risk Indicators, Perceived Risk and Consumer's Choice of Information Sources', *Swedish Journal of Economics*, LXXIV, 2 (1900) 246.

the consumer and the producer is more or less excluded. The control by the consumer affects the technological as well as the economic responses of the supply. As the consumer is kept ignorant, does there exist a similar control by decision-makers over decision-makers and by producers over producers? Under the prevailing conditions such control cannot be expected. Also, it may not be correct to expect, as is normally supposed, that the monopolistic supply, which is insensitive to consumer preferences, will tend to destroy its position.[1]

(2) *The Input*

Is the kind of input the consumer protection represents, with all its side-effects, suitable in respect to the characteristics wanted?

(a) The separation of ownership and control and the substitution of the consumer liability lessen the independence of the consumer, without ensuring the guarantees intended. Thus, consumer protection may prove to be a deceptive practice.

(b) The strengthening of the physician's rights induces his incentives to dominate. The mutual dependence of the pharmaceutical industry and the physician produces for the industry the incentives to extend this dependence. The institutional framework of the D.M. causes the opposite of the effects expected. The incentives to combine protective objectives (prescription regulation and one or the other security scheme) with allocative effects have so far been operating in a situation biased towards under-compensation for the consumer.[2]

What seems to be overlooked or underrated is the importance of incentives induced by the regulation. The incentives which are now effective on the side of the supplier tend to maintain the prevailing weak economic position of the consumer. It is a not too encouraging result which is to be observed in the D.M. (as in other markets): consumer protection tends to impair consumer sovereignty. Consumer choices are restricted, and induced to go astray. Nobody knows if a protection, like the prescription for ethical drugs, results in a technologically more perfect or more imperfect protection, a more efficient provision. This is very well shown by the arguments offered in the discussion which started at the beginning of 1973 concerning the costs of consumer protection in the market for ethical drugs (by Peltzman, Friedman, Müller and others). There exist many more indications that the protection of the supply has become more

[1] R. A. Jenner 'An Information Version of Pure Competition', *Economic Journal*, LXXVI (1966) 799, 801, 803.

[2] O. E. Williamson, D. G. Olson and A. Ralston, 'Externalities, Insurance and Disability Analysis', *Economica*, XLIII (1967) 252.

perfect. The reaction to this fact may – in the future as in the past – lead to new protection, especially in the form of more restrictions of choice, more public authorities and more use of power. Such a chain of protectionism may have more expansion effects, introduced and justified by the argument that the public interest, i.e. the consumer, needs such protective measures. Nevertheless, these may be a façade behind which the protégés unconsciously support the protectors and are paying the costs for these protections.[1] Therefore, 'it will be important to learn how to regulate better by keeping appropriability in mind, for regulation may well become one of our fastest-growing industries'.[2]

Until today, drugs have been treated as special goods because they may have more or less dangerous side-effects. But there are also other goods with similar side-effects, like alcohol, tobacco, cosmetics, cars, gasoline, etc., which may destroy health and cause medical expenditures. The consumer of these goods is generally not protected, with one special exception – alcohol. There has existed something like a consumer protection against alcohol – prohibition (e.g. in the United States and Sweden) – but these measures were abandoned after a while. Such experiences refer to the fact that (with some exceptions) the problem may not only be a regulation to protect against the loss of health, but a problem of the professionals in the regulated area. What may be important is not a restriction of demand, but more services and other incentives. As the costs of drugs are steadily rising, the discussion about the D.M. is also rising. Such questions as over-medication may become more vital. Doubts may be expressed in respect to the consequences of the growing use that results in a mere shifting from one illness (the infectious disease) to another (the chronic disease), the stagnation of the life expectancy (for males) in the highly industrialized countries, etc.

The final conclusion is, therefore: the prevailing regulation which results in a special protection of the appointed protectors (the mediators and the producers) poses anew the problem of the protection (of the consumer). This consumer protection is one of the most urgent subjects of modern health economics.

---

[1] The interdependence between the different medical services may result in higher costs for the services of the physician and the hospital caused by e.g., inappropriate prescription.

[2] McKean, 'Property Rights', p. 52.

Summary Record of Discussion

Of the three papers allocated to this session, those of Mr Cooper and of Messrs Culyer and Cullis were considered together as being concerned with problems arising in the British National Health Service (N.H.S.) system. The third paper, by Professor Liefmann-Keil, was concerned with the regulation of drugs and was considered separately.

A. *Mr Cooper's and Messrs Culyer and Cullis's papers*
Professor Atkinson introduced the Cooper paper on 'The Economics of Need' by pointing out that the subject transcends Britain and covers any free system. The resources available for health care are less than the 'needs' assumed by the medical profession or the patients themselves. There is a need for rationing, formal or informal. In the British system, the physicians are the main micro-level decision-makers, under the rubric of 'clinical freedom', but leave to others responsibility for the decentralized allocation of resources at the macro-level. Mr Cooper would like to see some restrictions on clinical freedom and somewhat more hierarchical control at the center.

This analysis needs further development, Professor Atkinson stated, on three lines:

1. How *do* doctors behave? Mr Cooper believes they apply, in each case, an absolute concept of 'correct' treatment, completely without external controls. There are, however, constraints which Mr Cooper underestimates, some imposed by central authorities and others by patient expectations. (An example of the latter is surgery to extend the patient's life-span in terminal cases.)
2. Mr. Cooper is looking at a quite general planning problem, the division of authority between the center and local managers. By going as far as he does in the direction of centralization, Mr Cooper may be inconsistent with experience elsewhere in other branches of planning. As an alternative, Professor Atkinson suggested that in theory there are a wide range of institutional alternatives, including pricing – market-price incentives to doctors to locate in undesirable areas, shadow-prices put on expensive types of treatment, etc.
3. The paper does not discuss the redistributive effect of the N.H.S. by income classes. Variations in treatment generate horizontal inequalities, as Mr Cooper shows, between areas of Britain, but perhaps these also reflect vertical inequalities between income classes, with working-class areas like Sheffield getting shorter shrift than middle-class ones like Oxford. Professor Atkinson referred to Hart's 'inverse care law', by which availability of care was inverse to need, and wished Mr Cooper's suggestions had included specific offsets to this tendency.

In contrast with Mr Cooper's focus on a grand and universal issue, *Professor Evans* said that the Culyer – Cullis paper focused on a specifically British problem, the special hospital-bed reservation privileges of physicians in their private practices, and their effects on the waiting lists for beds in general. Yet, in a way, the problem is more general: namely, the role of private markets in a generally public system. The arguments against the retention of private-sector enclaves are partially ideological, but also involve costs to the public sector in the form of delayed access and sometimes also of concealed subsidy of the private practitioner. The Culyer–Cullis waiting list problem involves the first, namely access cost; it is also alleged that the public system may be subsidizing private hospital patients.

However, the paper presents no alternatives to the present British practice. The private enclave is only about 2 per cent of the total hospital throughput. If, when this enclave is abolished, the private patients would emigrate, die or evaporate, there would be a gain to the public patients. On the other hand, if the private patients would join the public system and act like other public patients, the problems might well get worse. After all, the concept of 'waiting list' is not easy to define. Only 85 per cent of hospital beds are occupied at any given time, suggesting that the constraint on admissions lies elsewhere. Moreover, more than half of all hospital patients are discharged within two weeks, so that average waiting periods may not be long. Furthermore, when the waiting period is long, the responsible factor may be the personal preferences of patients and physicians for particular hospitals or surgeons. The waiting lists may even be maintained artificially by some physicians to encourage the use of private beds and, if so, they are not measures of scarcity at all. If private practice is restricted or abolished. the main result might be increased physician emigration to North America.

Professor Evans suggested a more formal model of physical behavior in terms of such factors as income, leisure and waiting lists. On the issue of subsidy, he would also like to see distinctions made between the average and marginal cost to the N.H.S. of maintaining private beds.

Mr Cooper expressed some measure of diagreement with Professor Atkinson's interpretation of his paper, which he had intended primarily as a plea for research. We know little, he said, about either the demand or the supply sides. Clinical freedom is, he agreed, less than absolute, but the restraints are almost entirely implicit and we do not know their starting-points. Expectations of treatment and waiting are, he agreed, bound up with class background, persistence, and personal relations of patient and physician, but we do not know the importance of this factor.

Help to terminal patients? Certainly, psychological aid is justified on humanitarian grounds, but surgical aid is another matter. Line management may be necessary for the system as a whole, although it may be out of place in an individual hospital.

There may also be a logical pattern to the inequalities of patient treatment, Mr Cooper agreed, but what should be done about them? Should the 'good' areas be brought down to the average, or the 'poor' ones brought up to it? It is unfortunate that economists must still fight what Mr Cooper called 'the battle of the need to ration', against the doctors and administrators of the N.H.S. These folk have maintained that resources should be increased indefinitely to eliminate any need to ration N.H.S. services. This view, according to Mr Cooper, underlies whatever is wrong with the N.H.S.

In Mr Cullis's absence, *Mr Culyer* spoke to the Evans criticisms. Where would private patients go if private beds were eliminated? Mainly to the private hospitals, which Professor Evans did not consider, and so elimination of private practice would probably reduce waiting time in the public system. Do physicians use waiting lists to encourage their own private practices and 'queue-jumping'? Patients think so; doctors deny it; nothing is really known.

A formal model of physician behavior? Messrs Culyer and Cullis had tested several econometric models of the system but, with waiting lists as the dependent variable, had found little evidence that excess demand (lists) and supply of hospital resources were negatively related. Mr Culyer, a non-econometrician, was skeptical of formal models of physician behavior – the data were so limited. He thought it more important for priorities to be set centrally with a maximum waiting time imposed. At the moment, behavior was as hard to explain as it was diverse in similar objective circumstances.

Professor Robinson, chairman of this session, suggested that comments from the floor be concerned initially with the related subjects of centralization versus decentralization, and with the role of clinical freedom. *Professor L. Lave* opened the general discussion by pointing out the relations between micro-incentives and macro-behavior. Clinical freedom for physicians and the absence of price rationing for patients make the N.H.S. act as it does, and it is almost impossible to impose from above a macro-system contradicting that system's own micro-incentives.

In reply, *Professor Perlman* pointed to the great variety of rationing systems not involving price. Doctors ration patients by time (waiting) or by expertise (the most popular physician seeing only the most desirable patients). It is also quite possible that clinical freedom may involve exploitation of the patient.

Mr Kaser maintained that clinical freedom has great value in itself, but that it should operate in a regime where resource limitations are stated explicitly, and where there is some evaluation after the fact.

Dr Phelps pointed out that where time is economically valuable, waiting is itself a form of price discrimination, insofar as the rich man's time is more valuable than the poor man's. This is why, in a public system, one would expect 'queue-jumping by income', with the rich patronizing the private enclave.

Professor L. Lave re-entered the discussion with a fragmentary model rationalizing both American and British physician behavior. In each system, the physician is to do his best to cure those patients whom he decides to see, but no others. Each system, therefore, works like a lottery, with probabilities often less than 1 of being seen at all. The alternative, according to Lave, would be to spread some given level of care equally among all patients; both physicians and patients oppose anything of this sort.

Dr Kleiman asserted that, whereas in market systems of health care the income distribution dominates the health services, the preferences of physicians dominate most public systems. He cited a British 'scandal' at Neasden, where rules were formalized and posted, including a refusal of resuscitation equipment to cardiac patients above a certain age, and the tumult caused when the facts were known.

Mr Pole interposed a factual comment on the British scene. He claimed that most private medicine and, particularly, private hospitals are maintained by firms for the saving of their executives' valuable time, and not by the executives themselves, as per the Phelps view of the world.

Dr Davis was surprised at the lack of consideration given to price-system alternatives in the Cooper paper. She also felt that such rationing can be combined quite easily with other sorts. She wondered whether differentials in the *length* of hospital care in Britain could be explained on grounds related to patients' income .She doubted that the rich man's time is more valuable economically than the poor man's, inasmuch as the rich tend to have more sick leave at full pay.

Professor Robinson suggested that the most important element of waiting time is not waiting for hospital admission, but delaying, voluntarily, one's first approach to a doctor. This is especially true, at least in Britain, for rural patients. There are also miscellaneous personal factors operating; for example, some people appear to enjoy visiting the doctor . . . Then resuming his chairman's role, Robinson suggested concentration upon the redistributive effects, if any, of the N.H.S.

Mr Culyer proposed that redistribution be considered in terms of the marginal utility of income, not of income itself. A given waiting time, if associated with the same income loss, is harder for a poor man to bear than for a richer one – if you believe in these interpersonal comparisons.

Dr Davis and *Mr Culyer* then engaged in factual colloquy. Dr Davis inquired whether the charges to private patients in public hospitals were on a *per diem* basis. On receiving an affirmative answer, she said that, in the United States, short stays mean higher cost per day. Does this factor add to the subsidy in Britain? Mr Culyer believed not. Rather, the size of the subsidy of the private beds by the N.H.S. depends mainly upon the case-load mix. Since the subsidy was on the capital side, it was lower *per patient* the shorter the stay.

Professor Rosett suggested that the charge on the private 'queue-jumper' in the public hospital be related to the costs his behavior imposes on other patients, rather than to the costs imposed upon the hospital itself.

Professor Robinson pointed out that such patients also pay higher taxes.

Professor L. Lave, drawing on technical economics, felt that Professor Rosett was 100 per cent right if the supply function for hospital beds was vertical, but 100 per cent wrong if it was horizontal. He also suggested another possibility, namely that the British government has reduced its N.H.S. contribution as private funds have come in a s payment for, e.g., private hospital beds.

Mr Cooper, dealing with the Culyer-Cullis paper rather than his own, felt that the 'queue-jumping' problem is overstressed in British discussions, and for ideological reasons. He felt that such patient activity added to the country's total supply of medical services. It diverted physicians, he said, not from public N.H.S. patients but from the golf course. *Mr Culyer* agreed that the effects of private practice on waiting lists are probably small in either direction. He added that, if Britain decides to eliminate it nevertheless, a Pandora's box of new problems will result.

Professor Evans repeated his previous argument about waiting lists being short, the turnover of hospital beds rapid and individual cases of long waits being due to shortage of other resources. This led to some disagreement between *Professors Robinson* and *J. Lave* as to whether physicians' decisions as to the length of patients' hospital stay varied with the length of the waiting list in the hospital concerned. (Professor Robinson felt that it did, while Professor J. Lave cited a study by Professor Feldstein to show that it did not.) Under all circumstances, it appears that British physicians are concerned primarily with patients already admitted to hospitals, and keep them hospitalized longer than in private systems. She cited normal childbirth as an example. *Professor Liefmann-Keil* added that experience in Germany pointed to cost considerations, including social insurance schemes paying daily lump sums, and physicians' preferences as biasing them in favour of over-long stays. Public patients, for example tend to remain longer for general observation.

Dr Hartwell noted that, in the recent slowdown and partial strike of non-medical hospital employees in Britain, queues did not lengthen and the quality of service did not decline. These results were contrary to expectation.

Professor Intriligator expressed an interest in other factors than waiting time as determining the quality of care, and asked whether no other distinctions were made in Britain as between private and public patients. *Mr Culyer* replied that private patients get more 'hotel' facilities, more consulting time, more nursing care and also more *choice* of admission time. *Mr Cooper* added that a 'perk' for executives in the private system is a freer choice of consultant. This enables one to avoid registrars, junior people and the 'wrong' schools of psychiatry.

Professor J. Lave harking back to the Hartwell comment, recalled that, in both Britain and Canada, mortality rates improved as doctors went off to war. She wondered how one decides between, say improved housing and more medical care as aids to the poor or to anyone else. In her own view, it is no favor to operate on terminal cases, as well as being a waste of resources. More important may be information. Also, in the Neasden case referred to by Dr Kleiman, it may be better for the elderly patient himself *not* to be resuscitated after a heart attack. The euthanasia issue should not be overlooked completely.

B. *Professor Liefmann-Keil's paper*

Mr Jinushi introduced and discussed this paper. The drug industry is peculiar, according to Professor Liefmann-Keil, in that goods are produced by A (drug industry) for B (the consumer) on the basis of prescriptions by C (the physician) and usually paid for largely by D (a public agency). Professor Liefmann-Keil believes that a multitude of legal restrictions upon A to assist B primarily benefit C instead. She refers particularly to the requirement that prescriptions be obtained before drugs can be purchased, and claims that such restrictions generate 'unwanted externalities' for consumers. Granted that consumers are presently ignorant of such matters as dosages, dangers and side-effects, Professor Liefmann-Keil prefers consumer sovereignty in this market as in others, because of the danger (connected with differentials in information) that the uninformed may be axploited by the informed. She would like to see the present restrictions supplemented and/or replaced by independent and effective information for the consumer as well as for the physician.

Dr Jinushi himself, disagreed quite sharply. In his view, consumer sovereignty does not work in the drug and medical industries, and social sovereignty is much to be preferred. It is unreasonable to expect consumers to be given adequate information in pharmacological matters. Consumer education would be prohibitively expensive, to say the least, as a matter of social cost; at best, it can only supplement a set of legal restrictions.

The side-effect problem is due to imperfections of the prescription system rather than to the lack of consumer sovereignty. The real desideratum (in Japan) is the removal of physicians' incentives to overprescribe. Rather than moving towards consumer sovereignty, more restrictions should be put upon B, and fewer drugs made available without prescription.

Mr Jinushi also wished that the paper had said more about the structure and functioning of the drug industry. In his view, more social sovereignty is required here too, in the form of price and/or quality control, not to mention restraints upon monopolistic tendencies.

Opening discussion from the floor, *Professor Rosett* pointed out that the medical profession does not benefit from a *drug* but from a *prescription* monopoly, and referred to scandals in the American system as a result of doctor – pharmacist collusion, with doctors owning interests in pharmacies or even in drug-manufacturing firms.

Professors Perlman and *Evans* disagreed as to the educational services of the drug companies to the medical profession. Professor Perlman gave the industry credit for educating physicians rapidly in both the positive and the negative effects of its products, as well as for introducing new products rapidly and re-educating physicians accordingly. Professor Evans, on the other hand, maintained that the quality of this 'education' is genuinely bad, and referred to studies showing inverse correlation between the quality of prescriptions by physicians and the attention these physicians paid to drug company salesmen or 'detail men'. He felt that the system is to send physicians too much information rather than too little. Diminishing or negative returns set in, channels are effectively blocked, and provision of information is left to the detail man.

Dr. Christiansen discussed conditions in Denmark, and gave the industry credit for providing the bulk of the research on new drugs. In Denmark, he said, 80 per cent of the population pay little or nothing for prescriptions. Far too many sleeping pills, tranquillizers, etc., are consumed. He suggested discriminatory fees for such types of medication.

Mr Cooper supplied institutional information for Briatin. There, he said, the moral responsibility for drug abuse is on physicians rather than on the drug industry. Doctors respond to advertisements, not to medical journals. This may be because medical education, aimed at producing specialists rather than general practitioners, places too little stress upon pharmacology. At the same time, the British physician does not benefit from prescriptions, contrary to the situation in many other countries, except when a prescription permits him to break off a consultation without offending a patient. In Britain, also, clinical testing is more severe for N.H.S. drugs than for such remedies as 'bed rest'. There is, in fact, a double standard here, and the British trade-off between progress and risk is such that, had aspirin been invented fifty years later than it was, it could not have passed the N.H.S. screening procedures.

Professors Moriguchi and *Emi* commented upon the situation in Japan. There is a double-price system, according to Professor Moriguchi, with the doctor charging the patient half the price and the remainder being paid by the insurance system. Doctors overdose, and patients discard freely. The rising trend of drugs in total medical expenditure has already been stressed in Dr Kawakami's paper. Professor Emi said that 80 per cent of drugs are dispensed through doctors who sell drugs themselves, and that study of the Japanese drug market should include both professions. Such study should include problems of eligibility to enter, quality of products and content of advertising. Professor Moriguchi added that there was an urgent problem of consumer protection in Japan, since 'health drug' preparations, like hormones and vitamins, are advertised and sold freely, without prescriptions or testing. As a secondary point, the pharmaceutical industry subsidizes university-related research scientists and their conferences.

Professor Liefmann-Keil then entered into the discussion actively. The main source of abuse, in Japan as elsewhere, she found in the medical profession. (She has not been concerned with over-the-counter drugs. – The industry, she felt, is profiting indirectly from the medical monopoly. The problem remains one of information supply, where there is no alternative to the drug companies as information sources for medical men.)

Professor Fuchs made two points relative to the United States. There is, in America, a neutral newsletter concerning drugs, which, although cheap, is not popular among physicians. The problem, in his view, is primarily one of incentives and not of information. In the Seattle Group Health co-operative, for example, prescription costs were included in patients' fees, instead of being charged separately. This removed physicians' incentives to over-prescribe, and prescription costs fell.

Professor J. Lave added a sceptical note on the information available even in scholarly journals. In the thalidomide case, she recalled, propaganda by drug company representatives was published under respected 'neutral' names in reputable journals, and she did not know how many similar abuses occurred.

Professor Robinson, as chairman, closed the discussion, except for summaries by authors of the papers. He also raised the question of how the supposed 'drug monopoly' works, and what the basis may be of whatever monopoly power it possesses. He noted that the problem of drug abuse is common to many varieties of medical system, and wondered what might be done by pressure for generic rather than brand-name prescriptions.

Mr Cooper said that his paper had had two objects: to inspire more research on how doctors and patients behave, and also on how resources (including medical expertise) are allocated by the N.H.S. He felt that economists should worry more about 'need' than they do, not shrugging it off as meaningless or leaving it to other disciplines. On management, he repeated, doctors want to have their cake (control) and eat it too (freedom from responsibility). All sorts of rationing go on – time on kidney machines and in operating rooms. The Neasden resuscitation case is unusual only in its dramatic aspects. The N.H.S. does not yet correct in any systematic way for inequalities in income, location, persistence or relationships with doctors.

Mr Cooper then answered, specifically, the various intimations from the floor that the N.H.S. should rely more fully on market mechanisms. The only alternative he saw was private insurance, which, he said, has all the problems of the N.H.S., plus others related to the loss of the monopoly power which the N.H.S. can exercise over cost. The health insurance company is really a doctor's surrogate. While ability to pay has some role, it should not depend on wealth *at the time of illness*, as it does in a private system.

Turning briefly to private practice in Britain, Mr Cooper said that its main benefit was freer choice of consultant. As evidence, he claimed that the waiting list *for preferred consultants* is longer in private hospitals than in the N.H.S. itself.

Mr Culyer began his own summary by stressing the arbitrariness of decisions in the hospital area, even those involving the valuation of human life. In connection with British road programs, life is evaluated by the transport authorities at £17,000 per head for investment decisions.

Like Mr Cooper, Mr Culyer objected to more reliance on market prices, insisting that the N.H.S. system can plausibly be argued to be Pareto-preferred to the market system by the consuming public.

Mr Culyer agreed that waiting lists could be reduced by improved management, but what are the parameters of administrative and physician choice here? Some hospitals manage lists more efficiently than others, but we are not sure how to set about improving the performance of the laggards. He thought, in view of the difficulty of explaining the variation in waiting list length from hospital to hospital, that an alternative (not mutually exclusive) research approach might be appropriate, namely devising a uniform priority system for assigning patients to lists.

Professor Liefmann-Keil repeated that her main interest had been the monopoly of the medical profession, exercised through the prescription mechanism. She would prefer a system in which doctors have interest only in curing patients, and can disinterestedly supplement information available to consumers and physicians from other sources. She would like to see the medical profession unrelated to the drug industry. As for the government role, she would prefer it limited to quality control and regulations, giving incentives to lessen the different abuses by B and C, as above.

Under the present system, doctors have imperfect information as well as economic interests in prescribing drugs. The doctors are related too closely to the drug industry, which seeks to strengthen the dependence on it by those physicians. Governments have introduced a number of reforms which operate mainly to increase the doctor's incentive to exploit the patient.

Professor Liefmann-Keil disputed Mr Jinushi's claim that the doctor knows best, and pointed out that public agencies may have their own self-interests and make mistakes too, even in a regime of 'social sovereignty'. In her view, the solution is to give consumers more adequate information and more responsibility for their own decisions – in other words, another kind of 'division of labor' in the pharmaceutical market.

9 Price and Income Elasticities for Medical Care Services[1, 2]

Joseph P. Newhouse and Charles E. Phelps

(*with the assistance of David J. Weinschrott
and Mark S. Thompson*)

RAND CORPORATION, SANTA MONICA, CALIF.

*This paper develops a framework for estimating demand for
medical care, expanding Grossman's 'investment model' in
three significant ways: multiple medical inputs are allowed in
production of health, reimbursement insurance is introduced
(altering the net price of care) and choice of different
'styles' of care is allowed.*

*Demand curves are estimated from 1963 United States
household survey data, with the analysis limited to those with
positive observed quantities of service. Use of explicit parameters from insurance policies to defined net price is a unique
empirical aspect of the paper. Price elasticities of demand for
hospital, physician office and hospital outpatient services are
found to be small, all lying below 0·2 in absolute value. Wage
income elasticities are positive and non-wage income is found
to have no effect on demand, both as hypothesized by the
model. Insurance coverage is also shown to influence price of
services used, as does wage income and the quantity of
services demanded.*

I. THEORY

In this paper we estimate price and income elasticities for medical
care services. Our effort is guided by an underlying theory which is
a generalization of Michael Grossman's work (1972). Grossman

---

[1] This is a revised version of the paper given at the Tokyo Conference. Care
has been exercised to retain the trenchancy of the commentators' views.

[2] We should particularly like to thank Ronald Andersen of the Center for
Health Administration Studies at the University of Chicago. Without him this
paper would truly have never come into being, since he graciously made the
data from the 1963 Center for Health Administration Studies' survey available
to us. David Weinschrott provided us with most of our computational assistance
and spent a great deal of effort to ensure the accuracy of our insurance policy
parameters. Mark Thompson gave us assistance in a preliminary draft of this
paper which used data from families. We should also like to thank Michael

postulates two models, the 'investment model' and the 'consumption model'. He prefers the former because: (1) It generates the strong prediction that non-work-related income has no effect on demand. (2) There is an unambiguous positive sign on the effect of wage income. In the consumption model, if medical care is sufficiently time-intensive, the sign of wage income may be negative. (3) The investment model leads to a simpler prediction on the effect of education.[1] Grossman finds empirical support for the investment model, most notably that non-wage income does not appear to be related to the stock of health.

We generalize Grossman's investment model in three significant ways: (1) We drop the assumption that medical care goods are a homogeneous commodity. Since medical care services have neither fixed relative prices nor are they consumed in fixed proportions, they do not satisfy the conditions required of a composite commodity. Consequently, we introduce specific medical services, such as hospital days, for which we estimate demand equations. Separate demand equations are also helpful in understanding where excess demand is likely to arise if there is an exogenous reduction in the price of medical care services, as, for example, might occur if a public health insurance program were enacted or modified. (2) We explicitly introduce health insurance into the analysis, so that the prices facing the consumer are net of insurance. We allow for the possibility that individual insurance is endogenous, that is, affected by *expected* medical care consumption. In doing so, we build on Phelps's (1973) theory of demand for insurance. To treat insurance as exogenous could result in overestimating the price elasticity.[2] (3) We explicitly take account of 'style' phenomena, for example, differences in amenities among various providers.

Under certain assumptions (most notably that investment in health and other commodities is produced by linear and homogeneous

---

Grossman, Bridger Mitchell and Richard Rosett for general advice and counsel, but we assume responsibility for any errors.

This investigation was supported by the United States Public Health Service Grant No. HS00840 from the National Center for Health Services Research and Development. The views expressed herein do not represent the views of the National Center for Health Services Research and Development.

[1] The investment model also predicts a difference between the effect of a change in wage and a change in the amount of time necessary to consume medical services on the consumption of those services. In the consumption model, these effects are identical in elasticity form (see Acton, 1973).

[2] This is always true if premiums are divorced from *individual* expected health status (and set on the basis of population characteristics). We assume this to be the case. The same result holds under many circumstances if insurance is priced by individuals' characteristics (see Phelps, 1973).

production functions), it can be shown (Newhouse and Phelps, 1973) that $\eta_{i p_j}$, the price elasticity of the ith medical service with respect to the jth service's price, equals:

$$\eta_{i p_j} = k_j(\sigma_{ij} - \eta), \tag{1}$$

where k_j is the budget share of the jth service in gross investment between the ith service in gross investment $(p_j M_j/I)$, σ_{ij} is the Allen partial elasticity of substitution between the ith and jth input (Allen, 1938, pp. 502–9), and η is the elasticity of the marginal efficiency of health capital schedule, which is positive (Grossman, 1972). If i and j are substitutes, σ_{ij} is positive, if they are compliments, negative, and σ_{ij} is always negative if $i=j$. The effect of a change in time or goods required to produce medical care due to technological change is analogous to a change in price.

The effect of a change in the wage rate (of price of time) is more complicated. Grossman derives the result for the two-factor case that:

$$\eta_{i w} = (1 - K)\eta + K\sigma, \tag{2}$$

where σ is the elasticity of substitution between goods and time in a two-factor gross investment production function and K is the budget share of time in gross investment.

This result can be generalized to the many-factor case by using the result from Allen stated in (1). A change in the wage rate changes a subset of factor prices and also the product of price, since the value of the time saved per unit is w (Newhouse and Phelps, 1973). A change in the product price in a perfectly competitive market with linear and homogeneous production functions changes the demand for each factor by η, the price elasticity of demand for the product. (This is the source of the η term in (2).) Since each time input has the wage rate as a price, and since the wage rate changes equally for each price, we can simply sum the right-hand side of (1) over all time inputs and add the η term just derived to reach:

$$\eta_{i w} = (\sum_j K_j \sigma_{M_i T M_j}) + (1 - \sum_j K_j)\eta \tag{3}$$

where K_j is the budget share of the jth time input in gross investment and $\sigma_{M_i T M_j}$ are Allen partial elasticities of substitution between the ith good and the jth time input.

A number of implications follow. Since σ_{ii} is negative and η is positive, own-price elasticity is always negative. Second, cross-partial elasticities of substitution are equal, $\sigma_{ij} = \sigma_{ji}$. This restriction, imposed by the theory, can be taken account of. Third, the sum of σ_{ij}, weighted by budget shares, equals zero. Since our data do not give TM_i, we cannot compute all budget shares. Hence, we cannot take account of this restriction, and η is underidentified. There is also the restriction that η is identical across services, and greater than zero; we account for this only indirectly, in requiring the own-price elasticity be negative.

For policy purposes we are interested in any possible interactions between price elasticity and income. (One should distinguish between wage and non-wage income: Newhouse and Phelps, 1973.) We test for such interactions. Other price elasticity interactions are also of interest, especially the interaction with health status and/or size of loss. This would show whether 'quite sick' individuals responded to price differently from individuals who were not 'seriously ill'. This interaction is beyond the scope of this paper. We have also not explored how price elasticity changes through the range of price. We anticipate examining these hypotheses in subsequent work.

Another major generalization of Grossman's model is the introduction of insurance parameters. We have reduced each insurance policy to three parameters: a deductible, a coinsurance rate and a limit. Between the deductible and the limit, the marginal price equals the coinsurance rate times the gross price; otherwise it equals the gross price. We shall focus on the effect of a change in the *marginal* price (net of insurance).[1] This is consistent with the theory, which focuses on marginal changes. This treatment ignores any phenomena which result from the non-convexity of the price line, due, for example, to deductibles. As we develop in another paper, such non-convexity implies that the entire schedule of prices is relevant to the decision of how many medical care services to purchase (Phelps and Newhouse, forthcoming). The effect of ignoring it is to bias our estimated elasticities toward zero. For simplicity, we assume here that the bias introduced by dealing only with the marginal price is small, although we have no evidence that this is so. In one case where this approximation is known not to hold, the choice of hospital when the policy pays up to a fixed price per day, we modify our specification.

Inclusion of a number of other variables follows from Grossman's model. Grossman hypothesizes that the depreciation rate on an individual's health stock increases with age after some point. This increases gross investment, if η is less than 1, which he estimates it to be. We enter age in dummy variable form to allow for non-linear depreciation rates by age, and we expect consumption of medical services to rise with age.

Following Michael (1972), Grossman postulates that education is

---

[1] The asymmetry between a change in the coinsurance rate and a change in the gross price is empirically too small to attempt to measure (see Phelps and Newhouse, 1973).

An exception is made for demand for hospital admissions, which has an all-or-nothing character about it.

an environmental variable which enters household production functions. Specifically, the more educated are assumed to be more efficient producers of commodities and of gross investment in health. This will serve to increase their demand for health stock; however, if η is less than 1, demand for medical services will fall with education (in the investment model). Grossman does not find empirical support for this proposition, the one instance of a 'wrong' sign in his empirical results, but he has not controlled for variation in price which individuals in his sample face. Since we shall be working with the same data base as Grossman, but controlling for price, we can attempt to determine whether the positive sign Grossman finds on education is due to the more educated having more complete health insurance in this sample. We therefore enter education and expect to find a negative sign.

The investment model predicts that non-wage income will have no effect on the amount of health stock demanded or medical goods purchased. Grossman estimates that the effect of non-wage income on the demand for health stock is not significantly different from zero.[1] If non-wage income exerts no effect, one of the two possible reasons for including family size as an explanatory variable is eliminated, namely that family size measures the family's control over real resources. Another reason for including family size is that health stock and child services are complements in a utility function; however, Grossman does not find significant family size effects on the purchase of medical services. We therefore do not expect to find a significant effect of family size on individuals' quantity of services consumed.

Grossman shows that under weak assumptions, purchase of medical services rises with health stock loss.[2] His model does not treat health stock loss as stochastic, but to do so will lead to the same conclusion (Phelps, 1973). Thus, precision is improved if such loss is well measured, and we include variables which should be associated with health stock loss. We expect health stock loss to be positively related to the consumption.

Finally, Grossman does not consider the supply of services in a local market area. Implicitly, in his model there is no variation in market supply opportunities faced by individuals, either because all individuals are in the same market or all markets are identical. But

---

[1] Note that, to the extent health stock loss is random, assets or non-wage income will not be determined simultaneously with health stock and expenditures on medical services. Hence, non-wage income can be treated as exogenous. Even if an individual planned his asset accumulation and medical care expenditure simultaneously, the operational implication would be to control for age, which we do.

[2] Grossman (1972) appendix B.

markets are local and the supply of services across local market areas varies markedly. It is unreasonable to suppose that the degree of excess demand does not also vary as a result. This could be because of disequilibrium, due to a differential mobility between consumers and factors of production. It could also be an equilibrium situation, if consumers and labor factors of production have different locational preferences. Regardless, variation in excess demand may lead to certain kinds of non-price rationing.[1] For example, there may be substantial waits for an appointment with a physician or for elective procedures at hospitals if excess demand is high. If the self-limiting nature of much illness outweighs a tendency to progressive deterioration individual utilization will fall as excess demand rises. Similarly, physicians may use various other types of non-price rationing devices, such as varying the revisit rate or the case-mix seen if excess demand is high. Thus, it is desirable to include measures of the supply of services, for which we use the physician/population ratio and the bed/population ratio. Although these measure supply of services imperfectly, we have no better measures readily available. We expect the physician/population ratio to be positively related to office visits, and the bed/population ratio to be positively related to hospital length of stay. These 'cross-non-price effects' cannot be signed *a priori*. Note that these variables can be assumed to be exogenous to the individual, thus avoiding the identification problem plaguing most studies using areal data.

II. STYLE PHENOMENA AND PRICE VARIATION

In the American medical system, there are numerous independent providers, often charging nominally different prices. This means that analysis of expenditures will lead to different results from analysis of physical quantities, and raises the question of which variable is appropriate.

There are at least four possible aspects of price variation. Higher prices could simply reflect higher quality (differences in marginal productivity). If so, one should analyze expenditures rather than physical quantities, since expenditures measure quantity in efficiency units.

Higher prices could represent various kinds of product differentiation. One type is less queueing. In this case, one would expect substitution of higher-priced for lower-priced medical services by those with a high opportunity cost for time. If the entire difference in prices among providers is attributable to queue differences, one

---

[1] Thus, we allow for the possibility of non-price as well as price rationing. Why non-price rationing should exist in addition to price rationing is an issue we do not consider.

should analyze utilization of services separately from choice of provider. Choice of provider would be determined by the price of time and the price of using that provider (which could vary across individuals because of differences in insurance coverage), while utilization of services (in physical units) would be determined by all the factors heretofore analyzed.

Third, some of the price variation could reflect other kinds of product differentiation, such as better food in a hospital or more tasteful office decoration. Such amenities are produced jointly with investment in medical services and can be treated analytically as any consumption commodity. Like reduced queueing time, this implies a separate choice-of-provider equation. It also implies that work-related income, non-work-related income and possibly family size should affect the price of the provider selected. The distinction with queueing time is that non-work-related income is relevant in this case. If price differentials are solely due to amenity differences, utilization may be measured in physical units.

Finally, some of the price differential may be due to differences in search costs. We would expect individuals with higher values per unit of time to engage in less search and hence use more expensive providers, although this effect is blurred if other members of the family with lower prices of time perform the search function. We would also expect those individuals with more generous insurance to search less, since the return from search is less for them. The effect and conclusions are similar to price variation attributable to varying queue length.

This analysis suggests that we disaggregate utilization of medical services into three components: (1) the pure quantity of services; (2) the usual source of care, measured by an average price index for that source across the entire sample; (3) the price paid, given the usual source of care.[1] If price differences do not reflect differences in productivity, the first dimension should be measured in physical units. If price differences do reflect differences in productivity, the situation is more complicated. Since variation in price could reflect the other factors outlined above, the theory does not apply to consumption measured in physical units and applies in only a partial way to consumption measured by expenditures.

We adopt a middle course; we assume that different sources of physician care (specialists, general practitioners) have different productivities and so multiply visits by the average price of the usual source of care (across the sample) to obtain a utilization variable for the physician equation. Similarly, we assume that different types of

[1] This disaggregation has been suggested to us by Michael Grossman.

hospital care (ward, semi-private) have different productivities, reflected by their average prices across the sample. Hence, the dependent variable in the hospital length-of-stay equation is length of stay multiplied by average price for that type of care.

Price differences among similar usual sources of care are assumed *not* to reflect differences in productivity. This assumption derives by considering the extent of consumer knowledge about productivity; the aspect of productivity which the consumer can readily judge is the credential possessed by his usual source of care, so that price variation among similar usual sources is assumed to be uncorrelated with marginal productivity, and instead to reflect the second, third and/or fourth factors. We have not yet tested the sensitivity of our results to these assumptions.

There remains the problem of specifying an equation to explain price, given the usual source of care. We measure this price deviation by a difference rather than a ratio, since returns from further search are measured in absolute, not relative, terms. For reasons just outlined, we expect individuals with a high price of time and a low money price (net of insurance) to use providers with a high gross price.

Non-wage income permits us to distinguish the third reason for price variation from the second and fourth. If amenities are the sole cause of price variation, non-wage and wage income should have the same coefficient in the price-of-provider equation. If price is higher solely because of less queueing or because individuals with a higher price of time search less, then wage income should be positively associated with price, but non-wage income should not be associated with price. Family size is entered and we expect a negative sign, because larger families have fewer resources per person, and lower information costs within the family permit more efficient search.

Individuals who anticipate using many services will have an incentive to search for cheaper providers. We enter actual services used (as an endogenous variable) as a measure of anticipated use; we expect a negative relation with the deviation of actual price from the average price of the usual source of care.

We also enter a number of variables to control for possible nominal price variation; these include four regional dummy variables to control for regional differences in medical prices and the physician/population ratio of this area, which previous work has found positively related to price in an area (Newhouse, 1970).

If education improves efficiency of searching for medical services differentially from other non-market activities, education should also be entered as a control variable. If, for example, education raises medical care search efficiency by less than an average amount, we would expect a positive sign on the education variable.

III. PROBLEMS OF ESTIMATION AND OPERATIONAL SPECIFICATION OF THE MODEL

Because of the endogenity of individual insurance and price, simultaneous equation methods are appropriate. Also, it is particularly important in analyzing hospital utilization to take account of the constraint that consumption cannot be negative. Since most individuals are not hospitalized in a year, the bias introduced by failing to account for this constraint could be substantial.

We view the hospital admission and hospital length-of-stay decision as made sequentially. Therefore, logit methods should be applied to explain hospital admissions. Such an equation is beyond the scope of this study.[1] Nor have we estimated the analogous equation for physician use, although this is much less limiting, since most individuals use physicians. Hence, the results we present are conditional on usage. We have excluded non-participants in the labor force, since we do not now have data which would permit us to estimate a time price for these individuals.[2] The exclusion of non-labor-force participants results in an unknown bias in our elasticity estimates, depending on non-labor-force participants' price of time and any interaction between the price of time and money price elasticity (Phelps and Newhouse, 1973).

To derive our estimates of price and income elasticities, we use the 1963 survey of the Center for Health Administration Studies (C.H.A.S.) at the University of Chicago, which is described in Andersen and Anderson (1967). The advantage of these data is that the detail available is sufficient to calculate the marginal price. As outlined in the previous section, we assume that the marginal coinsurance rate is the relevant rate to a first approximation.

The coinsurance rates were computed from the corresponding coinsurance rates reported in the policy. We first checked to see which policy would apply to the marginal expenditure (in cases in which the family held more than one policy), then to see if a deductible had been exceeded (if it had not, the marginal coinsurance rate was 1·0); if it had, we used the coinsurance rate reported in the policy.[3] We have entered the room and board coinsurance rate times mean

[1] The admission decision has an all-or-nothing character about it; in general, admission to a hospital implies some kind of prolonged stay. Therefore, some kind of expected total cost figure is relevant to this decision. To derive the expected total cost, one must account for the entire price schedule, this being an exception to working with marginal price.

[2] We expect to obtain such data and include these individuals in later work.

[3] A detailed description of these calculations is available from the authors.

expenditure[1] as the cross-price term in the outpatient visit equation, and the M.D. office coinsurance rate times physician office price as the cross-price term in the length-of-stay equation. In equations explaining price of provider selected, only the coinsurance rate applicable to that provider is entered.

The 1963 survey attempted to verify charges for all inpatient utilization, as well as the health insurance policies the individuals held. No verification was received for at least one policy for 788 families, members of which we have excluded. Missing verification tended to be from large firms, which have systematically better insurance than smaller firms (Phelps, 1973), thus biasing upward the mean level of coinsurance held in our (unweighted) sample. We have therefore weighted our sample by income and work group size so that it is representative of the population.[2] This prevents a potential bias away from zero in our elasticities as estimates of the population mean. Additionally, if elasticities fall as coinsurance falls, our estimates are biased away from zero relative to what changes in current insurance might produce, since insurance has generally improved since 1963.

We have excluded individuals who exceed the limits of their insurance policies, because of our imperfect ability to measure health status. For example, if an individual's insurance policy paid only for 30 days of hospitalization, and the severity of his illness meant that he had to remain 60 days, we would observe an individual with a very long stay and a 100 per cent marginal coinsurance rate. It is even possible (we do not know) that if these individuals were included, a positively sloping demand curve would result. The effect of this exclusion is to bias our elasticity estimates away from zero, if there is no interaction between size of loss and elasticity. The reason is that we attribute some of the variation in length of stay and office utilization to price which properly belongs to variation in health status. More severely ill individuals, who will use more services, are more likely to exceed a deductible or move to a range of a policy with a lower coinsurance rate. In so far as our health status measures control for this imperfectly, there is a bias away from zero. Although

---

[1] Mean expenditure in the outpatient visit equation refers to the mean room and board expenditure across the sample. We were forced to use mean expenditure, since most individuals who used outpatient services did not use hospital services; the effect is simply to rescale the room and board coinsurance rate variable.

[2] The sample is weighted according to the national distribution of income and work group size relative to sample proportions.

There is very little evidence on how elasticities change with the coinsurance rate. From evidence presented in Phelps and Newhouse (1973), one can infer that elasticities fall as coinsurance falls in the range of 25 to 10 per cent coinsurance.

we cannot show it (since we cannot measure health status well), we conjecture that this bias is small, and is almost certainly small relative to the downward bias which we would have observed had we not made this exclusion.

We have also excluded all individuals whose wage income exceeded $500 per week, on the grounds that there may have been reporting errors and that if there were not, our functional form was likely to be inappropriate for them.[1] The wage rate is measured per week, since we do not have hours worked per week available to us to compute an hourly rate. In so far as labor supply adjustment takes place in weeks worked rather than hours per week, this is the appropriate variable.[2] Non-wage income also has some extreme values. Because we did not wish to impose a functional form on this variable, we split the value at $3,000 per year, so there are two non-wage income one variables, with a coefficient for those with non-wage incomes greater than $3,000 per year, another with incomes less than $3,000 per year. (An intercept shift is also allowed for.)

Health status is measured in two ways. Respondents were asked whether they would characterize their health status as excellent, good, fair or poor. Their response was entered in dummy variable form. The second measure was the number of self-reported disability days the individual suffered in 1963. These variables measure different phenomena than a clinical examination would, but they are relevant measures.[3]

A table of all included variables, the units in which they are measured, and their expected sign is shown in Table 9.1. The means, standard deviations, minima and maxima of all variables are contained in Newhouse and Phelps (1973).

IV. RESULTS OF ESTIMATION

(1) Hospital Length of Stay

The length-of-stay equations (Table 9.2) show negative own-price elasticities of demand, negative cross-price elasticities with physician price, and positive wage income elasticities. In both the two-stage least squares (T.S.L.S.) and the ordinary least squares (O.L.S.)

---

[1] For computational reasons we have not attempted to exclude transitory components from either our wage or non-wage income measures.

[2] It is appropriate if the average weekly wage equals the marginal weekly wage, which would not be true in seasonal industries.

[3] In part, the difference between these measures and a clinical examination has to do with prognosis; a patient may have terminal cancer but feel well and be unaware of it; he may also feel nauseous with a common cold but be well the next day. In so far as this is the difference, it is the individual's perception of his health status which motivates some utilization.

TABLE 9.1

Explanatory variable	Units	Expected sign, comments
Utilization equations:		
Marginal own price	$	Negative
Marginal cross-price	$	Not signed, depends on sign of σ_{ij}
Wage rate	$/week	Positive
Non-wage income	$/year	Zero
Education	Highest grade completed (dummy variables for intervals)	Negative (if $\eta < 1$)
Age	Years (dummy variables for intervals)	Positive (if depreciation increases with age)
Family size	Individuals	Zero
Sex	1 = female, 0 = male	No prediction
Race	1 = non-white, 0 = white	No prediction
Health status, self-perceived	Dummy variables	Negative
Disability days	Days	Positive
Beds/population	Population in 1,000's	Positive in length-of-stay equation
Physicians/population	Population in 1,000's	Positive in office visits equation
Price equations:		
Own coinsurance rate, if defined	Proportion; 0 if not defined	Negative
Internal dollar limit per day, hospital equation only	$; 0 if not present	Positive
Full semi-private room dummy, hospital equation only	1 if insurance policy is of this type; 0 otherwise	No prediction
Wage income	$/week	Positive
Non-wage income	$/year	Positive if amenities play a role, otherwise zero; elasticity less than wage income
Education	Highest grade completed	No prediction (control for possible non-neutrality of education's effect on non-market productivity)
Family size	Individuals	Negative
Race	1 = non-white, 0 = white	No prediction; non-whites may face different market
Regional dummy variables	—	No prediction; control for regional price variation
Physicians/population	Population in 1,000's	Positive in M.D. price

TABLE 9.2

DEPENDENT VARIABLE = HOSPITAL DAYS;
$n = 122$ (WEIGHTED BY AVERAGE PRICE
OF TYPE OF ROOM)

Explanatory variable coefficient (t-ratio) (Elasticity)	Eq. (1) T.S.L.S. (no interaction)	Eq. (2) O.L.S. (no interaction)
Hospital coinsurance × Price of bed	−0·020 (0·22) $\eta = -0.03$	−0·062 (1·73) $\eta = -0.10$
M.D. office coinsurance × Price	0·125 (0·28) $\eta = 0.05$	−0·241 (1·25) $\eta = -0.10$
Wage income/week	0·011 (1·13) $\eta = 0.11$	0·008 (0·74) $\eta = -0.08$
Non-wage income	−0·876E-03 (1·31) $\eta = -0.05$	−0·001 (1·20) $\eta = -0.07$
Non-wage income if greater than $3,000	0·158E-03 (0·09)	0·990E-03 (0·44)
Dummy = 1 if non-wage income > $3,000	−3·390 (0·39)	−7·863 (0·74)
Education 9–11 years	1·814 (1·44)	1·514 (0·84)
Education 12 years	−0·380 −0·28)	−0·285 (0·14)
Education 13–15 years	−2·149 (0·95)	−3·088 (1·03)
Education 16+ years	0·825 (0·41)	1·029 (0·34)
Age 25–34	2·784 (0·75)	3·760 (0·70)
Age 35–54	6·567 (1·88)	7·051 (1·34)
Age 55–64	9·013 (2·33)	10·296 (1·88)
Age 65+	10·780 (2·76)	12·142 (2·22)
Family size	−0·535 (1·76)	−0·451 (1·03)
Sex (= 1 if female)	0·760 (0·57)	0·593 (0·30)
Race (= 1 if non-white)	0·679 (0·41)	0·743 (0·32)
Disability days	0·026 (4·10) $\eta = 0.18$	0·029 (3·43) $\eta = 0.19$
Health status good	−0·109 (0·08)	−0·256 (0·12)
Health status fair	0·924 (0·56)	0·575 (0·24)
Health status poor	−1·858 (1·06)	−1·667 (0·63)
M.D.s/100,000	−0·024 (2·32) $\eta = -0.30$	−0·022 (1·47) $\eta = -0.28$

TABLE 9.2—*continued*

DEPENDENT VARIABLE = HOSPITAL DAYS; $n = 122$ (WEIGHTED BY AVERAGE PRICE OF TYPE OF ROOM)

Explanatory variable coefficient *(t-ratio)* *(Elasticity)*	*Eq.* (1) T.S.L.S. *(no interaction)*	*Eq.* (2) O.L.S. *(no interaction)*
Beds/1,000	0·358	0·250
	(1·54) $\eta = 0.19$	(0·85) $\eta = 0.13$
Married (=1)		
Constant term	1·644	3·132
	(0·38)	(0·53)
R^2		0·345
Corrected R^2		0·191
Dhrymes F (d.f.)	4·811	
	(23·8)	
t-ratio adjustment factor	0·635	
Asympototic F (d.f.)	1·917	2·243
	(23·98)	(23·98)

TABLE 9.3

DEPENDENT VARIABLE = PHYSICIAN OFFICE VISITS; $n = 842$ (WEIGHTED BY AVERAGE PRICE OF TYPE OF PROVIDER)

Explanatory variable coefficient *(t-ratio* *(Elasticity)*	*Eq.* (5) T.S.L.S. *(no interaction)*	*Eq.* (6) O.L.S. *(no interaction)*
Hospital coinsurance	−0·043	−0·034
× Price of bed	(0·88) $\eta = -0.13$	(2·83) $\eta = -0.10$
M.D. office coinsurance	−0·017	−0·054
× Price	(0·10) $\eta = -0.02$	(2·02) $\eta = -0.06$
Wage income week	0·004	0·004
	(0·97) $\eta = 0.06$	(1·58) $\eta = 0.08$
Non-wage income	−0·70E-04	−0·76E-04
	(0·31) $\eta = -0.01$	(0·28) $\eta = -0.01$
Non-wage income if	0·347E-03	0·357E-03
greater than $3,000	(2·10) $\eta = 0.03$	(1·89) $\eta = 0.03$
Dummy =1 if non-wage	−0·504	−0·552
income > $3,000	(0·46)	(0·44)
Education 9–11 years	0·218	0·267
	(0·46)	(0·53)
Education 12 years	0·147	0·177
	(0·32)	(0·34)
Education 13–15 years	0·294	0·396
	(0·42)	(0·63)
Education 16 + years	−0·849	−0·765
	(1·30)	(1·20)

TABLE 9.3—*continued*

DEPENDENT VARIABLE = PHYSICIAN OFFICE VISITS;
$n = 842$ (WEIGHTED BY AVERAGE PRICE
OF TYPE OF PROVIDER)

Explanatory variable coefficient (t-ratio (Elasticity)	*Eq. (5)* T.S.L.S. *(no interaction)*	*Eq. (6)* O.L.S. *(no interaction)*
Age 25–34	−0·707 (0·86)	−0·722 (0·75)
Age 35–54	−0·844 (1·07)	−0·815 (0·89)
Age 55–64	−0·407 (0·43)	−0·403 (0·41)
Age 65+	−0·878 (1·02)	−0·818 (0·84)
Family size	−0·079 (0·72)	−0·070 (0·59)
Sex (=1 if female	0·377 (0·90)	0·405 (0·87)
Race (=1 if non-white)	1·653 (3·09)	1·616 (2·84)
Disability days	0·007 (2·06) $\eta = 0·02$	0·008 (1·86) $\eta = 0·02$
Health status good	1·663 (4·67)	1·671 (3·99)
Health status fair	3·677 (8·02)	3·683 (6·83)
Health status poor	6·879 (9·55)	6·824 (8·52)
M.D.s/100,000	0·005 (1·04) $\eta = 0·11$	0·006 (1·53) $\eta = 0·13$
Beds/1,000	−0·104 (1·42) $\eta = −0·09$	−0·105 (1·22) $\eta = −0·09$
Married (=1) Constant term	3·983 (2·80)	3·804 (3·28)
R^2		0·181
Corrected R^2		0·158
Dhrymes F (d.f.)	10·224 (23·8)	7·857 (23·818)
t-ratio adjustment factor	0·845	
Asympototic F (d.f.)	7·733 (23·818)	

results the interaction of price with wage income was not significant (*t*-statistics around 0·5). Hence, we present the equations which do not include the interaction terms.

The estimated elasticity using T.S.L.S. is smaller than the O.L.S. estimate and insignificant. The O.L.S. estimated own-price elasticity

TABLE 9.4

PRICE-OF-CARE EQUATIONS

	Hospital room and board (n=122)		Physician office visit (n=854)	
	T.S.L.S.	O.L.S.	T.S.L.S.	O.L.S.
Room and board coinsurance rate	-18.520 (-2.278) η = -0.46	-5.317 (-1.959) η = -0.13		
Number of hospital days	-0.171 (-1.019) η = -0.10	-0.217 (-1.529) η = -0.13		
Maximum payment per hospital day	-0.139 (-0.601)	0.131 (0.876)		
Dummy (=1 if no limit on $/day)	2.093 (0.261)	5.778 (0.873)		
Physician office visit coinsurance			-2.988 (-1.024) η = -0.38	-0.958 (-1.283) η = -0.12
Number of physician office visits			-0.561E-01 (-2.266) η = 0.05	-0.530E-01 (-2.175) η = -0.05
Wage income	-0.030E-01 (-1.332) η = -0.14	-0.109E-01 (-0.644) η = -0.05	0.857E-02 (2.219) η = 0.10	0.973E-02 (2.787) η = 0.11
Non-wage income	0.144E-02 (0.905) η = 0.06	0.162E-02 (1.194) η = 0.07	0.183E-03 (0.557) η = 0.01	0.194E-03 (0.593) η = 0.01
Non-wage income greater than $3,000	0.483E-02 (1.267) η = 0.08	0.538E-02 (1.655) η = 0.09	0.283E-03 (1.172) η = 0.02	0.256E-03 (1.077) η = 0.02
Dummy (=1) if non-wage income > $3,000	-24.040 (-1.344)	-23.492 (-1.536)	-1.190 (-0.710)	-0.771 (-0.493)
Education 9–11 years	3.284 (1.063)	3.604 (1.367)	0.560 (0.880)	0.598 (0.946)

	(1)	(2)	(3)	(4)
Education 16+ years	5·630	5·208	0·846	0·813
	(1·039)	(1·125)	(1·047)	(1·113)
Family size	-0·444	-0·658	-0·250E-01	-0·475E-01
	(-0·661)	(-1·162)	(-0·176)	(-0·345)
North-east	-2·109	-0·279	-1·319	-1·502
	(-0·486)	(-0·775E-01)	(-1·639)	(-1·976)
North-Central	-7·271	-5·819	-0·278	-0·643
	(-1·878)	(-1·798)	(-0·303)	(-0·844)
South	-6·334	-7·136	-0·773	0·458
	(-1·613)	(-2·139)	(-0·857)	(0·583)
Mountain	-3·058	-4·099	1·134	0·888
	(-0·471)	(-0·742)	(0·787)	(0·637)
Physicians/population			0·246E-01	0·241E-01
			(4·505) $\eta = 0·40$	(4·471) $\eta = 0·40$
Constant	16·478	8·250	5·873	4·258
	(2·273)	(1·739)	(2·575)	(1·256)
R^2		0·243		0·075
Corrected R^2		0·120		0·057
Dhrymes F (d.f.)	1·579		2·463	
	(17·20)		(16·23)	
t-ratio adjustment factor	1·056		1·301	
Usual asymptotic F (d.f.)	0·470	1·968	3·748	4·245
	(17,104)	(17,104)	(16,837)	(16,837)

is -0.10 ($t = 1.73$), 95 d.f.[1] The mean coinsurance rate for hospital room and board in our sample is 0.39, with a standard deviation of 0.43. Both estimates of the price elasticity of length of stay are close to estimates for lower coinsurance rates which we have made from other data (Phelps and Newhouse, 1973). The estimated elasticities are substantially smaller than the price elasticity found by Feldstein (1971) or Davis and Russell (1972) using areal data. The cross-price elasticity is estimated to be -0.10 ($t = 1.25$) using O.L.S. and 0.05 ($t = 0.28$) using T.S.L.S. Although the t-statistics are not large, the negative sign using O.L.S. is reinforced by the findings to be reported below for physician office visits. The coefficients on non-wage income are insignificant in accordance with the Grossman model, although the wage income coefficient is also insignificant, contrary to hypothesis.

The supply variables are of marginal significance and their elasticities are of moderate size using both O.L.S. and T.S.L.S. The elasticity with respect to the beds/population ratio is 0.19, using T.S.L.S. The elasticity of length of stay with respect to the physician/population ratio is -0.30, indicating that more physicians in an area reduces length of stay.[2]

Most of our other hypotheses are supported. Education has no systematic effect, which is quite plausible. The efficacy with which hospital days are used to produce a 'cure' (once the patient is admitted) may be much more a function of the physician's skill than the patient's stock of human capital. Age variables show the expected increasing demand with age. Disability days are quite significant. Since use of disability days poses the danger of being tautological in an equation estimating hospital days, we estimated the equation omitting this variable; the results were hardly affected at all.

(2) *Hospital Price*

The divergence between O.L.S. and T.S.L.S. in the estimated effect of the coinsurance rate (Table 9.4) is striking; T.S.L.S. estimates show a much larger effect, implying that adverse selection is not a significant problem. Because we expected the O.L.S. bias to be away from

[1] We report the absolute value of t-statistics, The t-ratios we report in T.S.L.S. are computed by the Dhrymes technique (Dhrymes, 1969). The degrees of freedom in this test are equal to the extent of overidentification in the equation. The conventional statistic, an asymptotically normal variate, can be derived by multiplying the Dhrymes t's by an adjustment factor reported with each equation.

[2] This finding is not inconsistent with a negative cross-price elasticity, as might appear at a first glance. If the cross-price elasticity is negative, we know that σ must be less than η, but σ may still be positive, as this result appears to imply. Alternatively, non-price rationing may work through a different mechanism than price rationing so that the two coefficients would bear no relationship to each other.

zero, we suspect the T.S.L.S. result is an artefact. Hence, we discuss the O.L.S. results. The principal result of interest is the elasticity of room and board price with respect to the coinsurance rate, -0.13 ($t = 1.96$). The coefficient indicates that those with complete coverage chose hospitals which had room and board rates $5.32 above those chosen by individuals with no insurance. While this may appear to be a small difference, the mean room and board rate in 1963 (in our sample) was $15.58. Thus, choice of hospital price (holding constant type of accommodation) is sensitive to the coinsurance rate, as conjectured by Newhouse and Taylor (1970). The other insurance policy parameters do not appear to exert a significant effect.

Of the remaining results, only one is of note. Those who remained in the hospital longer tended to stay in lower-price hospitals as hypothesized (the elasticity is -0.13, $t = 1.53$). Most of our other hypotheses were weakly supported..

Note that we have not estimated an equation with admissions or inpatient ancillary services as a dependent variable, so that our current estimates cannot be used to derive an elasticity for all hospital services.

(3) *Physician Office Visits*
As with the hospital days equation, the interaction terms of price and income were not significant in explaining physician office visits (Table 9.3). Hence, we present the equations omitting the interaction terms. The T.S.L.S. elasticity is again closer to zero than that estimated by O.L.S.; the estimated precision, however, is again considerably better using O.L.S.

The own-price elasticity is estimated to be -0.06 ($t = 2.02$, 819 d.f.) using O.L.S., and 0.02 ($t = 0.10$) using T.S.L.S. These estimates are lower than those found by us in other data (Phelps and Newhouse, 1973), although those estimates pertained to the 25 per cent to zero coinsurance range. The range is quite different here. The mean coinsurance rate is 0.882, suggesting that around 90 per cent of the sample had no effective insurance for outpatient services. The cross-price elasticity estimated by both O.L.S. and T.S.L.S. is negative, thus agreeing with the sign of the cross-price term in the O.L.S. hospital length-of-stay equation. We have not, in this paper, imposed the constraint that $\sigma_{ij} = \sigma_{ji}$.

The estimated wage income elasticity is 0.06 in T.S.L.S. ($t = 0.97$) and 0.08 in O.L.S. ($t = 1.58$), weakly supporting Grossman's hypothesis. Grossman reports a representative income elasticity of 0.7 for total medical *expenditures*, considerably larger than what we find for either physician office visits or hospital days. Our corresponding expenditure elasticity can be found by adding the utilization income elasticities and choice-of-price income elasticities for each service. As discussed further below, we estimate a wage income elasticity of 0·1 for physician office visit price, so that the expenditure elasticity for physician services would be between 0·15 and 0·2. We feel that a major reason for the discrepancy between Grossman's estimate and ours is his omission of insurance, which is known to be a positive function of income (Phelps, 1973).

The physician/population ratio has the hypothesized effect. The elasticity is 0·11 in T.S.L.S. ($t = 1·04$). The bed/population ratio has a negative elasticity of $-0·09$ ($t = 1·42$), consistent with the negative elasticity of the physician/population ratio in the length-of-stay equation. There is thus some weak evidence to support a pattern of non-price rationing of services.

There was no consistent pattern in the age and education variables. Other hypotheses were generally weakly supported.

(4) *Physician Office Visit Price Equation*

These equations differ from the corresponding hospital price equations in that there are typically no 'internal limits' in the policies regarding the price of the physician selected. Hence, the only insurance policy parameter in the equation is the coinsurance rate. Again, the T.S.L.S. estimates are much larger than the O.L.S. estimates, contrary to expectation. Because of this, we focus on the O.L.S. results.

The elasticity of price with respect to the coinsurance rate is $-0·12$ ($t = 1·28$, 837 d.f.). The coefficient suggests that those with complete coverage would select a physician costing $0·96 more per visit than those with no insurance. (The mean price per visit in 1963 was $6·86.) The relatively large standard error may be because our sample is clustered at a coinsurance rate of 1·0; as noted above, around 90 per cent of the sample paid full price for their outpatient visits.

The estimated elasticity of physician price with respect to additional visits is $-0·05$ ($t = 2·18$), confirming the hypothesis that higher returns to search lead to a lower price of care. The magnitude of the elasticity is stronger for hospital price than for office price, consistent with the hypothesis that more intensive search will be carried out for more expensive items. Additionally, we find a wage income elasticity of physician price of 0·11 ($t = 2·79$), whereas the non-wage income elasticity is effectively zero and insignificant. This implies that the higher price paid for physician office visits by income is to avoid queues, and to shorten time spent obtaining services in general, rather than simply being an income elasticity for amenities. An additional factor, not discussed in the theory section, is possible price discrimination by physicians by income. The insignificance of the non-wage income variables tends to suggest that there was rather little price discrimination by income.

One of the more striking findings is the positive elasticity of 0·40 ($t = 4·5$) with respect to the physician/population ratio. This corroborates a finding using data across cities (Newhouse, 1970) and casts doubt upon the notion that an increase in the number of physicians will mitigate physician price increases.

V. CONCLUDING REMARK

In this paper we have presented estimates of price and income elasticities, which we regard as preliminary. Nevertheless, we have more confidence in these estimates than we do in most existing estimates of price and income elasticities in the economics literature because of the precision with which we have been able to measure the parameters of the insurance policy. In particular, our price elasticities are substantially below those of Rosett and Huang (1973), Feldstein (1971) and Davis and Russell (1972), but the estimates in this paper support estimates we have made using other data (Phelps and Newhouse, 1973). In subsequent work we shall attempt to exploit more fully the implications of our theoretical framework (for example, imposing the constraint that $\sigma_{ij} = \sigma_{ji}$) and extend our results (for example, to include hospital admissions and ancillary services), and to include non-labor-force participants and non-users of services in the sample.

REFERENCES

Acton, Jan P., 'Demand for Health Care among the Urban Poor, with Special Emphasis on the Role of Time' (Santa Monica: RAND Corporation, 1973) (R-1151-OEO/NYC).

Allen, R. G. D., *Mathematical Analysis for Economists* (London: Macmillan, 1938).

Andersen, Ronald, and Andersen, Odin, *A Decade of Health Services* (Univ. of Chicago Press, 1967).

Davis, Karen, and Russell, Louise, 'The Substitution of Hospital Outpatient Care for Inpatient Care', *Review of Economics and Statistics*, LIV (May 1972).

Dhrymes, Phoebus, 'Alternative Asymptotic Tests of Significance and Related Aspects of 2S.L.S. and 3S.L.S. Estimate Parameters', *Review of Economic Studies*, XXXVI (Apr 1969).

Feldstein, Martin S., 'Hospital Cost Inflation: A Study of Nonprofit Price Dynamics', *American Economic Review*, LXI (Dec 1971).

Grossman, Michael, *The Demand for Health: A Theoretical and Empirical Investigation* (New York: Columbia Univ. Press, 1972).

Michael, Robert T, *The Effect of Education on Efficiency in Consumption* (New York: Columbia Univ. Press, 1972).

160　　　　　　　　*The Economics of Health and Medical Care*

Newhouse, Joseph P., 'A Model of Physician Pricing', *Southern Economics Journal*, xxxvii (Oct 1970).
—— and Phelps, Charles E., 'Price and Income Elasticities for Medical Care Services' (Santa Monica: RAND Corporation, 1973) (R-1197-NC).
—— and Taylor, Vincent, 'The Subsidy Problem in Hospital Insurance', *Journal of Business*, xlii (Oct 1970).
Phelps, Charles E., 'The Demand for Health Insurance: A Theoretical and Empirical Investigation' (Santa Monica: RAND Corporation, 1973) (R-1054-OEO).
—— and Newhouse, Joseph P., 'The Effects of Coinsurance on the Demand for Physician Services' (Santa Monica: RAND Corporation, 1972) (R-976-OEO).
—— and ——, 'Coinsurance and the Demand for Medical Services' (Santa Monica: RAND Corporation, 1973) (R-964-OEO/NC).
—— and ——, 'The Theory of a Consumer Facing a Variable Price Schedule under Uncertainty' (Santa Monica: RAND Corporation, forthcoming).
Rosett, Richard N., and Lien-Fu Huang, 'The Effect of Health Insurance on the demand for Medical Care', *Journal of Political Economy*, lxxxi, 2 (1) (Mar–Apr 1973).

APPENDIX

SUMMARY DATA STATISTICS

Exogenous variables	Mean	Standard deviation
M.D.s/100,000	114·174	50·8661
Beds/1,000	4·25832	2·15688
Married	0·705545	0·456068
Net room and board price	15·2915	15·2245
Net M.D. office price	5·88964	6·58853
M.D. office visits	5·05004	5·38867
Dummy: non-wage income > $3,000	0·681775E–01	0·252200
Disability days	14·5358	47·0871
Non-wage income	424·520	711·822
Wage income/week	88·1354	79·5548
Sex	0·234025	0·423640
Family size	3·14421	1·76085
Race	0·110568	0·313782
Size of work group	5·01065	2·84476
Age 25–34	0·173313	0·378743
Age 35–54	0·423886	0·494466
Age 55–64	0·160447	0·367238
Age ⩾65	0·199909	0·400169
Education 9–11 years	0·211888	0·408889
Education 12 years	0·228797	0·420308
Education 13–15 years	0·118795	0·323739
Education 16+ years	0·132791	0·339551
Professional	0·188927	0·391683
Manager	0·168658	0·374672
Sales	0·160156	0·366969
Foreman	0·299055	0·458116
Agriculture–mining–construction	0·207484	0·405746

SUMMARY DATA STATISTICS (*contd.*)

Exogenous variables	Mean	Standard deviation
Manufacturing	0·233272	0·423165
Finance	0·610183E–01	0·239506
Public administration	0·195050	0·396474
Entertainment	0·733193E–02	0·853629E–01
Health status good	0·397636	0·489700
Health status fair	0·184931	0·388472
Health status poor	0·824960E–01	0·275282
Non-wage income if over $3,000	374·109	1660·85
Beds/1,000	4·54781	2·42312
Married	0·741566	0·439579
Room and board net price	13·8899	19·8586
M.D. office net price	3·46742	3·72900

Dependent variables	Mean	Standard deviation
Hospital ($\eta = 122$):		
Weighted days	8·50	7·77
Gross price	15·58	12·42
Marginal coinsurance	0·39	0·43
Net price	13·89	19·86
Physician office ($\eta = 842$):		
Weighted visits	5·05	5·39
Gross price	6·86	6·75
Marginal coinsurance	0·88	0·31
Net price	5·89	6·59
Clinic ($\eta = 216$):		
Visits	3·78	4·92
Net price	1·36	4·20

10 Supplier-Induced Demand: Some Empirical Evidence and Implications[1]

Robert G. Evans
UNIVERSITY OF BRITISH COLUMBIA

The professional relationship arises from the significant information differential between physician and patient, and permits the physician to exert direct, non-price influence on the demand for his own services. If the economic status of the physician affects the level and direction of such influence exerted, then models of the demand for care which do not include explicit consideration of supplier behavior are incompletely specified.

This paper outlines the effect on demand analyses of two alternative specifications of physician behavior, and notes that each can lead to 'perverse' response of price to increases in supply, or of quantity demanded to price. It then examines several pieces of empirical evidence from Canada and the United States which are consistent with substantial demand influence by physicians, with responses of generated output to physician stock around 80 per cent through increases in supply of physician-initiated services. The conclusion is that policy to limit price inflation, correct 'shortages' or restrain unnecessary utilization cannot be based on conventional supply and demand models.

Everyone knows that physicians exert a strong influence over the quantity and pattern of medical care demanded in a developed economy. The professional status of the physician and the peculiar 'doctor–patient relationship' are rooted in the dual roles which the physician must perform. He acts as the agent of the patient, providing expert direction or assistance in the interpretation of the patient's health status, the identification of the capacity of current medical technology to improve that status, and the skilled application of that technology. But at the same time he is a supplier of a particular class of services whose income and work satisfaction are related to the

---

[1] This is a revision of the paper given in Tokyo. Care has been exercised to retain the trenchancy of the commentators' observations.

volume of services he supplies and the price he receives for them. In this role the interests of the physician tend to conflict with those of the patient, particularly if medical practice is organized on an entreprenurial fee-for-service basis. Such a setting creates strong economic incentives for the physician to overemphasize the supply of his own services to the exclusion of substitutes and to bias the patient's 'choice' of services towards those which yield the highest net revenue per time unit for the physician. One purpose of the professionalization of the physician role is the formation of a set of attitudes which will counteract these incentives.

If physicians were simply entrepreneurs supplying a particular good, 'medical care', then one could analyze the behaviour of the medical market using the conventional theoretical tools of supply and demand analysis. The demand side of the market could be treated as a function of price and consumer characteristics such as age, sex, income, insurance status, and so on with efforts made to define and measure demand curves for aggregate or sub-markets. Shifts in demand due to such 'policy instruments' as types of insurance coverage could be studied without reference to supply-side behaviour. At the same time the supply side could be handled in a conventional manner, assuming perfect competition or monopoly and investigating the implications of each with or without recognition of the fact that the entrepreneur running the firm is also a principal factor supplier with his own income–leisure trade-off.[1]

What is neglected, however, is the theoretical significance of the other aspect of the physician's role, the patient's agent. The physician can exert direct influence on the demand function of the consumer by altering the patient's perceptions of his needs and of the capacity of medical technology to satisfy them. Thus, the medical service market cannot be simply dichotomized into demand side and supply side, with price serving as the only nexus between the two; rather we must allow for shifts in the demand curve itself in response to supplier

[1] A variety of analyses of demand, some with quite sophisticated analyses of consumer motivation, are surveyed by Cliff Lloyd, 'The Demand for Medical Care: A Selective Review of the Literature', Univ. of Iowa Working Paper Series No. 71–9 (Apr 1971). The physician's income–leisure trade-off may be handled by estimating demand curves simultaneously with a rising supply curve in which the source of rising marginal cost is the increasing marginal disutility of labour to the physician; this appears to be the rationale for J. P. Newhouse, 'A Model of Physician Pricing', *Southern Economic Journal*, xxxvii, 2 (Oct 1970), as corrected by H. French and P. Ginsburg, 'Physician Pricing: Monopolistic or Competitive', *Southern Economic Journal*, xxxvii, 3 (Dec 1970). Similarly, M. Feldstein, 'The Rising Price of Physicians' Services' *Review of Economics and Statistics*, lii, 2 (May 1970) develops a supply curve embodying a physician work–leisure trade-off which appears to be backward-bending.

behaviour. Market clearing may take place directly through the information which suppliers pass to consumers as well as by adjustments in price.

In such a market, it may no longer be taken for granted that conventional economic propositions hold. If, for example, physicians respond to increases in price by exerting a stronger positive influence on patient's perceptions of their 'need' for service, then it is not impossible for the total response of quantity demanded to price to be positive. The *partial* response may be negative as consumer theory predicts, but the *ceteris* do not remain *paribus*. Instead they vary in a systematic way with price.

Similarly an increase in the physician stock, if physicians have discretionary power over demand, may lead to increases in both output and prices. This is because the power to sell more at the current price (by increasing each consumer's demand) is equivalent to the power to sell the current output at a higher price (by increasing demand and simultaneously raising price). An increase in number of suppliers at a given volume of demand and price will lead to a fall in each supplier's income; he can respond to this change by expanding his effort on demand generation and then either working more or raising prices, or both.[1]

Of course, demand cannot be expanded indefinitely at any given price level. There undoubtedly comes a point where continued increases in supply will lead to the re-emergence of price-competitive behaviour. The usefulness of discretionary models depends on an assumption that such a point is significantly far from where we now are, and that the social costs of reaching it would be relatively large in terms of the negative health impact of 'over-doctoring' and quality dilution as well as the economic costs of public investment and subsidy.

A further implication of the same argument has to do with deterrent charges as a device for reducing utilization and moderating cost increases under medical insurance plans. Insofar as such charges are successful in lowering workloads at current prices, they will lower physician incomes. If physicians have discretionary power over demand, they will respond by shifting the demand curve rightward

---

[1] Such a reaction by physicians should not be interpreted as the deliberate provision of unnecessary care. If physicians as a group believe that the public 'needs' more care than it now receives (and there is evidence that they do, e.g. interviews by H. Schonfeld *et al.*, 'Number of Physicians Required for Primary Medical Care', *New England Journal of Medicine*, no. 286, 16 Mar 1972), then they may well react to lowered workloads resulting from increased density of physicians by attempting to take better care of their patients through more frequent recalls and follow-ups, more extensive testing, consultations, and more services generally.

and either raising price of increasing output back to previous levels.[1] The distribution of care may change, but overall expenditures are unlikely to fall.

Thus, the possibility that suppliers can individually or collectively exercise influence over the demand curve can have rather radical implications for the role of prices as market signalling devices on the effects of exogenous shifts in supply and demand on expenditure and price.

By itself, however, the notion that suppliers influence demand does not vitiate any of the conventional propositions of market analysis. If suppliers took no account of economic data in the information which they provided to consumers, e.g. if physicians disregarded prices, their own incomes and their workloads in making recommendations to patients, then the demand function as a relation between quantity and price could be treated as stable and negatively sloped because the other parameters of the utility function would still be exogenously determined.[2] Unfortunately, the literature on physician behaviour abounds with references to the responsiveness of physician practice behaviour to economic factors.[3] At the other

---

[1] The emphasis on physician responses to overall workload changes indicates that the results of partial and general deterrent charges may be quite different. A small insured group which does not account for a large part of the income of its local medical community may indeed respond to deterrents by reducing utilization. On the other hand, a deterrent fee introduced in a national or provincial insurance plan is much less likely to affect overall utilization and more likely to exert upward pressure on medical prices. R. G. Beck, 'An Analysis of the Demand for Physicians' Services in Saskatchewan', unpublished doctoral dissertation (Univ. of Alberta, Edmonton, Spring 1971) emphasizes the reactions of physicians as well as patients to the province-wide deterrent fee introduced in 1968, and points out that this fee happened to coincide with a significant upward revision in the provincial fee schedule, as well as apparently *increasing* utilization by certain classes of patients.

[2] If the full information assumption for patients is relaxed, one can still insulate the non-price variables in the demand function from indirect supplier price and income effects by hypothesizing a purely professional physician who considers only technical factors in informing his patients, then wears his entrepreneurial hat when responding to the resulting demand. It is hard to see how an economist could regard such behaviour as either rational or optimizing.

[3] For example, G. Monsma, 'Marginal Revenue and the Demand for Physicians' Services', in H. Klarman (ed.), *Empirical Studies in Health Economics* (Baltimore: John Hopkins Press, 1970) surveys data on the response of physician practice patterns to rates of payment. U. Reinhardt, 'An Analysis of Physicians' Practices', unpublished doctoral dissertation (Yale Univ., 1970) calculates rates of payment per minute for several types of common activities and notes how these bias activities. The *Task Force Reports on Costs of Health Services in Canada* (Ottawa: The Queen's Printer, 1970) note instances of specific responses to fee schedule revisions – sharp increases in activities whose relative price had risen – as well as general 'over-doctoring' in areas with relatively large physician stocks as procedures were multiplied to maintain incomes. The list could go on indefinitely.

extreme, if physicians are pure income-maximizers it is clear that each individual physician will always exert as much influence as he can to increase demand for his own services. In this case, analysis of the medical services market becomes merely a version of the monopolistic competition model with advertising and a rather peculiar advertising cost function.[1] The assumption of income maximization assures that *unexerted* discretionary influence over the demand curve does not exist, hence the demand curve can be treated as exogenous.

In a real world lying between these two extremes, however, discretionary power by physicians may persist. If it is a significant feature of the medical care supply process, then it must be incorporated into models of the medical market; and there appear to be two basic ways of doing this. One can retain the maximizing framework and postulate that physicians have some broader objective function including the exercise of discretion as well as income and/or workload. Alternatively, one can abandon the maximizing framework for some general 'target' model, in which physicians are assumed to have rough targets for both income and leisure (the origin of such targets is unclear, but no more so than the origin of the utility function!) and to adjust prices and/or discretionary behaviour so as to approach these moving targets.

The extended maximizing model can be applied to any market in which *some* price responsiveness by consumers exists due to full or partial self-payment; it cannot explain market behaviour in a full-insurance system such as Canada's Medicare Plan. Such a model might specify each physician's utility as a positive function of his income (Y) and a negative function of his workload (W) and the extent to which he exerts discretionary influence (D) to increase demand. D may also be interpreted as a positive preference for non-price rationing. If we regard each physician as a monopolistic competitor whose market share depends on the population/physician ratio (R), and each of whose patients demands an amount of care negatively related to the price charged and positively related to demand-expanding behaviour, then we may write:

$$U = U(Y,W,D)$$
$$W = R \cdot f(P,D)$$

where W is the physician's workload, $f(P,D)$ is the demand for care by his 'representative' patient, and R allows for shifts in workload

[1] An advertising model with costless advertising is essentially rather uninteresting, while the usual explicit cost function for demand generation through advertising is implausible in this context.

arising from shifts in the exogenous population/physician ratio. The problem is to maximize *U* subject to the workload constraint *W*, by setting price level, workload and discretionary behaviour. Income is equal to the product of price level and workload, assuming a constant proportion of overhead expense.

The comparative statics of such a model are relatively straightforward, if somewhat tedious, and it turns out that the conditions for a maximum are 'reasonable' *a priori*. But predicted responses to exogenous shifts are not determinate; in particular, an exogenous increase in supply (a fall in *R*) may well result in a *rise* in price. If the *D* variable is suppressed, a fall in *R* for *P* given lowers both income and workload. The marginal utility of income rises and the marginal disutility of work falls, so the physician cuts price so as to increase workload and income. (Of course, the elasticity of demand for care faced by each physician must be greater than unity to make this model work.) But in the more general model, the physician may increase both *P* and *D* to get back to equilibrium. In general, the difficulty is that the *D* variable introduces an extra off-diagonal term from the Hessian matrix of the constrained maximization problem into each shift-response equation, and nothing is determinate.[1]

A maximizing model extended to include physician discretion is thus able to break the conventional association between rising prices and scarcity of excess demand, but at the cost of giving up all definite predictions about pricing behaviour. A further source of weakness in such models is the structure of the patient demand equation; conditions for a maximum require that the price elasticity of demand faced by each physician must be greater than unity. As noted below, this requires either that most measurements of the elasticity are erroneous, or that physicians are price-competitive with one another. *A fortiori*, such a model will not explain pricing behaviour in a fee-for-service market under comprehensive, universal medical insurance such as the Canadian Medicare system. The fact that such markets do indeed function, with price behaviour roughly similar to the United States self-paying market, suggests that the maximizing model may be inadequate.

A less formal, non-maximizing model may be constructed if we hypothesize that physicians have rough targets with respect to income and workload, based on their training, expectations and previous experience. Discrepancies between these targets and actual experience lead to adjustment behaviour; if income and workloads are below targets, demand generation may take place. If physicians

---

[1] This is a general problem with extended maximising models, analyzed by G. C. Archibald, 'The Qualitative Content of Maximizing Models', *Journal of Political Economy*, LXXIII, 1 (Feb 1965).

feel overworked and underpaid, upward pressure on prices may develop either collectively (revision of fee schedules) or individually (independent adjustments in billing behaviour).

In Canada, revision of fee schedules requires that a large enough number of physicians in any province find target incomes unattainable and seek to put through a uniform schedule revision; the physician whose targets run ahead of his colleagues' can only work harder. In the United States, where individual physicians have more power over their own prices, the factors limiting short-run adjustment are less clear. Nevertheless, there is considerable evidence that price adjustment is only one of several possible strategies a physician may employ in meeting his practice objectives.

The implications of such a model have been developed in more detail elsewhere,[1] but in general they include upward pressure on prices when supply increases, as well as relatively little response of income per physician. Increases in regionwide fee schedules are likely to lower output per physician (although not unambiguously), and thus rising prices are ineffective as a rationing device for clearing markets. The primary function of price is (in conjunction with workloads) to achieve physician income targets. A model of this sort is distressingly fuzzy in its failure to explain the formation of target incomes or the distribution of target shortfalls between price increase and demand generation. It does, however, have the capacity to interpret a number of empirical observations which are anomalous in a conventional supply/demand framework.

If physician influence over demand is a significant feature of the medical service market, we would expect to find relatively little relationship between physician workload and physician density per capita. On the other hand, if demand is exogenous to the physician, workload should vary inversely with density. Within each of the provinces of Canada, physicians are now paid according to a standardized fee schedule; thus, one can use annual incomes of physicians within the same province as indicators of their relative workloads. In British Columbia, annual gross receipts of each physician from the provincial medical insurance plan are published by physician name, and it is thus possible to link up gross receipts with data on physician specialty, length of practice, location, form of practice (solo or group by size) and place of training. Furthermore, since each physician is located by school district and hospital district (the latter being aggregations of continuous school districts forming a single catchment area for purposes of regional hospital planning), it is possible to

[1] R. Evans, *Price Formation in the Market for Physician Services in Canada 1957–69* (Ottawa: The Queen's Printer, for the Prices and Incomes Commission, 1973) chap. 2.

measure demographic and other aggregate variables by region and to investigate their significance as predictors of physician gross income and workload.

This data base has been investigated for both 1969 and 1971 in order to determine *inter alia* the influence on physician workload of relative physician densities by region.[1] The procedure employed in both surveys has been to reduce the total physician census to a subset assumed to be in full-time medical practice, and then to relate the average incomes of these physicians to a set of independent dummy variables representing professional characteristics. This data base consists of 2,279 physicians in 1969 and 2,457 in 1971. Dummy variables are used to control for each of the characteristics listed above, thus enabling one to estimate for any particular set of characteristics the total amount by which the income of the physician which they represent would have exceeded that of the base reference physician (a general practitioner who graduated from the University of British Columbia within the last five years and is in solo practice in Vancouver). Details on data file are available from the author.

With physician workload (gross receipts) standardized for the characteristics of the physician, it is then possible to introduce measures of the relative availability of medical care in each region. These are unfortunately conceptually fuzzy, for several reasons. Availability is a relation between the exogenous 'demand' for medical care (in a fully insured population) and the exogenous 'stock' of care in each region. The crudest measures of each are total populations by region and total physician stock. But clearly, people are not homogeneous in their health characteristics; the exogenous demand of a population depends on age, sex, fertility, climate, occupation, socio-economic status, etc. Out of all these factors we carried out a rough standardization for age alone, using relative utilization weights for four different age groups to derive a standardized population for each region. Nor are physicians homogeneous; we therefore calculated physician/ (standardized) population ratios for all physicians, general practitioners, and general practitioners and 'practicing specialists',[2] and

[1] R. Evans, E. Parish and F. Sully, 'Medical Productivity, Scale Effects and Demand "Generation" ' (mimeo), Univ. of British Columbia, Department of Economics Discussion Paper No. 79 (June 1972) reports investigations with the 1969 data.

[2] 'Practicing specialists' is a concept borrowed from D. Anderson and A. Clough, 'The Location of British Columbia Physicians', *British Columbia Medical Journal*, II, 5 (Sep 1960). It excludes radiologists, pathologists, anesthesiologists, public health physicians and rehabilitation specialists, in an attempt to focus only on specialists who are or might be in direct primary contact with patients. The substitution between general practitioner and practicing specialist is obvious in the case of a paediatrician: it becomes more strained in the case of a neuro-surgeon.

fitted separate equations for each group. The problem of course is to define a subset of physicians who are substitutes for one another (more or less), and there exists no precisely correct procedure. Regional boundaries are a further problem, since one may choose small regions such as school districts, in which case referral across boundaries leads to mis-specification of available supply, or large regions such as hospital districts which may span several medical 'markets'. We chose the latter to minimize the referral problem: tertiary referrals to the university-affiliated hospitals in Vancouver are missed, but secondary referrals to urban centres are in general within regions.

The coefficients on these physician/population density variables are as follows (*t*-statistics in brackets):

	AMD	GP	GPPS	PS
1969	-0·158	-0·125	-0·179	0·013
	(2·68)	(1·46)	(2·75)	(0·27)
1971	-0·087	-0·274	-0·070	0·061
	(1·27)	(2·28)	(0·88)	(1·06)

AMD is the equation fitted for all physicians of whatever speciality, *GP* are general practitioners only, *PS* are selected specialties (see footnote 2, p. 169) and *GPPS* is fitted on sums from *GP* and *PS*. Equations are double-log, so coefficients represent elasticity. The *PS* equation suggests that interaction among specialists has a positive effect on workload; all other equations indicate weak negative effects from density to workload. This is consistent with the hypothesis that physicians can to a large extent generate enough activity to insulate their workload against supply shifts. Adjustment is not complete, however, so a target income model would also suggest that supply increases generate upward price pressure. Moreover, the incomplete adjustment is consistent with increasing marginal disutility of demand generation.

Shifting 'demand' in response to changes in the effective supply of physicians is not of course the only interpretation of these results. One could argue that British Columbia has a physician shortage such that all physicians are working at full capacity regardless of the number available and that some patients are turned away. The plausibility of this argument is weakened by the fact that British Columbia (B.C.) has far and away the highest ratio of physicians to population in Canada, about 25–30 per cent above the national average (depending on definition). Many regions of B.C. have still higher ratios. Alternatively, one could argue that demand is a function of the shadow price of time and other access costs which are reduced when physician density increases; moreover, demand may vary from region to region due to shifts in non-measured variables and physicians have simply distributed themselves in response to income differentials in such a way as to even out incomes. Neither of these arguments can be tested directly with aggregate data, since they appeal to unmeasured shadow prices and demand shifts, but they can be indirectly tested by evidence on the particular patterns of medical services supplied as physician density changes.

Data on the mix of services by physician and region in B.C. were not available for this study. However, a set of data on the operations of the Canadian non-profit private insurance plans which predated the universal federally initiated Medicare program is available from 1957 to 1967. These data indicate that across provinces the relative frequency of physician-initiated services such as consultations tends to be more closely correlated with physician availability than does the frequency of patient-initiated services such as first office or home visits.[1] Moreover, the rapid increases in physician availability in Canada during the period 1957 to the present, due both to increases in manpower and to increases in services per physician,[2] have likewise been associated with increases in the mix of total services accounted for by physician-initiated services. Consultations and diagnostic tests per capita have increased much faster over time than home or office calls; this is not consistent with either the argument that patients are responding to shadow prices or that medical services are merely reducing a backlog of unmet need. In the same context, it is notable that the shift from house to office calls in Canada over the past fifteen years has not been associated with any change in their relative prices. Thus, what evidence we have on inter-regional and intertemporal patterns of service mix is consistent with supplier generation of demand rather than consumer response to implicit prices or exogenous demand-side effects.[3]

---

[1] Evans, *Price Formation*, chap. 4. It must be confessed that data points are scanty and correlations are not perfect; data cover B.C., Alberta, Manitoba, two Ontario plans and the Maritime Provinces, with one observation for each.

[2] Ibid., chap. 1. The problem is that price data are thoroughly unreliable, while data on increases in gross income per physician are drawn from taxation statistics and are quite good. The increases in gross receipts must be allocated between output per man and price, allowing for some quality change. Between 1957 and 1970 gross receipts per physician have risen 144·3 per cent, or 7·1 per cent per year. Regardless of how it is split up, this yields very high rates of increases in price or output or both. Over the same period, the Consumer Price Index rose about 2·5 per cent per year, and the stock of physicians per capita (in active fee practice) rose 1·5 per cent per year.

[3] Of course, all such evidence can be rationalized in a conventional supply and demand framework. Inter-regional differences in physician availability may lead to differences in implicit costs of physician access, hence different demand patterns. Changes in service mix may be due to changes in patient tastes,

If, in fact, discretionary influence over demand is a significant feature of the market behaviour of physicians, then we should expect to find it reflected in price behaviour. And we do discover a general tendency for physician prices to be relatively higher in regions where physicians are plentiful than where they are scarce. While data are sketchy and relative levels are hard to establish owing to the discontinuous jumps which take place in listed fees, there is a clear tendency for medical care prices to be higher in those provinces of Canada with high physician/population ratios (Ontario, British Columbia) than in those with low (Saskatchewan, the Maritimes). The direction of causality in such an association is by no means obvious: higher prices per unit of output could as easily be the magnet which attracts more physicians. But the problem with this argument is that *income* relationships are much less clear: high prices are associated with both high (Ontario) and low (British Columbia) relative incomes. There is some evidence that higher than average increases in physician density are associated with lower than average increases in income; but the mechanism is clearly not through slower rates of price increase. Rather it appears to be incomplete ability to adjust quantity of work-load per physician, perhaps operating with a lag.[1]

If the demand relationship is made subsidiary to supplier behaviour, then one ought to be able to use similar models to interpret United States and Canadian physician behaviour in spite of the differences in medical care financing. Patterns of organization on the supply side remain relatively similar. The existence of physician discretionary power is indicated by such United States results as Feldstein's inability to derive any sort of 'reasonable' demand curve with a negative price term even in the context of a simultaneous market model under several different price adjustment specifications.[2] His conclusion that physicians may hold prices below market clearing levels to enjoy the utility of non-price rationing is the inverse of the notion that demand generation at given prices is possible but involves disutility. Similarly, Newhouse[3] finds systematic positive correlations between physician density and price in the United States, rejecting both 'competitive' and 'monopolistic' models of the market which use price as the only nexus between supply and demand. He notes

---

operating through the physician as intermediary. Inter-regional variations in 'health' or tastes for medical care may lead to bidding up of prices in high-demand regions and drawing in of more physicians, hence a positive correlation between physician density and price. But a model rescued by a succession of *ad hoc* unobservables is an irrefutable and uninteresting model.

[1] Evans, *Price Formation*, chap. 3.

[2] Feldstein, *op. cit.*

[3] Newhouse, *op. cit.*

that rationing by physicians may explain his results. Reinhardt[1] finds that the internal organization of physician practices is inconsistent with income maximization in that the shadow prices of physician time implicit in fee schedules are much higher than those implicit in physician/aide mixes. He suggests that a state of generalized excess demand creates a 'price umbrella' permitting this form of discretionary 'inefficiency by preference', but discretionary power over demand is an equally good umbrella. It permits the physician whose preference for income is strong to organize a fast throughput 'shop' without squeezing out his less aggressive competitors. Finally, the numerous studies which measure elasticities of demand for medical care at between −1 and zero are rendered plausible: if physicians wer income- or income/leisure-maximizers, they should always seek higher prices to raise income and lower workload, and the observed market result would depend on their having insufficient ability to collude so as to raise prices all round. But if in fact each physician generates his own demand, then no stable exogenous demand curve exists to be measured. Price being correlated with demand-generation effort will lead to a reduction in the measured response of demand to price, but the partial response of demand to price, *everything* else held constant, is not being tested.

Thus, there exists a wide range of empirical evidence that the market for physicians' services is not self-equilibrating in the usual sense, that price does not serve primarily to balance supply and demand because there are important alternative channels of information which perform this function. The primary role of price is instead as an input to supplier incomes, which are not themselves the product of explicit maximizing behaviour but rather of target-seeking through the manipulation of several different control variables. In this context, as noted above, the explanation of supply, 'shortages', utilization and price and cost behaviour may be very different from the usual market models. To the extent that shortages, prices or costs are objects of public policy, policy prescriptions must take account of these differences.

[1] U. Reinhardt, 'A Product Function for Physician Services', *Review of Economics and Statistics*, LIV, 1 (Feb 1972).

11 Some Economic Aspects of Mortality in Developed Countries[1]

Victor R. Fuchs

CENTER FOR ADVANCED STUDY IN THE BEHAVIORAL
SCIENCES, PALO ALTO, CALIF., AND NEW YORK UNIVERSITY

Three types of data – cross-section within countries, cross-section among countries, and some time series – reveal that the traditional negative association between mortality and income per capita is disappearing in developed countries. The marginal contribution of medical care to life expectancy, holding the state of the art constant, is also very small. Improvements in medical science (primarily new drugs), however, have had significant effects during the period 1930–60.

Current differences in mortality across, and within, developed countries are primarily related to 'life-style' – diet, exercise, smoking, drinking, psychological stress, etc. The 'demand' for a long life, and the ability to 'produce' it, differ greatly among individuals and populations. A major research task is to gain a better understanding of these demand and production functions.

I. INTRODUCTION

Death is the result of a complex set of interacting physiological, behavioral and environmental factors; its social and economic consequences are frequently profound. In most countries considerable resources are devoted to postponing death, and the success achieved in developed countries over the past two centuries is generally regarded as one of the outstanding benefits of economic development. It is well to recall that, at the beginning of the eighteenth century, life expectancy in Western Europe was scarcely higher than it had been under the Romans. Not one infant in ten could expect to reach the Biblical 'threescore and ten'. Today, in developed countries, close to three-fourths of the female and over half of the male infants can expect to reach the age of seventy.

[1] This paper was written while I was a Fellow at the Center for Advanced Study in the Behavioral Sciences. I am grateful to the Carnegie Corporation for financial assistance, to Carol Breckner for research assistance and to Perry Gluckman for advice concerning the appendix.

Despite its importance, economists have not had much to say about death. At one time the problem may have appeared too trivial – mortality rates depended upon per capita income and upon not much else. Now, the problem may be too complex – variations in mortality across and within developed countries are still substantial, but their relationships to economic variables are not well understood.[1]

It is widely believed that increased life expectancy is an inevitable consequence of economic growth. Over the broad sweep of economic development there is ample justification for this belief. Among developed countries currently, however, some new bits of evidence suggest that the negative association between mortality and income is disappearing. Three types of data – cross-section within countries, cross-section among countries, and some time series – do not reveal the expected association. Thus, a major subject of interest in this paper is the relationship between mortality and income. How has it changed over time? Why has it changed? In the course of the inquiry, consideration is also given to the role of medical care and scientific advances. Some additional insights concerning economic aspects of mortality are obtained by an examination of differentials associated with sex, marital status and 'way of life'.

II. INCOME PER CAPITA

It seems intuitively reasonable to assume that 'life' is a normal good, and to predict a negative relation between mortality and real income per capita. For about two centuries, from the middle of the eighteenth to the middle of the twentieth, there was ample confirmation of that prediction. Indeed, it is now believed that until this century most of the reduction in death rates was due to increases in real income rather than to improvements in medical care.[2]

In 1963 Irma Adelman seemed to go so far as to argue that the role of real income in life expectancy increases as income rises. She wrote:

... once the major benefits from these improvements [basic public health measures] have been reached it may well be that economic conditions play the primary role in determining the subsequent rate of progress in mortality, for it stands to reason that such factors as better nutrition, improved housing, healthier and more humane working conditions, and a somewhat more secure and less care-worn mode of life, all of which accompany economic growth, must contribute to improvements in life expectancy. ([1] p. 324)

---

[1] For a concise discussion of some of the difficulties encountered in analyzing mortality differentials, see [3].

[2] See [8]. For a contrary, but not particularly convincing, argument see [10].

In 1965 I reported that income no longer seemed to have any favorable effect on interstate mortality differentials for United States whites except at young ages [4]. This finding was confirmed by Auster, Leveson and Sarachek using a much more comprehensive model employing both ordinary least squares and two-stage least squares estimating procedures [2]. Michael Grossman provided additional insights concerning income and health using survey data on individuals instead of state averages, and measuring ill-health by disability days abd restricted activities days instead of by mortality [6].

More importantly, Grossman developed a model of the demand for health which shows how rising income could lead to higher death rates. The essence of his argument is that the consumption of some goods (e.g. rich foods, motor-cars) may adversely affect health. If the income elasticity for such goods is very high, the 'shadow price' of health rises, and the quantity of health demanded falls. Rising incomes could, therefore, actually raise mortality. Grossman's model shows how this might happen but does not predict that it will, or even that the favorable effect of income diminishes as income rises. The following discussion indicates why there is a tendency for this to occur.

Let us suppose that the elasticity of mortality with respect to income varies for different causes of death. For instance, the death rate from malnutrition or tuberculosis is likely to have a large negative income elasticity, while the death rate from aircraft accidents is likely to have a small elasticity, or may even be positively related to income. The overall elasticity of mortality with respect to income is a weighted average of the elasticities for different causes where the weights are the fraction of deaths accounted for by each cause (see appendix). As income rises, *ceteris paribus*, the causes with small negative elasticities or positive elasticities become relatively more important, and the overall elasticity *must move toward zero or even turn positive*. Assuming initial values and constant mortality functions of income for each cause, the overall elasticity at any subsequent time is a function of the level of income. The following analysis of cross-sectional differences in infant mortality provides a good illustration of this process at work.

(1) *Infant Mortality*
Age of death is usually reported more accurately than cause, and in infant mortality there is a rough correspondence between time of death and cause. Neonatal deaths (within 28 days of birth) are usually attributable to congenital anomalies, prematurity and complications of delivery. Post-neonatal deaths (after 28 days but within one year) are frequently the result of infectious diseases or accidents, although,

admittedly, correspondence between time and cause is not perfect. Separate regressions of the form $LnM = a + b_1 Ln Y$ were fitted across the states of the United States and across developed countries for 1937 (average of 1936–8) and 1965 (average of 1964–6) for neonatal and post-neonatal mortality. Because of data limitations, the country set includes only fifteen developed countries with market-type economies. The income series in 1965 are the United Nations estimates of G.N.P. per capita in U.S. dollars. For 1937, Colin Clark's estimates of 'international units' are converted to U.S. 1965 dollars by the U.S. G.N.P. price deflator.

The results presented in Table 11.1, Part A, show that the income elasticity for neonatal deaths is significantly lower than for post-neonatal deaths. Within each category, the elasticities do not vary as much as they do between states and countries or between time periods. There is some tendency for the elasticities to fall over time,

TABLE 11.1

REGRESSION OF NEONATAL AND POST-NEONATAL MORTALITY ON INCOME PER CAPITA ACROSS STATES AND COUNTRIES, 1937 AND 1965

Part A

		Neonatal		Post-neonatal		
Units of observation	*Year*[a]	*Income elasticity* b_1	*Standard error of* b_1	*Income elasticity* b_1	*Standard error of* b_1	*N*
States	1937	−0·17	(0·04)	−0·53	(0·11)	48
States	1965	−0·19	(0·04)	−0·49	(0·12)	48
Countries	1937	−0·24	(0·13)	−1·03	(0·27)	15
Countries	1965	−0·02	(0·18)	−0·49	(0·33)	15

Part B

		Income elasticity b_1	*Standard error of* b_1	*Shift coefficient* b_2	*Standard error of* b_2	*Effect of change in knowledge*[b] %	*N*
Neo:							
States	1937 and 1965	−0·18	(0·03)	−0·50	(0·02)	−39	96
Countries	1937 and 1965	−0·15	(0·11)	−0·60	(0·11)	−45	30
Post:							
States	1937 and 1965	−0·52	(0·08)	−0·96	(0·06)	−62	96
Countries	1937 and 1965	−0·82	(0·21)	−1·02	(0·21)	−64	30

Note: All state regressions weighted by population.

[a] Death rates based on three-year averages centered on year shown.
[b] Equals (antilog $b_2 - 1$) (100).
Sources of country data: [S-2], [S-16], [S-17].
Sources of state data: [S-3], [S-5], [S-6], [S-7], [S-8], [S-11].

TABLE 11.1A

MEANS AND STANDARD DEVIATIONS OF VARIABLES IN COUNTRY AND STATE REGRESSIONS

	1937		1965	
Countries ($N=15$)	Mean	*Standard deviation*	Mean	*Standard deviation*
Income per capita (1965 $)	1,024	375	1,954	623
Neonatal mortality (per 1,000 live births)	29·41	6.72	14·52	3·32
Post-neonatal mortality	32·63	18·09	6·45	2·94
Death rates per 1,000				
Males 15–19	2·69	1·66	1·05	0·17
Males 45–49	8·70	2·55	5·66	1·22
Males 65–69	42·33	8·07	38·74	5·36
Females 15–19	2·35	1·82	0·34	0·06
Females 45–49	6·55	1·27	3·34	0·48
Females 65–69	32·96	4·28	21·33	2·39
States ($N=48$)[a]				
Income per capita (1965 $)	1,589	457	2,880	401
Neonatal mortality	29·38	2·80	15·95	0·80
Post-neonatal mortality	19·83	6·94	5·30	0·74

[a] State variables weighted by population.
Sources: See Table 11.1.

probably for the same reason that the overall elasticity tends to fall as income rises. An attempt was made to fit a curvilinear function by adding $(Ln Y)^2$, but this term was never significant. Given the size of the standard errors we cannot, with confidence, reject the null hypothesis that the elasticities within each category were the same in 1965 as in 1937.

(2) *Advance in Knowledge*
Assuming constant elasticities for 1937 and 1965, we can pool the observations for the two time periods and obtain an estimate of the shift in the mortality–income function with regressions of the form $LnM = a + b_1 Ln Y + b_2 T$, where T is a dummy variable with a value of 1 for 1965 and 0 for 1937.

This shift can be attributed to the advance in knowledge of medical science *per se*, plus other knowledge that contributes to a reduction in infant mortality. To be sure, the shift coefficient is also affected by variables other than income that are related to infant mortality and that changed between 1937 and 1965. Where data were available, the number of physicians per capita and years of schooling were tried in the single-year regressions, but their inclusion did not have any significant effect on the results.

Part B of Table 11.1 shows the income elasticities (b_1) obtained with the pooled regressions and the shift coefficients (b_2). By taking the antilog of b_2, subtracting 1 and multiplying by 100, we obtain the percentage decline in mortality that can be attributed to advance in knowledge. The results for the states and countries are quite similar. They indicate that, holding income constant, the neonatal death rate declined about 40 per cent and the post-neonatal declined about 60 per cent. The differences between the two shift coefficients are statistically significant. These shifts are very substantial relative to the gains that can be attributed to the increase in income alone. They suggest that between two-thirds to three-fourths of the decrease in infant mortality between 1937 and 1965 was due to shifts in the mortality–income function, and only from one-fourth to one-third to movement along the function.

It should be noted that differential shifts in the functions also affect the income elasticity of total infant mortality by changing the relative importance of the different causes (see appendix). As it happens, the differential shift due to advances in knowledge and the difference in elasticities both work in the same direction: namely, to decrease the weight of post-neonatal deaths in total infant mortality over time. If the shift differential was the opposite of the elasticity difference, the prediction of an overall elasticity that constantly approaches zero or becomes positive as income rises would have to be modified.

It is possible to predict the income elasticity of total infant mortality in 1965 given the elasticities and the shift coefficients for neonatal and post-neonatal mortality reported in Table 11.1, Part B. This prediction can then be compared with the actual elasticities obtained from regressions. The predicted value for the states is the same as the observed. A sharp decline is predicted for the countries but it falls short of the observed decline because the prediction assumes constant elasticities within each category over time, whereas in fact these also tended to decline.

Income elasticity of infant mortality

	1937	Predicted 1965	Actual 1965
States	−0·32	−0·27	−0·27
Countries	−0·64	−0·37	−0·17

(3) *Adult Mortality*

In 1936–8, other age-specific death rates were also negatively related to income per capita, as indicated by the regression results presented in Table 11.2. The elasticities were particularly high for adolescents and tended to decline as age increased. By 1965 the negative relation had disappeared. Although there is still considerable variability in age-specific death rates (coefficients of variation are around 15 per

TABLE 11.2

REGRESSION OF AGE-SPECIFIC DEATH RATES
ON INCOME PER CAPITA ACROSS
DEVELOPED COUNTRIES, 1937 AND 1965 ($N = 15$)

	Age	1937[a]		1965[a]	
		Income elasticity b_1	Standard error of b_1	Income elasticity b_1	Standard error of b_1
Males	15–19	−0·72	(0·21)	+0·12	(0·13)
	45–49	−0·32	(0·17)	+0·05	(0·17)
	65–69	−0·18	(0·11)	−0·01	(0·12)
Females	15–19	−0·93	(0·23)	+0·04	(0·12)
	45–49	−0·19	(0·11)	+0·05	(0·12)
	65–69	−0·13	(0·08)	−0·06	(0·09)

[a] Death rates based on three-year averages centered on year shown.
Sources of data: See Table 11.1.

TABLE 11.3

MALE MORTALITY INDEXES,
ENGLAND AND WALES, 1949–53
(all = 100)

Part A

Age-adjusted 20–64

Social class	All causes	Coronary disease, angina
I	98	147
II	86	110
III	101	105
IV	94	79
V	118	89
VI	124	60

Part B

Occupation	35–44	45–54	55–64
Higher administrative, professional and managerial	80	92	102
Other administrative, professional and managerial	73	85	88
Shopkeepers	91	97	104
Clerical workers	115	119	104
Shop assistants	85	86	84
Foremen	74	77	91
Skilled workers	97	100	107
Semi-skilled workers	103	98	96
Unskilled workers	134	125	112
Personal service	135	122	106
Farmers	78	66	68
Agricultural workers	79	71	72

Sources: Part A [S-14]; Part B [S-16, 1967].

cent), income is no more useful in explaining variability across developed countries than it is in explaining variability of United States whites across states.

Because the elasticities change so much over time we cannot measure the effect of advance of knowledge by pooling the data and looking at the shift coefficient. If it were possible to divide death rates into different causes, however, we might find some consistency in elasticities over time. Once these are identified, shift coefficients could be estimated for each cause.

Within developed countries, the relationship between mortality and income for adults is also tending to disappear, except for those at the lowest income levels. This can be seen in the data for English male mortality by social class and occupation, presented in Table 11.3. For the first four social classes there is no systematic relation between class and mortality for males 20–64, age-adjusted. The bottom two classes do show slightly higher rates, but at least part of this relationship probably reflects a causality running from health to occupation (and, hence, to social class) rather than the reverse. Mortality from coronary disease actually increases with social class, providing a good example of a death rate with a positive income elasticity. Across occupations the relationship between income and age-specific death rates is also very mixed, with several comparisons showing a positive correlation.[1]

III. MEDICAL CARE

The extent to which medical care affects mortality is a subject of considerable controversy. A realistic appraisal requires distinguishing between changes in the quantity of medical care holding the state of the art constant (movement along the mortality–medical care function) and improvements in the state of the art (downward shifts of the function). A further complication arises because these improvements do not come at a steady rate through time, nor are they some simple function of the volume of resources devoted to medical research.

Studies at the National Bureau of Economic Research on inter-state differences in mortality [2, 4, 5, 6] all show that variations in the number of physicians per capita, expenditures for physicians' services (deflated or not) and other medical care inputs have only slight effect on mortality, frequently fading into insignificance. Inclusion of the number of physicians per capita in the age-specific mortality regressions across developed countries in 1956 produces similar results. In

---

[1] It was noted at the Conference that there are probably many errors in the reports of occupation on death certificates. I agree with this caveat.

the absence of contrary evidence it would seem that the marginal
contribution of medical care to reductions in mortality, holding the
state of the art constant, is small in developed countries.[1]

Changes over time in what medical care can do, however, have had
a very large effect on mortality. This was particularly true for the
period beginning in the 1930s and extending through the 1950s. The
acceleration in the rate of decrease in mortality after 1930 can be seen
clearly in Fig. 11.1, which shows the average annual percentage rate

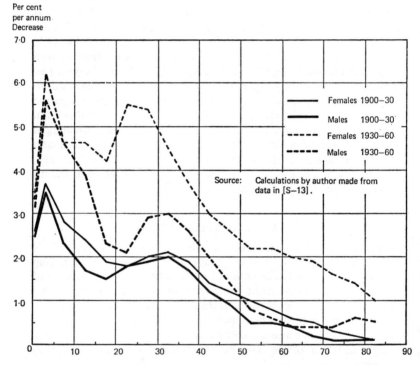

FIG. 11.1   Rates of decrease in mortality rates, United States whites by
age and sex, 1900–30 and 1930–60.

Source: Calculations by author made from data in [S-13].

of decline by age and sex for 1900–30 and 1930–60. For every age–
sex group the rate of decrease was greater in the more recent decades.

[1] This conclusion applies, of course, only over the observed range of variation.
Were inputs of care to be reduced significantly below the lowest levels now
observed, the marginal contribution might be much larger.

According to Walsh McDermott, this was attributable to the development in medicine for the first time of a 'decisive technology' [7]. Medical improvements in those years took many forms, the most noticeable being the discovery of sulfonamide, penicillin and the modern antibiotics. The broad picture portrayed in Fig. 11.1 of more rapid decrease after 1930 than before, of more rapid decreases for females than for males, and of a tendency for the rate of decrease to be smaller at older ages, is characteristic of the pattern in developed countries generally.

Recent Trends

By 1960 the really effective improvements in medicine were widely diffused throughout developed countries. Subsequent advances, such as organ transplants and other complex types of surgery, seem to have had only small impact on death rates and in some countries have actually been offset by adverse changes in the environment and in personal behavior. In most countries adult death rates are leveling off, and in the United States, Sweden and Norway age-specific death rates for males 25–60 have actually been rising slowly since about 1960 (see Table 11.4). This adverse trend could be reversed at any

TABLE 11.4

RECENT CHANGES IN MALE DEATH RATES
(per cent per annum)

Age	United States[a] (whites)	Sweden[b]	Norway[c]
25–29	+ 0·9	+ 0·1	− 2·0
30–34	+ 0·8	+ 0·1	+ 0·2
35–39	+ 0·5	+ 0·2	+ 0·7
40–44	+ 0·3	+ 0·2	+ 1·0
45–49	− 0·2	+ 0·1	+ 1·5
50–54	− 0·4	+ 0·1	+ 0·7
55–59	+ 0·3	0	+ 0·8

[a] 1959–61 to 1967–8.
[b] 1959–61 to 1967–9.
[c] 1956–60 to 1967–9.

Sources: Calculations by author made from data in [S-1], [S-12], [S-15].

time, but such a reversal is not likely to come about simply from the growth of income per capita or the allocation of more resources to medical care. If it comes, it is likely to be the result of the application of new knowledge or or a profound change in behavior.

Recent trends in infant mortality show precisely such a reversal. Consider the following average rates of change in United States infant mortality (per cent per annum):

	Neonatal	Post-neonatal	Total infant mortality
1935–50	−3·0	−6·6	−4·3
1950–65	−1·0	−1·4	−1·1
1965–71	−3·6	−5·9	−4·2

After a drastic leveling-off from 1950 to 1965, infant death rates started to drop dramatically again, achieving rates of decline equal to the record decreases of 1935–50.

The reasons for this recent rapid decline are not known. Some observers believe that special programs of maternal and child care aimed at disadvantaged groups are the principal explanation. Without denying that these programs may have had some effect, it seems to me that improvements in birth control (the pill, intra-uterine devices and liberalized abortion laws) probably deserve a great deal of the credit. The infant mortality rate for 'unwanted' children is undoubtedly many times higher than for wanted children.

A related point is the sharp drop of births of higher order in recent years. Babies of birth order four or higher are at greater risk than those of lower order. Between 1950 and 1965 the higher-order birth rates actually increased by 17·5 per cent, while the lower-order birth rate declined by 15·5 per cent. Since 1965 the lower-order birth rates have continued to decline moderately, but the birth rates of fourth order or above have dropped drastically, probably by as much as 50 per cent by 1971, although the detailed statistics are not yet available. To be sure the change in the distribution of births by order is not, in itself, large enough to explain the huge decrease in infant mortality since 1965, but it is indicative of the general improvement in birth control that has been achieved in recent years.

One piece of relevant evidence is that rapid decreases in infant mortality after 1965 were experienced in most developed countries. In half of them the rate of decrease was more rapid than in the United States. The special health programs were the result of United States legislation, whereas the pill and the I.U.D. became available generally in developed countries.

IV. WAY OF LIFE

If mortality in developed countries is relatively independent of income, and if the marginal contribution of medical care is small, what does make a difference? In brief the *way* people live has considerable effect on *how long* they will live.[1] Both the 'demand' for life, and the ability to 'produce' life (i.e. to postpone death), seem to vary considerably among individuals and groups. The differentials examined in this section are suggestive of the importance of such variation.

[1] The influence of genetic factors on longevity is not considered in this paper.

(1) *Sex*

In all developed countries, male deaths rate considerably higher than those of females of comparable age. At young ages the differential is of the order of one-third and seems to be fairly constant for different developed countries and for different parts of the United States, suggesting that some inherent biological difference is the primary explanation. After age 15, however, the size of the differential varies considerably, both within the United States and among developed countries. This variation is probably related to an interaction between biological and socio-economic factors.

Some idea of the extent of the sex differential in mortality, and how it varies with age and from one population to another, can be obtained from Fig. 11.2. In the United States among young white adults, the male death rate is triple the female rate; in Sweden the ratio is

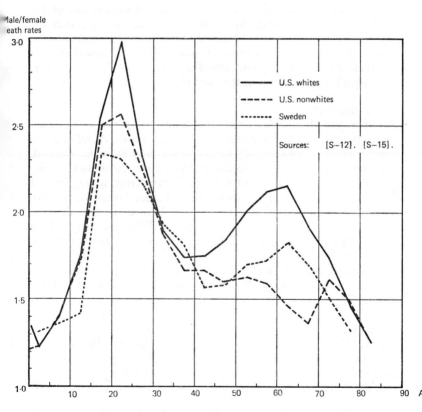

FIG. 11.2   Male/female death rate ratios, 1967–8.

only 2·3. Again, at age 45–65 the ratio is appreciably lower in Sweden than for United States whites. In both cases the high ratio for the United States whites is attributable to relatively high death rates for males, while females rates approach those found in Sweden. Among young males the excess deaths in the United States over Sweden are primarily the result of *accidents*. For the 45–65 age group the excess is primarily due to *heart disease*. Although attempts are frequently made to link the lower mortality in Sweden to their system of medical care, it seems unlikely that this system acts differentially for males and females, or that it plays a significant role in the lower incidence of accidents and heart disease in Swedish men.

Among United States whites the largest sex differentials are in small southern towns and the smallest in the suburbs of large northern cities. For 15–64 age-adjusted, the male excess is 137 per cent in non-metropolitan counties of the South Atlantic division, and only 82 per cent in metropolitan counties without a central city of the Middle Atlantic division. Again, it is extremely unlikely that the *difference* in the differential is related to medical care, income or the like. The most promising hypothesis is that sex-role differentiation in production and consumption varies from one population to another, with significant implications for mortality.

(2) *Marital Status*
Another type of mortality differential which is common to all developed countries is that associated with marital status. At all ages the unmarried have substantially higher death rates than the married. This may be the result of a selective marriage market with the causality running from health to marital status. Alternatively, it may be that life is produced more efficiently in a husband–wife household. Finally, it may be that married persons have a stronger demand for life. An examination of variations in the differential may help to shed a little light on these competing (but not mutually exclusive) hypotheses.[1]

Table 11.5 presents unmarried/married death-rate ratios and percentage unmarried by sex for thirteen developed countries *c.* 1965. The males are age 45–54, while the females are age 45–64, a comparable group from the point of view of death rates. We see that the mortality differential associated with marital status is much greater for men than for women in every country. This may be viewed as giving some support to the 'production of life' hypothesis, if it is assumed that life is primarily produced by non-market activities and that the female tends to specialize in such activities. It may also be

---

[1] For some of the hazards of speculating about marital status differentials, see [9].

TABLE 11.5

MORTALITY INDEXES AND PERCENTAGE UNMARRIED, DEVELOPED MARKET COUNTRIES, *c.* 1965

	Unmarried mortality index[a] (married = 100)		Percentage unmarried	
	Males	*Females average of*	*Males*	*Females*
	45–54	*45–54 and 55–64*	*45–54*	*45–54*
Japan	349	174	4·3	30·6
Canada	235	139	10·7	24·6
West Germany	227	129	7·1	34·8
United States	223	146	13·2	28·7
Australia	201	124	15·0	26·2
Sweden	198	138	18·3	25·8
France	194	124	15·9	29·0
Finland	183	138	14·7	37·2
Netherlands	174	130	8·6	22·2
Denmark	167	130	15·9	26·8
New Zealand	160	111	17·0	26·3
Norway	155	123	18·9	26·0
England and Wales	153	129	11·1	25·2
Median	194	130	14·7	26·3

[a] Weighted average of death rates for single, widowed and divorced with weights equal to United States distribution in 1970.

Source: Calculations by author made from data in [S-16, 1967].

TABLE 11.6

MARITAL STATUS MORTALITY INDEXES, UNITED STATES WHITE MALES 45–54, BY CAUSE OF DEATH, 1959–61

Cause of death[a]	*Single*	*Widowed* (married = 100)	*Divorced*	*Widowed* (single = 100)	*Divorced*
Arteriosclerotic heart disease	136	164	211	121	155
Malignant neoplasms, respiratory	114	174	263	153	231
Malignant neoplasms, digestive	148	162	199	109	134
Vascular lesions–C.N.S.	201	224	274	111	136
Other accidents	253	299	540	118	213
Suicide	174	352	395	202	227
Motor accidents	157	292	393	186	250
Cirrhosis of liver	276	508	784	184	284
Diabetes mellitus	221	188	298	85	135
Leukemia and aleukemia	107	101	129	94	121
Tuberculosis	520	669	1,062	129	204
Homicide	195	269	721	138	370

[a] Listed in descending order of importance.

Source: [S-9].

viewed as supporting the selectivity argument because unmarried males are a much smaller fraction of their age cohort than are females, and might be presumed to be more atypical with respect to health. For males there is a slight negative correlation between percentage unmarried and the unmarried/married mortality ratio, again suggesting some selectivity at work. No such correlation is evident for females.

Within the unmarried male category there is a fairly consistent pattern, with divorced men showing the highest death rates, widowed the next highest, and single men coming closest to the married rate. The median ratios to married for the thirteen countries are 221, 187 and 167 respectively. This pattern is also evident in Table 11.6, which shows marital status mortality ratios for United States white males 45–54 by cause of death.

Why should the rates of widowed and divorced be so much higher than for single men? One hypothesis is that of adverse selection. It has been suggested that widowed and divorced males (who do not remarry) constitute an 'inferior' group. An examination of earnings and hours of work by marital status shows that such men do earn less and work fewer hours than do married men (holding color, age and schooling constant) (see Table 11.7). Compared to single men, however, there is no support in the earnings and hours data for the adverse-selection hypothesis. There is, apparently, some extra factor raising mortality for the widowed and divorced that does not as

TABLE 11.7

EARNINGS AND HOURS, UNITED STATES
WHITE EMPLOYED 45–54, BY SEX, MARITAL
STATUS AND YEARS OF SCHOOLING, 1959

Variable by years of schooling	Males indexes (married = 100)			Females indexes (married = 100)		
	Married	Single	Widowed and divorced	Married	Single	Widowed and divorced
Hourly earnings:						
5–8	$2·60	90	81	$1·43	109	97
9–11	2·85	79	81	1·62	111	100
12	3·22	75	78	1·81	113	98
Annual hours:						
5–8	2,044	93	91	1,566	118	108
9–11	2,142	90	95	1,617	119	118
12	2,219	92	91	1,603	124	118
Annual earnings:						
5–8	$5,313	83	74	$2,239	129	104
9–11	6,103	71	77	2,617	132	118
12	7,152	68	71	2,900	141	115

Source: Calculations by author made from [S-4].

strongly affect single men. This may well be a weaker demand for life.

When we compare mortality ratios for widowed and divorced to single by cause of death, the highest ratios are recorded for suicide, motor accidents, cirrhosis of the liver, homicide and lung cancer. These are all causes where a self-destructive behavioral component is very significant. At the other end of the scale, the widowed and divorced death rates come closest to the single for vascular lesions, diabetes, leukemia and aleukemia, and cancer of the digestive organs – all causes in which identified behavioral decisions play a smaller role.

(3) *A Tale of Two States*

A startling illustration of the mortality differentials that can result from differences in way of life can be found in a comparison of Nevada and Utah, two contiguous western states. Infant mortality is 40 per cent higher in Nevada and comparable differentials exist at most other ages for both males and females (see Table 11.8). The

TABLE 11.8

MORTALITY INDEXES AND RELATED
VARIABLES, NEVADA AND UTAH

Part A: Nevada Mortality Indexes
(Utah = 100)

	<1	*1–19*	*20–29*	*30–39*	*40–49*	*50–59*	*60–69*
All causes							
Males	142	116	144	137	154	138	126
Females	135	126	142	148	169	128	117
Cirrhosis of the liver and malignant neoplasms of the respiratory system							
Males				690	211	306	217
Females				543	396	305	327

Part B

	Nevada	*Utah*
Median income	$10,942	$9,356
Physicians per 10,000	11·3	13·8
Per cent rural	19·1	19·4
Paramedicals per 1,000	16·1	18·0
Median schooling	12·4	12·5

Part C

	Nevada	*Utah*
Per cent 20+ born in the state	10	63
Per cent 5+ in same residence 1970 and 1965	36	54
Per cent males 35–64 unmarried or not married to first spouse	47·4	25·5

Sources: Calculations by author made from [S-11], [S-12], [S-18], [S-19].

states are similar in many respects, including availability of medical care, schooling and climate. Income is slightly higher in Nevada. Why, then, the huge differential in mortality?

The most likely answer is that Utah is inhabited primarily by Mormons, who eschew tobacco and alcohol and, in general, lead a quiet, stable life. Nevada, by contrast, is a state with high rates of cigarette and alcohol consumption, and very high indexes of marital instability and geographical mobility.

This comparison points up some confusion in contemporary economic thought about mortality. In an interesting paper, Dan Usher argued that an imputation should be made for increases in life expectancy to be added to the conventional measures of economic growth [11]. If such an adjustment is justified for intertemporal comparisons, it would presumably also be appropriate for cross-section comparisons. According to this view, we should significantly scale down the estimates of real income per capita in Nevada relative to Utah.

But what if the mortality differentials are the result of deliberate, informed choices by all parties concerned? What if Nevadans place a higher value on tobacco and alcohol and a smaller value on longevity than do the people in Utah? Or, to put the matter even more strongly, suppose someone discovers or invents a new activity or a new good which affords a great deal of pleasure but has unfavourable implications for life expectancy? If a substantial number of people avail themselves of the new opportunity, and average life expectancy falls, it would be absurd to say, *ceteris paribus*, that real income has fallen.

There is, however, a case for adjustment for mortality differentials when the differential is attributable to the way income is produced. If the inhabitants of one state have more hazardous occupations, an adjustment would be in order, just as if hours of work were much longer in one state than in the other.

As a practical matter, it is exceedingly difficult to separate consumption patterns from production. Are bartenders heavy drinkers because of their occupation, or do they become bartenders because they like alcohol? Consumption and production are frequently linked and for the present we fall back on the more comprehensive, albeit general, notion of 'way of life'.

V. CONCLUDING COMMENT

At one time, economic growth was both a necessary and sufficient condition for increasing life expectancy. Now it is neither. Although substantial differences in mortality persist within and between developed countries, they are the result, primarily, of differences in the demand for life and the ability to produce life which are un-related to income. A major task for health economists is to gain a better understanding of these demand and production functions.

APPENDIX

Let A =age-specific death rate from causes A
B =age-specific death rate from causes B
$M = A + B$ =age-specific death rate from all causes
a =elasticity of A with respect to income per capita
$b = (a + k)$ =elasticity of B with respect to income per capita
m =elasticity of M with respect to income per capita
$\alpha = A/M$ =share of causes A in total death rate
Y =income per capita
subscript 0 =initial period
$g = Y \div Y_0$

$$m = \alpha a + (1 - \alpha)b \tag{1}$$

$$m(Y) = \frac{\alpha_0 a Y_o^b Y^a + (1 - \alpha_0)b Y_o^a Y^b}{\alpha_0 Y_o^b Y^a + (1 - \alpha_0) Y_o^a Y^b}. \tag{2}$$

This can be rewritten:

$$m(g) = \frac{\alpha_0 a + (1 - \alpha_0)(a + k)g^k}{\alpha_0 + (1 - \alpha_0)g^k}. \tag{3}$$

As income per capita grows, the B cause gets more weight if $k > 0$ and less if $k < 0$. Either way, the entire term becomes less negative or more positive.

If we let $c = A_1 \div A_0$ and $d = B_1 \div B_0$ where A_1 and B_1 are the death rates in period 1, holding income constant but taking account of the shifts, we can rewrite equation (3) to take account of the shifts as follows:

$$m(g, t = 1) = \frac{c\alpha_0 a + d(1 - \alpha_0)(a + k)g^k}{c\alpha_0 + d(1 - \alpha_0)g^k}. \tag{4}$$

REFERENCES

[1] Adelman, Irma, 'An Econometric Analysis of Population Growth', *American Economic Review*, LIII, 3 (June 1963) 314–39.
[2] Auster, Richard, Leveson, Irving, and Sarachek, Deborah, 'The Production of Health; an Exploratory Study', *Journal of Human Resources* (Fall, 1969), reprinted in V. Fuchs (ed.), *Essays in the Economics of Health and Medical Care* (New York: Columbia Univ. Press, for the National Bureau of Economic Research, 1972).
[3] Benjamin, B., *Social and Economic Factors Affecting Mortality* (Paris: Mouton, 1965).

[4] Fuchs, Victor R., 'Some Economic Aspects of Mortality in the United States, mimeo (N.B.E.R., 1965).

[5] ——, and Kramer, Marcia, *Determinants of Expenditures for Physicians' Services in the United States, 1948–68* (Washington: U.S. Government Printing Office, forthcoming).

[6] Grossman, Michael, *The Demand for Health: A Theoretical and Empirical Investigation* (New York: Columbia Univ. Press, for N.B.E.R., 1972).

[7] McDermott, Walsh, 'Demography, Culture, and Economics and the Evolutionary Stages of Medicine', in Edwin D. Kilbourne and Wilson G. Smillie (eds.), *Human Ecology and Public Health*, 4th ed. (London: Collier–Macmillan, 1969).

[8] McKeown, Thomas, and Record, R. G., 'Reasons for the Decline of Mortality in England and Wales during the Nineteenth Century', *Population Studies*, XVI (Nov 1967) 94–122.

[9] Sheps, Mendel C., 'Marriage and Mortality', *American Journal of Public Health*, LI, 4 (1961).

[10] Stolnitz, G. J., 'A Century of International Mortality Trends', *Population Studies*, IX, 1 (1955); X, 1 (1956).

[11] Usher, Dan, 'An Imputation to the Measure of Economic Growth for Changes in Life Expectancy', N.B.E.R. Conference on Research in Income and Wealth, 4–6 Nov 1971.

SOURCES FOR TABLES AND FIGURES

[S-1] Central Bureau of Statistics of Norway, *Statistical Yearbook of Norway*, 1969.

[S-2] Clark, Colin, *The Conditions of Economic Progress* (London: Macmillan, 1960).

[S-3] U.S. Department of Commerce, Bureau of the Census, *U.S. Census of Population*, 1960, vol. I, part 1.

[S-4] U.S. Department of Commerce, Bureau of the Census, *U.S. Census of Population and Housing, 1960*, 1/1000 sample.

[S-5] U.S. Department of Commerce, Bureau of the Census, *Vital Statistics of the U.S.*, 1937, 1938.

[S-6] U.S. Department of Commerce, Bureau of the Census, *Vital Statistics Rates in the U.S., 1900–1940* (U.S. Government Printing Office, 1943).

[S-8] U.S. Department of Commerce, Office of Business Economics, *Personal Income by States since 1929* (Washington, D.C., 1956).

[S-9] U.S. Department of Health, Education and Welfare, National Center for Health Statistics, 'Mortality from Selected Causes by Marital Status, United States', part A, *Vital and Health Statistics*, series 20, no. 8A (Rockville, Md., Dec 1970).

[S-10] U.S. Department of Health, Education and Welfare, Public Health Service, *Vital Statistics of the U.S.*, 1959, 1960, 1961, vol. II: *Mortality*.

[S-11] U.S. Department of Health, Education and Welfare, Public Health Service, *Vital Statistics of the United States*, 1964, 1965, 1966, vol. II: *Mortality*.

[S-12] U.S. Department of Health, Education and Welfare, Public Health Service, *Vital Statistics of the United States*, 1967, 1968, vol. II: *Mortality*.

[S-13] U.S. Department of Health, Education and Welfare, Public Health Service, *Vital Statistics of the U.S.*, 1968, vol. II, Section 5, Life Tables.

[S-14] Kilpatrick, S. J., 'Occupational Mortality Indices', *Population Studies*, XVI, 2 (Nov 1962).
[S-15] *Statistical Abstract of Sweden*, 1971.
[S-16] United Nations, *Demographic Yearbook*, 1967, 1966, 1957, 1951.
[S-17] United Nations, *Statistical Yearbook*, 1967.
[S-18] American Medical Association, Department of Survey Research, *Distribution of Physicians in the United States, 1970* (Chicago, 1971).
[S-19] U.S. Department of Commerce, Bureau of the Census, *Census of Population, 1970*, U.S. Summary, *General Social and Economic Characteristics* and *Detailed Characteristics*, vol. 30 (Nevada), vol. 46 (Utah).

Summary Record of Discussion

This session returned to the three-disparate-paper format of the second session. The papers discussed were by Drs Newhouse and Phelps on the price and income elasticities of demand for medical services, by Professor Evans on supplier-induced demand for these services, and by Professor Fuchs on mortality rates in advanced countries. The first two papers were considerably more technical and quantitative than most of those considered previously.

A. *Drs Newhouse and Phelps's paper.*[1]
Dr Grossman introduced and criticized the Newhouse–Phelps paper, which he considered an excellent example of a small-scale model estimated from household data for a group of related decisions. It extends his own work and model of demand for health and medical service by allowing for separate inputs and health production functions for several types of medical service. It treats the role of health insurance in a novel way, by viewing it as endogenous to its own expected utilization, and using details of insurance arrangements to compute relevant coinsurance rates for different demand functions. It analyzes variations in the nominal prices of health care services between individuals, allowing, for example, for the fact that a visit to a specialist is more expensive than a visit to a general practitioner. It treats the prices of different sorts of care as endogenous, and as products of search processes. It derives empirical demand curve for hospital care (various lengths), for office visits and for outpatient care, using more data than has been available to previous students. Fortunately for mainstream economics, most theoretical anticipations are borne out by the results.

Dr Grossman went on to develop three criticisms and qualifications:

1. The paper argues that higher wages should make the demand for medical care less elastic.[2] It is true that a given degree of medical care forms a smaller part of the consumers' budget as his wage rate rises, but another consumer cost (in addition to money) is his own time. An hour of his time becomes more, not less, valuable as wages rise, so that the conventional effect on elasticity is to some extent, counteracted.

2. Drs Newhouse and Phelps use the losses from an initial hypothetical 'stock of health' as variables in their demand functions, whereas Grossman would himself prefer the flow of depreciation on a 'health, variable'; the Newhouse–Phelps variable also relates to actual health, which is an endogenous variable in the system. Of course, it is prob-

---

[1] This paper appears in a reduced version; the condensations do not affect the trenchancy of the comments.

[2] Dr Grossman amplified his remark by stressing that 'the share of medical care would fall only if the elasticity and substitution between medical care at the own time if the consumer in the production of health were less than 1. Moreover, a reduction in the share of medical care would lower the wage elasticity only if the price elasticity of demand for health exceeded the elasticity of substitution in production between medical care and own time.

ably not possible to measure the depreciation rate, which Dr. Grossman had associated with age.

3. While wage income has its expected positive effect upon the demand for health in the Newhouse–Phelps model, non-wage income seems to have no significant effect at all. This result may be due to measurement error, but Dr Grossman believed it was a statistical artefact. There seems to be a positive correlation between wage and non-wage income, but greater variance in the non-wage component. In multiple regression analysis, this results in the entire weight being put on the wage income variable and almost none on the non-wage income variable.

Dr Newhouse was unable to attend the Conference, so that only *Dr Phelps* replied to these comments. He agreed that the stock of health is related to health status; in fact, age is expected to be a proxy for the systematic component of health stock and health state for the more variable remainder. Very crudely, then, health stock is a compound of age and the state of health.

Dr Phelps also discussed future research plans, which involved an extension to a larger sample, including non-employed people. This change, he believed, would result in a greater stress on non-wage income.

Dr Friedman suggested that the Newhouse–Phelps model does not allow for dynamic changes, i.e. for the fact that a visit to a doctor or a hospital may be a part of a longer program. He found in the model no allowance for preventive care, or for building up health 'reserves' against future strain. Perhaps, he thought, the model might move in these directions. *Dr. Phelps* thought it impossible to dynamize in this way on the basis of his data, or to distinguish one motivation from another.

Professor Intriligator had compared the numerical values of the Newhouse–Phelps elasticities with those obtained by his colleagues and himself. He found the two sets of values 'in the same ball park' if one considered only his own results for *surgery*; the results for *medicine* were higher. The Phelps–Newhouse income elasticity was positive, however, while his own was negative; in the special case of outpatient services, also, the two results were quite inconsistent with each other. *Dr Phelps* felt that his own results were generally lower than Intriligator's with regard to both price and income elasticity estimates. He could not explain the inconsistencies out of hand, but pointed out that the two studies were based on completely different samples.

Mr Kaser objected to the Newhouse–Phelps model's stress on price, which enters at every point. In many public schemes there is no price or cost. He also did not see why one should always have a coinsurance rate (whose size varies with the patient's stock of health), and wondered whether the patient's education might not be an additional variable in his demand for health.

Dr Davis pointed out that, while the original Newhouse–Phelps sample included some 7,800 cases, exclusions lowered its size to 122 for hospital care, 842 for medical care and 246 for outpatient care; perhaps bias was introduced here. As a second caveat, she said the study fails to consider people not already in the health care system. That is to say, it does not consider original decisions to seek medical or hospital assistance. Neither does it consider substitutions among medical, hospital and outpatient care in any satisfactory way. Cross-elasticities are computed, but only some sort of average price is used for the service not used, whereas the actual price is estimated for the service actually employed.[1] Finally, the model's predictive power seems weak, as measured by the coefficients of multiple correlation.

Dr Phelps replied to both these comments simultaneously. His reply to Mr Kaser stressed the point that insurance rates are endogenous in the Newhouse–Phelps model and not given in advance. They can therefore work out to be zero in public systems. As for the several Davis objections, he said that while the sample will be expanded for future studies, past reductions in sample size represented attempts to standardize for quality, and that the correlation was not at all bad when one considers that each observation is related to a single consumer unit rather than to a larger group.

Dr Friedman believed that care for dependants responded to price changes to a greater extent than care for family heads, and that an employee normally has little choice in the nature of the insurance package secured on his behalf by his employer. *Dr Grossman* replied (primarily to Dr Friedman's earlier interpellation) that preventive medicine was eligible for inclusion in the observations. He went on to argue that the health stock included the results of past investment in health, and that the method used in the model was much like that used for physical capital and for many types of human capital unrelated to health.

Mme Sandier inquired whether the Newhouse–Phelps model, had it been available earlier, could have been used to forecast the results of the Medicare and Medicaid programs in the United States.

Professor Rosett said that Drs Newhouse and Phelps had allowed for quality differences by the distinction between general practitioners and specialists. This was good as far as it went, but ignored variations within particular specialties. Furthermore, he felt that in any investment model the effect of non-wage (i.e. investment) income must be of some importance. Otherwise the results are hardly believable, as is the case here.

B. *Professor Evans's paper*[2]
Dr Kehrer, introducing the paper, felt that its purpose was to develop the implications of the dual role of the physician as both the patient's agent and the supplier of services to him. There is, thus, a certain conflict of interest, especially in a private system; it is more serious in medicine than in other professions, because of the patient's higher degree of ignorance.

---

[1] *Dr Phelps*, in a postscript, believes Dr Davis misunderstands the Phelps argument: the cross-elasticities in question are computed from each consumer's coinsurance rate *times* the price of outpatient care (the average price being used only if no outpatient care was actually purchased). Hence, the own-price and cross-price variables are conceptually identical.

[2] The paper was printed in a revised form; the intent to protect the trenchancy of the commentator's views was manifest.

This means that the medical care market cannot be divided neatly into demand and supply sides; rather, supply influences demand and prices no longer signal exogenous shifts in demand or in supply alone. However, Professor Evans's numerical results suggest that demand can still be treated as (almost) exogenous.[1] At least, the results of such treatment are more plausible than those of a rival model, which uses a target income for the physician achieved by generating demand. (Demand generation is not a desired or approved activity for physicians.) But there is still some ambiguity as to the meaning of exogenous shifts in supply: are they 'really' exogenous, or the result of physicians' operations on the demand side?

The empirical hypothesis which forms the basis of Professor Evans's study is the relationship between physicians' workloads and the density of practicing physicians in various areas of British Columbia. If there were an inverse relationship, then the conflict of interest would not be significant. Actually, 'weak negative effects from density to workload' are 'consistent with the hypothesis that physicians can generate enough activity to insulate their workload against supply shifts', but do not, in fact, do so since the effects concerned are so weak.

Dr Kehrer went on to make a number of critical comments upon the paper:

1. The assumption of conflict of interest may be valid only in the short run. In the longer term, demand generation by a physician may induce patient distrust of his advice.
2. There are probably limits to whatever demand generation is possible, but the Evans's paper assumes there are none.
3. Professor Evans's empirical analysis uses an equilibrium model, which *assumes*, but does not prove, the absence of any overall excess demand for physicians' services.
4. Professor Evans does not measure the physician's workload directly, but uses his income as a proxy. But the physician's income will reflect his product mix, and variations in product mix, with workload constant, may account for observed differentials in physicians' incomes. In fact, however, it might be better to use income instead of workload as the stated dependent variable.
5. Income data may be influenced by price changes, and the price of these services may be influenced by such relations as (alternatives):
   (i) urbanization leading to higher cost of living and larger demand for medical care, which combine to cause high medical incomes; *or*
   (ii) greater concentration of doctors leading to demand generation, which leads to high medical incomes.
6. If there is a target-income system, the choice of target value is now exogenous. It may even vary, via the emulation process, with physician density.
7. Professor Evans uses the terms 'low' and 'high' without adequate explanation.
8. Professor Evans confines any allowance for heterogeneity within his model by dealing only with different age classes of the population, but heterogeneity may have nothing to do with age.

[1] *Professor Evans* disclaims any such inference.

9. Professor Evans believes that the fact that physician-initiated medical services have increased faster than patient-initiated ones is evidence of demand generation. But this may be only the result, assuming it to be true, of technical changes in the mix of services available.

10. Is not the malpractice suit by the disgruntled patient (or his heirs) an important omitted variable?

In his reply, *Professor Evans* stressed the specifics of Canadian practice and data. Under the British Columbia system, the individual physician cannot set the prices of his services. Therefore, the exigencies of pricing set no limits on the British Columbia physician's demand generation, and income can be used as a measure of workload. The British Columbia system does not produce the statistical data required to test Dr Kehrer's hypotheses about conflict between the long-run and short-run motivations of physicians, about the possible variability of target incomes by areas within British Columbia, or about the effects of variations of individual physicians' mixes of service. Education would not appear a significant determinant of consumers' demand for physicians' services, and malpractice suits are not 'big business' anywhere in Canada as they are in some parts of the United States. The great attraction of the target-income model, however, is a simplistic one. It corresponds with what physicians tell us they are doing.

Professor Sloan expressed the view that Evans's results were not surprising, whether or not one recognized any significant conflict of interest within the physician's decision-making process. His regressions are probably correct, and the results confirm those of similar work he (Sloan) has done himself. However, the study does not yield many results useful for policy-makers. How are targets set? How are they policed against price-cutting? Should there be more physicians? Should they be directed where to practice their profession? We need different tests which could distinguish more directly between supply-created demand and the more ordinary phenomenon of excess demand.

Professor Fuchs then suggested that physicians' services not be treated quite so aggregatively as in the Evans model. He (Fuchs) believed there was a quite ordinary excess demand for house calls (with no 'stimulation' by the physician himself), but at the same time the services of some types of surgeons were in excess supply.

Dr Kleiman wondered whether the problem of supply-induced demand for physicians' services did not have counterparts in many other professions regulated by various forms of professional ethics. (Answer by *Professor Evans*: The force of professional ethics – the Oath of Hippocrates – is stronger in medicine than are similar rules in other professions.) Dr Kleiman also wondered whether the incomes of patients, as well as of physicians, should not be considered as important causative factors in the Evans model, particularly in considering physician density. (Answer: Overall income levels did not seem important in fitting regressions for the province of Saskatchewan.)

M. Foulon noted a rapid rise in consultation and teaching by physicians rather than in house calls, and felt that the substitution involved higher overall costs to consumers of medical care. He agreed with Professor Evans that supply is leading and influencing demand in a kind of feedback relation. Such feedback relations, however, are not uncommon in the service industries; they should always be taken into account in forecasting future demands for services. He (Foulon) was looking for a usable answer to the general question of how public policy could best influence physicians' behavior.

Professor Lévy felt that the division of physicians into general practitioners and specialists was less relevant for most purposes than a division into innovators and traditionalists. He also hoped this could be investigated with special reference to physicians' widely varying choices as to the particular innovations they press for and are willing to accept.

C. *Professor Fuchs's paper*

Professor L. Lave retitled the paper 'Mortality Parables', and traced through a number of the problems collected by Professor Fuchs in his paper. He agreed that Professor Fuchs had opened up an interesting set of factors, but was uneasy at the number of 'uncontrolled factors' involved in many of the Fuchs relations, which related only two variables at a time and did not employ a formal model.

Professor Fuchs felt that, while Professor Lave had summarized his individual points and conclusions correctly, he had somehow missed the spirit of the paper as a whole. He maintained that, in developed countries, income no longer has its presumptive effect on mortality. (This is something new, and addition of additional variables to his regressions will not change it.) In dealing with the effects of medical care on mortality, Professor Fuchs felt one must distinguish between movements along a given curve relating medical care to mortality and shifts in that curve. He reasserted his belief that, while the marginal contribution of more medical care (of the same kind) is now small, it may have been important in 1930–60; what matters is shifts in the curve as a result of technical improvements of various sorts. Another factor which makes a difference is one's choice of life-styles; here Professor Fuchs cited the two neighboring American states of strait-laced Utah and wide-open Nevada. (Utah has the higher life expectancy, Nevada the higher mortality rate.) Should the government, in this last sort of situation, intervene, concentrating medical care in Nevada to the neglect of Utah until the two life expectancies were approximately equal? He himself thought the 'equality of outcomes' version of marginal analysis decidedly out of place in this context.

Professor J. Lave discussed the effects of income levels on infant mortality rates specifically. She felt that both income levels and the number of physicians practicing affect the results in individual S.M.S.A.s, but that the differences wash out, somehow, in larger areas. The conventional causality is still working, but only in micro-measures. *Professor Fuchs* wondered how much of Professor J. Lave's income effects (within individual S.M.S.A.s) were not actually racial, and recalled the agreement in his paper that higher incomes reduce mortality at sufficiently low initial income levels.

Professor Atkinson believed that some of Professor Fuchs's results may have been biased, in so far as they were based on reports by widows and other survivors, of patients' incomes and social classes. He said widows, in particular, tended to locate their late husbands higher on both social and economic scales than a more objective report might have done.

Dr Grossman suggested that the differential life expectancy of married over single, widowed or divorced men was concentrated in those diseases over whose progress the patient himself has some degree of control, e.g. by moderation of his eating, drinking and smoking habits.

Urbanization, in addition to income, is an important mortality-rate determinant, according to *Dr Hartwell*. Another related variable is occupational. Perhaps the occupational mix has shifted in recent years in the direction of more high-mortality occupations.

Commenting upon the recent upturn in mortality rates, *Dr Friedman* felt this was due largely to 'self-destructive behavior', such as addictions, which are less important among married persons. Passing to policy, Dr Friedman questioned the wisdom of permitting people to indulge themselves in self-destructive behavior, and also added that, in some cases, this behavior may be due to frustrations. Among the world's frustrations are many traceable to income or wealth inequality. (*Professor Machlup* pointed out at this stage that divorce, in particular, may be either the cause or the effect of some self-destructive behavior.)

Professor J. Lave reminded the audience that epidemiologists know more than do economists about why people die, and that their knowledge of the causes of death has improved over the years. What economists call income is no longer as good a surrogate for long-term and non-specific causes of death as it once may have been, and the real issue may be to find and measure actual variables rather than mere surrogates. These may be found in personal habits and life-styles, but the evidence for extreme 'self-destruction' theories is not good. What other speakers have called 'self-destruction' is largely a matter of a short-run attitude toward one's health, and not self-destruction in anything like a suicidal sense.

Dr Christiansen expressed his personal view that policy should concentrate on keeping single males alive through the crises of their middle years. Divorce and widowhood, he said, need not be permanent for either sex in the age group 45–54. He also questioned the attribution of death in some cases in some countries; what is reported as accidental or apoplectic death may be due to alcoholism, venereal disease or suicide.

Professor Fuchs and *M. Dupuy* continued the discussion of the Fuchs paper with a brief exchange. Professor Fuchs claimed that many people no longer place great value on long life *per se*. He did not know whether this change was exogenous or endogenous to either the medical or the economic system, and doubted that anyone else knew either. M. Dupuy wondered what the use of marginal health expenditures might be if Professor Fuchs were correct, and received the reply that patients want 'care, not cure', meaning (in sociological terms) social identity and validation as well as comfort and companionship.

Professor Liefmann-Keil raised two hypotheses relative to the greater life expectancies of the female sex and of married persons generally. She said that women use medical care more readily than men, and wondered whether this might not explain lower female mortality rates. She also wondered whether the lower mortality of the married might not rather be related to the size of their households (referring particularly to the number of generations in the household). The social system, she thought, might be responsible for smaller and fewer-generation households, and thus, perhaps, for lower life expectancies. *Professor Fuchs* was skeptical on both counts. For some reason not covered by the Liefmann-Keil interpellation, the female one-person household lives longer (relative to females generally) than does the male one-person household relative to all males. One cannot rule out a biological theory of the lower female death rate, but its effects, if any, are probably modified in modern society by sex differentiations of activity.

Dr Kleiman inquired whether there might be some inverse correlation between infant mortality rates and mortality at higher age groups, reflecting, perhaps, different concentrations of medical expenditure and, perhaps, the survival beyond infancy of physically weak individuals. *Professor Fuchs* replied that there was some evidence of such correlation, but only at very advanced ages.

Returning to the Liefmann–Keil question of sexual differentiation in mortality rates, *Professor J. Lave* said that her hypothesis will be tested in the near future, as the result of the greater professionalization of women. *Professor Evans* felt that results from the Teachers' Insurance and Annuity Association in the United States indicate thus far that professionalization is making little difference.

Final comments were now made, closing the session, by the authors of each of the papers presented. *Dr Phelps* addressed himself to the question whether health care demand estimates for 1963, such as he and Dr Newhouse had used, would hold today, after substantial changes in the American medical system. He felt that they would remain valid for movements along the demand function, but that there might have been shifts in the entire curve. The results of additional studies, he said, would be forthcoming soon.

Professor Evans undertook to answer the question: what might medical economists usefully tell policy-makers? For one thing, that demand estimates will vary with the specifications imposed by different researchers and investigators. For another, that incentives to consumers will not operate to reduce shortages, because physicians may be expected to work against them. Neither, for the same reason, can they be eliminated by providing more doctors. There is, of course, some evidence of long-term technical change, but technical change seemed to Professor Evans a frail reed to rely upon for avoidance of his pessimistic outlook. *Professor Fuchs*, in lieu of restating his own position on his own paper, closed the discussion by suggesting that policy-makers decide how they desire physicians to behave and then adjust economic constraints accordingly.

Part Three

The Impact of Demand for Health Services

12 Health, Hours and Wages[1]

Michael Grossman and Lee Benham

NATIONAL BUREAU OF ECONOMIC RESEARCH, NEW YORK

This paper has two purposes. The first is to obtain structural health parameters in wage and labor supply function based on a completely specified model of the determination of these two variables. The second is to examine how the estimated effects of health on labor market behavior are altered when health is made an endogenous variable. We hypothesize that an increase in health should raise market productivity, measured by the wage rate, and should also increase the amount of time available for work in the market. Health, it- self, should respond in a positive fashion to increases in variables associated with efficiency of production within the household, such as schooling, and to increases in utilization of market goods which enter into the production of good health. We examine three variables related to the level of medical utilization: physicians per capita in the county of residence; health insurance coverage; and utilization of preventive medical services.

I. INTRODUCTION

Several recent studies have indicated that health has significant effects on labor supply and wage rates (Greenberg and Kosters, 1970; Boskin, 1971; Fleisher, 1971; Hall, 1971; Luft, 1972). Although these studies have increased our understanding of the role of health in the labor market, they have not estimated health parameters in the context of fully specified structural equations for labor supply and wage determination. Moreover, they all treat health as an exogenous variable, whereas previous work by Grossman (1972a, 1972b)

[1] Research for this paper was supported by P.H.S. Grant No. 5 P01 HS00451 and by P.H.S. Grant No. HS00080 from the National Center for Health Services Research and Development. We should like to thank Ronald Andersen for generously making the data available for this study; Yoram Ben-Porath, Barry Chiswick, Linda Nasif Edwards, Lee Lillard and Jacob Mincer for helpful comments and suggestions; and Phyllis Goldberg, Harold Pashner and Janice Platt for diligent research assistance. This paper is not an official National Bureau of Economic Research publication, since the findings reported have not yet undergone the full critical review accorded the National Bureau's studies, including approval of the Board of Directors.

suggests that health, itself, is an endogenous variable. Luft (1972) confines his entire analysis to reduced-form health effects. Greenberg and Kosters (1970) and Fleisher (1971) use the observed wage rate to estimate the labor supply function. Since there are likely to be errors of measurement in this wage variable, its regression coefficient and the coefficients of variables that are correlated with the true wage rate, such as health, would be biased.[1] Boskin (1971) and Hall (1971) use instrumental variables, including health, to estimate the wage, but exclude health from their labor supply equations.

This paper has two purposes. The first is to obtain structural health parameters based on a completely specified model of the determination of wages and hours of work. The second is to examine how the estimated effects of health on labor market behavior are altered when health is made an endogenous variable. The household production function approach to demand theory (Becker, 1965; Lancaster, 1966; Muth, 1966; Michael and Becker, 1973; Ghez and Becker, 1972; Michael, 1972) serves as the point of departure for both out two-equation model (wage and hours of work endogenous) and our three-equation model (wage, hours and health endogenous). This approach assumes that consumers produce their basic objects of choice with inputs of market goods and their own time. Within the context of the household production function framework, wage rates depend on investments in various forms of human capital, health depends on the resources that the household allocates to its production, and the amount of time supplied to the market depends on the amount of time demanded for non-market, or household, production. Clearly, observed wage rates, hours of work and health reflect a set of interrelated decisions made by the household.

In its most complete version, our specific model consists of a wage-generating function, a supply curve of hours of work in the market, and a health function. The health function contains variables that affect both the demand for health and the production of health. It is hypothesized that an increase in health should raise market productivity, measured by the wage rate, and should also increase the amount of time available for work in the market. Health, itself, should respond in a positive fashion to increases in variables associated with efficiency of production within the household, such as schooling, and to increases in utilization of market goods which enter into the production of good health. Three variables are examined which are related to the level of medical utilization: physicians per capita in the county of residence, health insurance coverage, and utilization of preventive medical services. Section II of this paper describes the data

---

[1] Special problems arise when the wage is computed from data on earnings and hours. For a discussion of this point, see section III.

source that is used to estimate the model and discusses the measurement of the endogenous variables. Section III outlines the model, and section IV presents the results of estimation by two-stage least squares.

II. DATA AND MEASUREMENT OF ENDOGENOUS VARIABLES

The data source that is employed to estimate the model is the 1963 health interview survey conducted by the National Opinion Research Center and the Center for Health Administration Studies of the University of Chicago. The N.O.R.C. sample is an area probability sample of the civilian non-institutionalized population of the United States in which each family had the same probability of inclusion. Data were obtained from 2,367 families, comprising 7,803 persons.[1]

The empirical analysis is restricted to white males who were at least 18 years old, had completed their formal schooling and did not reside on farms.[2] The sample size of this group is 1,228. Many of the estimates are limited to the subsample of this group, comprised of men with positive earnings in 1963. The sample size of this group, termed the labor force in the subsequent analysis, is 1,049. These subsamples are used because more is known about the factors affecting the earnings and labor force behavior of white males than is the case for other groups in the population. Moreover, by examining only white males we avoid problems associated with low labor force participation rates of married women, discrimination against nonwhites and women, and variations in the true parameters of the earnings and labor supply functions among groups in the population.[3]

The number of weeks worked in 1963, the weekly wage rate and an index of ill-health are the empirical proxies for the endogenous variables in the model. The number of weeks worked is used as the sole measure of labor supply, since the sample contains no information on the number of hours worked per week. The weeks worked variable includes paid vacation time, but specifically excludes sick time, even if the respondent was paid for it.[4] The weekly wage rate is computed as annual earnings in 1963 divided by weeks worked, since the sample does not contain a direct measure of the wage rate.

---

[1] For a complete description of the sample, see Andersen and Anderson (1967).

[2] The sample is described in more detail in section (1) of the appendix.

[3] For evidence that these parameters do differ among groups, see, for example, Mincer (1962), Heckman (1971), Leibowitz (1972) and Smith (1972).

[4] In this respect, the N.O.R.C. weeks worked variable is a better measure of labor supply than weeks worked reported in the Census of Population and the Survey of Economic Opportunity. Both these data sources include paid sick time in weeks worked.

Two measures of self-evaluation of health status are included in the data: (1) the number of symptoms which individuals reported having, from a checklist of twenty common symptoms,[1] and (2) individuals' self-evaluation of their general health as excellent, good, fair or poor. To incorporate the independent information contained in each of these variables, a composite index of ill-health (IH) has been constructed through principal components analysis of four variables: the number of symptoms reported (S) and three health status dummy variables (HS_1, HS_2 and HS_3), where $HS_1 = 1$ if health status is good, fair or poor; $HS_2 = 1$ if health status is fair or poor; $HS_3 = 1$ if health status is poor. The index is defined as the first principal component of these four variables when they are normalized to have zero means and unitary standard deviations.[2]

Note that IH is a negative health index, so that an increase in it will be associated with a reduction in health. Note, also, that the scaling scheme dictated by the principal components analysis is essentially arbitrary. Therefore, the estimated effects of IH on wages and weeks and the effects of variables in the health function on IH are fundamentally qualitative in nature rather than quantitative.

III. THE MODEL

(1) *Structural Equations*

The three-equation model consists of a wage-generating function, a supply curve of weeks worked and a health function. These three structural equations are as follows:[3]

$$LNWAGE = a_1IH^* + a_2SCH + a_3EXP + a_4EXPSQ + a_5UNION + a_6SOUTH + a_7SMSA + a_8OCITY \qquad (1)$$

---

[1] Examples of the symptoms included are persistent cough, swelling in joints, frequent backaches, unexplained loss of weight and repeated pains in or near the heart.

[2] That is, the characteristic vector associated with the largest characteristic root of the correlation matrix of these four variables provides a set of weights to aggregate the four variables into an index of ill-health. The actual index is

$$IH = 0 \cdot 5242s + 0 \cdot 4264hs_1 + 0 \cdot 5567hs_2 + 0 \cdot 4833hs_3$$

where lower-case letters refer to normalized variables. The weights used maximize the variance of IH, subject to the constraint that, if they are squared and then added, this sum must be equal to 1. The mean number of symptoms for men in each of the four health status categories is as follows: excellent, 0·98; good, 1·75; fair, 3·34; poor, 6·25. For a more complete discussion of the relationship between symptoms and health status, see section (1) of the appendix, esp. Table A.2.

[3] Intercepts are not shown. An asterisk next to a variable means it is endogenous. Table 12.1 defines all variables, and Table A.1 in the appendix gives their means and standard deviations.

$$LNWEEK = b_1 LNWAGE^* + b_2 IH^* + b_3 EXP + b_4 SOUTH + b_5 SMSA$$
$$+ b_6 OCITY + b_7 MAR + b_8 KIDLE6 + b_9 OTINC \qquad (2)$$

$$IH = c_1 LNWAGE^* + c_2 SCH + c_3 EXP + c_4 OTINC + c_5 MAR$$
$$+ c_6 MD + c_7 LLPRE + c_8 POLIO + c_9 GI + c_{10} NGI. \qquad (3)$$

In the two-equation model, health is treated as exogenous, and only equations (1) and (2) are estimated. The two-equation model is referred to as Model 1, and the three-equation model is referred to as Model 2 from now on.

TABLE 12.1

DEFINITION OF VARIABLES

Variable	Definition
LNWAGE	Natural logarithm of weekly wage
LNWEEK	Natural logarithm of weeks worked
IH	Index of ill-health
SCH	Years of schooling completed
EXP	Years of experience in the labor force
EXPSQ	Square of years of experience
UNION	Union member = 1
SOUTH	Reside in South = 1
$SMSA^a$	Reside in one of ten largest S.M.S.A.s = 1
$OCITY^a$	Reside in a city other than ten largest S.M.S.A's = 1
MAR	Married = 1
KIDLE6	Youngest person in family under six years old = 1
OTINC	Non-earnings income of the family adjusted for individual's years of experience
MD	Doctors per capita in county of residence
LLPRE	Length of time in months since person had a physical exam because he thought it was time to have an exam, or because the exam was required in order to get a job or a life insurance policy
POLIO	Polio vaccine received = 1
GI	Covered under group health insurance = 1
NGI	Covered under non-group health insurance = 1

[a] Omitted class in residence is a rural non-farm area.

(2) *Wage-Generating Function*

The wage generating function is based on the definitive work on wage determination by Mincer (1970, 1972). Using the theory of investment in human capital, he shows that the natural logarithm of annual earnings or the natural logarithms of the weekly wage rate should be positively related to investment in formal schooling, measured by years of schooling completed,[1] and to investment in on-the-job

[1] Mincer proves that, under certain conditions, the regression coefficient of schooling in equation (1) can be interpreted as the rate of return to an investment in formal schooling.

training, measured by years of experience in the labor market.[1] Mincer's model predicts that the amount invested in on-the-job training should decline over the life-cycle. Therefore, the wage–experience profile should be concave to the origin, and the square of years of experience should have a negative regression coefficient in the wage function.

Our wage equation adds health to Mincer's basic set of human capital variables. Health capital, as one component of human capital, should raise market productivity and the wage rate. Therefore, the regression coefficient of *IH* in equation (1) should be negative. A second reason for expecting a positive health effect is that experience is imperfectly measured in the sample. Suppose that current and past health are positively correlated. Then, if poor health reduces the amount of time spent in the labor market, the health variable might reflect, to some extent, past investment in on-the-job training.

Our wage equation contains several variables, in addition to health, that are not considered by Mincer. These are dummy variables for residence and, membership in a labor union. The wage equation should relate the *real* wage rate to human capital variables. It is well known that the cost of living is not the same in all parts of the United States. It is lower in the South than in other regions, lower in rural areas than in cities, and higher in large cities than in small cities. Consequently, all other things being equal, the regression coefficient of *SOUTH* should be negative, and the coefficients of *SMSA* and *OCITY* should be positive.[2] Finally, there is considerable evidence that labor unions raise wage rates. Therefore, the regression coefficient of *UNION* should be positive.

[1] There is no direct measure of years of experience in the sample. Therefore, we use Mincer's procedure (1972, Table 1) of computing this variable as current age minus an independent estimate of age at entry into the labor market by years of schooling completed. This is similar to, although not identical with, a definition of experience as current age minus years of schooling completed minus age, say six years, at the beginning of schooling.

[2] Let w be the money wage rate, p be an index of the cost of living and x be a vector of exogenous variables in the wage equation.
Then
$$\ln (w/p) = ax$$
or
$$\ln w = ax + \ln p.$$

Let an equation for the cost of living be
$$\ln p = d_1 SOUTH + d_2 SMSA + d_3 OCITY$$

where $d_1 < 0$, $d_2 > 0$ and $d_3 > 0$. Substitution of the cost of living equation into the wage equation gives
$$\ln w = ax + d_1 SOUTH + d_2 SMSA + d_3 OCITY.$$

(3) *Supply Curve of Weeks Worked*

The supply curve of weeks worked is derived from the household production function model of consumer behavior.[1] In this model, consumers produce the commodities that enter their utility functions with inputs of market goods and their own time. An increase in the wage rate raises the price of non-market time and generates a substitution effect in favour of the time spent in the market.[2] There is also an income effect associated with an increase in the wage rate. This should increase consumption of commodities and the derived demand for non-market time. Therefore, the sign of the coefficient in the supply curve of weeks worked is ambiguous.[3] It would be positive if the substitution effect outweighed the income effect and negative if the reverse were true.

The preceding analysis pertains to changes in the real wage rate. Therefore, the three residence dummy variables are included in the supply curve to control for differences in the cost of living. With money wage rates held constant, residents in the South, for example, should have higher real wage rates. If the substitution effect dominates, then they should supply more weeks to the market.

An increase in property income exerts a 'pure' income effect on labor supply that should lower the number of weeks worked.[4] Difficulties arise in measuring this effect, because observed non-earnings income might be an endogenous variable that depends on weeks worked. In the context of a model of life-cycle labor supply, consider the effects of variations in preferences for future consumption among otherwise identical individuals. Those with relatively strong preferences for future consumption would spend more time at work and would have more savings in the current period than others. This

---

[1] Many previous studies have used this model to derive labor supply functions. See, for example, Becker (1965), Heckman (1971), Ghez and Becker (1972), Leibowitz (1972) and Smith (1972).

[2] This substitution effect has two components. The first consists of substitution of goods for time in the production of commodities. The second consists of substitution in consumption away from 'time-intensive' commodities (those whose production requires relatively large amounts of the consumer's time).

[3] Since the supply curve relates the logarithm of weeks worked to the logarithm of the weekly wage, the wage coefficient is an elasticity. The logarithm of the weekly wage is used because Mincer's work indicates that this is the relevant form of the dependent variable in the wage function. The logarithm of weeks worked is used for convenience.

[4] By a pure income effect, we mean an income effect due to a change in income that is not accompanied by a change in the value of time. Property income would be positively related to the value of time for people who are not in the labor force. For such individuals, an increase in property income would raise the ratio of market goods to consumption time, the marginal product of consumption time, and its 'shadow price'.

would tend to create a positive relationship between property income (return on assets) and weeks worked.[1] A factor that goes in the opposite direction is that the *NORC* non-earnings income variable includes transfer payments as well as property income. An increase in the number of weeks worked should reduce such payments.

In theory, the most appropriate variable for measuring the pure income effect is property income that accrues to initial (inherited) assets. Since this variable is not available in the data, the non-earnings income variable ($OTINC$)[2] in the supply function is adjusted for experience. If $OTINCR_k$ is reported non-earnings income of someone who completed k years of formal schooling, then

$$OTINC_k = OTINCR_k + \alpha_k(21 - EXP)$$

where 21 is the mean number of years of experience in the sample and where α_k is estimated from a regression of $OTINCR_k$ on EXP by years of schooling completed.[3] This adjustment raises non-earnings income for people with fewer than 21 years of experience and lowers it for people with more than 21 years. It should reduce, although not completely eliminate, the dependence of non-earnings income on weeks worked.

Previous estimates of labor supply functions have included age, marital status and family composition, either as standardizing variables or as variables that measure relative non-market productivity of various groups. In the context of a life-cycle model of labor supply, if the rate of interest is positive, then consumption of commodities and time spent producing these commodities should rise with age.[4] Since students spend little or no time in the market, the life-cycle allocation of working time should be more closely related to experience than to age. The coefficient of experience in equation (2) should be negative. It is often argued that women are relatively more productive in the household than men.[5] Therefore, married men should reallocate their time in favor of the market, and the coefficient of the marital status dummy variable should be positive. Leibowitz (1972)

---

[1] For more complete discussion of this point, see Greenberg (1972) and Smith (1972).

[2] The arithmetic value of this variable, rather than its logarithm, is employed because it is often equal to zero.

[3] Regressions were run for three schooling groups: 0 to 8 years of formal schooling completed, 9 to 12, and 13 and over. The procedure for adjusting non-earnings income for experience is based on a method used by Michael (1971).

[4] More formally, consumption would rise with age if the rate of interest exceeded the rate of time preference for the present. For a proof, see Ghez and Becker (1972).

[5] See, for example, Mincer (1962), Becker (1973) and Leibowitz (1972).

and Smith (1972) propose that the presence of small children in the household raises the wife's relative non-market productivity and should cause a substitution of her non-market time for her husband's. This suggests that the coefficient of the dummy variable *KIDLE6*, which is equal to 1 if the youngest person in the family is under six years old, should be positive.[1]

Grossman's treatment of health capital (1972*a*, 1972*b*) assumes that an increase in the stock of health increases the total amount of available time for work in the market and for household production during any specified time interval, say a year. With the market wage rate and non-market productivity held constant, it would not be optimal for a consumer to allocate all this additional time to household production. If such a plan were followed, then the ratio of consumption time to market goods would rise, which would cause the wage rate to exceed the value of the marginal product of consumption time.[2] Based on this argument, health should have a positive effect on the amount of time supplied to the market, and the regression coefficient of *IH* in equation (2) should be negative.

If health is viewed as an exogenous variable, then its effect on labor supply reflects a pure income effect. With the wage rate and non-market productivity held constant, an increase in health would raise 'full income', defined as earnings plus property income plus the monetary value of time spent in consumption. Since healthier persons would have more full income, their demand for commodities and their derived demand for market goods would expand. In order to purchase additional goods, they would spend more time at work in the market.[3] Although both property income and health influence hours

---

[1] In a complete model of household decision-making, marital status and family composition would be treated as endogenous variables. Such a treatment is beyond the scope of this paper.

[2] Suppose that the linear homogenous production function of some househhold commodity (z) is

$$z = f(c,t)$$

where c is a goods input and t is a time unit. If w/p is the real wage rate, then in least-cost equilibrium

$$(w/p) = (MP_t/MP_c)$$

where MP_t is the marginal product of time and MP_c is the marginal product of goods. The variable $p(MP_t/MP_c)$, which is negatively related to t/c, may be interpreted as the value of the marginal product of time or the 'shadow price' of time.

[3] In theory, health could reduce time spent in the market if 'goods-intensive' commodities (those whose production requires relatively large amounts of market goods) were sufficiently inferior. This condition would imply that total consumption of market goods would have a negative income elasticity and can be ruled out for all practical purposes.

of work by means of a pure income effect, these effects go in opposite directions. This difference arises because an increase in property income has no effect on the amount of consumption time associated with a *given* amount of working time. On the other hand, an increase in health has no effect on the amount of consumption of market goods associated with a *given* amount of working time.

(4) *Health Function*

The health equation is based on Grossman's health model (1972a, 1972b). It consists of variables that affect the demand for health and the production of health. Both demand and production variables are included, because it is difficult to specify completely the demand curve or the production function and to measure all the relevant variables.[1]

The actual health equation contains two basic sets of variables: a set (*SCH, EXP, LNWAGE, OTINC, MAR*) that influences the demand for health and the household production of health, and a set (*MD, GI, NGI, POLIO, LLPRE*) that indirectly measures the hypothesized positive effect of medical care on health. It would be inappropriate to measure this effect directly by entering the actual quantity of medical care consumed in the health function. In a cross-section of individuals, it is not unlikely that sicker people will demand more medical care than do others. Put differently, the observed relationship between health and medical care reflects causality running both from medical care to health and from health to medical care. Of course, we could have treated medical care as an endogenous variable, but this would 'tax' the data and is beyond the scope of the present paper.

Most of the variables in the second set can be interpreted as lowering the price of medical care. Under this interpretation, the estimated function would be primarily a demand curve for health. Alternatively, the wage rate and non-earnings income can be viewed as proxies for inputs, besides medical care, that affect health.[2] Under this interpretation, the estimated function would be primarily a production function of health. Instead of emphasizing one of these two extreme interpretations, we view the health equation as a mixture of a demand

[1] Grossman's work contains a fairly well-specified demand curve for health. When this demand curve is estimated, most of the *a priori* predictions are verified, but a significant amount of the variation in health is 'unexplained'.

[2] Examples of these inputs include the own time of the consumer, diet, housing services, cigarette smoking and alcohol consumption. The last two inputs have negative marginal products in the health production function. They are purchased because they also produce other commodities in the utility function. Therefore, joint production occurs in the household. For an analysis of this phenomenon, see Grossman (1971).

curve and a production function. For this reason, we do not discuss predicted effects in great detail.[1]

Grossman's health model suggests that health should rise with years of schooling completed if schooling raises the efficiency with which health is produced, and should fall with age if the rate of depreciation on health capital rises with age.[2] Since a married man has the benefit of his wife's time, as well as his own, for the production of health, married men should have higher health levels than others. It has already been indicated that the wage rate and non-earnings income can be interpreted as proxies for non-medical inputs in the production function. Given this interpretation, their effects on health should reflect the net impact of these inputs.

Our full model contains one, and only one, simultaneous relationship: that between health and the wage rate. For this reason, it is worthwhile to consider the effects of the wage on health in somewhat more detail. On the production side, consumers with relatively high wage rates would have an incentive to substitute medical care for their own time in the production of health. With medical care held constant, an increase in the wage rate would reduce the amount of time spent producing health, which would cause the quantity of health produced to fall.[3] A factor that goes in the same direction is that, with schooling and experience fixed, the wage might be positively correlated with the amount of time spent in occupations that are hazardous or otherwise detrimental to health. On the demand side, the rate of return to an investment in health should be positively correlated with the wage rate. Therefore, the quantity of health demanded should rise with the wage.[4]

Physicians per capita in the county of residence and the health insurance dummy variables should be negatively correlated with the price of medical care and, therefore, positively correlated with the quantity of medical care demanded. Consequently, to the extent that medical care improves health, these variables should be negatively associated with *IH*. Physicians per capita would be negatively correlated with price if most of the variation in this variable were due to

[1] For a complete discussion of the effects of variables in the health function, see Grossman (1972*a*, 1972*b*).

[2] With schooling held constant, age and years of experience in the labor market are almost perfectly correlated. Therefore, the regression coefficient of experience in the health function shows the effect of age on health.

[3] This conclusion assumes that market goods and services, besides medical care, that effect health are also held constant. It would have to be modified if these inputs were not held constant and if, on balance, they had a positive effect on health.

[4] This prediction assumes that health is primarily an investment commodity. See Grossman (1972*b*, chaps. 2–3) for a discussion of the difference between the investment demand curve for health and the consumption demand curve.

shifts in the county supply curve of physicians around a fairly stable demand curve. Another factor that should produce a negative correlation between the *MD* variable and the true price of medical care is that the travel waiting and inconvenience costs of obtaining physicians' services should fall as the number of physicians per capita rises. A standard proposition in the medical economics literature is that, since health insurance is reimbursement, rather than indemnity, insurance, it lowers the price of medical care from the point of view of the consumer.[1] Benefits provided by group health insurance typically exceed those provided by non-group insurance. Thus, the regression coefficient of the group insurance dummy variable should exceed that of the non-group dummy variable.[2]

The health equation contains two variables that serve as proxies for preventive medical services, *POLIO* and *LLPRE*. An individual who obtained a polio vaccine should have a propensity to obtain other types of preventive medical services, so that the vaccine variable should be positively related to health. An increase in the length of time that has elapsed since a person had a preventive physical examination, which is measured by *LLPRE*, should lower health.

(5) *Estimation Techniques and Contents*

The two-equation model, in which health is exogenous, represents a recursive system rather than a full simultaneous equations model. First, the wage rate is determined independently of the number of weeks worked, and then the number of weeks worked is determined from the wage rate and other variables. Estimation of a recursive system by ordinary least squares is equivalent to estimation by the method of full-information maximum likelihood (Johnston, 1963). There is, however, a good reason for not estimating the supply curve of weeks worked by ordinary least squares. Recall that the natural logarithm of the weekly wage rate is computed as the difference between the natural logarithm of annual earnings and the natural logarithm of weeks worked. It can be shown that, if there are errors of measurement in weeks worked, then the probability limit of the estimated wage elasticity would tend toward -1.

To avoid the bias that is introduced by errors of measurement in weeks worked, the Model 1 labor supply function is fitted by the method of instrumental variables. Specifically, the wage-generating

[1] See, for example, Andersen and Benham (1970), Feldstein (1970) and Phelps (1972).

[2] Phelp's work on health insurance (1972) suggests that the demand for health insurance is positively related to the size of the potential loss that is being insured. Therefore, the estimates of the insurance parameters in our health equation are biased toward zero. To take account of this simultaneity problem by making insurance endogenous is beyond the scope of this paper.

function is fitted by ordinary least squares, the predicted value of the wage rate is obtained, and this predicted value, rather than the actual value of the wage rate, is used to calculate the labor supply function. The only difference between this estimation technique and two-stage least squares is that exogenous variables which enter the labor supply function alone are not used to predict the wage rate.

The Model 1 wage and weeks equations have been estimated for the sample of 1,049 white men in the labor force (i.e. with positive earnings) who were at least 18 years old in 1963. In addition, separate regressions have been run for a sample of 1,006 men in the labor force between the ages of 18 and 64. The second set of regressions has been obtained to explore the possibility that health has a different and, perhaps, a larger effect on weeks and wage rates at older ages. The ideal way to examine this issue would be to fit the model for men beyond the age of 64, but the sample size of this group is too small.

The most important effect of poor health on labor supply might be to drive men out of the labor force entirely. Therefore, supply functions have also been obtained for all men who were at least 18 years old and for all men between the ages of 18 and 64. The sample sizes of these two groups, both of which include men with no earnings and no weeks of work in 1963, are 1,228 and 1,042 respectively. Their labor force participation rates are 85·4 per cent and 96·5 per cent respectively.

Since it is not possible to compute a wage rate for men with no earnings and no weeks of work, separate wage functions are not estimated for the last two groups described. The labor supply function of all men between the ages of 18 and 64, for example, is estimated by predicting wage rates from the wage function for men in the labor force between these ages. This technique supplies us with a set of potential wage rates for men who are not in the labor force. It suffers from the defect that the shadow price of time of these men exceeds their potential wage rate.[1] On the other hand, it does allow us to partition the gross effect of health on labor supply into a direct effect and an indirect effect that operates via the effect of health on the wage rate.

The three-equation model, in which health is endogenous, is estimated by two-stage least squares for members of the labor force only. Certain difficulties arise in estimating the supply curve of weeks worked in this model. Moreover, it is not entirely clear how to interpret the role of an endogenous health variable in the weeks equation.

[1] Heckman (1972) has proposed an extremely interesting method for estimating the shadow price of time and the market wage rate simultaneously. We do not employ this technique because only a small fraction of our sample is out of the labor force.

For these reasons, the Model 2 labor supply function is presented in section (2) of the appendix, where the difficulties of estimation and interpretation are discussed in detail. Here it should be noted that there is no causality in the model that runs either from weeks to the wage rate or from weeks to health. Therefore, the wage and health functions can be estimated independently of the weeks equation. Put differently, exogenous variables that enter the weeks function alone would not appear in the reduced-form equations for the wage and health.

IV. EMPIRICAL RESULTS

(1) *Model 1: Labor Force*

Table 12.2 presents estimates of wage-generating functions for the two samples of men in the labor force, and Table 12.3 presents instrumental variables estimates of supply curves of weeks for these two groups.[1] In both wage functions in Table 12.2, ill-health has negative effects on the weekly wage rate. For men between the ages of 18 and 64, the regression coefficient of *IH* is statistically significant at the 0·10 level of confidence on a one-tail test, but not at the 0·05 level. When men over the age of 64 are included, the regression coefficient of *IH* increases in absolute value and is significant at the 0·05 level. This suggests that the negative effect of ill-health on wage rates is larger in absolute value for older men.[2] The signs of the regression coefficients of the other variables in the wage equations are consistent with a *priori* expectations.

In the two supply curves of weeks worked, the regression coefficients of ill-health are negative. The estimated effect of health on weeks worked for younger men is nearly double that for the combined sample. For the former group the regression coefficient of *IH*

---

[1] When either the instrumental variables or the two-stage least squares estimation technique is employed, the ratios of the regression coefficients to their standard errors do not have Student's *t*-distribution. These ratios do, however, approach the normal distribution as the sample size becomes large. Since there are over 1,000 observations in each regression, statements made about statistical significance in the text assume an infinite number of degrees of freedom. The unadjusted coefficients of multiple determination (R^2) in Table 12.3 should be interpreted with extreme caution. We forced the R^2 to fall between 0 and 1 by using the variance of the logarithm of the predicted wage rate, rather than the variance in the logarithm of the actual wage rate, in computing them. We employed this procedure to get a rough approximation of 'explanatory power'. This statement is also relevant to the R^2 in Tables 12.7, 12.8 and 12.9.

[2] In the pooled sample, the regression coefficient of *IH* depends on the coefficient for men between the ages of 18 and 64, the coefficient for men over age 64, and the mean differences in health and wage rates between these two groups. Therefore, conclusions reached in the text with regard to differences in health effects for older men compared to younger men should be viewed as tentative.

TABLE 12.2

ORDINARY LEAST SQUARES ESTIMATES OF WAGE FUNCTIONS, MODEL 1, LABOR FORCE[a]

Variable	Ages 18–64		Ages 18 and over	
	Regression coefficient	t-ratio	Regression coefficient	t-ratio
IH	−0·016	−1·57	−0·19	−1·78
SCH	0·072	15·55	0·067	14·04
EXP	0·027	6·56	0·031	9·38
EXPSQ	−0·0003	−4·10	−0·001	−8·51
UNION	0·100	3·46	0·119	3·90
SOUTH	−0·070	−2·31	−0·064	−1·98
SMSA	0·085	2·25	0·089	2·24
OCITY	0·048	1·56	0·043	1·24
R^2	0·241		0·242	

[a] Intercepts are not shown. R^2 is the unadjusted coefficient of multiple determination

TABLE 12.3

INSTRUMENTAL VARIABLES ESTIMATES OF SUPPLY CURVES OF WEEKS WORKED, MODEL 1, LABOR FORCE[a]

Variable	Ages 18–64		Ages 18 and over	
	Regression coefficient	t-ratio	Regression coefficient	t-ratio
LNWAGE*	0·166	4·12	0·218	5·39
IH	−0·017	−2·50	−0·009	−1·23
EXP	−0·001	−1·24	−0·002	−2·80
SOUTH	0·042	2·13	0·053	2·47
SMSA	0·012	0·48	0·012	0·45
OCITY	−0·010	−0·51	−0·008	−0·35
MAR	0·020	0·52	0·051	1·25
KIDLE6	0·025	1·19	0·017	0·75
OTINC	−0·000003	−0·81	−0·000005	−1·32
R^2	0·043		0·071	

[a] An asterisk next to a variable means it is endogenous.

is significant at most conventional levels, while for the latter group it is not significant at the 0·10 level. This difference arises, in part, because the effect of experience on weeks worked also varies between the two groups. An increase in experience causes weeks worked to fall, but the magnitude of the decline for younger men is one-half as large as for the combined sample. When this variable is deleted from the regressions, the regression coefficient of ill-health for younger men is only one and a half times as large as the coefficient for all men.[1]

[1] With experience omitted, the coefficients of IH are 0·018 ($t = −2·80$) and 0·012 ($t = −1·61$) for those under 65 and all men, respectively.

Of the other variables in the labor supply function, nearly all have the predicted effects, although statistical significance is sometimes lacking.[1] The effects of the wage and non-earnings income variables merit discussion in some detail. Estimated wage elasticities are positive, significant at all conventional levels of confidence, and approximately equal to 0·2 for both groups. This implies that the substitution effect associated with a change in the real wage rate dominates the income effect. The coefficient estimates of *OTINC* indicate a weak negative income effect for men in the labor force in 1963. Given the problems of measuring the pure income effect that were discussed in section III, these results should be interpreted with caution.

TABLE 12.4

ESTIMATES OF PURE INCOME AND
SUBSTITUTION ELASTICITIES, LABOR
FORCE, AGES 18–64

Full income	Pure income elasticity	Pure substitution elasticity
$5,000	−0·015	0·180
10,000	−0·030	0·194
15,000	−0·045	0·208
20,000	−0·060	0·223
30,000	−0·090	0·251

Table 12.4 shows estimates of pure income elasticities of weeks worked at various levels of full income for men between the ages of 18 and 64.[2] It also shows estimates of pure substitution elasticities of weeks worked, i.e. the elasticity of labor supply with respect to the real wage rate when utility is held constant.[3] For example, if full in-

[1] Given that the substitution effect of an increase in the real wage rate is positive, the regression coefficient of *SMSA* should be negative.
[2] Full income is defined as

$$F = w\Omega + v$$

where w is the wage rate, Ω is the constant amount of time available in the period and v is non-earnings income. Since $df = dv$, the pure income elasticity is defined as

$$\eta = \frac{\partial t}{\partial v} \frac{F}{t} = \frac{\partial \ln t}{\partial v} F$$

where t is a measure of labor supply and where the wage rate is held constant.
[3] According to the Slutsky budget equation,

$$\hat{\epsilon} = \epsilon + k\eta$$

where $\hat{\epsilon}$ is the elasticity of labor supply with respect to the wage rate, with non-earnings income held constant; ϵ is the pure substitution elasticity of labor supply with respect to the wage rate, with utility held constant; and k is the share of earnings income in full income. Since our measure of labor supply is weeks worked, the computations in Table 12.4 assume that k is equal to the ratio of mean come equals \$15,000, the pure income elasticity equals -0.045, and the pure substitution elasticity equals 0.208.

There is a tradition in labor economics literature that the supply curve of labor for men is backward-bending. This means that, in the relevant income range, the income effect of a change in the wage rate dominates the substitution effect. Our results indicate otherwise. One reason for this discrepancy is that the use of instrumental variables reduces the negative bias in the parameter estimate of the wage elasticity due to measurement error in weeks worked. For example, the ordinary least squares estimate of the supply curve for men between the ages of 18 and 64 is as follows (*t*-ratios in parentheses):

$$LNWEEK = 0.010 \; LNWAGE - 0.023 \; IH - 0.001 \; EXP + 0.028 \; SOUTH + 0.036 \; SMSA$$
$$(0.57) \qquad (-3.26) \quad (-1.31) \qquad (1.52) \qquad (1.53)$$
$$+ 0.005 \; OCITY + 0.021 \; MAR + 0.008 \; KIDLE6 - 0.000002 \; OTINC \quad R^2 = 0.026.$$
$$(0.26) \qquad (0.55) \qquad (0.39) \qquad (-0.48)$$

Another reason for the discrepancy is that the income effect of a change in the wage rate might be much weaker in a cross-section than over time. In a cross-section, most of the variation in wage rates is due to variation in investment in human capital. Several factors suggest that these investments might be weakly correlated with *total* wealth. First, there might be a negative correlation between efficiency in investing in human capital and efficiency in investing in physical capital. Second, Becker (1967) argues that there should be a negative correlation between inheritances invested in human capital and inheritances invested in physical capital. Finally, since borrowing rates on financing investments in human capital typically exceed lending rates, self-financing becomes an important source of funds, If inherited wealth were the same for everyone, persons with relatively strong preferences for future consumption would have more funds available for investment. On the other hand, in a time series, physical and human capital should be highly correlated, and tastes should be fairly stable. Therefore, changes in the wage rate should be more closely correlated with changes in wealth over time, which explains the observed dominance of the wealth or income effect over time.[1]

Since the wage elasticity is positive in the supply curve, ill-health has an indirect negative effect on weeks worked as well as a direct effect. The indirect effect arises because ill-health lowers wage rate,

---

weeks worked to 52 weeks, or 0.94. Of course, k will vary with full income and with the wage rate. Therefore, the computations should be regarded as approximations to the true substitution elasticities.

[1] We should like to thank Jacob Mincer for suggesting this interpretation of our results.

which, in turn, lowers weeks worked. Table 12.5 shows estimates of the direct, indirect and total effects of ill-health on weeks worked for

TABLE 12.5

ESTIMATES OF DIRECT, INDIRECT AND
TOTAL EFFECTS OF ILL-HEALTH ON
WEEKS WORKED, LABOR FORCE

	Ages 18–64	Ages 18 and over
Direct effect	−0·017	−0·009
Indirect effect	−0·003	−0·004
Total effect	−0·020	−0·013

the two groups of men.[1] For men between the ages of 18 and 64, the indirect effect is approximately one-sixth as large as the direct effect. For all men, the direct effect is approximately two-fifths as large as the indirect effect. These results indicate that, while the major impact of ill-health on weeks worked operates via its increase in the shadow price of time, the channel that reflects the reduction in the market wage rate is also important.

(2) *Model 1: All Men*
Table 12.6 compares mean health characteristics of men in the labor force to those of men not in the labor force. The table reveals dramatic differences in ill-health between the two groups of men. It suggests that, among men, ill-health is a crucial determinant of labor force participation.

This implication is supported by Table 12.7, which presents supply

TABLE 12.6

MEAN HEALTH CHARACTERISTICS
BY LABOR FORCE STATUS

Variable	Labor force, ages 18–64	Labor force, ages 18 and over	Not in labor force, ages 18–64	Not in labor force, ages 18 and over
Symptoms	1·592	1·615	4·249	3·177
Excellent health[a]	0·500	0·494	0·129	0·158
Good health[a]	0·368	0·368	0·282	0·382
Fair health[a]	0·112	0·118	0·141	0·241
Poor health[a]	0·020	0·020	0·448	0·219
IH	−0·097	−0·076	2·756	1·602
Sample size	1,006	1,049	36	179

[a] Per cent.

[1] The direct effect equals the regression coefficient of IH in the labor supply function. The indirect effect equals the coefficient of IH in the wage function multiplied by the wage elasticity of weeks worked. The total effect equals the sum of the direct and indirect effects and is an estimate of the reduced-form ill-health parameter.

TABLE 12.7

INSTRUMENTAL VARIABLES ESTIMATES OF
SUPPLY CURVES OF WEEKS WORKED,
MODEL 1, ALL MEN

| | Ages 18–64 | | Ages 18 and over | |
Variable	Regression coefficient	t-ratio	Regression coefficient	t-ratio
LNWAGE*	0·149	4·27	0·400	10·68
IH	−0·048	−9·06	−0·037	−5·86
EXP	−0·002	−3·27	−0·012	−15·75
SOUTH	0·024	1·42	0·042	1·90
SMSA	−0·004	−0·17	−0·046	−1·65
OCITY	−0·015	−0·90	−0·045	−2·00
MAR	0·030	0·89	0·129	3·41
KIDLE6	0·020	1·09	−0·027	−1·07
OTINC	−0·0001	−2·84	−0·00002	−6·21
R^2	0·155		0·487	

functions of weeks worked for all men.[1] When men who are not in
the labor force are included in the regressions, the negative effects of
ill-health and of experience on weeks worked rise dramatically. As in
Table 12.3, the parameter estimates of *IH* indicate a larger impact of
ill-health on weeks worked for younger men than for the combined
sample. Once again, this finding can be traced to a differential impact
of experience on weeks worked between the two groups.[2] These results imply that, at older ages, the retirement motive, measured by
the regression coefficient of experience, is the most important determinant of labor force status. On the other hand, at younger ages,
health is the most important determinant of labor force status.
Even at older ages, however, health has a significant impact on
labor force participation, with experience and other variables held
constant.

Problems arising in estimating supply curves that include men who
are not in the labor force because the shadow price of time exceeds
the market wage rate for these men. Owing to these problems, the
regression coefficients in Table 12.7 should be interpreted with
caution. It is worth noting that, for men between the ages of 18 and
64, the coefficients of most of the variables besides ill-health and
experience are not greatly affected by including those who did not

---

[1] In the regressions in Table 12.7, the dependent variable is weeks worked,
not the natural logarithm of weeks worked. All regression coefficients are multiplied by the reciprocal of the mean of weeks worked to make them comparable
to those obtained for men in the labor force.

[2] When experience is deleted from the regressions, the coefficients of *IH* are
− 0·053 (*t* =−10·19) and − 0·053 (*t* =−7·73) for men under 65 and all men, respectively.

work at all in 1963.[1] Although more refined estimation methods are
clearly called for in the future, we do not believe that these methods
would radically alter the conclusions that emerge from Tables 12.6
and 12.7. Our results show that, for men in most age groups, ill-
health is the best predictor of labor force status. This finding is in
sharp contrast to the results of studies of labor force participation of
women, which show that marital status and the presence of young
children are the best predictors of women's participation in the
market.

(3) *Model 2: Labor Force*
Table 12.8 presents two-stage least squares estimates of wage-
generating functions for the two groups of men in the labor force, and

TABLE 12.8

TWO-STAGE LEAST SQUARES ESTIMATES OF WAGE FUNCTION, MODEL 2, LABOR FORCE

| | Ages 18–64 | | Ages 18 and over | |
| | Regression | | Regression | |
Variable	coefficient	t-ratio	coefficient	t-ratio
IH*	−0·265	−3·55	−0·282	−3·38
SCH	0·054	7·02	0·050	6·22
EXP	0·031	6·11	0·039	8·06
EXPSQ	−0·0004	−3·80	−0·001	−7·42
UNION	0·114	3·13	0·142	3·65
SOUTH	−0·048	−0·123	−0·043	−1·04
SMSA	0·040	0·80	0·054	1·07
OCITY	0·029	0·75	0·023	0·57
R^2	0·254		0·253	

Table 12.9 presents two-stage least squares estimates of health functions. When health is treated as endogenous, striking changes occur
in the wage function coefficients of this variable. For men between
the ages of 18 and 64, for example, the regression coefficient of *IH*
increases in absolute value from −0·016 ($t = −1·57$) to −0·265 ($t = −3·55$). At the same time, the coefficient of schooling falls from
0·072 ($t = 15·55$) to 0·054 ($t = 7·02$). This suggests that one source of
the expansion in ill-health effect is multicollinearity between schooling and predicted ill-health. Although these two variables are more
highly correlated than schooling and actual ill-health, multicollinearity is not overly destructive: both variables exert significant
partial effects on the wage rate.

[1] One exception is that the coefficient of *OTINC* indicates a much stronger
non-earnings income effect than the one estimated in Table 12.3. This finding
is likely to reflect the greater frequency of transfer payments to men who did
not work at all in 1963.

TABLE 12.9

TWO-STAGE LEAST SQUARES ESTIMATES OF HEALTH FUNCTIONS, MODEL 2, LABOR FORCE

Variable	Ages 18–64		Ages 18 and over	
	Regression coefficient	t-ratio	Regression coefficient	t-ratio
LNWAGE*	0·550	0·79	0·794	2·03
SCH	−0·102	−2·19	−0·108	−4·07
EXP	0·002	0·28	0·003	0·62
OTINC	−0·00002	−0·85	−0·00002	−1·19
MAR	−0·338	−1·72	−0·273	−1·47
MD	−0·002	−1·29	−0·002	−1·73
LLPRE	0·001	4·05	0·001	4·34
POLIO	−0·260	−2·76	−0·259	−2·86
GI	−0·143	−0·71	−0·189	−1·18
NGI	−0·066	−0·33	−0·077	−0·47
R^2	0·109		0·104	

There are two other reasons for the increase in the size of the ill-health coefficient in the wage function. First, the wage rate has a positive effect on ill-health in the health function. Therefore, the ordinary least squares estimate of the health parameter in the wage function is biased downward. Second, there might be measurement error in the ill-health variable, which would also bias the ordinary least squares parameter estimate downward. This bias, as well as the simultaneous equations bias, should be reduced by the use of a set of instrumental variables.

In the health functions in Table 12.9, the coefficients of all the proxy variables for medical care (*MD, LLPRE, POLIO, GI, NGI*) indicate positive impacts of these variables on health. Other things being equal, an individual's health is worse, the fewer the number of physicians per capita in his county of residence, and the greater the length of time since he had a preventive physical examination. In addition, persons with non-group health insurance are in poorer health than those with group insurance, persons with no insurance are in poorer health than those with non-group insurance, and persons who have not had a polio vaccine are in poorer health than those who have had a vaccine. These results demonstrate that, by measuring medical services indirectly, one can uncover the presumed positive effect of these services on health in a cross-section of individuals. The findings may be viewed as extensions of those of Auster, Leveson and Sarachek (1969) to data for individuals. Using states of the United States as the unit of observation, these authors found a weak negative effect of medical care on the age-adjusted death rate of whites.

Our results tentatively imply that government policies that are designed to increase the availability of medical care, such as national health insurance and subsidies for physicians' training, would also improve the health of the population. This is a tentative implication because the physician variable and the insurance variables are significant only at low levels of confidence. Furthermore, Newhouse and Phelps (1973) and Benham (work in progress) find only a weak positive association across individuals between the number of physicians per capita in the county of residence and utilization of physicians' services. In addition, the length of time since an individual had a preventive physical examination and whether he received a polio vaccine are highly correlated with experience. These intercorrelations are partly responsible for the statistically insignificant experience coefficient in the health equation.[1] Finally, the estimated effects of *POLIO* and *LLPRE* are subject to more than one interpretation.[2] Before results such as ours can serve as a guide for government policies in the medical care sector, research with other measures of health and medical care clearly is necessary.[3]

The endogenous wage rate has positive effects on ill-health for both men between the ages of 18 and 64 as well as for the entire sample of all men in the labor force. In the latter case, the parameter estimate is significant at the 0·05 level of confidence on a two-tail test. It should be realized that the wage effect is estimated with years of formal schooling completed and proxies for medical care held constant. When schooling is deleted from the health functions, the coefficients of the wage rate are $-0·903$ ($t = -4·18$) and $-0·555$ ($t = -2·74$) for those under 65 and all men, respectively. Possible explanations of the positive wage coefficient in the health function include an increase in the consumption of market goods that are harmful to health, a reduction in the time spent producing health, and a greater tendency to choose a hazardous occupation as the wage rate rises.

Table 12.9 reveals that ill-health is negatively related to years of formal schooling completed and to the presence of a wife. These results are consistent with the hypotheses that schooling is an important determinant of the efficiency of household production and that the presence of a wife is an important determinant of the resources available for household production. They are also consistent with other hypotheses. For example, Grossman (work in progress) has argued that schooling might be a function of health at early ages.

---

[1] It should be noted, however, that experience is also highly correlated with the predicted wage rate. When the latter variable is omitted from the health function for men under age 65, the coefficient of experience is $0·008$ ($t = 2·08$).

[2] For example, a person whose health is very poor probably had his last physical examination because he was ill. Therefore, he would report a relatively high value of *LLPRE*. This suggests that *LLPRE* is, at least in part, a proxy index of health.

[3] For one effort along these lines, see Benham (work in progress).

Therefore, the relationship between these two variables might reflect causality running from health to schooling, as well as causality running from schooling to health.[1] Although future research in this area is required it is unlikely that the entire schooling effect in the health function is due to causality from health to schooling.

If one assumes that the effect of schooling really reflects causality from this variable to health, then our findings have a number of interesting implications. Since schooling is an important policy variable from the point of view of both the individual and society, it is useful to examine the reduced-form wage and ill-health parameters of schooling. Table 12.10 shows estimates of these two parameters for men between the ages of 18 and 64. It also decomposes each parameter into a direct component and an indirect component.[2] The reduced-form wage parameter of schooling indicates a rate of return

TABLE 12.10

ESTIMATES OF DIRECT, INDIRECT AND
TOTAL EFFECTS OF SCHOOLING ON THE
WAGE RATE AND ILL-HEALTH,
LABOR FORCE, AGES 18–64

	Wage effects	Ill-health effects
Direct effect	0·047	−0·089
Indirect effect	0·024	0·026
Total effect (reduced-form parameter)	0·071	−0·063

to investment in schooling of 7·1 per cent. The indirect component, which is because schooling raises health and health raises market wage rates, is approximately one-half as large as the direct component. The reduced-form ill-health parameter of schooling indicates that a small part of the negative direct effect of schooling on ill-health is offset by the positive effect of the wage rate on ill-health.

Although the positive relationship between schooling and wage rates is well documented, many persons have wondered about the

---

[1] Along similar lines, selective mating in the marriage market can explain why married men are healthier than other men (see Fuchs, 1973).

[2] Let a_1 and a_2 be the regression coefficients of ill-health and schooling in the wage function, and let c_1 and c_2 be the regression coefficients of the natural logarithm of the wage rate and schooling in the health function. Then the reduced-form wage parameter of schooling, which is obtained by expressing the natural logarithm of the wage rate as a function of all the exogenous variables in the model, equals $(a_2 + a_1c_2)/(1 - a_1c_1)$. The term $a_2/(1 - a_1c_1)$ gives the direct component, and the term $a_1c_2/(1 - a_1c_1)$ gives the indirect component. Similarly, the reduced-form ill-health parameter of schooling is $(c_2 + c_1a_2)/(1 - a_1c_1)$, where $c_2/(1 - a_1c_1)$ is the direct component and $c_1a_2/(1 - a_1c_1)$ is the indirect component.

specific mechanisms by which schooling raises wage rates.[1] Our results suggest that one important mechanism operates via an increase in health with schooling. Future research is necessary to ascertain whether the health effect on market productivity reflects physical energy, capacity for hard work, a positive effect of weeks worked on the wage rate, or other factors.

V. SUMMARY AND CONCLUSION

In this paper we have used the household production function model of demand theory to examine the effects of health on wages and weeks worked. The estimated structural equations for wage determination and labor supply indicate that health has positive effects on these two components of earnings. We have also used the household production function model to treat health as an endogenous variable. In this case, the impact of health on market productivity is strengthened. Some additional results of our empirical analysis are as follows. The cross-sectional labor supply function of white men is not backward-bending. Health is positively related to physicians per capita in the county of residence, health insurance, and two crude measures of preventive medical care: whether a person had a polio vaccine and the frequency with which he has a preventive physical examination. With medical care and schooling held constant, the endogenous wage rate has a negative effect on health. Schooling and the presence of a wife have positive impacts on health. An important mechanism by which schooling raises wage rates may operate via its effect on health.

We view the present paper as work in progress on the two-way relationship between health and various aspects of consumer behavior, such as labor force participation, investment in schooling, wage determination and marriage. In a sense, it represents a sub-sector of a complete model in which all these variables are determined simultaneously. Owing to the preliminary nature of our work, we have not hesitated to suggest alternative interpretations of certain findings and areas for future research. These areas include (1) the use of estimation methods that take account of the inequality between the shadow price of time and the market wage rate for men who do not participate in the labor market, (2) a more detailed study of the effect of medical care on health, and (3) studies that would establish the direction of causality implied by the relationship between schooling and health and between marital status and health.

During the past two decades, empirical research in economics has moved in the direction of the estimation of large-scale econometric models. Partly as a result of this trend, a number of interesting and

[1] See, for example, Welch (1970) and Taubman and Wales (1973).

TABLE A.1

MEANS AND STANDARD DEVIATIONS

Variable	Labor force, ages 18–64		Labor force, ages 18 and over		All men, ages 18–64		All men, ages 18 and over	
	Mean	Standard deviation	Mean	Standard deviation	Mean	Standard deviation	Mean	Standard deviation
SYMPTOMS	1·592	2·086	1·615	2·119	1·685	2·196	1·843	2·342
EXCELLENT HEALTH[a]	0·500		0·494		0·487		0·445	
GOOD HEALTH[a]	0·368		0·368		0·365		0·370	
FAIR HEALTH[a]	0·112		0·118		0·113		0·136	
POOR HEALTH[a]	0·020		0·020		0·035		0·049	
LNWAGE[c]	4·815	0·467	4·792	0·502				
LNWEEK[b]	3·861	0·254	3·849	0·281	46·958	11·811	41·236	18·765
IH	−0·097	1·300	−0·076	1·317	0·000	1·462	0·169	1·606
SCH	11·636	3·258	11·549	3·333	11·549	3·309	11·070	3·577
EXP	20·575	12·267	21·857	13·571	21·046	12·525	26·279	17·156
EXPSQ	573·650	564·910	661·750	709·090	599·630	586·710	984·670	1,105·600
UNION[a]	0·315		0·310		0·309		0·293	
SOUTH[a]	0·260		0·258		0·263		0·260	
SMSA[a]	0·224		0·228		0·221		0·222	
OCITY[a]	0·497		0·496		0·499		0·503	
MAR[a]	0·950		0·947		0·950		0·932	
KIDLE6[a]	0·373		0·357		0·365		0·310	
OTINC	483·570	2,439·200	504·910	2,429·700	520·300	2,422·800	662·500	2,453·200
MD[d]	120·270	45·438	120·520	46·146	119·770	45·350	119·200	46·630
LLPRE	172·940	228·690	182·880	243·660	175·430	231·780	242·810	282·650
POLIO[a]	0·615		0·602		0·610		0·549	
GI[a]	0·741		0·724		0·728		0·662	
NGI[a]	0·097		0·110		0·102		0·147	

[a] Per cent. Standard deviations of dummy variables not shown.
[b] For the two samples of all men, the mean of weeks worked, rather than the mean of the natural logarithm of weeks worked, is shown.
[c] Not shown for the two samples of all men.
[d] Per 100,000 population.

fairly large-scale models of various sectors of the medical care market have been constructed. Although we welcome these models, we believe that their existence should not detract from the need for small-scale econometric models of the household. Our results suggest that such models will be extremely useful, particularly if they are constructed in the context of the household production function approach to demand theory and emphasize the relationship between health and consumer behavior.

APPENDIX

(1) *Sample and Variables*

The empirical analysis in this paper is restricted to white males who were at least 18 years old in 1963, had completed their formal schooling and did not reside on farms. In addition to these restrictions, men were excluded from the analysis if there was no information on their symptoms, health status, earnings, weeks worked, schooling, or work-loss weeks due to illness. Finally, men who said they were unmarried non-heads of households were eliminated. In cases where there were unknown values of variables other than the ones just listed, the mean value of the relevant variable was substituted.

Table A.1 shows means of all variables and standard deviations of continuous variables for four groups of men: labor force, ages 18 to 64; labor force, ages 18 and over; all men, ages 18 to 64; and all men, ages 18 and over. Note that the index of ill-health, IH, was estimated for all men between the ages of 18 and 64. Therefore, it has a mean of zero for this group and non-zero means for the other three groups.

TABLE A.2

REGRESSIONS OF SYMPTOMS ON HEALTH
STATUS DUMMY VARIABLES[a]

| Group | Intercept | Regression coefficient of: | | | R^2 |
		HS_1	HS_2	HS_3	
Labor force, ages 18–64	0·944	0·726	1·675	3·155	0·238
	(11·64)	(5·83)	(8·57)	(7·15)	
Labor force, ages 18 and over	0·956	0·692	1·756	3·311	0·248
	(11·85)	(5·61)	(9·26)	(7·64)	
All men, ages 18–64	0·951	0·732	1·690	3·155	0·290
	(11·57)	(5·83)	(8·67)	(8·96)	
All men, ages 18 and over	0·978	0·771	1·592	2·909	0·290
	(11·58)	(6·16)	(8·92)	(9·79)	

[a] *t*-ratios in parentheses.

Table A.2 presents regressions of symptoms on three health status dummy variables for the four groups of men.[1] The intercept of the regres-

[1] The health status dummy variables are coded as follows: $HS_1 = 1$ if health status is good, fair or poor; $HS_2 = 1$ if health status is fair or poor; and $HS_3 = 1$ if health status is poor.

sion for men in the labor force between the ages of 18 and 64 indicates that the mean number of symptoms for men in this group in excellent health equals 0·9. The regression coefficient of HS_1 indicates that men in good health have 0·7 more symptoms on average than men in excellent health. Similarly, men in fair health have 1·7 more symptoms than men in good health, and men in poor health have 3·2 more symptoms than men in fair health. These differences in symptoms by health status, as well as those in the other three regressions, are all statistically significant at the 0·01 level of confidence on a two-tail test.

(2) *Model 2 Labor Supply Function: Labor Force*
The first regression in Table A.3 shows the Model 2 labor supply function for men in the labor force between the ages of 18 and 64. In this regression, both the wage rate and ill-health are endogenous variables. The main difference between this supply function and the Model 1 supply function is that the endogenous ill-health variable has a positive effect on weeks

TABLE A.3

TWO-STAGE LEAST SQUARES ESTIMATES OF SUPPLY CURVES OF WEEKS WORKED, MODEL 2, LABOR FORCE, AGES 18–64

Variable	*Regression 1* Regression coefficient	t-ratio	*Regression 2[a]* Regression coefficient	t-ratio	*Regression 3[b]* Regression coefficient	t-ratio
LNWAGE*	0·291	5·24	0·241	5·75	−0·001	−0·05
IH*	0·076	1·69	−0·017	−2·53	−0·080	−2·62
EXP	−0·003	−2·27	−0·001	−1·18	0·001	0·49
SOUTH	0·044	1·96	0·045	2·27	0·032	1·66
SMSA	0·012	0·40	0·001	0·06	0·023	0·92
OCITY	−0·012	−0·53	−0·016	−0·79	−0·001	−0·07
MAR	0·017	0·36	−0·002	−0·06	0·003	0·07
KIDLE6	0·029	1·19	0·029	1·38	0·015	0·72
OTINC	−0·00001	−1·87	−0·00001	−2·01	−0·000002	−0·70
R^2	0·060		0·063		0·020	

[a] In this regression, *IH* is exogenous.
[b] In this regression, *LNWAGE* is exogenous.

worked.[1] This finding arises, in part, because schooling is the most important predictor variable of either the wage rate or ill-health in the first stage. Therefore, the predicted values of *LNWAGE* and *IH* are highly correlated.

The second and third regressions in Table A.3 show that the multicollinearity problem is alleviated, to some extent, by treating either the wage rate or ill-health as an exogenous variable. In the second regression, *IH* is exogenous, while *LNWAGE* is predicted from all the exogenous variables in the wage and health functions. The regression coefficient of the exogenous ill-health variable is negative and statistically significant,

[1] Ill-health also has a positive effect on weeks worked in the Model 2 supply curve for all men in the labor force (not shown).

and the coefficients of the other variables are similar to those obtained in Model 1. In regression 3, *IH* is endogenous, while *LNWAGE* is exogenous. The coefficient of *IH* is negative and, compared to regression 2, much larger in absolute value. The estimated wage elasticity is zero, which reflects the downward bias due to measurement error in weeks worked.

Given the multicollinearity problem and the downward bias that arises when the actual wage is used, more weight should be given to the co-efficients in regression 2 than to those in the other regressions. Regression 2 also merits emphasis because there is no causality in the model that runs from weeks to the wage rate, or from weeks to ill-health. Consequently, it is not entirely clear how much one gains by estimating the labor supply function with an endogenous ill-health variable.

REFERENCES

Andersen, Ronald, and Anderson, Odin W., *A Decade of Health Services: Social Survey Trends in Use and Expenditure* (Univ. of Chicago Press, 1967).
——, and Benham, Lee, 'Factors Affecting the Relationship between Family Income and Medical Care Consumption', in Herbert E. Klarman (ed.), *Empirical Studies in Health Economics* (Baltimore: Johns Hopkins Press, 1970).
Auster, Richard D., Leveson, Irving, and Sarachek, Deborah, 'The Production of Health: An Exploratory Study', *Journal of Human Resources*, IV, 4 (Fall 1969) 411–36, reprinted in Victor R. Fuchs (ed.), *Essays in the Economics of Health and Medical Care* (New York: Columbia Univ. Press, for the National Bureau of Economic Research, 1972).
Becker, Gary S., 'A Theory of the Allocation of Time', *Economic Journal*, LXXV, 299 (Sept 1965) 493–517.
——, *Human Capital and the Personal Distribution of Income: An Analytical Approach*, W. S. Woytinsky Lecture No. 1 (Ann Arbor: Univ. of Michigan Press, 1967).
——, 'A Theory of Marriage: Part I', *Journal of Political Economy*, LXXXI, 4 (July/Aug 1973).
Benham, Lee, 'Resource Allocation and Health Status' (in progress).
Boskin, Michael J., 'The Economics of the Labor Supply', unpublished paper (1971).
Feldstein, Martin S., 'The Rising Price of Physicians' Services, *Review of Economics and Statistics*, LII, 2 (May 1970) 121–33.
Fleisher, Belton M., 'The Economics of Labor Force Participation: A Review Article', *Journal of Human Resources*, VI, 2 (Spring 1971) 139–48.
Fuchs, Victor R., 'Some Economic Aspects of Mortality in Developed Countries', pp. 174–93 above.
Ghez, Gilbert R., and Becker, Gary S., 'The Allocation of Time and Goods over the Life Cycle', mimeographed (New York: National Bureau of Economic Research, 1972).
Greenberg, David H., 'Problems of Model Specification and Measurement: The Labor Supply Function', mimeographed (Santa Monica, Calif.: RAND Corporation, 1972).
——, and Kosters, Marvin, 'Income Guarantees and the Working Poor: The Effect of Income Maintenance Programs on the Hours of Work of Male Family Heads', mimeographed (Santa Monica, Calif.: RAND Corporation, 1970).

Grossman, Michael, 'The Economics of Joint Production in the Household', mimeographed (Center for Mathematical Studies in Business and Economics, Univ. of Chicago, 1971).

——, 'On the Concept of Health Capital and the Demand for Health', *Journal of Political Economy*, LXXX, 2 (Mar/Apr 1972a) 223–55.

——, *The Demand for Health: A Theoretical and Empirical Investigation* (New York: Columbia Univ. Press, for the National Bureau of Economic Research, 1972b).

——, 'The Correlation between Health and Schooling' (in progress).

Hall, Robert E., 'Wages, Income and Hours of Work in the U.S. Labor Force', unpublished paper (1971).

Heckman, James J., 'Three Essays on the Supply of Labor and the Demand fo Goods', unpublished Ph.D. dissertation (Princeton Univ., 1971).

——, 'Shadow Prices, Market Wages, and Labor Supply', unpublished paper (1972).

Johnston, J., *Econometric Methods* (New York: McGraw Hill, 1963).

Lancaster, Kelvin J., 'A New Approach to Consumer Theory', *Journal of Political Economy*, LXXV, 2 (Apr 1966) 132–57.

Leibowitz, Arleen S., 'Women's Allocation of Time to Market and Nonmarket Activities: Differences by Education', unpublished Ph.D dissertation (Columbia Univ., 1972).

Luft, Harold S., 'Poverty and Health: An Empirical Investigation of the Economic Interactions', unpublished Ph.D dissertation (Harvard Univ., 1972).

Michael, Robert T., 'Dimensions of Household Fertility: An Economic Analysis', *1971 Proceedings of the Social Statistics Section of the American Statistical Association*, pp. 126–36.

——, *The Effect of Education on Efficiency in Consumption* (New York: Columbia Univ. Press, for the National Bureau of Economic Research, 1972).

—— and Becker, Gary S., 'On the New Theory of Consumer Behavior', *Swedish Journal of Economics* (1973).

Mincer, Jacob, 'Labor Force Participation of Married Women', in *Aspects of Labor Economics*, a Conference of the Universities–National Bureau Committee for Economic Research (Princeton Univ. Press, for the National Bureau of Economic Research, 1962).

——, 'The Distribution of Labor Incomes: A Survey with Special Reference to the Human Capital Approach', *Journal of Economic Literature*, VIII, 1 (Mar 1970) 1–26.

——, 'Schooling, Experience and Earnings,' mimeographed (New York: National Bureau of Economic Research, 1972).

Muth, Richard, 'Household Production and Consumer Demand Function', *Econometrica*, XXXIV, 3 (July 1966) 699–708.

Newhouse, Joseph P., and Phelps, Charles E., 'Price and Income Elasticities for Medical Care Services', pp. 139–61 above.

Phelps, Charles E., 'The Demand for Health Insurance: A Theoretical and Empirical Investigation', unpublished Ph.D. dissertation (Univ. of Chicago, 1972).

Smith, James P., 'The Life Cycle Allocation of Time in a Family Context', unpublished Ph.D dissertation (Univ. of Chicago, 1972).

Taubman, Paul J., and Wales, Terence J., 'Higher Education, Mental Ability, and Screening', *Journal of Political Economy*, LXXX, 1 (Jan/Feb 1973) 28–55.

Welch, Finis, 'Education in Production', *Journal of Political Economy*, LXXVII, 1 (Jan/Feb 1970) 35–59.

13 A Test of Alternative Demand-Shift Responses to the Medicare Program[1]

Bernard Friedman

BROWN UNIVERSITY, PROVIDENCE, R.I.

Introduction of the Medicare program in the United States in 1966 has been associated with an acceleration in the rise in price of health services, particularly hospital care. In part, this reflects large increases in real resources used per patient treated. This paper reviews the aggregate evidence, and examines some data on possible changes in the diagnosis, treatment and survival of women with breast cancer. The data lend some support to a model in which increased employment of resources offers utility benefit to health professionals who have considerable discretionary decision power.

I. INTRODUCTION

Medicare is a recent United States government program which partially reimburses certain providers of health services for their expenses on behalf of elderly persons. The total reimbursement by the government was more than $7 billion in 1971. Since the program began in July 1966, it has had a strong impact on the overall allocation of resources to the health sector, and on the relative prices of health services.

This paper begins with a review of some of the aggregate evidence on the impact of Medicare. From aggregate data it may be inferred that the lowering of consumer out-of-pocket cost has been associated with rising prices and utilization of services. Economists have been concerned, however, with the need for better understanding of the decision-making of physicians and other service providers who often have a direct role in determining utilization and costs.

Evidence on the microeconomics of demand behavior is presented below. A study was made of possible changes in the early diagnosis and treatment of breast cancer, comparing years before and after the Medicare program began. The results lend some support to a model

---

[1] Grateful acknowledgement is made to Dr Paul Parker and the Massachusetts Tumor Registry for the use of case records, and to Martin Feldstein for criticism of an earlier version of this paper.

in which physicians make decisions reflecting their own preferences, though constrained by out-of-pocket cost to the consumer. The direct role of consumer actions, in particular the shortening of delay in diagnosis, does not seem to be a major source of the inflationary impact of Medicare.

Section II gives a brief description of the Medicare coverage and financing as compared to prior health insurance coverage of elderly persons. The rationale of the program is discussed.

Section III presents some aggregate data on Medicare reimbursement experience. The overall experience of short-stay hospitals is examined for price, quantity and quality changes, associated in time with the introduction of Medicare.

Section IV contains a formal model of professional decisions. The preferences of the service providers are assumed to be only partially determined by the quantity of service and the money income received. These decisions are constrained by the quantity of service demanded by consumers as a function of out-of-pocket cost.

Section V provides some statistical analysis of changes in the early diagnosis and treatment of breast cancer, comparing 1967 with 1965 experience in six major Boston area hospitals.

II. MEDICARE REIMBURSEMENT PROVISIONS AND PRIOR HEALTH INSURANCE COVERAGE OF THE ELDERLY

Medicare provides reimbursement for hospital expenses for virtually all persons aged 65 and over, according to the following current formula: After a deductible (per episode) of $52, the first 60 days of hospital care are fully reimbursed. The next 30 days are subject to a 20 per cent copayment (or 'coinsurance' or 'direct cost') by the enrolled consumer. This same population is reimbursed fully for the first 20 days of care in an Extended Care Facility. The next 80 days are subject to 20 per cent copayment. Costs of purely custodial care are not reimbursed.

The above coverage is supplemented by a voluntary program for reimbursement in the event of other medical expenses. More than 90 per cent of eligible persons have elected the supplementary coverage for which they pay one-half of the actuarial cost. Reimbursement is made according to the following formula: After a deductible of $50 per year, 80 per cent of expenses are reimbursed.

Medicare reimbursement is made directly to the providers of health service, using criteria of 'reasonable and customary' costs. More than 20 million persons are currently enrolled.

Table 13.1 shows the annual portion of personal health expenditures paid directly by consumers, together with the payments made by third parties for fiscal years before and after the introduction of Medicare.

TABLE 13.1

A COMPARISON OF HEALTH INSURANCE
COVERAGE BEFORE AND AFTER THE
INTRODUCTION OF MEDICARE

($ million)

Year	Total expenditures	Direct payments	Private insurance reimbursement	Government payments	Medicare only
Age 65+					
Fiscal 1966	8,242	4,382	1,309	2,460	none
1967	9,990	3,681	589	5,644	3,172
1971	17,863	4,661	1,030	12,082	7,478
Age <65					
Fiscal 1966	27,974	14,286	7,627	5,432	none
1971	47,269	19,601	15,585	11,209	none

Source: Cooper and Worthington [1].

In fiscal year 1966, elderly persons were paying directly about one-half of all costs incurred on their behalf, while five years later they were paying directly one-fourth of total costs.[1] During the same period, the share of direct payment by those under age 65 fell roughly from 50 per cent to 40 per cent.

The table reflects other changes in public provision and reimbursement for health services. At the same time that Medicare began, a program was established for the federal government partially to reimburse state and local governments for expenses on behalf of families with low income relative to their medical expenses (the so-called Medicaid program). For persons under age 65, this program represented $3,170 million of the increase in all government payments to 1971. The rest of government expenditure reflects chiefly military-related health expenses and other local government assistance largely for care in long-stay institutions. This paper will restrict further attention to civilian, non-veteran health services and short-stay institutions only.

III. AGGREGATE EXPERIENCE ASSOCIATED WITH THE INTRODUCTION OF MEDICARE

By lowering the share of expenses paid directly by the consumer of medical care, the Medicare program is believed to have increased the

---

[1] The comparison would probably be made more striking if the amount of free care given before and after Medicare were properly counted.

demand for care by the elderly. Although economists have not developed a close consensus on the size of the sensitivity of demand to consumer net prices, important studies have been made by Feldstein [5], Phelps and Newhouse [9], Rosett and Huang [10], and others.

The results of increases in demand are not as transparent for the health sector as they seem to be in other industries. Entry is severely limited. Because of the special nature of the product, social institutions weigh against profit-maximizing behavior. The special nature of supply responses in the health sector has been examined by many authors. Of key interest in the evaluation of the current impact of Medicare is analysis of expenditure increases that result from the interaction of consumer and supplier decisions, into quantity, 'quality' and pure price changes.

During 1960–6 the medical care component of the Consumer Price Index (C.P.I.) rose at 3·5 per cent per year, as compared with 1·5 per cent for the overall C.P.I. For 1966–9 the rates of rise were 8·0 per cent and 4·1 per cent respectively.

When expenditures are adjusted for the changes in the medical care price index, the average real increase in the volume of service during the 1967–71 period was 2·4 per cent per year for those aged 19–64, and 6·0 per cent for those aged 65 and over.

If the measurement of pure price changes were accurate, an argument could be made that further distinctions between quantity and 'quality' changes are irrelevant for the discussion of economic efficiency and welfare. The argument is not acceptable, however, when the 'quality' changes provide utility primarily to the suppliers of service and motivate their behavior. The presence of this sort of quality change has been discussed by Newhouse [7], and some recent evidence of its importance is given by Davis [2]. The restriction of competition allows health institutions to follow criteria other than consumer preferences. If, by stimulating demand for health services, a predictable transfer of welfare to suppliers is generated, a change of the regulatory rules may be a desirable supplementary action.

The quantity of care is not an obvious concept. As a simple example, a physician who works shorter hours may be able to give more efficacious treatment per hour, in which case it would seem inappropriate to measure quantity by hours worked or number of visits.

The difficulty of assessing quantity is further illustrated in Table 13.2. The aggregate experience of Medicare has not been a strongly rising trend in the number of hospital admissions, but rather in the total charges per case. This reflects partly longer stays and partly increased use of resources per day. A longer stay may give more efficacious treatment, a quantity change. The total value of the longer

TABLE 13.2

HOSPITAL INPATIENT CLAIMS
PROCESSED UNDER MEDICARE

	Number of claims (million)	Total charges per claim ($)
July 1966–Dec 1967	7·25	634
Calendar 1968	5·94	746
1969	6·08	845
1970	6·19	939
1971	6·16	1,039

Source: Social Security Administration.

stay may be an overestimate of gain in well-being, however, to the extent that there is substitution away from cheaper home care. Increased real cost of resources per day is the more germane problem for the present analysis, where the question is over who benefits from higher input cost.

Table 13.3 separates the input components of cost inflation in short-stay hospitals. The accelerated inflation of wages and the

TABLE 13.3

ANALYSIS OF COST INCREASES PER PATIENT-DAY
IN SHORT-STAY COMMUNITY HOSPITALS, 1960–70

	Average annual percentage increase	
Item[a]	1960–6	1966–70
Compensation per employee (W)	4·1	9·8
Number of employees[b] (L)	2·5	2·8
Price index of non-labor inputs (P)	1·5	4·8
Quantity index of non-labor inputs (N)	6·0	11·0
Consumer Price Index	1·6	4·9

[a] Average cost per patient-day $= W \cdot L + P \cdot N$.
[b] Full-time equivalent units.
Source: Social Security Administration, Research and Statistics Note No. 4 (Feb 1972).

volume of non-labor input after 1966 is dramatic. Again, more skilled workers and more advanced equipment, in so far as the efficacy of treatment is improved, do not represent the kind of 'quality' change which solely affects the preferences of the suppliers. Indirect evidence of changes in health status of those treated would seem to be essential for further decomposing the real increases in services. One such measure is used in section v below, which supports the importance of the quantity/quality distinction discussed here.

IV. MICROECONOMICS OF DEMAND

For an industry under competitive supply conditions, an important tool for economic analysis is the demand function relating quantity demanded to the price paid by consumers. When there is no non-price rationing of commodities or services, observed price and quantity movement often allow quantitative insight about this function.

The insurance provisions of Medicare offer reimbursement for the

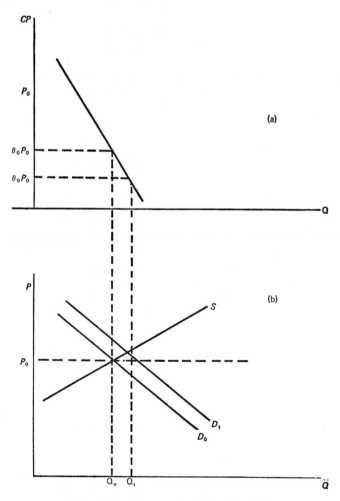

FIG. 13.1   Consumer direct cost model

services that depends on the total value received. A consumer direct cost (C.D.C.) model of demand would analyze the effect of such a reimbursement program in the context of a simple demand model widely used for other products.

Fig. 13.1, in its upper portion, gives the quantity demanded of health services, Q, as a function of direct consumer price CP. Suppose the initial market price per unit is P_0 and, because of insurance, the consumer must pay only the fraction θ_0 of this price directly. Notice that at the time illness occurs, any previous insurance premium is a sunk cost that would not be considered by the individual consumer.

The bottom portion of Fig. 13.1 shows the relationships observed in the market in terms of gross prices, P, and the quantity, Q. For a fixed θ_0, movement along the consumer demand function in (a) generates the locus of points D_0 in (b).

Now the effect of Medicare for the average experience in the event of illness is to reduce the direct cost fraction, or copayment rate, from θ_0 to θ_1. At any previous gross price, the quantity demanded is now greater. A new locus of points D_1 in (b) may be drawn, and its intersection with the supply function S would yield a new equilibrium combination of higher gross price and higher quantity purchased.

If, in fact, the rationale of the competitive market does not underlie the relationships observed in (b) of the C.D.C. model, it would be misleading to use estimates of these relationships for making welfare judgments.

A second model in which professional preference plays a strong role in generating the observed data is being discussed by the authors mentioned above, and, as an approximation, the model may be better appreciated in the following formal framework.

Suppose that a health professional desires to maximize a function expressing his preferences, such as $V(Q, Z)$, where a new variable, Z, is meant to represent the quality of care that may be of little concern to the patient. It is quite crude to assume that there is some single scalar variable for this concept, but it is hoped that the model may be fruitfully applied to smaller-scale decision-making with more precision.

The professional is constrained in the choice of Q and Z which he chooses to maximize $V(Q, Z)$. First, there is the cost function $C = C(Q, Z)$, where C is the cost per unit of service output. Additionally, there is the willingness to pay, or the demand function, of the consumer $Q = Q(\theta \cdot C)$ where θ is the rate of copayment dictated by reimbursement coverage.

The feasible boundary between Q and Z for a given θ_1 is determined by the above constraints, and depicted in Fig. 13.2 (a) by F_1. Formally, the boundary is given by

$$\frac{dQ}{dZ} = \frac{\theta \dfrac{dQ}{d(\theta C)} \dfrac{\partial C}{\partial Z}}{1 - \theta \dfrac{dQ}{d(\theta C)} \dfrac{\partial C}{\partial Q}} < 0. \tag{1}$$

The slope is negative, due to the negative slope of the demand function $Q(\theta P)$. The curve is also drawn convex to the origin, reflecting a conventional assumption of increasing costs per unit of each output with the amount of the other held constant.

From (1) it can be seen that a lowering of θ_1 to θ_2 leads to a less steep trade-off between Q and Z as depicted by the boundary F_2 in Fig. 13.2 (a). More of both Q and Z will be attained, and if the preferences embodied in the function $V(Q, Z)$ are homothetic, it follows that the expansion in Z will be relatively greater than the expansion of Q.[1]

The importance of professional preference has been suggested in the context of choice of specialty by physicians, and the response of physicians to the growth of malpractice claims. The next section examines whether the simple insights of the professional preference model may be relevant to observed changes in the diagnosis, treatment and consequences of breast cancer.

V. CHANGES IN THE EARLY DIAGNOSIS AND TREATMENT OF BREAST CANCER

The female breast is the most common primary site of cancer and one of the most accessible to self-diagnosis. The disease is believed to spread from a single mass of cells. If treated before there is evidence of cells in other regional tissues or lymph nodes, the five-year relative survival rate[2] is estimated at 82 per cent. When regional tissues are involved, the survival rate drops to 53 per cent. Spread of the disease to distant organs makes a cure virtually hopeless.

The average human capital value of saving one death due to breast cancer was estimated at $37,000 in 1970, using the age distribution of victims. Despite the obvious gains from early diagnosis and public education efforts, the proportion of cases treated while still localized has remained less than 50 per cent.

The Massachusetts Tumor Registry receives abstracted information on new cancers examined at various hospitals and clinics in

[1] Homothetic preferences have the property that if the relative feasibilities are unchanged, the equilibrium ratio Q/Z would remain unchanged, as along the line R_1 in Fig. 13.2 (b).
[2] This is the number surviving, divided by the number who would be expected to survive, given a standard population with the same age distribution.

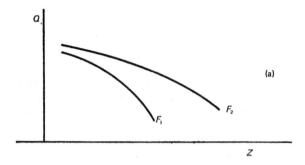

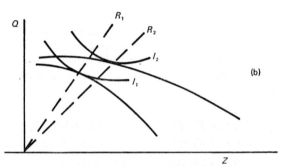

FIG. 13.2   The professional preference model

Massachusetts. Patients are followed-up at regular intervals after diagnosis and treatment. For the present analysis, all the abstracts of new cases for women first treated in 1965 and 1967 at six major Boston area hospitals were selected. There were approximately 200 cases each for the years 1965 and 1967. The data include date of initial diagnosis, demographic information, characteristics of the tumor at the time of original diagnosis and first treatments.

The seeking of early diagnosis of disease, or the frequency of routine examinations, is a consumer activity of the type that under-lies the C.D.C. model. Between 1965 and 1967 there was a small increase in the proportion of cases which had localized extent at the time of first treatment. Table 13.4 shows a higher gain in the propor-tion of localized cases for the elderly than for women under age 65.

The type of case treated may have changed during the period, and it is necessary to use a multivariate analysis to test for significance of the pure time change associated with the changes in reimbursement

TABLE 13.4

BREAST CANCERS AT TIME OF FIRST TREATMENT,
CLASSIFIED BY AGE OF PATIENT AND
EXTENT OF DISEASE

	1965		1967	
	Number	% localized	Number	% localized
Under age 65	107	33·6	144	38·2
Age 65+	66	33·3	82	42·6
Total sample	173	33·5	226	39·8

coverage. Two methods will be used here. First, a linear multiple regression may be calculated with each case as an observation. the *t*-tes tfor significance of an individual coefficient, when all the variables are dichotomous dummy variables (taking the value 1 or 0), is equivalent for large samples to the chi-square test for dependence in contingency tables.

The linear model is not constrained to guarantee that fitted values of the dependent variable lie in the interval (0, 1). In addition, the use of a dichotomous dependent variable implies that the variance of the random error in the model will not be constant among observations.

Alternative tests are calculated for grouped data using the logit transformation of observed frequencies (see [11] pp. 632–6).

A previous study of the determinants of early cancer diagnosis [6] gave attention to age, marital status, tumor characteristics and housing values as variables related to the proportion of localized cases. In the current sample, housing value or other measures of family financial resources are unknown. In Table 13.5 the remaining variables offer little explanation for the variation in extent of disease. In particular, it is not possible to distinguish the small improvement in

TABLE 13.5

DEPENDENT VARIABLE: LOCALIZED
(value 1 if extent localized at time of first treatment)

Variable[a]	Coefficient	t-value
Age <65 Histology Code 006[b]	0·11	(1·8)
Previous cancer occurrence	0·12	(1·0)
1967 dummy	0·06	(1·0)
Intercept = 0·27 $R^2 = 0·02$ d.f. = 247		
Age 65+ Histology Code 006	0·04	(0·5)
Previous cancer occurrence	0·32	(2·2)
1967 dummy	0·06	(0·8)
Intercept = 0·31 $R^2 = 0·04$ d.f. = 144		

[a] Marital status and age were also insignificant.
[b] American Cancer Society code for intraductal carcinoma.

early diagnosis as a pure time change, rather than the result of changes in measured case characteristics. This should not prejudge the consumer behavior with respect to other serious illness that may be attended with less fearful attitudes.[1]

The patients in this sample have been followed long enough to determine the proportion surviving at least three years from the date of diagnosis. Table 13.6 gives the percentage mortality for the first,

TABLE 13.6

THREE-YEAR SURVIVAL EXPERIENCE
OF SAMPLE CASES

	Number	% dead within 3 years	% dead within 2 years	% dead within 1 year
1965: Under age 65	107	30·0	22·4	14·0
Age 65+	66	51·5	39·3	22·7
Total sample	173	38·2	29·9	17·3
1967: Under age 65	144	32·6	24·3	11·1
Age 65+	82	54·2	43·9	18·3
Total sample	226	40·7	31·4	13·7

second and third years. Both age groups show no improvement in three-year survival. Over the first year there is a reduced mortality rate in 1967. This improvement, however, cannot be judged significant when other variables are held constant.[2]

Table 13.7 indicates that surgical treatment is the variable having the largest independent association with reduced mortality. For neither age group is the addition of radiation therapy significantly associated with reduced mortality. For older persons, a localized disease has a significant independent effect in reduced mortality, in addition to any indirect effect in determining the choice of treatment.

The interpretation of Table 13.7 is clouded by the possibility of bias due to correlation of the treatment choice with the unobserved random variation in survival. One way of approaching this problem is to replace both surgery and radiation with instrumental estimates based on prior regressions of each treatment variable on the list of exogenous variables. When this was done, neither variable could be judged significant. This certainly does not imply that patients would survive as long without treatment. The instrument variables do not give a satisfactory close fit to the treatment variables, which themselves are weak measurements due to variation in the procedures that are

---

[1] There would also be expected an increase in the number of diagnostic visits where suspicions of cancer were proved groundless.

[2] Table 13.7 uses three-year death rate as a dependent variable. When a one-year rate was used, the 1967 dummy remained insignificant.

TABLE 13.7

DEPENDENT VARIABLE: *DEAD3*
(value 1 if patient dead within three years of diagnosis)

Variable	Coefficient	t-value
Age <65 Surgery[a]	−0·55	(−7·9)
Radiation[b]	0·04	(0·7)
Localized	−0·07	(−1·3)
Age	0·001	(0·5)
Histology Code 006	−0·05	(−0·9)
1967 dummy	−0·01	(−0·2)
Intercept = 0·73	R^2 = 0·27	d.f. = 244
Age 65 + Surgery	−0·31	(−3·5)
Radiation	−0·11	(−1·3)
Localized	−0·26	(−3·1)
Age	0·008	(1·9)
Histology Code 006	−0·05	(−0·6)
1967 dummy	0·05	(0·7)
Intercept = 0·23	R^2 = 0·20	d.f. = 141

[a] Value 1 if some surgery during first admission.
[b] Value 1 if some radiation therapy during first admission.

classified as surgery or radiation, particularly the latter. Underlying influences, i.e. localized extent and intraductal histology, however, are judged as significantly reducing mortality.

A national survey for 1969 gives some notion of the relative costs of surgery and radiation. For all cancer sites, first hospital admissions had an average cost of $1,584 if surgery was the only procedure. Cases having both surgery and radiation cost an average of $1,931.[1]

The proportion of cases treated by surgery and radiation changed between 1965 and 1967, as shown in Table 13.8. The proportion of cases treated by either method alone fell, while the proportion of

TABLE 13.8

CLASSIFICATION OF SAMPLE CASES BY
TYPE OF INITIAL TREATMENT

	Number	% surgery only	% radiation only	% surgery and radiation
1965: Under age 65	107	55·1	11·2	24·3
Age 65+	66	40·9	25·8	19·7
Total sample	173	49·7	16·8	22·5
1967: Under age 65	144	30·0	10·4	50·0
Age 65+	82	40·2	12·1	32·9
Total sample	226	33·6	11·1	43·8

[1] *Preliminary Report, Third National Cancer Survey*, D.H.E.W. Publication No. (NIH) 72–128.

cases treated by both methods rose dramatically. For the entire sample, the proportion of cases treated by both surgery and radiation was approximately doubled in two years. This rise occurred at each of the six reporting hospitals, three of which are operated by the Massachusetts Department of Public Health.

According to Table 13.8, the proportion of cases treated with some radiation grew sharply for the group under age 65, but did not grow for the older group. This result would not be anticipated for a true random sample in view of the aggregate experience of larger gains in reimbursement for the elderly group than for the rest of the population. The nature of the actual sample helps to explain the observation. For cases treated at the three hospitals not operated by the state, the proportion having some radiation rose from 33·0 per cent to 46·1 per cent for the younger group, and from 35·3 per cent to 42·5 per cent for the older group.

At state hospitals, which accounted for about 30 per cent of the sample in 1965, but 50 per cent of the 1967 sample, younger women experienced a much greater rise in radiation treatment than did older women. Changes in the degree of state subsidy to all patients at these hospitals do not permit inferences about the independent influence of the Medicare program.

Even at the private hospitals, some unanalyzed forces were at work to increase the use of radiation for all patients. Part of the rise for younger persons may still be due to lower cost to older patients, according to the manner in which 'standards' of care become applied.

The general impression given by these data is that the amount of treatment increased substantially in two years, with little, if any, improvement in the three-year survival rate. The Medicare program may not have been the only important new influence on treatment choice. With some reservations, the results argue against the C.D.C. model for making welfare comparisons.

The analysis has ignored the possibility that radiation achieves substantial palliative benefits. Since radiation was often previously used as a later course of therapy, technological development may have improved the desirability of radiation even in the initial treatment. The notions of professional preferences are, in any case, challenged to provide additional insight as to why technological change of this sort might have meaningful utility benefits to providers.[1]

---

[1] One may speculate on benefits of stimulating scientific activity in developing new equipment, the relief of taking more direct action against the disease enemy, and a game of establishing hierarchies of prestigious institutions. Further, the adoption of a new trial technique for some cases may change the 'standards' of care for all others.

VI. CONCLUDING OBSERVATIONS

Some evidence, on both the aggregate and the micro-levels, that is emerging after the introduction of Medicare does not support the adequacy of conventional demand analysis for evaluating the welfare impact of health expenditure reimbursement programs.

Models in which physicians and health institutions make decisions reflecting their own non-monetary preferences seem to provide implications that are fruitful for quantitative analysis. Further research is needed to examine alternative regulatory controls that may serve the public interests.

REFERENCES

[1] Cooper, Barbara S., and Worthington, Nancy, 'Medical Care Spending for Three Age Groups', *Social Security Bulletin* (May 1972).
[2] Davis, K., 'Economic Theories of Behavior in Non-Profit Private Hospitals', *Economic and Business Bulletin* (Aug 1972).
[3] Feldstein, M. S., *The Rising Cost of Hospital Care* (Washington, D.C.: Information Resources Press, 1971).
[4] ——, 'The Rising Price of Physicians' Services', *Review of Economics and Statistics*, LII (May 1970) 121–33.
[5] ——, 'Hospital Cost Inflation: A Study of Nonprofit Pricing Behavior', *American Economic Review* (Dec 1971).
[6] Friedman, B., Parker, P., and Lipworth, L., 'The Influence of Medicaid and Private Health Insurance on the Early Diagnosis of Breast Cancer' (forthcoming in *Medical Care*).
[7] Newhouse, J. P., 'Toward a Theory of Nonprofit Institutions: An Economic Model of a Hospital', *American Economic Review*, LX (Mar 1970) 64–74.
[8] Pauly, M. V., 'The Economics of Moral Hazard', *American Economic Review*, LVIII, 4 (1968).
[9] Phelps, C. E., and Newhouse, J. P., 'The Effects of Coinsurance on Demand for Physical Services', *Social Security Bulletin* (June 1972).
[10] Rosett, R. N., and Lien-Fu Huang, 'The Effect of Health Insurance on the Demand for Medical Care', mimeographed (1970).
[11] Theil, H., *Principles of Econometrics* (New York: Wiley, 1971).
[12] U.S. Public Health Service, *End Results in Cancer*, Report No. 3 (Washington, D.C., 1968).
[13] U.S. Department of Health Education and Welfare, Office of the Assistant Secretary for Program Coordination, *Program Analysis: Cancer, October 1966* (Washington, D.C., 1966).
[14] U.S. Senate, Committee on Finance, *Medicare and Medicaid: Problems, Issues and Alternatives* (Washington, D.C., 1970).

14 Demand for Emergency Health Care and Regional Systems for Provision of Supply[1]

Ulf Christiansen

DANISH BUILDING RESEARCH INSTITUTE, COPENHAGEN

In 1971 a proposal for a new emergency care system for Greater Copenhagen (1·3 million inhabitants) was submitted to the local authorities in the area by a committee of experts. The proposed system would contain emergency wards with beds, centers for traumatic surgery, coronary units, modern emergency ambulances, a central referral office with wireless connections to all ambulances for the purpose of giving medical advice, and clinics for light casualties.

The proposal was based upon a casualty survey in the area during November 1968, covering all hospitals, to which 16,500 patients were admitted through the casualty departments. For each patient, extensive information was collected; identification; time, place and type of accident; diagnosis; ambulance response and trip time.

The proposal was evaluated by a model assigning patients to the new system and a linear simulation model for the location and number of ambulances based upon an evaluation of the value of the patient's time and condition. The location and number of hospitals were determined by political decisions, dating back to the beginning of the 1960s.

The system is in the process of implementation.

In 1967 the three integrated hospital administrations in Greater Copenhagen set up a committee for the planning of the casualty services. Planning data of a sufficient quality were not available, although the need for statistics concerning hospital use and demand going beyond the hospital statistics currently published had long been recognized. Owing to this lack of data a one-month survey of the demand for casualty services was undertaken during November 1968.

[1] The investigation and the proposed system described in the paper are the results of a collective enterprise in which Lars Bostrup, M.A., Niels Stephenson, M.D., and Gunnar Schiøler, M.D., took part, together with the author. A regional advisory committee for emergency care has submitted the proposal to the relevant authorities.

I. THE DEMAND FOR CASUALTY SERVICES 1960–7: SYSTEM AS OF 1968

For many years the emergency care system has consisted of hospitals with casualty departments, ambulance stations and ambulances. Some of the hospitals are highly specialized, e.g. have departments for neuro-surgery and advanced cardiology. They may be classified as medical centers or university hospitals. The others are general hospitals, mostly of large size (over 500 beds).

Casualty departments in the hospitals receive surgical and medical emergencies of all kinds, and of very differing degrees of seriousness. The casualty department proper is manned with either young on-duty surgeons from a surgical inpatient department, or with permanent staff. They are not, however, qualified to perform major operations, and may call upon senior staff as well as other specialists. The casualty department has no beds, except for the purpose of observations of a few hours' duration.

The area is served by four different ambulance administrations, three of them municipal and one private. Each administration is allotted its own geographical area of operations. This may in some cases add to the transportation for patients who are picked up on the edge of administrative boundaries.

The ambulances are manned by two drivers, who are trained in first-aid and resuscitation techniques, but who are not, in any sense, qualified nurses. The ambulances are equipped with two-way radios. Ambulance calls are handled by a municipal central alarm office which orders ambulances belonging to municipal fire-brigades to proceed to the place of the accident, if it is situated in the inner metropolitan area (Copenhagen, Frederiksberg, Gentofte). In the outer area the calls are transferred from this office to a county office operated by a private ambulance company (Falk-Zonen), which sends out its own ambulances. During ths 1960s 10 hospitals in Greater Copenhagen operated casualty departments. In November 1968, 23 emergency ambulances, located at 22 ambulance stations, were available (see Fig. 14.1).

From 1960 to 1967 the number of patients received at the casualty departments rose steadily (see appendix, Table A.1). In the fiscal year 1964–5, 169,800 patients, or 126 patients per 1,000 inhabitants per year, were admitted. In the fiscal year 1967–8, the number had increased to 189,400, or 141 patients per 1,000 inhabitants per year. This corresponds to a monthly average of 11·75 patients per 1,000 inhabitants – not considering seasonal variations and normal annual increases. The number of patients measured in relation to the number of inhabitants may be taken as a rough indicator of the demand

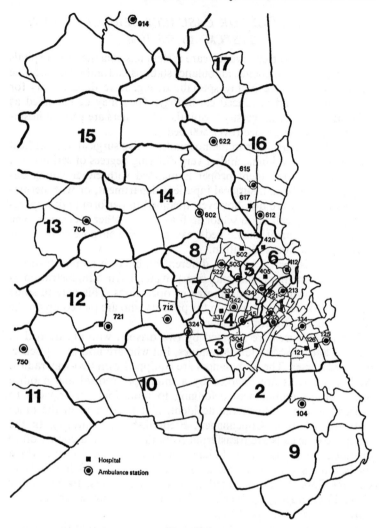

FIG. 14.1

in the whole area, but is of limited value for forecasting. This becomes clear when looking at the relationship for smaller geographical areas. An illustration of this fact is given in Fig. 14.2, where the annual number of patients admitted to seven of the ten departments for the fiscal years under consideration has been related to the population in the districts from which each department receives ambulances.[1] It is evident from the figure that no simple relationship exists between the resident population and the expected number of

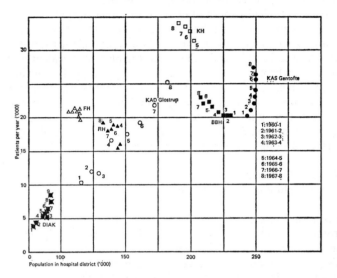

FIG. 14.2

casualty cases. This ambiguity may be explained by various factors, among them:

1. There is no complete correspondence between the actual catchment area and the ambulance district.
2. The population at risk is the population present in the area and, thus, not identical with the resident population during working hours and the early evening.
3. The tendency to use the casualty clinics is subject to an annual variation due to exogenous factors such as employment, residential density, traffic conditions, etc.

II. THE NOVEMBER 1968 SURVEY

The investigation lasted from 8 a.m. on 1 November to 8 p.m. on 2 December 1968. All patients who came into contact with the casualty departments, or who were admitted directly as inpatients from accidents involving traumatic injuries, were registered. Six types of questionnaire were used.

[1] This corresponds roughly to the catchment area.

(1) *Areas and Zones*

One of the purposes of the investigation was to evaluate the location of the casualty departments (and, thus, of the hospitals) in relation to the geographical pattern of demand. Another purpose was to estimate ambulance transportation times in relation to distances travelled, leading to judgments about the location of ambulance stations.

In order to be able to do this, both the place of accident and the place from where the patient came had to be registered, using an area code. When choosing the area code, compatibility with other relevant data classified by area (especially population data) was necessary. This restricted our choice to the zones or sub-areas used by the Regional Planning Authority of Greater Copenhagen and Northern Zealand, although the size of these zones ranges from 0·1 sq. km to 35 sq. km from the city center outwards. The total number of sub-zones in Greater Copenhagen is 161. The sub-zones may be added together to form ambulance districts (hospital districts) and main zones.

(2) *Incidence of Casualties in November 1968*

A total of 16,509 patients were admitted to the casualty departments. The total population in the area was 1,345,000 as of 1 November 1968. This gives an average incidence of cases for November 1968 of 11·8 per 1,000 inhabitants. 4,342 (27 per cent) arrived in emergency ambulances. The distribution of patients according to residence is shown in Table 14.1.

TABLE 14.1

DISTRIBUTION OF PATIENTS
AMONG MUNICIPALITIES

Place of residence (municipality)	Number of cases	Referred to inpatient departments	Population (1 Nov. 1968)
Copenhagen	8,543	1,149	649,200
Frederiksberg	1,236	178	104,500
Copenhagen County	6,031	853	591,800
Total number of patients resident in region	15,810	2,180	1,345,500
From outside region, address unknown	699	132	
Total	16,509	2,312	

The number of patients per 1,000 inhabitants was as follows:

Copenhagen	13·2 per 1,000 inhabitants
Frederiksberg	11·8
Copenhagen County	10·2
Region	11·8

250 patients left the casualty departments without treatment and 16,253 received treatment. After treatment, 13,791 were sent home and 2,312 admitted as inpatients. In 28 cases a diagnosis was not made. Of the remaining 16,225 patients, 13,519 were traumatic cases (including poisonings) and 2,706 (16 per cent) were sudden illness. Table 14.2 shows the variation between the traumatic and the non-

TABLE 14.2

NUMBER OF TRAUMATIC AND NON-TRAUMATIC CASES
RECEIVED AT CASUALTY CLINICS IN
GREATER COPENHAGEN, NOVEMBER 1968

Casualty clinic	Traumatic cases	Non-traumatic cases	Total	Percentage non-traumatic
Rigshospitalet	1,355	355	1,710	20·8
Kommunehospitalet	2,477	546	3,023	18·1
Bispebjerg hospital	1,536	371	1,907	19·5
Sundby hospital (casualty dept.)	1,140	273	1,413	19·3
Frederiksberg hospital	1,419	276	1,695	16·3
Diakonissestiftelsen	572	87	659	13·2
Københavns amts sygehus, Glostrup	2,185	307	2,492	12·3
Københavns amts sygehus, Gentofte	2,014	369	2,383	15·5
Sgt. Elisabeths hospital	422	89	511	17·4
Ortopædisk hospital	191	11	202	5·4
Statshospitalet i Glostrup (psychiatry)	1	16	17	94·1
Sundby hospital (surgical dispensary)	207	6	213	2·8
Total	13,519	2,706	16,225	16·7

traumatic cases. The percentage of non-traumatic cases varies significantly between the clinics (as it does also when the last three very specialized departments are omitted).

(3) *Incidence Related to Sub-zones and Zones*
The 161 sub-zones were added together to form 17 zones using, *inter alia*, employment criteria, so that type of employment and employment/resident ratio varied among them. The number of cases in each main zone is shown in Table A.2 in the appendix, together with the incidence per zone unit. The highest incidence was found in area 5, Nørrebro, which is among the most densely populated parts of the metropolitan area, and the second highest in the central business district (zone 1). Both were above 200 per sq. km. In the outer districts we find much lower incidences, the highest being in areas 12, 14

and 16, where the figure is around 20 per sq. km. These differences between the casualty densities reflect differences in densities of built-up areas and industries in the main zones. They are, however, averaged out, flattened so to say, in several of them, owing to the fact that the built-up areas are restricted to a few of the sub-zones which make up the zones in question.

The zonal incidence in Copenhagen and Frederiksberg is shown in Fig. 14.3. There is a large variation from zone to zone of the activities

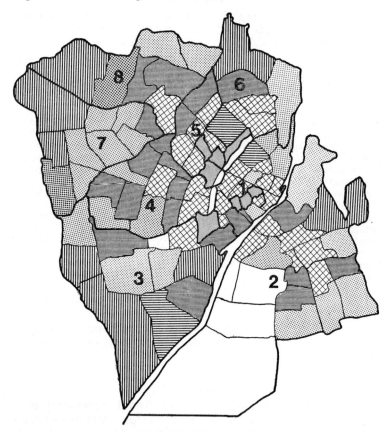

FIG. 14.3   Inner zones

that the patients were engaged in at the time of accident (see appendix, Table A.2). On the face of it, this variation might be ascribed to differences in the structure of population and employment. However, there is no such simple explanation. For example, the number of casualities originating in the home varies from 231 to 496 per 100,000 inhabitants per zone, and the number at workplaces from 223 to 952 per 100,000 employees per zone.

(4) *Transportation by Ambulance*

4,342 patients (27 per cent) were transported by emergency ambulance to the hospitals. The number of trips as a percentage of the patients received at the casualty departments does not vary significantly between main zones except for main zone 3. We feel that this percentage may be regarded as fairly high, considering that 1,781 of the patients using ambulances suffered from superficial wounds, eye lesions and bruises.

Between 5 and 10 per cent of these patients were admitted as inpatients after referral at the casualty departments. However, 70 per cent of all ambulance trips originate outside the patients' homes and, very often, the third party calling the ambulance may not know how serious the patient's condition is. He may also call the ambulance out of sheer convenience or have a high risk-aversion, as can be the case with schools, etc.

(5) *The Time Factor*

The response time is defined as the interval elapsing between the ambulance's departure from an ambulance station (or any other place where it is reached by a call for service) until it reaches the place of the accident. The transportation time is defined as the time interval elapsing from the arrival of the ambulance at the place of the accident until the arrival at the casualty department. The transportation time, thus, includes the time spent at the place of the accident (Fig. 14.4).

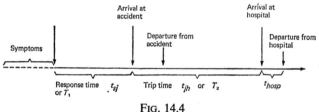

FIG. 14.4

The response and transportation times have been submitted to statistical analysis. A stratified sample of 950 trips was taken. The distribution of response times gives a crude indication of how well the ambulance stations are located in the Greater Copenhagen area. Cumulative distribution functions of response times are shown in Fig. 14.5 (a), (b) and (c). Fig. 14.5 (a) relates exclusively to ambulances going to hospitals in the county of Copenhagen, i.e. in the less densely populated outer districts, while 14.5 (b) and 14.5 (c) relate to

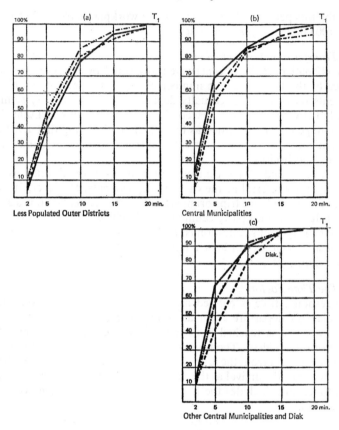

FIG. 14.5   Response times for different groups of hospitals

the central municipalities (the curve marked 'Diak.' excepted). In the outer districts, between 40 and 50 per cent of the response times are below 5 minutes. In the inner districts, between 55 and 70 per cent lie below 5 minutes. Only 5 per cent lie above 15 minutes. If we compare these results with conditions in other large cities, we may consider them as quite good.

For example, in London, Warren (1970) finds an average response time of 8·5 minutes for accidents and an average transportation time of 18·3 minutes. In Copenhagen the average response time was on the order of 7 minutes. For Brooklyn, New York, Savas (1969) finds a response time of 11·9 minutes. 10 per cent of the trips had a response time of more than 20 minutes. In Copenhagen this was true of 5 per cent of the trips.

The trip times are, naturally, longer than the response times, as 22 ambulance stations and only 10 casualty departments were available at the time of investigation. On average, only 20 per cent of the trip times lie below 5 minutes, while 12 per cent lie above 15 minutes. The distributions of trip times indicate how well the hospitals are

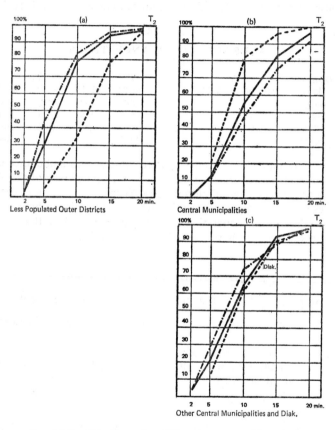

FIG. 14.6   Trip times for different groups of hospitals

located in their catchment areas and how large these areas are. Trip times are particularly long in the outer districts and especially so in the western parts of the county of Copenhagen (served by the hospitals KAS Gl. and Diak.) and in the northern and northwestern parts of Copenhagen proper (served by BBH) (see Fig. 14.6).

As to the distribution of the ambulance trips during the day, more than 40 per cent occur between 12 noon and 6 p.m. and only 7 per cent from 12 midnight to 6 a.m.

The accidents have been grouped according to their average distance to the casualty departments. The means in the sample of response and trip times have been cross-classified according to distance and time of day in Table 14.3. *A priori*, there is no reason for the response times to correlate with the distance to hospital, but there does

TABLE 14.3

AVERAGE AMBULANCE TIMES
(minutes)

Distance (km)	T_1 00–06	T_1 06–24	T_2 00–06	T_2 06–24	T_2 12–18	$T_1 + T_2$ 00–06	$T_1 + T_2$ 06–24
0·625	5·4	5·1	5·8	6·7	4·9	11·2	11·8
1·875	5·6	6·0	9·0	8·5	8·8	14·5	15·0
3·750	7·5	8·1	10·7	11·6	11·3	18·2	19·7
7·500	–	7·1	–	13·7	13·0	–	20·0

exist a correlation in the outer districts, where both ambulance and hospital districts are much larger than in the central part of the city, owing to the lower population density. Surprisingly enough, neither the response nor the transportation times vary significantly with the time of day. Traffic congestion as well as peak periods in the ambulance service seem to have exerted no appreciable influence.

III. THE PROPOSED NEW SYSTEM

The proposed system will contain the following new elements:

1. Emergency wards (E.W.) for emergencies and acutely ill patients (with beds).
2. Centers for traumatic surgery.
3. Central referral office (C.R.O.) with immediate access to cardiological advice. (The C.R.O. is permanently staffed with one physician or surgeon.)
4. Coronary units.
5. Ambulances equipped with E.C.G.-transmission sets, resuscitation equipment, defibrillator, etc., and staffed with two drivers and one nurse.
6. Clinics for light casualties.

The system is illustrated in Fig. 14.7.

The existing type of casualty department can be therefore discarded.

In the proposed new system, all patients going by emergency ambulance are sent either to an emergency ward, to a coronary unit

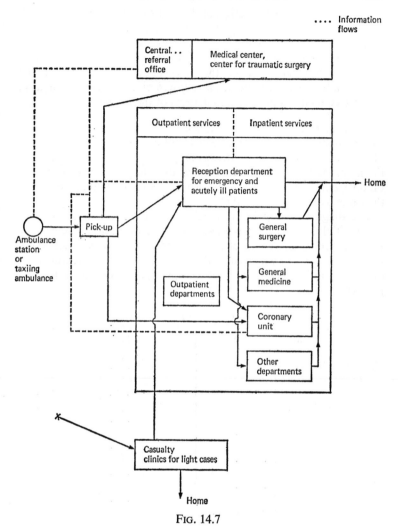

FIG. 14.7

or to a center for traumatic surgery, after consultation between the ambulance nurse and the referral office. All other patients are initially only received at a clinic for light casualties. More serious cases may be sent along from there to an emergency ward, etc., after consultation between the clinic and the referral office. When deciding on the necessary number of ambulances and their bases, we must remember that not more than 5 per cent of the emergency calls should be answered with a response time exceeding 5 minutes.

The most important function of the C.R.O. is to advise the ambulance crews on difficult cases and, for all cases, to direct the ambulance to the nearest system component with free capacity, where the patient may receive adequate treatment. The component chosen receives immediate information from the office about the arrival and the likely condition of the patient. The office receives current information about free facilities in the various parts of the system.

Assignment of Patients to the System

The evaluation of the system begins with an estimate of the number of patients assigned to the various component parts of the system, on the assumption that the total number of patients, their distribution on different diagnoses, and their propensity to use ambulances were the same as in November 1968.

The diagnoses have been classified in 248 groups based on the three initial digits of the modified W.H.O. classification. For each of these groups, the surgeons of the working party have determined the units of the system which are sufficient for either final treatment or diagnosis and referral, without compromising the result for the patient.

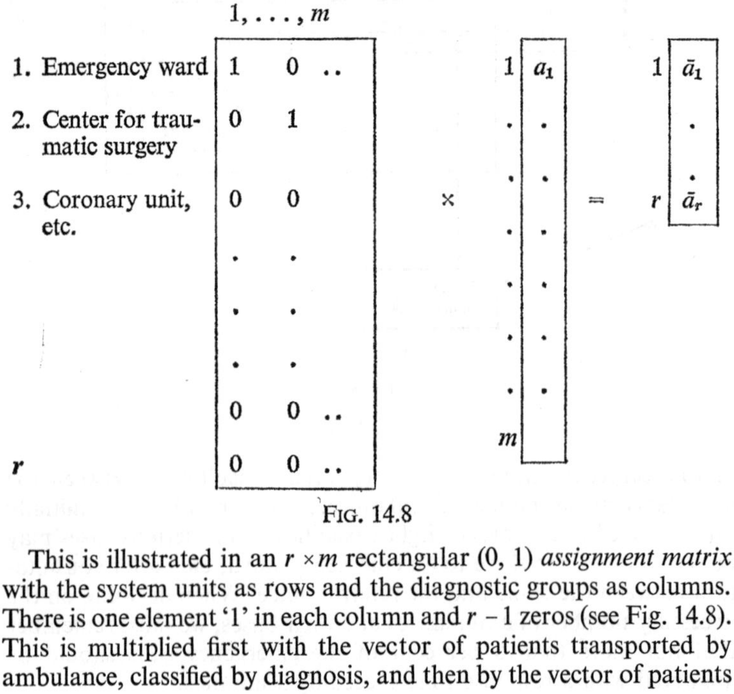

Fig. 14.8

This is illustrated in an $r \times m$ rectangular $(0, 1)$ *assignment matrix* with the system units as rows and the diagnostic groups as columns. There is one element '1' in each column and $r - 1$ zeros (see Fig. 14.8). This is multiplied first with the vector of patients transported by ambulance, classified by diagnosis, and then by the vector of patients not transported by ambulance. By suitably arranging the resulting vectors, we obtain the patient flows in Table A.3 of the appendix.

IV. EVALUATION OF THE EMERGENCY CARE SYSTEM

The purpose in this section is to develop a location policy for ambulance stations and emergency wards. This can be done on a single simulation model. The model should be able to say something about:

1. Satisfactory locations and numbers of ambulance stations or, eventually, a relaxation of the location concept.
2. A distribution of ambulances between stations (or in the area) and a total satisfactory number of ambulances.
3. A way of assessing the effects on system performance of altering the number and location of emergency wards in the area.

(1) *Variables and Indices*

The metropolitan area is subdivided with p sub-zones. For each sub-zone, the number of calls $A_j(j = 1, \ldots, p)$ is known. The total number of calls is given by the vector.

$$\mathbf{A} = \{A_1, \ldots, A_p\}.$$

The area is served by $N(N < p)$ ambulance stations, each having n_s ambulances at its disposal. Each ambulance station serves a given set of sub-zones unless all ambulances at a neighboring station are already in use. For the duration of the use it will have to serve the sub-zones of this station as well. The total number of ambulances is given by the vector.

$$\mathbf{n} = \{n_1, \ldots, n_N\}.$$

Initially, each zone is allotted to a definite hospital (emergency ward). This does not entirely correspond to the new system in which the C.R.O. decides the allocation of the patients, but is, in most cases, a good approximation.

The variable A_j is indexed in different ways. A_{sj} represents the number of ambulance calls from station s to sub-zone j. A_{jh} refers to the number of ambulances travelling to hospital h from zone j. The mean travel time from every ambulance station s to every zone j is known, i.e. we have a rectangular $N \times p$ matrix T_{sj} of 'response times'. Further, we know the mean travel time from every zone j to every hospital h and, thus, have a rectangular $p \times M$ matrix T_{jh} of 'trip times'. The mean duration of stay of an ambulance at a hospital is called T_{hosp}. T_{hosp} is assumed to be independent of station and hospital.

An ambulance is considered free for service as soon as it leaves the hospital after having discharged a patient. The total amount of time an ambulance is occupied will be the sum of elements from the matrices T_{sj} and T_{jh} plus T_{hosp}.

Generally, low values of T_{sj} and T_{jh} will be favorable to the patients in need of immediate treatment. Low values of T_{sj} signify that ambulance stations must be widely dispersed over the metropolitan area in 'median' locations and, further, that the number of ambulances must be high enough at each station to secure low probabilities of rejection of demand for service. This dispersion and provision of relatively high immediate capacity must be balanced against the resulting costs, which consist mainly of station site costs, depreciation and maintenance costs of ambulances and costs of necessary personnel on a duty rota. Low values of T_{jh} result from a wide dispersion and a larger number of hospitals with possibly, but not invariably, small emergency wards. A smaller size of department may be staffed by less experienced personnel, fewer specialists, and a definite or low risk of providing insufficient treatment for the patient. Thus, we may well get a significantly better system by accepting somewhat higher values of T_{jh} than otherwise, if ambulances are well equipped with life-saving equipment and well-trained paramedical personnel.

C denotes the cost per unit of time per ambulance incurred by the ambulance administration. The financial cost of the emergency wards, coronary units, etc., will not be introduced into the model and variables associated with this cost are, thus, not necessary.

A distinction between operating costs and users' costs will be made.[1]

Total cost K is further specified by

$$K = D + B \tag{1}$$

where D is operating cost, including maintenance and depreciation, and B is users' cost. In the model, D is very straightforward. All the problems are related to the specification of B.

(2) *Indicators of System Performance*

Disregarding behavior and costs incurred by the hospitals, the total mean response time T_{sj} and the total mean trip time T_{jh} give two separate measures of performance of the ambulance system and, partly, of the hospital system. At first sight, it seems impossible to add these variables together, particularly when it is recognized that a concentration of personnel and equipment in a small number of

---

[1] This distinction has a long tradition in the management of telephone equipment (see Jensen, 1950) and has lately gained acceptance in cost-effectiveness analysis.

hospitals may give substantial benefits to the patients, even though they must submit to somewhat larger, sometimes considerably larger, values of T_{jh}. An additional advantage of concentration is that it leads to a smaller total number of required beds and personnel in the emergency ward part of the hospital system, for a given level of service, than decentralization does.

In order to attach a monetary value to the patient's time, coupled with the seriousness of his condition, a weighting factor

$$w = [u\theta + z(1 - \theta)]$$

is introduced. This factor weights the total response and trip times, using either the proportion of cases where a short response time is considered essential, θ_1, or the proportion of cases for which a short trip time is essential, θ_2.

In the existing system, θ_1 and θ_2 may be considered approximately equal in the model, as life-saving procedures can, to any significant extent, first be instituted at the hospitals. In actual fact, θ_1 is likely to be slightly higher than θ_2.

In the proposed system, θ_1 should be significantly higher than θ_2, as the general philosophy is to bring adequate life-saving treatment to the patients at the place of accident or sudden illness. θ_1 and θ_2 may be directly estimated from the number of patients falling into certain critical diagnostic categories, compared with the ability of treating patients on the spot by the new ambulance system.

The term u is the cost associated with waiting 1 minute for a patient in the θ-category, and is time-dependent. For coronary cases with cardiac arrest occurring exactly at the time of alarm, the maximum response time is on the order of 2–3 minutes, since without

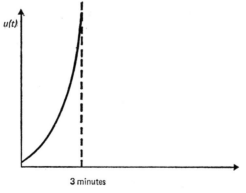

FIG. 14.9

oxygenation of the brain tissue irreparable brain damage occurs, on average after 4 minutes. This gives the shape of the u-function for cardiac arrests as shown in Fig. 14.9. Our specification does not take the time-dependence of u into account directly. In this, u is considered as an average, taken over a period of time, for all types of serious cases.

The term z is the cost associated with waiting 1 minute for all other cases (the $1 - \theta$ category). It will be much lower than u, but should still be taken into account.

(3) *The Model*
The model is based on the following specification of expression (1):

$$K = \Sigma D_s + \Sigma B_{sj} + \Sigma B_{jh} \qquad (2)$$

where ΣD_s is the total operating cost for ambulances, ΣB_{sj} the total users' cost associated with waiting for the ambulances in the zones, and ΣB_{jh} the users' cost associated with the transportation from zone to hospital.

For ambulance station s we may detail expression (2) as follows:

$$\begin{aligned} K_s &= D_s + B_{sj} + B_{jh} \qquad (3) \\ &= Cn_s + [u\theta_1 + z(1 - \theta_1)] \, [\Sigma A_{sj}\bar{t}_{sj} + \Sigma \hat{A}_{sj}f(E_1)] \\ &\quad + [u\theta_2 + z(1 - \theta_2)] \, [\Sigma A_{jh}\bar{t}_{jh}] \\ &= Cn_s + w_1 B_{sj} + w_2 B_{jh} \end{aligned}$$

The weighting factors w_1 and w_2 have been explained above, but B_{sj} and B_{jh} call for some explanation.

The first term, $\Sigma A_{sj}\bar{t}_{sj}$, in B_{sj} is the sum of all response times in one month for ambulance trips originating at station s. The second term, $\Sigma \hat{A}_{sj}f(E_1)$, is a calculated waiting time (see sub-section (4)) resulting from calls having to be served by ambulances from other stations owing to all ambulances at s being in use.[1] The calculation of this term will be further explained in the next sub-section. B_{sj} is thus the total response time per month for all calls (users) allotted to station s.

B_{jh} is the total trip time for all calls allotted to station s. A list of symbols is given in the appendix (Table A.4).

(4) *The Term* $\Sigma \hat{A}_{sj}f(E_1)$
Whenever a call for an ambulance cannot be responded to, owing to all ambulances at the station being in use, we shall have to call an ambulance from an alternative station. The probability of this event depends upon the demand in the zones allotted to the first station.

---

[1] Bars denote averages. T_{sj} is thus $\equiv t_{sj}$, etc.

In queuing terms the demanded occupancy is defined as the product of the number of calls during a given unit of time and the average time an ambulance is in use measured in the unit of time adopted.

The probability of directing calls to another station from s depends on the demanded occupancy and the number of ambulances available at s, n_s. We denote this probability E_1.

The demanded occupancy may be written

$$R_s = \hat{A}_s \times \hat{T}_s$$

where

$$\hat{A}_s = \Sigma \hat{A}_{sj}$$

and

$$\hat{T}_s = \Sigma \overline{T}_{sjh}.$$

The elements of the matrix T_{sjh} are given as

$$\overline{T}_{sjh} = \bar{t}_{sj} + \bar{t}_{jh} + t_{hosp}.$$

For the total metropolitan area we get the vector **R** of demanded occupancy:

$$\mathbf{R} = \{R_1, \ldots, R_N\}.$$

The probability E_1 is given by Erlang's loss formula[1]

$$E_{1,n}(R) = \frac{\dfrac{R^n}{n!}}{1 + \dfrac{R}{1!} + \ldots + \dfrac{R^n}{n!}}.$$

This probability is multiplied by the average response time associated with the alternative station but serving the zones of the first one, and we get $f(E_1)$.

(5) *Location and Size of Emergency Wards*

The possibilities for the location of E.W.s are limited by location of existing hospitals and decisions already made concerning the building activity in the hospital sector of the metropolitan area for the next ten to fifteen years. The locational problem is, thus, reduced to the selection of sites among known, well-defined alternatives. In principle, the number of E.W.s may vary from 1 to 11, as we have 11 possible sites and might choose a system from 1 to 11 E.W.s if the transportation time from the place of accident or other emergency to the E.W. were of no consequence for the service given to patients. However, this freedom of choice does not exist.

First of all, t_{jh} is important and, in some cases, vitally important. Furthermore, some solutions will not be technically feasible and

[1] See, e.g., Jensen (1950).

political factors must also be taken into consideration. It may even be that the number of feasible solutions is reduced to very few. For example, an operational policy of protecting the specialized departments of a general hospital from random disturbances as much as possible will entail that all such hospitals in the system must be equipped with an E.W.

Another problem is the capacity requirements of the E.W.s This is quite tricky, as it involves, among other things, decisions concerning treatment facilities, procedures for diagnosis, the choice between the possible cooperation with X-ray departments and an X-ray department specific to the E.W., rules for operating the department, etc. The demand is, in some way, dependent upon the size of the catchment area, no matter whether this is delimited by administrative boundaries or just by the factual operation of the centralized referral service. This may take transportation times into account, or may not, depending upon the presumed condition of the patient when he is picked up by the ambulance, or is reported to the referral service by a general practitioner as an acutely ill patient.

Some of the performance indicators necessary are the probability of all available beds being occupied at a given E.W., and the probability of all beds being occupied in the total E.W. system of the metropolitan area. By having a centralized referral service for patients brought to hospital by ambulance, it is possible to reduce the total number of beds in the E.W. system as compared with the number of beds required by a wholly decentralized system.

BIBLIOGRAPHY

Abernathy, W. J., and Hershey, J. C., 'A Spatial-Allocation Model for Regional Health Services Planning', *Operations Research*, II, 3 (May–June 1972) 629–42.

Bell, C., and Allen, D., 'Optimal Planning of an Emergency Ambulance Service', *Socio-Economic Planning Sciences* (Aug 1969).

Bostrup, G., Christiansen, U., Schiøler, G., and Stephensen, N., 'Skadeundersøgelsen i Storkøbenhavn', november 1968: I. Tilrettelæggelse og metodik; II. Forekomsten af tilskadekomne og pludseligt syge, som ankom til skadestuerne i Storkøbenhavn, november 1968', Ugeskrift for Læger, CXXXIV, 9 (1972).

Christiansen, U., 'Operationsanalyse og økonomiske modeller anvendt på hospitalsproblemer', *Nationaløkonomisk Tidsskrift*, CIX, 1–2 (1971).

Hogg, J. M., 'The Siting of Fire Stations', *Operations Research Quarterly* (Sept 1968).

Jensen, A., *Moe's Principle* (Copenhagen, 1950).

Larson, R. C., and Stevenson, K. A., 'On Insensitivities in Urban Redistricting and Facility Location', *Operations Research*, II, 3 (May–June 1972) 595–612.

Long, M. F., and Feldstein, P. J., 'Economies of Hospital Systems: Peak Loads and Regional Coordination', *American Economic Review*, LVII, 2 (May 1967) 119–29.

Morril, R., and Kelley, Ph., 'Optimum Allocation of Services: A Hospital Example', *Annals of Regional Science* (June 1969).

Revelle, Charles, Marks, D., and Liebman, J., 'An Analysis of Private and Public Sector Location Models', *Management Science*, XVI (1970) 692–707.

Savas, E., 'Simulation and Cost-Effectiveness Analysis of New York's Ambulance Service', *Management Science* (Aug 1969).

Schultz, George P., 'The Logic of Health Care Facility Planning', *Socio-Economic Planning Sciences*, IV, 3 (Sep 1970).

Warren, K. E., 'Night Cover Provided by the London Ambulance Service for Emergencies', M.Sc thesis (Dept. of Mechanical Engineering, Imperial College, London, 1970).

Weinerman, E. R., Ratner, R. S., *et al.*, 'Determinants of Use of Hospital Emergency Services', *American Journal of Public Health*, LVI, 7 (July 1966) 1037–56.

APPENDIX

TABLE A.1

NUMBER OF PATIENTS AT CASUALTY DEPARTMENT IN GREATER COPENHAGEN
FOR THE FISCAL YEARS 1960–1 TO 1967–8

Casualty clinic	Fiscal year							
	1960–1	1961–2	1962–3	1963–4	1964–5	1965–6	1966–7	1967–8
Rigshospitalet	n.a.	15,777	15,548	18,937	18,971	18,291	18,010	19,315
Kommunehospitalet	n.a.	n.a.	n.a.	n.a.	31,728	33,012	33,781	34,200
Bispebjerg hospital	20,275	20,285	20,409	20,960	21,675	22,434	22,265	23,078
Sundby hospital	19,114	19,056	19,167	19,688	20,495	19,583	20,428	21,194
Frederiksberg hospital	19,761	20,608	20,419	21,293	20,930	21,480	20,990	21,021
Diakonissestiftelsen	3,636	4,245	5,251	5,623	5,962	6,243	7,297	8,296
Glostrup hospital	10,325	12,035	11,829	16,556	17,715	19,462	22,044	25,018
Gentofte hospital	20,267	21,269	22,338	23,252	24,253	25,819	26,590	27,676
Skt. Elisabeths hospital	3,636	4,015	4,360	4,262	4,915	5,801	5,947	6,660
Ortopædisk hospital	3,324	3,360	3,320	n.a.	3,193	2,974	2,675	2,942

TABLE A.2

NUMBER OF CASES DISTRIBUTED ACCORDING TO ZONE AND
TYPE OF ACCIDENT, NOVEMBER 1968

Main zone	Home		Work		Traffic		Leisure outside home		Other		Total	%
	No.	%	No.	%	No.	%	No.	%	No.	%		%
1. Indreby	243	18·9	348	27·0	237	18·4	349	27·1	111	8·6	1,288	100·0
2. Amager Nord	605	35·1	519	30·0	165	9·5	277	16·0	162	9·4	1,728	100·0
3. København Sydvest	450	29·9	461	30·6	194	12·9	272	18·0	130	8·6	1,507	100·0
4. Frederiksberg	462	33·8	262	19·2	207	15·1	263	19·2	173	12·7	1,367	100·0
5. Nørrebro	459	38·2	240	19·9	181	15·0	221	18·3	104	8·6	1,205	100·0
6. Østerbro	319	29·1	285	26·0	135	12·3	241	21·9	118	10·7	1,098	100·0
7. Brønshøj	232	34·9	111	16·7	102	15·4	138	20·8	81	12·2	664	100·0
8. Søborg	267	30·3	199	22·6	149	17·0	172	19·6	92	10·5	879	100·0
9. Amager Syd	202	35·5	140	24·6	66	11·6	86	15·1	75	13·2	569	100·0
10. Hvidovre	314	35·2	204	22·9	80	9·0	157	17·6	136	15·3	891	100·0
11. Greve–Tåstrup	65	35·0	62	33·3	21	11·3	19	10·2	19	10·2	186	100·0
12. Glostrup–Islev–Rødovre	386	32·7	345	29·2	114	9·7	186	15·8	149	12·6	1,180	100·0
13. Ballerup–Sengeløse	125	35·1	93	26·1	44	12·3	59	16·5	36	10·0	357	100·0
14. Herlev–Gladsaxe	477	33·4	384	26·8	144	10·0	241	16·8	187	13·0	1,433	100·0
15. Bagsværd–Lille Værlose	91	32·9	46	16·6	32	11·6	63	22·7	45	16·2	277	100·0
16. Gentofte	259	31·8	206	25·3	106	13·0	140	17·2	103	12·7	814	100·0
17. Lyngby–Søllerød	97	36·2	60	22·4	21	7·8	53	19·8	37	13·8	268	100·0
Total		32·2		25·2		12·7		18·7		11·2	15,711	100·0

TABLE A.3

PATIENT FLOWS IN THE PROPOSED SYSTEM

Receiving unit \ 'Sending' unit	Transportation unit		Treatment unit		Total
	Ambulance	Private transport	Reception department	Casualty clinic for light cases	
Casualty clinic for light cases	*	12,138 (854)	*	*	12,138 (854)
Emergency ward	4,139 (1,261)	*	*	1,632 (805)	5,771 (2,066)
Center for traumatic surgery	57 (52)	*	0	41 (29)	98 (81)
Coronary unit	145 (115)	*	0	33 (20)	178 (135)
Unit for treatment of poisonings	78 (78)	*	0	0	78 (78)
Unit for treatment of burns	19 (19)	*	0	0	19 (19)
Others	*	*	2,066 (2,066)	*	2,066 (2,066)
Sent home	*	*	3,588	10,429	14,017
Dead	*	*	117	3	120
Total	4,438 (1,525)	12,138 (854)	5,771 (2,066)	12,138 (854)	

* = impossible.

TABLE A.4

LIST OF SYMBOLS

j	Zone identification
s	Ambulance station identification
h	Emergency ward identification
n_s	Number of ambulances at ambulance station s
A_{sj}	Number of patients per month, picked up from zone j by ambulances from station s
A_{jh}	Number of patients per month, picked up from zone j and sent to emergency ward h
t_{sj}	Average response time from station s to zone j
t_{jh}	Average transportation time from j to h
t_{hosp}	Average time spent at hospital by ambulances (information not available but set at 10 minutes; Warren (1970) estimated it to 13 minutes)
0_1	Probability that a patient's condition is such that the response time is of vital importance

0_2 Probability that a patient's condition is such that the transportation time is of vital importance
($0_1 = 0_2$ in the old system without nurses in the ambulances, $0_1 = 0_2$ in the new system

u Cost for patients in categories 0_1 and 0_2 of 'waiting' 1 minute at the place of accident and 1 minute's transportation time to hospital

C Cost per month for one ambulance

z Cost per minute for waiting and transportation time for patients not vitally hurt or sick

A_{sj} A_{sj}, but only during the busy period of the day

Summary Record of Discussion

The three papers discussed at this session were by Drs Grossman and Benham on the effects of health upon the hours and wages of labor, by Dr Friedman on demand-shift responses to the American Medicare and Medicaid programs, and by Dr Christiansen on the location of emergency health care services in a large metropolitan area (Copenhagen). The first two papers were discussed before the mid-morning intermission.

A. *Drs Grossman and Benham's paper*

Dr Phelps introduced the paper with the view that effects on hours and wages were more appropriate measures of 'health output' than either mortality or life expectancy effects, or than expenditures on health inputs which might go for 'care' rather than 'cure'. In addition, study of wage and hour effects yields a more useful estimate of the effectiveness of medical services than study of either mortality or life expectancy.

Dr Phelps also praised Dr Grossman's 'investment' model of health care as having proved more susceptible than its alternatives to quantitative study, both as to the supply and the productivity of labor. This was because it combined the 'mortality' and 'morbidity' aspects of health problems. It was best to follow Grossman's example of including health variables in both labor supply and wage-generation equations. The effect of health seemed strengthened when these equations were combined in a simultaneous equation model. In their simultaneous equation model, Drs Grossman and Benham found the health effects on earnings roughly five times as strong as that on the labor supply measured in terms of hours on the job.[1] This result suggested to Dr Phelps more foresight on the employers' part, and more ability to estimate productivity of individual workers, than he would have been willing to assume in advance.

The provision of health, Dr Phelps continued, includes the market for medical services, but medical care has been exogenous in the Grossman and, now, the Grossman–Benham models.[2] It should be made endogenous, increasing the size of the Grossman–Benham model from three to five equations. The expansion would admittedly strain our data bases, but economists should be gatherers of data, rather than passive consumers of data gathered by others for purposes unrelated to economics.

---

[1] *Dr Grossman* replies in a postscript: 'The health effect that is strengthened in our simultaneous model is the effect of health on the weekly wage rate. That is, health has a much stronger effect on the wage when it (health) is treated as an endogenous variable compared to when it is treated as an exogenous variable. (Compare the coefficients of *IH* in Tables 12.2 and 12.8 of our paper.) It was my understanding that Charles Phelps was referring to this comparison rather than to a comparison of the effect of health on the wage versus its effect on weeks worked. The effects of health on weeks worked and the wages are about the same in our two-equation model (health exogenous). We do not estimate the effect of the endogenous health variable on weeks worked in the text of the paper.'

[2] *Dr Grossman's* view is that, in the Grossman–Benham paper, medical care is exogenous. Medical care, however, is *not* exogenous in his previous work.

In this case, the data we need to relate to health stocks and to shocks thereto.

Dr Phelps illustrated certain of his arguments by a diagram reproduced as Fig. 1. On this diagram, the health stock of a particular individual is

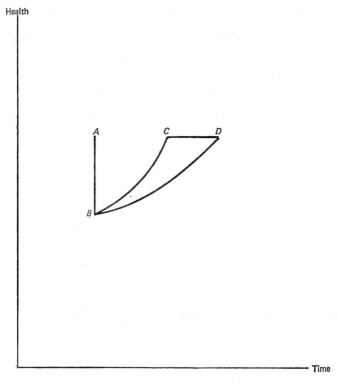

Health

Time

FIG. 1

measured on the vertical axis, and time on the horizontal axis. Suppose that an individual in position A becomes ill; his health stock falls at once to B. He recovers his previous health stock at C with the aid of medical care, but only later (at D) without such care. The course of his health is $ABCD$ with the aid of medical care and ABD without it. The area BCD may be regarded as the output of the medical system. It is reflected in fewer hours and days lost through illness, and in higher productivity on the job, even when it is not also reflected in lower mortality or higher life expectancy rates.

In Dr Benham's absence, *Dr Grossman* responded. He agreed with Dr Phelps that the model should be expanded so that medical care might be made endogenous, and that the change might be a significant one. As for the high effect of health upon wage rates (as compared with its effect on the crude labor supply variable), he felt that part of this may reflect error of measurement of his health variable, since health affects behavior and, hence, productivity even in the case of maladies too minor to be reflected in health statistics. It would be, Dr Grossman added, an improvement if health effects could be measured on people not in the labor force. This additional expansion could take account of the probable inequality between the shadow price of such people's time and the market wage which non-workers might have earned if employed.[1]

Professor Evans was puzzled by Dr Phelps's comment, as being to some degree inconsistent with Dr Phelps's own paper. He (Professor Evans) felt that depreciation rates on health status may be made negative for a considerable number of conditions, and that most people were motivated by their current health status and not by any long-term stock of health capital. Does this not undercut the human capital model as a whole? *Dr Grossman* replied that the human capital model treats a rise in the depreciation rate of health capital much like a rise in the price of such capital. The demand for health capital will, of course, fall if its depreciation rate rises, but if the elasticity of demand for health services is low, medical outlays will rise regardless. This framework, moreover, handles both preventive and curative aspects of the demand for health.

Professor Evans repeated his view that negative depreciation rates were inconsistent with the Grossman–Benham model, to which *Dr Phelps* replied (referring to Fig. 1) that the key variable of this model is the productive time *CD* gained by medical care, and not the depreciation rate. This technical discussion, however, was adjourned for private discussion outside the conference room after *Professor Rosett* had observed that an improvement in one's short-term health status should not be equated with depreciation in his health capital.

Dr Kleiman raised the issue of the Grossman–Benham health index. Why not, he inquired, include several health variables separately rather than any sort of composite index? He also wondered whether the components of the health index had been self-reported. If so, he felt there might be bias and reverse causation, as in the case of the malingerer reporting ill-health as an excuse for not working or of low productivity on his job. Dr Kleiman wondered, finally, whether such movements as Women's Liberation and other changes in the social fabric (weakening of the family system) might not affect health negatively. On this point, it was responded that the effects might depend upon the nature of the initial social system.

The discussion then turned to the measurement of the health variable. *M. Foulon* felt that the definition of 'health capital' was necessarily imprecise and approximate. It may be completely meaningless if based on reports of the individuals themselves, and quite unrelated to morbidity statistics, which he felt were more reliable. *Professor L. Lave* replied that objective measurement of morbidity is simply impossible, and that one

---

[1] *Dr Grossman* adds, after reviewing this summary: 'Our paper *does* measure health effects for a combined sample of people in the labor force and people *not* in the labor force. What I said was that, in measuring these effects. one should take account of the inequality between the shadow price of time and the market wage rate for people not in the labor force'.

must live with the subjective indices, as per the paper of which he was himself co-author. M. Foulon's proposal of objective measurement he dismissed as will-o'-the-wisp. *Professors Perlman* and *Fuchs* tended to agree that Professor L. Lave was basically right, Professor Perlman paraphrasing an aphorism, 'Health is what health does', and Professor Fuchs citing the accomplishments of Franklin D. Roosevelt under the handicap of poliomyelitis. (*Mr Pole* later introduced the counter-examples of such statesmen as Hindenburg and Churchill, who became senile while holding high office.) Professor Fuchs wondered whether one could distinguish the effects of health on productivity from those of absences unrelated to health. Absence, after all, was what mattered in many cases. *Dr Bell* expressed the view that all econometric results were weak because the health variables are so badly defined. In the American data files, he said, sick time was included in weeks worked, and symptomatology is related much more directly to work (occupational diseases) than to health generally. He also felt that men tend to work, or at least put in time on the job, regardless of poor health in cases where women would be more sensitive to their physical condition and remain home. *Professor Lévy* warned against confusing the number of one's symptoms with the state of one's health, arguing that self-evaluation of morbidity is only one measure and should not be relied on. (Most people claim, in France, to have from $2\frac{1}{2}$ to $3\frac{1}{2}$ diseases at any given time.) Professor Lévy also felt that preventive medicine had been more effective than many of the papers had been willing to admit, and cited polio vaccine as an example. He suggested more pressure in the preventive medicine direction.

Professor Sloan raised a question of economic theory. The Grossman–Benham paper had stated, as a more or less settled conclusion, that the labor supply was inversely related to wage rates. Actually, Professor Sloan said, the results were extremely sensitive to the specification of one's labor market model, particularly to the other variables included.

B. *Dr Friedman's paper*

Introducing this paper, *Professor Fuchs* praised its expository qualities. Dr Friedman's problem had been to analyze the effects of the massive infusion of new money upon the quality and quantity of medical care. He had, however, found it impossible to separate price from quantity effects, or 'strict' quantity effects from quality improvements, in the large, using a consumption model which attempted to include 'quantity changes as perceived by suppliers'. Dr Friedman had therefore concentrated upon the single and relatively more manageable problem of breast cancer. He found no significant effect of lower prices upon the speed of diagnosis among Medicare and Medicaid patients in the United States over the period 1965–71.[1] Neither did he find any significant increase in the three-year survival rate among the patients. He did find that, of three common modes of treatment (surgery, radiation, and a combination of the others),

[1] 'Medicare' relates to publicly assisted medical aid for those over 65; 'Medicaid' relates to publicly assisted aid for poverty patients regardless of age. 'Medicare' is national, while the details of 'Medicaid' vary between states.

the one which had most increased in popularity was the last and most expensive. This trio of conclusions led Dr Friedman to the conclusion that much of the expenditures for Medicare and Medicaid may have been wasted.

Professor Fuchs described this paper as useful and correct in its general conclusions, although Professor Friedman does not establish that the change in treatment from 1965 to 1967 was solely due to the increase in insurance coverage. Professor Fuchs's own term for the phenomenon Dr Friedman has isolated is 'physician's technological imperative': the physician wants to give all the care that is technicalyy possible and he clearly derives satisfaction from the exercise of skills that he has acquired at considerable cost. A similar phenomenon is found among many other sorts of specialists, including the econometricians. Physicians are not better or worse than others, but their opportunity to indulge their technological imperative is greater because of restrictions on entry, consumer ignorance and other limitations on competition.

Professor Fuchs noted that the 'restrictions on competition' referred to by Friedman, and mentioned by Mr Cooper in an earlier paper, are permitted if not encouraged) in all countries, regardless of political, economic or social system, and regardless of the methods used for financing medical care. Health economists would do well to do more than simply deplore such restrictions; they ought to try to explain why they arise. It may be related, Professor Fuchs suspects, to our basic attitudes toward illness and death.

The failure of breast cancer victims to obtain earlier diagnosis as the price of medical care fell was no surprise to Professor Fuchs. He referred to one experts' observation that 'physicians with cancer are just as likely to delay diagnosis as are laymen'. The barrier to earlier diagnosis is not primarily financial but psychological. Professor Fuchs wondered whether Dr Friedman had discussed this range of problems with physicians themselves.

He also noted that cancer is frequently fatal. After the patient dies, the physician is expected to tell the family: 'We did everything possible for him (her).' What connection, if any, is there between this expectation and the behavior described in the paper?

M. Dupuy agreed that it was most important to look at physician's behavior first and foremost, and had come to much the same conclusions as Dr Friedman with regard to the facts in the case. He expressed himself, however, as much less skeptical than Dr Friedman or than Professor Fuchs as regards the value of expenditures for medical care. They may still help the patient psychologically and sociologically when they do little for him medically. One can show waste only if the domination of physicians over the health care system actually injures patients. It is not enough, in M. Dupuy's view, to rely on mortality rates for pessimistic conclusions.

Professor Rosett agreed that technological imperatives were important in explaining physicians' behavior, but added that they could not be cured by preaching.

Dr *Bell* insisted that breast cancer is taken extremely seriously by patients, even though they delay seeking diagnosis. Perhaps the physician is acting purely as the patient's agent in seeking the most complex and expensive therapeutic methods.

Mr Pole argued that the shift of physicians to more complex medical technologies resulted from technological change itself, rather than from any technological imperatives. As to the effectiveness of the new technology, it is true that a New York study found it to be concentrated in the younger age groups, but Mr Pole suspected that the study may have involved some sampling bias, particularly since chronic and degenerative diseases may be less amenable than other diseases to these techniques. In any event, the advance of epidemiological knowledge is important in itself, and may enable the making of better estimates later on.

Like Mr Pole, *Professor J. Lave* was skeptical of technological-imperative explanations for physician behavior. The physician must make his decisions quickly and at the micro-level. It is only *ex post*, and in the aggregate, that the technological-imperative explanation is plausible. Also, with special reference to breast cancer, she reminded the group that the newest and most advanced method of treatment involved the removal of the tumor only, not the entire breast.

Radiologists, said *Dr Kehrer*, earn higher average incomes than practitioners of any other speciality. Yet they receive patients by referral only, and do not seek them out. It did not seem to Dr Kehrer that in their case the technological-imperative explanation had great validity. However, *Professor Rosett* claimed, most radiologists work in hospitals, and are in a position to determine quite arbitrarily the use of their own services.

Concluding the discussion of the Grossman–Benham paper, *Dr Grossman* began by replying to Professor Evans on the relation between health status and health stock as he saw it. Health status variables, he believed, relate to marginal changes in the health stock, and not to the average value of that stock over a period of time. Replying to Dr Kleiman, he continued, he and Dr Benham had been constrained to use a single health index, because it would be a dependent variable in certain of their mathematical and statistical formulations.

The measurement of the health stock is, of course, difficult, but something is better than nothing at all. Furthermore, the Grossman–Benham index correlates positively with other health variables.

Both wages and labor effort, Dr Grossman continued, are related to subjective rather than objective estimates of health. He did not consider the results weak, despite low coefficients of multiple correlation. (These are always low when one works with data for individuals rather than with group totals or averages.) They might, however, be improved if women had been considered separately from men, although the basic relationships were probably the same.

In summary, Dr Grossman believed, there were three important elements of novelty in the Grossman–Benham model: (1) labor market model was embedded in the health model; (2) the effect of poor health on the shadow value of time had been taken into account; and (3) the productivity and labor supply effects of health had been separated from each other.

Turning to his own paper, *Dr Friedman* ascribed much of the technical change in medicine to hospitals which compete for the services of eminent physicians by providing more advanced equipment for their use. In answer to a query by Professor Fuchs, he said he had indeed spoken to many physicians, and had been struck by the lag in knowledge as between the innovators and the general run of doctors. On Medicare and Medicaid, he felt that his study was only an interim and disequilibrium one, in that the dynamic effects of these programs would require much more time to work themselves out. He (Friedman) feared that the effects might not all be good. For example, the availability of these programs might induce people to take more risks in their youth, as well as making 'wrong' decisions about savings, family sizes and patterns of life.

C. *Dr Christiansen's paper*

Professor Uzawa introduced Dr Christiansen's plan for emergency services in Copenhagen as basically a cost-minimizing linear programming model, which includes in cost both the operation of centers and the operation of ambulances, but not the costs incurred by their users. This, said Professor Uzawa, is an unusual application of linear programming techniques, but it does not completely avoid elements of subjective value judgement. Professor Uzawa found in the Christiansen system two premises which he characterized as 'uncomfortable'. In the first place, he found no reference to the behavior patterns of hospitals, doctors or ambulance drivers. (In Tokyo, at least, patients use ambulances unnecessarily often when they are available without charge.) In the second place, the entire objective function appears to be the reduction of cost, but at the same time, no calculation is made of the patient's own opportunity cost. The optimum design for the entire emergency care system may vary with the estimate of such cost.

Professor Uzawa went on to sketch an alternative system based not directly on cost but on minimum time to get the emergency patient to a hospital or an aid station. Then, given this minimum time constraint, ordinary cost minimization may be acceptable. One should also see what the effect of varying the minimum time constraint would be, and seek balance by successive readjustments. Explaining why his alternative is preferable, Professor Uzawa argued that some minorities might suffer greatly under a standard linear programming system, and that this is why time constraints are required.

Professor L. Lave led off the floor discussion by asking how important time actually was. In Los Angeles, the only important interval ends with the arrival of someone knowing first aid. Secondly, a $10 charge for ambulance service, again in Los Angeles, caused a rapid decline in the demand for such services, especially by commercial establishments. Thirdly, where one emergency room was well equipped, it is often better to get to that emergency room than to the one nearest to the accident, which might be less well equipped. Fourthly, helicopters are of little use in meeting emergency medical crises. Fifthly, it is better to use cheap trucks as ambulances than the more comfortable Cadillac automobiles. Sixthly, and lastly, it is often better to use paramedical practitioners for first aid than to use full-fledged M.D.s.

Professor Williams also thought that response time might not be of first importance, and thought the Christiansen model should include some allowance for improvement in communications systems.

Mr Kaser added that the place of treatment is important. When, as in Belfast, there are special coronary-care ambulances available, it is not as necessary to reach a hospital so fast. In general, Dr Christiansen had not, in Mr Kaser's opinion, proved the efficiency of his proposed system, especially as compared with the alternative of having medical help available on premises near areas where emergencies may be expected to occur. *M. Foulon* raised questions about the definition of 'emergency', and questioned the wisdom of rushing patients to hospitals where no beds might be available. M. Foulon also agreed with Professer L. Lave on the importance of first aid, and suggested more general medical education on the subject. *Professor Liefmann-Keil* suggested that many 'emergency cases' result from little more than the unwillingness of physicians to leave their offices and make house calls. *Professor Perlman* noted the incongruity of removing internes from ambulance service (and replacing them with lightly trained first-aid technicians), whereas elsewhere the tendency is for doctors to decrease responsibilities given to highly trained nurses. *Dr Phelps* wondered whether, since fire-alarm boxes are so helpful, multiple-purpose alarm boxes might not also be installed for emergency medical aid as well as for firemen.

Dr Christiansen began his reply by commenting on Professor Liefmann-Keil's question about emergencies and house calls. No physicians in the Copenhagen inner city take house calls at all, except perhaps in coronary cases, but this is not true uptown and in the suburbs.

Replying to Professor Uzawa, Dr Christiansen denied that his model had been a standard linear programming one. Rather, it was derived by simulation, somewhat as Professor Uzawa had himself suggested it might be. The objective function had been hard to weight, and arbitrary methods were used. For example, a value of 15,000 kroner per minute was put on ambulance response time in u (true emergency) cases, and smaller amounts for z (less serious) cases. Also, time constraints of the sort proposed by Professor Uzawa had been included in Dr Christiansen's crude model. An ambulance must be able to reach 95 per cent of all cases within five minutes after receiving a call to the scene.

Replying to Professor L. Lave, Dr Christiansen repeated that the idea of the Copenhagen system is to get the patient as high as possible on the 'medical ladder' in as short a time as possible. This is why Copenhagen ambulances are so well equipped, and also why substations were so numerous. The essential time element is the resource time of the ambulance. In Denmark, ambulances have fibrillators and electrocardiogram units, but use no one beyond the level of a nurse. Agreeing with Mr Kaser,

Dr Christiansen felt that the role of huge ambulances of the Belfast type might be greater when the system is extended beyond the city limits rather than when, as in Copenhagen, operation is exclusively within an urban area.

At this point – after Dr Christiansen had finished – *Professor Fuchs* inquired whether account had been taken of any increased demand for medical care as a result of improved ambulance services. *Dr Christiansen* answered this question in the negative.

Part Four

The Quantitative and the Qualitative
Provision of Hospital, Physician and
Paraprofessional Services and Social
Control

15   The Role of Technology, Demand and Labor Markets in the Determination of Hospital Costs[1]

Karen Davis

BROOKING INSTITUTION, WASHINGTON, D.C.

This paper attempts to sort out the contribution of demand factors, labor market conditions and changing technology to the determination of hospital costs in the United States. Data on approximately 200 non-profit hospitals for the period from 1962 to 1968 are analyzed in a pooled time-series, cross-section regression estimation. Measures of sources of demand changes – such as insurance coverage, income and various demographic factors – proxy measures of composition of cases treated, hospital wage rates and a time-shift variable are used to explain variation in hospital expenses per admission and expenses per patient-day. Of the predicted increase in expenses per hospital admission, demand variables accounted for 45 per cent of the increase; case-mix variables added another 7 per cent. Increases in average earnings of hospital employees represented another 10 per cent of the overall increase, while shifts upward over time were responsible for the remaining 38 per cent. Labor and non-labor inputs, as well as the wage rate paid for labor, were also found to be responsive to demand, case-mix and technological factors.

I. INTRODUCTION

Numerous causes of inflation in United States hospital costs have been suggested. One view emphasizes the importance of increases in demand in inducing an upward shift in hospital costs.[2] Others point to specific factor inputs, such as excessive wage gains by hospital workers or duplication of capital facilities, as the major source of cost

---

[1] The work for this paper was funded by a contract with the Social Security Administration. The views expressed here are those of the author; they should not be ascribed to the Social Security Administration nor to the trustees, officers or the staff members of the Brookings Institution.
[2] For an exposition of a demand-oriented model of price and cost determination see Feldstein [5].

increases.[1] A more benign view of hospital inflation stresses the importance of changes in technology that lead to improvements in health status and reduce mortality, but at a high cost.

Understanding the contribution to cost inflation of each of these sources is important for a number of reasons. First, understanding the major cause of inflation in costs may help select more effective methods of combating inflation. For example, if the inflation is primarily demand-induced, it may be possible to restructure available insurance coverage to limit cost increases. On the other hand, if excessive wage increases are to blame, wage controls may be in order. Second, a model for predicting future trends in cost increases can be useful as a baseline from which to evaluate policies designed to curb inflation. Third, a model for predicting medical care costs should provide more reliable estimates of the costs of different types of national health insurance plans.

Since the primary purposes of this paper are to sort out the contribution of various causes of inflation and to provide a basis for predicting future changes, the paper develops a reduced-form estimation of hospital costs, rather than attempting to estimate a complete structural model of the hospital industry. In this way, both the direct and indirect effect of exogenous variables on hospital costs can be estimated. In addition to examining the impact of demand factors, labor markets and technology on average hospital costs, the paper examines various components of hospital costs, including both labor and real non-labor inputs per unit of hospital output.

Section II sketches a structural model of the hospital industry as a basis for construction of a reduced-form equation relating average hospital costs to exogenous factors. Section III describes the data base used in the study. Section IV presents some empirical results on the overall determinants of hospital costs, while section V investigates the contributing factors leading to increases in various components of hospital costs. Section VI summarizes the empirical results and discusses their implications for policies to curb inflation.

II. STRUCTURAL MODEL OF THE HOSPITAL INDUSTRY

A complete model of the hospital industry would encompass the demand for hospital care, the determinants of cost of providing hospital services, the relationship between prices charged for hospital services and their cost, and, perhaps, the long-run adjustment of

---

[1] For a discussion of several different views of the determinants of hospital cost inflation, see Davis and Foster [3].

hospital capacity.[1] If prices of factor inputs, particularly labor, are endogenous to the hospital, the model would include input determination relationships as well.[2]

Many different specifications of these key elements of the hospital industry lead to the same reduced-form specification of hospital costs.[3] One illustrative structural specification is sketched below as a basis for constructing a reduced-form equation.

(1) *Demand Relations*

The demand portion of the model consists of two functions: the per capita demand for hospital admissions and the mean length of stay of hospital patients. Explanatory variables consist of prices of hospital care, hospital insurance coverage, income, physician availability, hospital availability and demographic characteristics of the population:[4]

$$ADMPC = f(RP, INS, RINC, MDPC, \%GP, BEDSPC, DENS,$$
$$YOUNG, WHITE, EDYR)$$
$$MS = f(RP, INS, RINC, MDPC, \%GP, BEDSPC, DENS,$$
$$YOUNG, WHITE, EDYR)$$

where

$ADMPC$ = admissions per capita

MS = mean stay of hospital patients

RP = gross patient revenue per patient-day deflated by the consumer price index

INS = proportion of gross price paid directly by the patient

$RINC$ = disposable income per capita deflated by the consumer price index

$MDPC$ = patient care physicians per capita

$\%GP$ = ratio of general practitioners to patient care physicians

$BEDSPC$ = hospital beds per capita

$DENS$ = population per square mile

$YOUNG$ = ratio of population under age 65 to total population

$WHITE$ = ratio of white population to total population

$EDYR$ = median school years completed.

Economic factors affecting the demand for hospital care include price of hospital care, insurance coverage and income. Feldstein [4] has argued that a physician, making decisions as the patient's

---

[1] A complete model of the hospital industry is developed in Feldstein [5].

[2] For an empirical estimation of hospital wage determination, see Davis [2].

[3] Salkever [8] has taken a similar tack, estimating a quasi-reduced form of hospital costs for New York hospitals from 1961 to 1967. He includes a lagged average cost variable in the estimates on the assumption that hospitals adjust toward some level of desired costs gradually over time.

[4] The demand equations are taken from the specification proposed by Feldstein [5].

agent, may weigh patient's preferences – given income, gross price and insurance coverage – his own self-interest, pressures from professional colleagues, medical ethics and concern for making good use of hospital resources. When insurance coverage is extensive, concern for proper allocation of resources may weigh more heavily in physicians' decisions. If so, hospitalization may be more responsive to gross price than price net of insurance coverage. In addition, if the physician imperfectly perceives patients' income or insurance coverage or if the physician is guided by medical ethics to ignore differences in income or insurance in deciding upon treatment, the effects of insurance and income may be dampened. In the structural model, therefore, gross price and insurance are entered separately to allow for differences in demand responsiveness to these two factors. Insurance is measured by proportion of price paid directly by the patient and can be expected to reduce demand.

Two measures of physician availability are included in the demand equations: total physicians per capita and proportion of physicians in general practice. These measures are included to see if an increase in the number of physicians, particularly specialist physicians, will result in greater use of hospital services.

Hospital bed availability may affect demand, over and above any effect of hospital prices, by influencing physician decisions. If hospitals are crowded, physicians may decide to treat more patients on an outpatient or ambulatory basis. Consequently, for any given price of hospital care, inpatient demand may be less when hospital beds are at a premium.

Population density is included on the hypothesis that sparsely populated areas will make greater use of inpatient care, since repeat visits for ambulatory care may involve higher travel costs. If less serious cases tend to be hospitalized in sparsely populated areas, average stays may be somewhat shorter in those areas.

(2) *Pricing Behavior*

Several different hypotheses have been advanced about the relationship between hospital prices and costs. These range from the assertion that prices are equated to average costs, or are a mark-up over average costs where the mark-up is a function of the 'need' for investment, or a function of demand factors and monopoly position.[1] For illustrative purposes, a cost mark-up model where the mark-up is a function of demand factors and market position will be assumed here, although other specifications may lead to the same reduced-form specification of average costs:

---

[1] See Davis [1] for a test of several alternative models of hospital price determination.

$$RP = f(RAC, \ INS, \ MDPC, \ \%GP, \ BEDSPC, \ DENS,$$
$$YOUNG, \ WHITE, \ EDYR, \ BEDS, \ MDH/BED)$$

where

RAC = total expenses per patient-day deflated by the consumer price index

$BEDS$ = hospital bed size

$MDH/BEDS$ = active physicians on the hospital medical staff per hospital bed

and other variables are as defined above.

Explanatory variables include variables entering into the demand for hospital services, plus hospital bed size and physicians on the hospital staff per hospital bed. Various interpretations may be given to the inclusion of the latter two variables. Larger hospitals are likely to have a dominant market position, permitting them to charge higher prices relative to costs. In addition, such hospitals may be perceived by the community to provide high-quality care, again giving the hospital an opportunity to raise its charges, given average cost of providing care. A greater concentration of physicians on the hospital staff may enhance the hospital's market position, since it guarantees the hospital a wider range of patients for admission to a limited bed capacity. This variable may also capture the power relationship between hospital administrators and medical staff. When the hospital has many physicians on its staff relative to capacity, the hospital administrator may be able to ignore complaints of individual physicians, since loss of a few would not jeopardize the hospital. If the hospital has few physicians on its medical staff relative to its capacity, the administrator may be guided by physician wishes in setting a price policy. Pauly and Redisch [7] have argued that physicians always dominate hospitals' pricing policy and insist that hospitals equate prices to costs so that the physician component of the patient bill may be as high as possible. If this factor does not hold for all hospitals, but varies with the power relationship between the hospital administrator and medical staff, prices would be higher, given costs, the more physicians there are on the medical staff per hospital bed.

(3) Structural Unit Cost Relationship

Although an understanding of the relationship between hospital prices and costs is important for a number of purposes, the ability to predict prices, given trends in future average costs, is not completely helpful. To complete the structural model of the hospital industry, the underlying direct factors affecting hospital costs need to be investigated. Here it is assumed that the direct factors affecting hospital costs include level of output provided, case-mix, prices of variable inputs, quantities of fixed inputs and technology:

$$RTE/ADM = f(ADM/B, MIX, RWAGE, BEDS, PA/B, TIME)$$
or
$$RTE/PD = f(PD/B, MIX, RWAGE, BEDS, PA/B, TIME)$$

where

RTE/ADM = total expenses per admission deflated by the consumer price index

RTE/PD = total expenses per patient-day deflated by the consumer price index

ADM/B = case-flow rate or hospital admissions per bed

PD/B = patient-days per hospital bed (proportional to occupancy rate)

MIX = proxies for hospital case-mix (discussed below)

$RWAGE$ = payroll expenses per full-time equivalent employee deflated by consumer price index

PA/B = plant assets per bed

$TIME$ = time variable

Two units of hospital output are examined alternatively: hospital admissions and hospital patient-days. At the individual hospital level, it is extremely unlikely that the composition of patient types is the same for all hospitals. Unit costs may differ among hospitals as a result of differences in the types of cases treated, difficulty of treating patients of a given case type, and differences in the quality of care provided. Using hospital patient-days as a measure of output may adjust for some of these differences, since hospitals with more difficult types of cases and more difficult cases of a given type are likely to have longer mean stays. Higher-quality care, however, may shorten average stays resulting in higher costs per day of care, but not necessarily higher costs per admission.

Several proxies are used to adjust for differences among hospitals in case-mix. The first of these is residual mean stay, that is, length of hospital stay not explained by the various economic, socio-demographic and availability variables appearing in the demand equations. Such an adjusted mean stay variable should reflect the 'true' stay required strictly because of the nature of disease or illness. Affiliation with a medical school is also included in the cost equations, since such hospitals are more likely to treat the most difficult cases. If specialized personnel are required to treat more difficult patients, the composition of hospital personnel may also capture some aspects of case-mix. Included for this reason are the ratio of interns and residents to all hospital personnel, the ratio of registered practical nurses to all personnel, and the ratio of licensed practical nurses to all personnel. Finally, physicians on the hospital staff per hospital bed may also indicate the severity of cases admitted. If the hospital has many physicians on its staff per available bed, it may put pressures on physicians to admit only extremely serious cases. On the other hand, if the hospital serves only a few physicians relative to bed capacity, much less serious types of cases may be treated in the hospital. Beds and plant assets per bed may also be greater for hospitals with a greater complexity of case-mix. In summary, proxies for case-mix include:

RMS = residual mean stay (mean stay unexplained by variables in mean stay demand equations)
$MEDSCH$ = affiliation with a medical school
$\%INT\text{-}RES$ = ratio of interns and residents to full-time equivalent personnel
$\%RPN$ = ratio of registered practical nurses to full-time equivalent personnel
$\%LPN$ = ratio of licensed practical nurses to full-time equivalent personnel
MDH/BED = active physicians on the hospital medical staff per hospital bed as well as, possibly, beds and plant assets per bed.

Unfortunately, no direct measure of technology is available with which to capture the separate effects of changes in technology. A time variable is included in the model to capture the residual effect of increases in average costs over time, but such a variable may include not only changes in technology but basic shifts in patient, physician or hospital behavior. Plant assets per hospital bed, in addition to having a direct effect on costs as a measure of scale economies and an indirect effect on costs as a proxy for case-mix, may capture some changes in technology – particularly technology which takes the form of requiring more capital equipment for hospitals of a given size.

For purposes of prediction, the structural specification of hospital unit costs is inadequate, since policy-makers also need to know what will happen to hospital output under any given policy change, Hospital costs will be affected not only by those factors operating directly on costs, but also by factors which affect hospital output, such as price, income and other demand variables. In turn, factors which affect hospital prices, through their indirect effects on hospital output, will also affect hospital costs. After allowing for interactions among hospital output, price and unit costs, the direct and indirect determinants of unit costs may be represented by the following reduced-form equation:

$RAC = f(INS, RINC, MDPC, \%GP, BEDSPC,$ Demand
$\qquad DENS, YOUNG, WHITE, EDYR,$
$\qquad RMS, BEDS, PA/B, MEDSCH,$ Mix
$\qquad \%INT\text{-}RES, \%RPN, \%LPN, MDH/BED,$
$\qquad RWAGE, TIME).$ Wage, Technology

In the model presented here, hospital bed size and the ratio of plant assets to beds are treated as exogenous. A more complete model of the hospital industry would explain long-run adjustments in these variables as well. Insurance is also considered to be exogenous to the hospital, neglecting the feedback effect of hospital actions (such as price policy) on insurance coverage.

The variables in the reduced-form equation can be roughly characterized as demand variables ($INS, RINC, MDPC, \%GP, BEDSPC, DENS, YOUNG, WHITE, EDYR$), case-mix variables ($RMS, BEDS, PA/B, MEDSCH, \%INT\text{-}RES, \%RPN, \%LPN, MDH/BED$), wage rates ($RWAGE$) and technology ($TIME$). Several of the variables, however, have dual interpretations: for example, residual mean stay, RMS, as a proxy for the intensity of illness, also affects the demand for care, and plant assets per bed, PA/B, may represent technology case-mix or size.

III. DATA AND MEASUREMENT OF VARIABLES

Empirical estimation of the hospital cost model is based upon individual hospital data for seven years from 1962 to 1968. Hospitals included in the estimation are all non-profit, private hospitals submitting audited data from 1962 to 1966 in a sample survey conducted by the American Hospital Association under contract with the Social Security Administration. Of the 194 hospitals submitting pre-Medicare data, 159 hospitals submitted data to the Social Security Administration for 1967, and 149 of these submitted data for 1968. Total number of observations in the pooled cross-section time-series estimation, therefore, is 1,278.

All variables based on individual hospital data ($RAC, RP, ADM, MS, BEDS, PA/B, RWAGE, MEDSCH, \%INT\text{-}RES, \%RPN, \%LPN, MDH/BED$) are taken from Social Security Administration records. Data on specialized hospital personnel and physicians on the hospital staff are available only for 1967 and 1968. 1967 values, therefore, are used for the period from 1962 to 1968.

Data on the characteristics of the population and availability of medical resources in the area in which the hospital is located ($RINC, MDPC, \%GP, BEDSPC, DENS, YOUNG, WHITE, EDYR$) are based on the county in which the hospital is located. County data on racial composition, age composition and education are from the 1960

Census, while data on county hospital beds, physicians, population and income have been taken from annual American Medical Association publications.

Insurance is measured as the proportion of the gross price paid directly by patients. The variable is defined in the same way as developed by Feldstein, where the proportion of the population covered by hospital insurance is measured at the state level. Specifically, insurance is the ratio of the aggregate net expenditures on short-term hospital services by consumers to the aggregate total expenditure on short-term hospital services including net payments by consumers, insurance companies and the government. An increase, hence, in governmental programs, such as Medicare and Medicaid, will result in a reduction in insurance (that is, a reduction in the proportion paid out-of-pocket).

Residual mean stay is calculated by first estimating a double-logarithmic specification of the mean stay demand equation. All explanatory variables times their respective coefficients are then subtracted from actual log of mean stay ($LRMS = LMS - \Sigma\beta_i X_i$).

All regressions presented here are based on a double-logarithmic functional form. Exceptions are time, medical school affiliation and proportion of specialized personnel, which enter linearly. Estimates of linear regressions yielded substantially similar results, with slightly lower adjusted R^2 in some equations.

IV. EFFECT OF DEMAND, MIX, WAGES AND TECHNOLOGY ON AVERAGE HOSPITAL EXPENSES

Table 15.1 indicates the joint role of demand factors, mix of patients treated by the hospital, wage rates and technology in the determination of overall hospital expenses. Including all factors simultaneously explains a substantially higher proportion of average expenses than estimations based on just a few of the factors. For example, when all demand factors are omitted, the adjusted R^2 falls from 0·93 to 0·77 in the expenses per hospital admission regressions. Including demand factors, but omitting wage rates and proxies for case-mix (except for residual mean stay, which may also be interpreted as a demand variable), adjusted R^2 is 0·90. In the estimates of hospital expenses per patient-day, the adjusted R^2 similarly falls from 0·66 when all factors are included to 0·56 based on demand and technology variables, and to 0·58 using only mix, wage and technology variables. The combination of all factors, therefore, is required for a complete view of the determinants of average expenses.

Both insurance coverage and income are significant in explaining

TABLE 15.1

EFFECT OF DEMAND, MIX, WAGES AND TECHNOLOGY ON AVERAGE EXPENSES

(*t*-scores in parentheses)

	Expenses per admission			Expenses per patient day		
	(1)	(2)	(3)	(4)	(5)	(6)
Constant	−1·16	−1·37	0·22	−2·17	−1·99	0·33
	(1·58)	(1·66)	(0·93)	(2·06)	(1·71)	(1·55)
Demand						
INS	−0·21	−0·26		−0·03	−0·09	
	(13·29)	(14·49)		(1·12)	(3·73)	
RINC	0·21	0·21		0·05	0·06	
	(6·51)	(5·59)		(1·00)	(1·11)	
MDPC	0·10	0·10		0·16	0·16	
	(7·13)	(6·17)		(7·87)	(7·02)	
%GP	−0·0003	−0·06		0·06	−0·006	
	(0·02)	(4·25)		(3·29)	(0·29)	
BEDSPC	0·11	0·09		0·08	−0·09	
	(10·64)	(8·33)		(5·31)	(5·91)	
DENS	0·08	0·10		0·02	0·05	
	(21·14)	(24·94)		(4·12)	(8·37)	
YOUNG	0·10	0·41		0·35	0·72	
	(0·68)	(2·44)		(1·62)	(3·00)	
WHITE	0·03	0·09		0·06	0·14	
	(0·84)	(2·54)		(1·46)	(2·84)	
EDYR	0·11	0·14		0·36	0·42	
	(2·11)	(2·40)		(4·79)	(5·00)	
Mix						
RMS	1·01	0·99	0·90	0·02	−0·006	0·01
	(57·05)	(52·56)	(28·86)	(0·76)	(0·23)	(0·37)
BEDS	0·009		0·13	−0·004		0·04
	(1·54)		(14·74)	(0·49)		(4·78)
PA/B	0·05		0·05	0·06		0·05
	(10·64)		(7·06)	(9·33)		(8·01)
MEDSCH	0·06		0·12	0·08		0·07
	(5·27)		(6·51)	(4·94)		(4·43)
%INT-RES	−0·85		6·78	−0·41		1·89
	(1·38)		(6·43)	(0·46)		(2·01)
%RPN	−0·10		−0·11	−0·21		−0·08
	(2·24)		(1·44)	(3·30)		(1·18)
%LPN	−0·33		−0·60	−0·27		−0·45
	(5·39)		(5·60)	(3·15)		(4·74)
MDH/BED	0·07		0·15	0·08		0·14
	(9·85)		(13·59)	(8·36)		(14·81)
Wage						
RWAGE	0·15		0·34	0·24		0·33
	(8·85)		(11·96)	(10·15)		(13·11)
Technology						
TIME	0·02	0·03	0·04	0·03	0·04	0·03
	(9·81)	(10·44)	(12·13)	(9·55)	(10·40)	(10·42)
$\bar{R}^2$	0·93	0·90	0·77	0·66	0·56	0·58
S.E.	0·120	0·139	0·214	0·172	0·196	0·192

hospital expenses, with higher incomes leading to higher average costs and a greater proportion of out-of-pocket payments having a depressing effect on average expenses. Insurance coverage is particularly significant in the expenses per hospital admission estimates, with an elasticity of − 0·21 when all factors are included. When average cost is measured as total expenses per patient-day, however, insurance is insignificant, indicating that out-of-pocket payments affect costs primarily by reducing hispital stays, rather than by reducing the cost per day. Income is significantly positive in the expense per admission regressions, but, again, not in the expense per patient-day regressions. A 10 per cent increase in real per capita income increases expenses per admission by 2·1 per cent. Although the structural model of hospital cost determination stressed the importance of demand factors in influencing levels of output and, indirectly, costs, higher incomes may also give rise to higher costs of hospital care if residents of high-income areas demand higher-quality care.

An abundance of physicians in the area also tends to increase hospital costs, both in terms of number of admissions and in patient-days. Previous studies have indicated that the demand for hospital care is stimulated by the presence of physicians in the area. The hospital may be able to capitalize on this assurance of adequate demand to improve the quality of care or, at least, its expensiveness. Another interpretation of this result is that an abundance of physicians in the area gives the hospital administrator greater leeway in pursuing objectives of the hospital – rather than keeping costs and prices as low as possible, as suggested by Pauly, as being consistent with physicians' preferences.

Other demand variables which are important in the cost regressions are available hospital beds and population density, with both variables having a significantly positive impact on costs. Education also tends to increase hospital costs per admission, as well as on a per patient-day basis. In part, this may reflect the demand of more highly educated persons for higher-quality care.

Variables included in the cost regressions to capture the effect of composition of patients admitted to the hospital contribute significantly to the explanation of average costs. Residual mean stay is particularly important in the expenses per admission regressions, with longer stays dictated by non-economic or non-demographic factors leading to higher costs per admission but having little effect on average costs per patient-day.

Bed size has little independent effect on hospital costs when all factors are included. Higher levels of capital for hospitals of a given size, however, lead to slightly higher costs, with a 10 per cent increase in plant assets per bed yielding a 0·5 per cent increase in expenses per admission. These results might be interpreted as revealing that hospitals with more specialized equipment per bed treat more difficult cases or provide higher-quality care. Increases in plant assets per bed may also reflect changes in technology requiring greater capitalization, so that part of the increase in costs attributable to higher levels of capital may be a reflection of improved technology.

Affiliation with a medical school has a strong impact on hospital costs. Such hospitals tend to have costs per admission about 6 per cent higher than hospitals without such an affiliation. Greater proportions of interns and residents on the hospital staff do not tend to add significantly to hospital costs over and above that of affiliation with a medical school.

It was anticipated that higher proportions of registered and licensed practical nurses on the hospital staff would indicate a more difficult case-mix and that hospitals cost would be correspondingly higher. However, the regressions indicate that higher ratios of nurses to all personnel result in somewhat lower costs, with a higher ratio of licensed practical nurses having a greater depressing effect on costs than do registered practical nurses.

Presence of more physicians on the hospital medical staff per available bed, however, does result in fairly substantial increases in hospital costs. This is to be expected if hospitals with many physicians on the staff, relative to available bed capacity, put pressures on physicians to admit only the most difficult cases. It might also occur if hospital administrators feel free to increase the cost of care in situations where complaints of physicians about excessive costs can be largely ignored, that is, when the hospital is not dependent on all physicians to maintain desired levels of occupancy.

Increases in earnings of hospital employees also contribute to overall cost increases. A 10 per cent increase in annual earnings increases expenses per admission by 1·5 per cent and expenses per patient-day by 2·4 per cent. Although increases in wages cannot be held responsible for all the increase in hospital costs, wage rates exert fairly considerable, independent influence on hospital costs over and above that traceable to increases in demand, changes in technology or case-mix.

Holding constant for all other factors which plausibly affect hospital costs, costs continue to rise over time. Expenses per admission rise about 2 per cent annually. Although changes in behaviour on the part of patients, physicians or hospitals over time may account for part of this increase, it does suggest that the effect on costs of changes in technology has probably not exceeded this magnitude.

The relative importance of demand, mix, wages and technology in overall cost inflation may be summarized by calculating the contribution of each set of factors. Multiplying the percentage change for the nation as a whole in each of the variables by their respective elasticities gives the predicted change in average costs attributable to each variable. Of the predicted increase in expenses per admission, demand variables accounted for 45 per cent of the increase. Case-mix variables were responsible for another 7 per cent, while increases in average earnings of hospital employees represented another 10 per cent of the overall increase. Shifts upward over time were responsible for the remaining 38 per cent. These estimates should be treated with caution inasmuch as they assume that values obtained for individual sample hospitals can be applied to macro-trends.

V. COMPONENTS OF HOSPITAL COSTS

The preceding section indicated that all factors, including demand, case-mix, wages and technology, are required for a complete understanding of hospital cost inflation. It is possible, however, that some of these factors affect hospital costs primarily by affecting certain types of inputs. For example, changes in technology may take the form of requiring more non-labor input, while some of the impact of rising wage rates may be mitigated by substituting non-labor inputs for labor inputs. It is important, therefore, to disaggregate hospital costs by major components to reveal the way in which these basic sources of hospital cost inflation manifest themselves.

Table 15.2 examines the relationship of average annual earnings of hospital employees to demand, case-mix and technology variables, as well as an examination of their effect on labor input. Table 15.3 presents estimates of the determinants of non-labor inputs. Real non-labor inputs are defined as non-payroll expenses, deflated by the consumer price index. This assumes both that the consumer price index is representative of prices of non-labor inputs and that prices of non-labor inputs do not vary across geographical areas.

The previous section assumed that hospital wage rates could be considered as exogenous to the hospital. Feldstein [6] has suggested, however, that hospitals may engage in philanthropic wage behavior, paying hospital employees more than the minimal necessary to attract an adequate labor force. If the hospital's willingness to engage in philanthropic wage behavior depends upon the demand for its services, demand factors could be expected to increase wage rates. Case-mix variables, particularly those proxies which capture the need for specialized personnel to treat difficult cases, could also be expected to influence average wages. As indicated by the table, both demand and case-mix factors are important in determining wage rates. Not too surprisingly, hospitals in higher-income areas pay higher wages (elasticity of 0·09). This could occur because the hospital

TABLE 15.2

EFFECT OF DEMAND, MIX, WAGES AND TECHNOLOGY ON LABOR INPUT

(t-scores in parentheses)

	Wages	Personnel per admission			Personnel per patient-day		
	(7)	(8)	(9)	(10)	(11)	(12)	(13)
Constant	4·07	−1·45	−6·02	−1·24	−2·27	−6·76	0·24
	(2·96)	(1·34)	(4·26)	(1·95)	(1·73)	(4·39)	(0·23)
Demand							
INS	−0·10	−0·25	−0·22		−0·07	−0·05	
	(3·24)	(9·94)	(6·63)		(2·20)	(1·39)	
RINC	0·09	0·21	0·06		0·05	0·09	
	(1·77)	(5·04)	(1·11)		(0·98)	(1·56)	
MDPC	−0·02	0·11	0·14		0·17	0·20	
	(0·83)	(5·98)	(5·50)		(7·52)	(7·25)	
%GP	−0·005	+0·007	−0·03		0·07	0·02	
	(0·23)	(0·42)	(1·45)		(3·29)	(0·95)	
BEDSPC	0·02	0·09	0·09		−0·09	−0·10	
	(1·23)	(6·98)	(5·06)		(5·62)	(5·19)	
DENS	0·02	0·07	0·07		0·02	0·02	
	(3·25)	(15·46)	(11·88)		(3·27)	(3·19)	
YOUNG	0·28	−0·07	0·26		0·18	0·56	
	(1·10)	(0·37)	(0·97)		(0·73)	(1·94)	
WHITE	0·13	0·02	−0·07		0·06	−0·02	
	(2·50)	(0·53)	(1·28)		(1·16)	(0·29)	
EDYR	0·25	0·13	−0·007		0·38	0·27	
	(2·88)	(1·87)	(0·08)		(4·53)	(2·67)	
Mix							
RMS	0·04	0·96	0·99	0·86	−0·03	−0·01	−0·04
	(1·19)	(41·09)	(33·48)	(24·54)	(1·04)	(0·44)	(1·15)
BEDS	0·05	0·03		0·15	0·02		0·05
	(5·10)	(3·87)		(15·03)	(1·80)		(6·26)
PA/B	0·007	0·02		0·03	0·04		0·03
	(1·02)	(4·15)		(3·60)	(5·15)		(4·10)
MEDSCH	−0·02	0·05		0·11	0·07		0·06
	(1·26)	(3·37)		(5·31)	(3·91)		(3·39)
%F–R	1·75	−0·95		6·79	−0·53		1·87
	(1·68)	(1·16)		(5·75)	(0·53)		(1·80)
%RPN	0·67	−0·22		−0·22	−0·33		−0·19
	(9·38)	(3·89)		(2·59)	(4·75)		(2·62)
%LPN	0·19	−0·46		−0·75	−0·41		−0·60
	(1·86)	(5·79)		(6·28)	(4·24)		(5·74)
MDH/BED	0·04	0·08		0·16	0·10		0·17
	(3·77)	(8·85)		(13·14)	(8·70)		(15·20)
Wage							
RWAGE		−0·62		−0·42	−0·52		- 0·42
		(28·07)		(13·14)	(19·54)		(15·10)
Price of non-labour inputs							
CPI	0·001	−0·01	−0·01	−0·007	−0·01	−0·009	−0·02
	(0·24)	(2·42)	(1·47)	(1·12)	(2·32)	(1·16)	(3·96)
Technology							
TIME	0·002	0·03	0·03	0·04	0·04	0·04	0·06
	(0·51)	(2·80)	(2·09)	(2·52)	(3·37)	(2·50)	(4·76)
$\bar{R}^2$	0·35	0·85	0·72	0·66	0·49	0·23	0·38
S.E.	0·202	0·158	0·216	0·239	0·191	0·235	0·211

TABLE 15·3

EFFECT OF DEMAND, MIX, WAGES AND TECHNOLOGY ON NON-LABOR INPUT

(*t*-scores in parentheses)

	Non-labor input per admission			Non-labor input per patient-day		
Constant	-2·37	-2·86	-0·39	-3·19	-3·61	1·09
	(1·37)	(1·66)	(0·48)	(1·60)	(1·83)	(1·37)
Demand						
INS	-0·20	-0·18		-0·02	-0·007	
	(5·16)	(4·37)		(0·54)	(0·16)	
RINC	0·15	0·11		-0·009	-0·05	
	(2·27)	(1·62)		(0·12)	(0·59)	
MDPC	0·06	0·05		0·12	0·11	
	(2·11)	(1·57)		(3·54)	(3·09)	
%GP	-0·03	-0·06		0·03	-0·009	
	(0·96)	(2·38)		(1·11)	(0·30)	
BEDSPC	0·14	0·13		-0·05	-0·05	
	(6·52)	(6·24)		(1·83)	(2·23)	
DENS	0·08	0·08		0·02	0·03	
	(10·14)	(11·37)		(2·47)	(3·93)	
YOUNG	0·39	0·26		0·63	0·56	
	(1·21)	(0·82)		(1·73)	(1·54)	
WHITE	-0·04	-0·04		0·0006	0·02	
	(0·56)	(0·53)		(0·008)	(0·22)	
EDYR	0·19	0·14		0·44	0·41	
	(1·76)	(1·23)		(3·49)	(3·21)	
Mix						
RMS	1·05	1·00	0·93	0·05	-0·003	0·03
	(27·87)	(27·70)	(20·71)	(1·22)	(0·08)	(0·79)
BEDS	-0·006		0·12	-0·02		0·02
	(0·49)		(9·31)	(1·35)		(1·93)
PA/B	0·07		0·07	0·08		0·07
	(7·18)		(6·84)	(7·38)		(7·00)
MEDSCH	0·07		0·14	0·09		0·09
	(3·02)		(5·20)	(3·37)		(3·46)
%INT-RES	-1·59		5·78	-1·17		0·87
	(1·21)		(3·83)	(0·77)		(0·59)
%RPN	0·14		0·08	0·03		0·10
	(1·52)		(0·74)	(0·30)		(0·98)
%LPN	0·01		-0·24	0·06		-0·09
	(0·09)		(1·56)	(0·43)		(0·61)
MDH/BED	0·03		0·11	0·05		0·11
	(2·30)		(6·84)	(2·92)		(7·18)
Wage						
RWAGE	-0·23		-0·05	-0·14		-0·05
	(6·60)		(1·16)	(3·36)		(1·30)
Price of non-labor input						
CPI	0·02	0·03	0·03	0·02	0·03	0·01
	(2·96)	(3·50)	(3·20)	(2·36)	(3·20)	(1·38)
Technology						
TIME	0·006	0·0006	0·01	0·02	0·008	0·04
	(0·34)	(0·03)	(0·79)	(0·99)	(0·43)	(2·14)
$\bar{R}^2$	0·71	0·68	0·57	0·33	0·29	0·29
S.E.	0·253	0·263	0·307	0·291	0·301	0·300

translates greater ability of patients to pay into higher payments for personnel; it could also reflect higher going wage rates in high-income areas. More interestingly, wages are also significantly higher when patients pay a lower fraction of the hospital bill out-of-pocket. This provides somewhat more solid support of the philanthropic wage behavior contention. Wage rates are also higher in areas with greater population density and with high proportions of whites, presumably a reflection of labor market conditions.

Case-mix proxies which prove to be significant in the wage regression include size of hospital and composition of personnel. As bed size increases, say, from 300 to 400 beds, average annual earnings increase by about $60. A higher proportion of interns, residents, registered practical nurses and licensed practical nurses also raises average annual earnings, with the rate of increase being highest for interns and residents, next highest for registered nurses and lowest for licensed nurses.

Real wages do not shift up over time over and above that attributable to other factors, such as increases in real per capita incomes.

Virtually the same types of factors that affect overall hospital costs also affect quantities of labor and non-labor inputs, although demand factors tend to be more important in the determination of labor inputs than of non-labor inputs. A combination of demand, case-mix, wage rates and technology factors is required for the highest explanation of variation in personnel and real non-labor input per unit of output. Omission of either demand variables or wage and case-mix variables considerably lowers the explanatory power of these regressions. A higher proportion of out-of-pocket payments lowers both personnel per admission and personnel per patient-day, while higher incomes lead to greater employment of personnel per admission. A greater abundance of physicians in the area also tends to increase personnel. Out-of-pocket payments also reduce the use of non-labor inputs, but income has a somewhat weaker impact on increasing use of non-labor inputs.

Case-mix variables enter in the personnel and real non-labor input regressions in much the same way as in the overall regressions. Hospitals with more plant assets per bed also employ more personnel and non-labor inputs, as do hospitals affiliated with a medical school. A greater concentration of physicians on the medical staff also gives rise to an increase in personnel and non-labor inputs, both per hospital admission and per patient-day.

As might be expected, increases in wage rates lead to substantial reductions in personnel employed. A 10 per cent increase in real wages results in a 6 per cent decline in personnel per hospital admission. This could occur because the hospital substitutes other types of inputs for labor as labor becomes more expensive. Another explanation, however, is that the hospital has some given level of costs which it tries to achieve (or within which it tries to stay). Any increase in cost of one input must result in cutbacks in other areas – either in a reduction in the use of that input or in the use of other inputs. As indicated in Table 15.3, this latter explanation seems to be the correct one. Non-labor inputs are also reduced by increases in wage rates, although not so strongly (a 10 per cent increase in real wage rates causes a 2 per cent decline in real non-labor inputs per admission). The results, on the price of non-labor inputs, as measured by the consumer price index, however, are not completely consistent with this explanation. An increase in the consumer price index reduces the use of personnel, as predicted by the target cost hypothesis, but it also increases the use of non-labor inputs – which is not consistent with either the substitution view of input determination or the target cost hypothesis. Since the consumer price index and the time variable are closely related, it is possible that the consumer price index is picking up an acceleration in the rate of increase of non-labor inputs over time. The results, however, may indicate that the consumer price index is not an adequate proxy for price of non-labor inputs across geographical areas or over time.

VI. SUMMARY

Empirical estimation of a reduced-form equation of hospital costs has indicated that simultaneous consideration of a number of different determinants of hospital costs, including demand, case-mix, wage rates and changes in technology, is necessary for the best explanation of average costs. Omitting any of these important sources of cost increase substantially reduces the ability of the regression to explain overall variations in average costs, and in the various labor and non-labor components of average costs.

Demand variables of income, insurance and availability of physicians play particularly important roles in the determination of hospital expenses per hospital admission. These demand factors operate on expenses primarily through their effect on length of hospital stay. More comprehensive insurance coverage and higher incomes lead to longer hospital stays, but the increased length of stay induced by demand does not result in a reduction in the cost per day of caring for patients. The net effect of demand, therefore, is to increase the overall cost of caring for patients. Affiliation with a medical school and greater capitalization for hospitals of a given size both result in higher average costs – either because such hospitals treat more difficult cases, provide higher-quality care, or incorporate the latest advances in medical technology. Increases in average cost over time unaccounted for by changes in demand, case-mix or wage rates amount to 2 per cent annually.

In summary, of the predicted increase in expenses per hospital admission, demand variables accounted for 45 per cent of the increase; case-mix variables added another 7 per cent. Increases in average earnings of hospital employees represented another 10 per cent of the overall increase, while shifts upward over time were responsible for the remaining 38 per cent.

Demand and case-mix factors are also important in the determination of hospital wage rates, with hospitals paying higher wages in high-income areas and in areas where patients pay a small proportion of the hospital bill out-of-pocket.

Both labor and non-labor inputs per unit of hospital care are responsive to demand and case-mix factors, although demand factors tend to be somewhat stronger in the determination of labor input, while case-mix factors influence both types of inputs. Higher wages lead to a reduced use of both labor and non-labor inputs, suggesting that hospitals may be attempting to attain some target level of costs so that increases in one component of costs require cutbacks in other areas.

Many of these results should be viewed as tentative, because of the necessity of using proxies for hospital case-mix and the difficulties of obtaining characteristics on the exact population served by a given hospital. Insurance coverage, for example, was measured at the state level, and demographic composition of the population, physician and hospital availability were measured at the country level, which may not be relevant for all hospitals in the sample.

It does represent, however, a systematic attempt to pull together a number of different possible sources of increases in hospital costs and to make some rough estimates of the relative importance of these factors in overall hospital cost inflation. If these findings are supported by other studies, policy-makers should have some indication of the payoff to be gained in terms of tempering increases in hospital costs of policies directed toward controlling hospital wage rates, changing the structure of insurance coverage, influencing the availability of physicians, altering access of hospitals to capital funds, and redirecting research resulting in changes in medical technology. The desirability of pursuing any of these policies will depend upon a great many other criteria as well, but at least the impact of such policies on hospital costs can be roughly assessed.

REFERENCES

[1] Davis, Karen, 'An Empirical Investigation of Alternative Models of the Hospital Industry', paper presented at the American Economic Association meeting in Toronto, 30 Dec 1972.

[2] ——, 'Theories of Hospital Inflation: Some Empirical Evidence', *Journal of Human Resources* (Spring 1973).

[3] —— and Foster, Richard W., *Community Hospitals: Inflation in the Pre-Medicare Period* (Washington, D.C.: U.S. Government Printing Office, 1972).

[4] Feldstein, Martin S., 'Econometric Approaches to Health Economics', forthcoming in M. Intriligator and D. Kendrick (eds.), *Frontiers of Quantitative Economics*, vol. II (Amsterdam: North-Holland, 1973).

[5] ——, 'Hospital Cost Inflation: A Study of Nonprofit Price Dynamics' *American Economic Review*, LXI, 5 (Dec 1971) 853–73.

[6] ——, *The Rising Cost of Hospital Care* (Washington, D.C.: Information Resources Press, 1971).

[7] Pauly, Mark, and Redisch, Michael, 'The Not-for-Profit Hospital as a Physicians' Cooperative', unpublished paper (1971).

[8] Salkever, David, 'A Micro-econometric Study of Hospital Cost Inflation', *Journal of Political Economy*, LXXX, 6 (Nov/Dec 1972) 1144–66.

16 A Microanalysis of Physicians' Hours of Work Decisions[1]

Frank A. Sloan

UNIVERSITY OF FLORIDA

This study analyzes physician decisions regarding their work-week and the number of weeks worked per year, using data on 1,800 physicians from the Public Use Sample of 1960 United States Census. For several reasons, the demand that the physician faces is an endogenous variable. Therefore, wage equations in both the hourly and weekly wage are developed, in addition to two supply equations. The results indicate a positive supply response to the weekly, but a negative response to the hourly, wage. The latter result should be interpreted cautiously, since the pure income effect is very small and inconsistent with a backward-bending supply curve. In addition, income determines the impact of various demographic characteristics on physician supply. Female physicians with children work less than their colleagues do. The physician/population ratio in the area in which the physician practices affects individual physician supply negatively, especially in the week dimension.

I. INTRODUCTION

Evidence on trends in physician work patterns, though fragmentary, gives the present study of hours decisions some urgency. *Medical Economics*' data indicate a decline in total physician hours of work, from 64 in 1965 – prior to the introduction of Medicare–Medicaid – to 60 in 1968.[2] American Medical Association data show the patient care work-week declining slightly, from 45·3 in 1965 to 44·7 in 1969 and 1970.[3] The mean number of physician weeks worked in 1959 was 49·3, according to the U.S. Census. By 1969 the comparable figure

[1] This research was supported in part by a grant (HS00825), 'Analysis of Physician Price and Output Decisions', from the Center for Health Services Research and Development of the United States Department of Health, Education and Welfare, to the University of Florida.

[2] *Medical Economics* Continuing Surveys of Physician Practice. Conducted annually and published in various issues of the magazine.

[3] Theodore and Sutter (1967) and Center for Health Services Research and Development, A.M.A. (1971, 1972).

from an American Medical Association source ranged from 47·8 to 48·3, depending on the physician's type of practice.[1] Weeks and hours worked do not capture all facets of physician work patterns of concern to the public. Other dimensions include the supply of house and night calls, types of patients accepted for treatment, and physician willingness to take a second job, for example, in a neighborhood health center of a ghetto area. Unfortunately, data on these are even more fragmentary. Yet there are numerous published accounts suggesting trends in these areas quite similar to those in weeks and hours.[2]

This paper reports the results of statistical analysis of data from the Public Use Sample of the 1960 Census, a 1 per cent sample of the United States population. It is a valuable resource for an investigation of physician hours decisions as it contains detailed data on employment, both employment and non-employment income, and demographic information for both the physician and other members of his household. Many variables, in particular non-employment income and demographic characteristics, are difficult to obtain elsewhere. Physicians see little reason to respond to questions about their personal life in surveys of their practices, the usual data source on physicians. Moreover, unlike surveys of practices, the physician response rate to the Census is virtually 100 per cent. Thus, dangers of bias stemming from a low response rate do not exist.

Section II reviews features of physician practice that are pertinent to an analysis of physician work patterns. Section III presents the model. Since a physician wage predicted from a wage-generating equation is included as an independent variable in the supply equation, a wage as well as a supply equation is discussed. Section IV contains the empirical findings. The final section discusses the policy implications of this study and suggests some future research directions.

II. CONCEPTUAL CONSIDERATIONS

The theory of the household provides a powerful tool for empirical analysis of supply decisions. Nevertheless, in order for the results of the empirical work to be meaningful, it is necessary to recognize its limitations for the particular application under study. The theory assumes that prices are exogenous to consumers in both product and

---

[1] Center for Health Services Research and Development, A.M.A. (1972).

[2] When physicians have been asked in a recent year for their primary practice goal, the majority responds 'greater ease of practice' (see Reinhardt, 1970). For public statements on increased physician non-availability by non-physicians, see Carnegie Commission on Higher Education (1970) p. 36, and National Advisory Commission on Health Manpower (1967) pp. 1–2.

factor markets. The self-employed physician, 74 per cent of all active physicians in the 1960 Census sample, does not face exogenous prices for his own input. Rather his reward per work hour may depend in part on the number of hours he works for a least two reasons. Being the principal input to his practice, his marginal product most likely depends on his hours of work. Where large numbers of individuals in an input category are employed, the hours decision of a single individual will have only a minor effect on the aggregate number of hours worked by all labor and therefore only a minor effect on the marginal product for the input category as a whole. A self-employed physician, however, generally practices alone or in a small group. Increased work hours by an individual physician are likely to cause the marginal product for his input category to fall. Moreover, if the physician sets prices for his services, he faces declining marginal revenue per unit of output produced as his input increases.[1]

A modified form of the traditional model for analyzing hours of work patterns of the self-employed has appeared in several studies.[2] The fundamental difference from the traditional labor supply model is the budget constraint. Assuming that the self-employed physician sets prices for his services but not for the other inputs to his practice, the budget constraint is:

$$P_G \cdot G = Y + P_s(f(H, N, K; Z')) \cdot f(H, N, K; Z') - w \cdot N - r \cdot K \qquad (1)$$

where G is the number of goods purchased

$\qquad$ P_G is the price of consumer goods
$\qquad$ Y is non-employment income
$\qquad$ P_s is the price of the physician's services
$\qquad$ f is the production function for the physician's firm with inputs H, N, K representing his own input, other labor inputs and capital, respectively, and Z' exogenous characteristics of the physician and his work setting that affect productivity
$\qquad$ w is the wage

and

$\qquad$ r is the price of capital.

P_s depends on the quantity sold which, in the service industries, is synonymous with current production. Thus, $f(\cdot)$ may be substituted in (1) for the quantity sold.

---

[1] Although it is likely that the physician has some capacity to set prices, the evidence is not yet conclusive.

[2] See Horowitz (1970) for a review. This modified model dates back to Scitovsky (1943). Yett *et al.* (1970) and Reinhardt (1970) mention this model in the context of the physician, but do not implement it empirically.

Setting P_G equal to 1, total differentiating, and setting all differentials except dG and dH equal to zero,

$$\frac{dG}{dH} = \frac{\partial P_s}{\partial f(\cdot)} \frac{\partial f(\cdot)}{\partial H} \cdot f(H, N, K; Z') + P_s \cdot \frac{\partial f(\cdot)}{\partial H}. \tag{2}$$

The second term on the right is probably positive for any physicians one might observe.[1] The first is zero for product price-taking physicians. Otherwise it is negative. Manipulating (2), it is easily seen that dG/dH is positive if the decision-maker operates in the inelastic portion of his demand curve and is negative when he does not. Adding the tautology, $\bar{H} \equiv H + L$, available hours ($\bar{H}$) equal market work (H) plus leisure hours (L), and since $dH = -dL$, the relationship between G and H may be expressed graphically as in Fig. 16.1. Self-

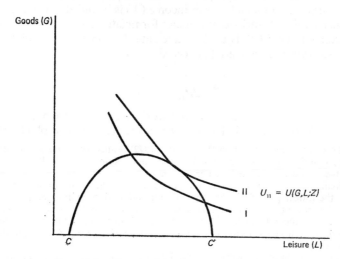

FIG. 16.1 The physician hours of work decision

employment *per se* only affects the transformation constraint, CC'. The allocation of time between market work and leisure is determined by the point of tangency of $U_{11} = U(G, L; Z)$ and CC', where Z represents a set of variables affecting the marginal rate of substitution between goods and leisure.

The fact that dG/dH varies may be the source of an identification problem in empirical work on supply, since hours worked affect average compensation per hour – the physician wage – negatively as

[1] According to Reinhardt (1972), $df(\cdot)/dH$ becomes zero at a physician input of 110 hours per week for general practitioners and is negative thereafter.

well as the reverse. A backward-bending supply curve may be mistaken for the negative impact of hours on the wage. Fortunately, $\partial f(\cdot)/\partial H$ appears to decrease slowly as hours increase.[1] Based on Reinhardt's (1972) production function parameter estimates for general practitioner visits, $\partial f(\cdot)/\partial H$ declines by between 0·05 and 0·06 per hour throughout the input range in which most physicians operate. Assuming P_s equalled $3 in 1959, the amount of decline in $P_s \cdot \partial f(\cdot)/\partial H$ per hour worked in 1959 was between $0·15 and $0·18.[2] If the physician sets prices, one must consider the first term of (2). Reinhardt also presents production function estimates with patient billings as the dependent variable. Unfortunately, neither this nor any other source of information is appropriate for assessing dG/dH when product prices are allowed to vary.[3]

Another consequence of physician self-employment appears to be more serious. Non-employment income (Y) is included in (1) as it is in the traditional work–leisure choice formulation. The coefficient of Y, expressing $\partial H/\partial Y$, is used to calculate the compensated price or pure substitution response (S) according to

$$S = \frac{dH}{dP_H} - H \cdot \frac{\partial H}{\partial Y} \qquad (3)$$

where P_H is compensation per hour worked. Since a large portion of the physician's assets is likely to be in medical practice plant and

[1] This statement is based on Reinhardt's (1972) results with a transcendental production function. For very low levels of hours, Reinhardt's results indicate that the physician's marginal product increases.

[2] Reinhardt's results for other physicians in other fields are quite similar. $3 is the lowest price for general practitioner office visits in 1959 reported in U.S. Department of Commerce, *Statistical Abstract of the United States, 1961*, p. 341. Since these data pertain only to S.M.S.A.'s one expects the mean P_s for the United States to be nearer to the lower estimate of all S.M.S.A.s than to the higher estimates.

[3] Reinhardt presents estimates of production function parameters with total patient billings by the physician as the dependent variable. These results are not useful for the present purpose, since the physician's customary fee for an initial office visit enters as an independent variable when billings is the dependent variable. If fees vary according to physician hours, the first office visit should do so as well. Cross-tabulations between hours worked per week and two fee measures, routine revisit price and average billing per visit, presented in Reinhardt (1970), show a negative relationship, but it is not possible to calculate $\partial P_s/\partial H$ from these grouped data, since means for each of the three hours categories are not given. It is possible that the price differences reflect an unspecified variable rather than work hours. In particular, physicians in rural areas are likely to work longer hours and charge lower fees. Maurizi (1969) presents a more detailed cross-tabulation for dentist hours and selected fees; no systematic relationship is apparent. Market demand curves for physician services have been estimated, but only a demand curve for the individual physician would be appropriate for the present purpose.

equipment, there is a good chance that a large percentage of returns to assets will be reported as earnings rather than non-employment income. Average hourly compensation has to be calculated from earnings and hours data, since no direct measure is available from the Census. Non-employment income may, thus, enter as part of P_H. Dividing earnings by hours to form P_H is one source of negative correlation bias; inability to separate earnings from non-employment income is another. The fact that 39·7 per cent of all physicians in the Census sample reported no non-employment income for 1959 is an indication that income from physician labor and capital sources is commingled in a number of cases.

An instrumental variable technique, whereby the physician wage is made a function of several exogenous variables, is employed to reduce the potential biases reviewed in this section. Use of a predicted rather than an actual physician wage in the supply equation should aid in identifying the supply relationship, because factors accounting for shifts in the transformation function CC' are included as instruments. Moreover, errors-in-variables bias in the wage parameter arising from inaccurate income reporting should be reduced. There is little to be done about errors in variables in Y. Unless an essentially different set of instruments for Y than for the wage could be found, serious multicollinearity in the supply equation would result if one attempted to correct for errors in Y. Thus, the actual Y is incorporated in the supply equation.

Consumer theory generally specifies utility as a function of goods and leisure. There are no special problems associated with this specification except the usual one that the decision-maker may not be completely free to vary the number of hours he works. Medical ethics may 'force' the physician to treat patients if no suitable physician or non-physician substitute is available. This consideration may be incorporated into the model by making utility from goods and leisure conditional on such variables as the physician/population ratio (a variable included in Z in the utility function given in Fig. 16.1).

The theory is completely unspecific about what is meant by leisure. Many, if not most, researchers have specified hours worked per year, the product of hours worked during the last complete work-week and the number of weeks worked last year as the supply measure. However, it would appear, *a priori*, that there are substantial differences between weeks and hours decisions. The discussion of declining marginal product with increasing hours is probably more relevant to hours than to weeks. Judging from empirical evidence, the two decisions are only weakly related. The simple correlation between physician weeks worked in 1959 and hours worked during a reference week (as defined by the Census) in March 1960 is 0·21. Given these considerations, weeks and hours supply equations are estimated separately.

The supply measures are specified as linear functions of the supply determinants. Non-linear terms are added to test for non-linear wage and income effects. Although dG/dH is not constant, the best available evidence suggests that it is nearly so. The gain from postulating a model whereby the physician maximizes a specific utility function subject to a constraint given by (1) and a time constraint is small relative to the additional computational cost. The only utility functions resulting in reduced-form equations appropriate for estimation are quite restrictive in any case. Given the constraint (1), which contains a production function that is probably non-linear, even simple utility functions result in highly non-linear first-order condition equations. And it is not possible to manipulate these equations into reduced-form equations, suitable for estimation. Alternative methods for obtaining the parameter estimates, such as simulation, exist. But then there is a problem of model validation. Since the physician's preference structure is not well understood, it is probably more fruitful at this point to obtain knowledge of physician work patterns from linear supply equations than from specific utility (and production) functions, although the latter approach has greater conceptual appeal.[1]

III. EQUATION SPECIFICATION

(1) Wage Equation

Predicted values from weekly and hourly wage equations are independent variables in the weeks and hours supply equations, respectively. Both wage equations are specified identically. Because of possible employer and patient discrimination, $SEX(=1$ if the physician is female) should have a negative impact on wages. Previous work on earnings-generating functions has found an inverted U-shaped relationship between experience and earnings. Data on experience are, unfortunately, not available from the Census. Though not a perfect measure, age is a reasonably good proxy for experience.[2] Four age dummy variables are included. $A2$ represents physicians in their thirties. $A3$, $A4$ and $A5$ are for physicians in their forties, fifties and

[1] Leuthold (1968), Kraft (1970) and Sloan (forthcoming) estimate supply equations derived from specific functional forms of the utility function.

[2] However, it is by no means perfect. Brown (mimeo) reports that about one-third of the physicians in his sample did not complete all their formal medical training before beginning practice. Returning to a residency program after a number of years in practice is surprisingly common. Given this variation in training patterns, one would expect some variation in practice experience within an age cohort.

the first five years of their sixties, respectively. The sample includes physicians aged 65 to 69, but excludes those under 30 and those who reported no work during the reference week and/or during 1959.

*FRN*1 equals 1 if the physician was born in an English-speaking country other than the United States or in Northern or Western Europe. Most (80 per cent) *FRN*1 physicians are from English- or German-speaking countries. Some patients and a larger proportion of referring physicians may consider medical education in many foreign medical schools to be below United States standards, and this factor may be reflected in earnings of foreign physicians. Moreover, foreign physicians may have language difficulties which may reduce earnings, or be subject to racial or ethnic discrimination. For these reasons, the coefficient on *FRN*1 is expected to be far less negative than *FRN*2's, which corresponds to all other physicians born outside the United States. Most numerous among the *FRN*2 physicians are those with native languages of Italian (19), Spanish (16), Yiddish (13) and Tagalog (12). *RACEN* equals 1 if the physician is black, 1·7 per cent of the 1,800 physician sample. The expected sign of *RACEN* is negative, reflecting both poor medical educational opportunities available to blacks until recently, as well as discrimination against the practicing black physician.

*WCL*1 and *WCL*2 are dummy variables for physicians employed by private companies (including voluntary hospitals and private medical schools) and governments, respectively. Parameters of both are hypothesized to be negative. Self-employed physicians have a greater entrepreneurial function and bear greater risks and uncertainties. *WCL*1 and *WCL*2 physicians constitute 14·8 and 11·4 per cent of the sample, respectively. Some physicians (15·2 per cent of the sample) are classified as self-employed, but report some earnings from employers. To allow for differential hours responses of physicians who derive earnings from both employment and self-employment sources, *EARNSAL* equals 1 if a self-employed physician receives some income from an employer. A negative coefficient for these semi-employed physicians, but smaller in absolute value than those for *WCL*1 and *WCL*2, was anticipated. But, as seen below, the parameter estimate of this variable is positive. Part-time physicians may have higher wages because other physicians cover for them during short-term absences, and sickness and disability pay is treated as part of earnings by the Census. Also, to some extent, dG/dH falls as hours of work rise. The variable *PT* equals 1 if the product of weeks worked in 1959 and hours worked during the reference week is 1,500 or less.

Improvement in life-cycle earnings is an incentive to migrate. However, the newcomer to an area will probably have lower earnings than his counterparts in the area until his practice is established. *M*1, *M*2 and $M3$ equal 1, respectively, if the physician lived in another county, another state or abroad in 1955. Physicians in this sample are surprisingly mobile. Between 1955 and 1960, 9·4 per cent changed counties but not states; 13·2 per cent changed states; 4·4 per cent moved to the United States from abroad.

The remaining explanatory variables pertain to the geographical area in which the physician is located. Some of these correspond to the physician's state and place of residence, either urban or rural. Others refer to the physician's state only. If the physicians' market were in equilibrium and if there were no non-pecuniary differences in alternative locations, the area would exert no independent effect on earnings. Entry by physicians would offset medical service demand differences. But, in fact, some areas are more attractive than others; thus, equilibrium differences in earnings are likely to exist. Moreover, at any point in time, one probably observes a market disequilibrium. *MEDY*, median income in the area, *SURINPOP* and *MEDINPOP*, the percentage of population with some basic surgical and medical insurance coverage, represent patient ability to pay for medical services. *AGLT5*, *AGT65* and *RAD*, percentage of the population less than age 5 and 65 and over, and the number of restricted activity days per capita population, represent patient need. *PHYPOP*, the physician/population ratio, measures the extent of demand pressure on individual physicians, One may anticipate that some parameter estimates of area variables will be biased toward zero because the geographical area encompassed by the variable is larger than the physician's market area. To test for potential biases, the observations have been aggregated into states, and wage regressions have been run with the state as well as the individual physician as the observational unit.

All variables in this study expressable in monetary units have been deflated by a state price index, but this does not exclude the possibility that intra-state wage differences might reflect the size of the community in which the physician practices. Binary variables have been specified to signify whether the physician works in a central city of a metropolitan area (S.M.S.A.), in the outer ring of an S.M.S.A., or in an urban, non-S.M.S.A. location. These variables were always insignificant and have been excluded from the results reported below.

(2) *Supply Equation*

Wage and income variables occupy central positions in the supply equation. Linear (*WAGEW* in the weeks and *WAGEH* in the hours equation) and squared wage variables are included; the latter permits a backward-bending supply curve, once a critical level of wages is reached. Non-employment income (Y) also enters Y as Y^2, thus permitting differential income effects over Y's range. Y is defined as the sum of income from children, persons living in the household other than the physician's spouse, and physician and spouse income from non-employment sources. Although data on such assets as house and some furnishings are available, no attempt is made to incorporate income flows from these assets, since there is no way of determining the physician's equity in these assets. Y covers a range of over $50,000, even though slightly under 93 per cent give Y as less than $5,000.[1] If leisure of the spouse and physician are substitutes, the parameter on spouse earnings (YS) should be more negative than Y's, since YS then incorporates a negative cross-substitution effect in addition to the 'pure' income effect which is common to the two. Conversely, if leisure of the two are complements, the cross-substitution effect is positive, and the YS parameter would be less negative. Only 16·9 per cent of physicians in the sample have spouses with earnings.[2]

The remaining variables account for inter-physician differences in the marginal rate of substitution between income and leisure. Given society's value system, females are recognized to be more productive than males in household work. This is likely to affect the marginal rate of substitution between goods and leisure so that there is less market work by female than by male physicians. The expected sign of SEX is, thus, negative. As individuals age, the value of further asset accumulation to them diminishes. Physicians in the higher age group thus may be expected to work less. $A2$ through $A5$ should have positive signs, but $A5$'s coefficient should be lower than the others. $FRN1$, $FRN2$ and $RACEN$ are included to measure taste differences based on ethnicity. Previous work by the author (reported in Sloan, forthcoming) found that foreign physicians spend less time in market work than do their peers. The shorter work-week of employed physicians is well established.[3] This pattern may reflect taste differences and/or differences in the marginal net revenue derived from extra effort. Employed persons on a fixed salary may obtain nothing for increases in market work above the amount required by the job.

[1] The mean is $1,476.

[2] An alternative is to estimate a spouse wage equation, using the parameter estimates of this equation to assign wages to each spouse in the sample. This was done in some preliminary work; however, the results are not reported here, since this approach assumes that the structure appropriate to a small number of spouses is representative of the entire group. On reflection, this assumption appears inappropriate.

[3] The evidence is reviewed in a paper on health manpower incentives, by the author, being written for the National Center for Health Services Research and Development, Economic Analysis Branch of the Department of Health, Education and Welfare.

Children have both negative substitution and positive income effects on market work. The negative effect arises from the increase in potential productivity in the household; the income effect derives from the fact that there are more mouths to feed. $C1$ and $C2$ equal 1 if there are children under age two and children over age two in the household, respectively. $SD \cdot C1$ and $SD \cdot C2$ equal 1 if the physician is female and is a parent. Married physicians may place a higher value on non-market time than their single colleagues. Thus, the expected sign on $MARRD (=1$ if the physician is married) is negative.

Feldstein (1970) hypothesizes that physicians' income aspirations vary directly with the level of income of persons in the upper tail of the income distribution. They will work harder if their reference group earns more. He measures reference income as the income corresponding to the 95th percentile of the income distribution. Reference income (YR) in this study is the mean income of physicians in the physician's state. If the marginal utility of money truly varies according to this argument, the coefficient of YR should be positive. Physicians in warmer climates may have greater opportunities for recreation and, thus, spend less time in medical practice. A climate variable, defined as the number of degree days, has been included.[1] Since colder climates have more degree days, the coefficient should be negative. As stated in the previous section, medical ethics dictate that a physician treat patients in emergencies who have no alternative source of care. In geographical areas with a low ratio of physicians to population, people have relatively few alternative sources of care. Physicians, in turn, will be forced to work longer and more irregular hours. The state physician/population ratio, thus, should have a direct, negative impact on the hours supplied by the individual physician.

IV. EMPIRICAL RESULTS

(1) Wage Equation

Table 16.1 contains the results for the weekly and hourly wage equations. Most of the coefficients are significant at the 5 per cent level or better. The first set of comments pertains to the significant coefficients. There is a substantial male–female difference in physician wages. In 1959–60 the female physician earned $153·2 less per week and $3·84 less per hour, *ceteris paribus*. These coefficients should be

[1] The degree day has been defined as follows: 'A unit, based upon temperature difference and time, used in estimating fuel consumption and specifying nominal heating load in the winter. For any one day, when the mean temperature is less than 65°F, there exist as many degree days as there are Fahrenheit degrees difference in the temperature between the average temperature for the day and 65°F.' U.S. Department of Commerce, *Statistical Abstract of the United States, 1970*, p. 160.

TABLE 16.1

WAGE EQUATIONS
(standard errors in parentheses)

Weeks – Micro / Hours – Micro

	SEX	A2	A3	A4	A5	FRN1	FRN2	RACEN	PT	WCL1	WCL2	EARNSAL	M1	M2
Weeks – Micro	-153·2* (33·4)	105·9* (38·5)	190·7* (38·1)	166·6* (39·1)	114·0* (45·8)	0·083 (33·5)	-69·7† (29·3)	-192·0* (57·7)	-68·9 (35·3)	-84·5* (23·2)	-160·8* (25·5)	310·5* (21·2)	-112·2* (26·5)	-91·4* (24·4)
Hours – Micro	-3·84* (0·81)	1·45 (0·93)	3·62† (0·92)	3·35* (0·94)	2·27† (1·10)	-0·21 (0·81)	-1·70 (0·70)	-3·80* (1·39)	8·32* (0·35)	-1·71* (0·56)	-2·38* (0·61)	5·79* (0·51)	-2·03 (0·64)	-1·72* (0·59)

Weeks – Micro (contd.) / Hours – Micro (contd.)

	M3	MEDY	AGLT5	AGT65	PHYPOP	SURINPOP	MEDINPOP	RAD	CONSTANT	
Weeks – Micro (contd.)	-157·8* (42·3)	0·017 (0·02)	-9·03 (5·70)	4·63 (6·48)	-11·22* (3·48)	-0·72 (1·40)	0·67 (1·43)	22·36* (6·93)	143·98 ‡	$R^2=0.27$ $\sigma_u=311.8$, $F=30.62*$
Hours – Micro (contd.)	-2·80* (1·02)	0·00056 (0·0050)	-0·11 (0·13)	-0·044 (0·15)	-0·15 (0·08)	-0·0074 (0·033)	0·016 (0·034)	0·523* (0·167)	0·81 ‡	$R^2=0.21$ $\sigma_u=7.53$, $F=18.48*$

Weeks – State / Hours – State

	%A2	%A3	%A4	%A5	%PT	MEDY	AGLT5	AGT65	PHYPOP	SURINPOP	MEDINPOP	RAD	CONSTANT	
Weeks – State	-3·55 (3·84)	-0·66 (3·98)	-1·99 (5·17)	-2·89 (4·54)	1·82 (2·98)	0·017 (0·043)	0·26 (17·61)	10·53 (11·61)	-13·75† (5·96)	-1·28 (2·24)	1·38 (2·56)	19·80 (11·18)	373·7 (606·0)	$R^2=0.47$ $\sigma_u=73.95$, $F=2.56†$
Hours – State	-0·047 (0·077)	0·011 (0·079)	0·026 (0·10)	-0·054 (0·094)	0·18* (0·06)	0·00024 (0·00087)	0·096 (0·036)	0·048 (0·23)	-0·19 (0·12)	-0·037 (0·045)	0·052 (0·051)	0·56† (0·23)	-0·21 (12·5)	$R^2=0.47$ $\sigma_u=1.48$, $F=2.43†$

* Significant at the 1 per cent level.
† Significant at the 5 per cent level.
‡ Computer program used does not give standard error of the constant term. Micro based on 1,800 observations, state based on 48.

compared to all-physician means of $432·84 and $8·04, respectively. Wages reach their peak for both weeks and hours within the 40–49 age group ($A3$). Male weekly wages for the 40–49 age group are 17 per cent higher than in the 30–39 and 15 per cent higher than in the 60–64 age group. Wages decline rapidly after age 64. The pre-age-40 wage increase is faster than the post-age-49 decrease until age 65. For the hourly wage, there is a relatively more rapid initial increase, $A3$ physicians having a wage 23 per cent higher than $A2$, and a relatively less pronounced decline, $A3$ being 14 per cent higher than $A5$'s hourly wage.

These life-cycle wage patterns reflect at least three factors. First, physicians at an early stage in their careers spend time building up their human capital and reputations. This time takes the form of reading, attending meetings and, in some cases, keeping the office open in an attempt to establish a practice. Time spent in these pursuits, unfortunately for purposes of this study, is recorded as work by the Census. This procedure has the effect of raising the length of the measured work-week and, simultaneously, depressing the hourly wage rate. Later in the physician's career, these investment activities decline.[1] The rather rapid initial increase in the hourly wage may reflect both the time young physicians devote to human capital accumulation as well as the effects of this accumulation, as reflected in the $A3$ hourly wage coefficient. Human capital accumulation is a potential source of measurement error in the wage. This error may not be fully removed by the instrumental technique as it is used here, since these investments are age-dependent. Yet to remove the age variables from the wage equation, if this error is not important (or not closely related to age), would reduce this equation's goodness of fit unnecessarily. Further research should concentrate on this issue, as this measurement error is a possible source of negative bias in the supply equation's wage coefficient. Vintage, a second determinant of life-cycle wage patterns, should generate a monotonic decline in wages over the life-cycle. Third, there are the effects of variables that were omitted from the equation for lack of data. These include specialty and board certification. Both variables should increase wages of the young relative to the older physicians. The patterns in Table 16·1 suggest that the first factor is the most important of the three.

Both $FRN2$ and $RACEN$ are negative and significant. $FRN1$ is not. $RACEN$ has approximately the same effect as SEX on hourly wages. On weeks, $RACEN$'s impact exceeds SEX's. As expected, the co-efficient of part-time physicians (PT) is positive in the hourly wage equation; PT enters negatively into the weekly wage equation, since

[1] On this point, see Peterson *et al.* (1956).

the higher wage per hour is offset by a shorter work-week. Physicians with private (*WCL*1) and government (*WCL*2) employers earn less per unit of time than self-employed physicians. *EARNSAL*'s co-efficients were unexpected. Semi-employed physicians may have unspecified characteristics that make them more valuable in the market-place; the return from working 'odd' hours for an employer may be high. Still another possibility is that the physician receives additional compensation to cover the transaction costs involved in holding two or more jobs. The coefficients of *M*1, *M*2 and *M*3 are negative, as expected. That the parameter estimate corresponding to physicians who recently moved to the United States from abroad is more negative than the other migration variables is also plausible. The physician/population ratio (*PHYPOP*) is significant in the weekly, and nearly so in the hourly, equation. Restricted activity days (*RAD*) is significant in both.

Most of the insignificant coefficients correspond to the area variables. With the exception of *PHYPOP* and *RAD*, all perform poorly. The individual observations have been aggregated into states for the purpose of running state wage regressions to test whether the zero coefficients reflect the errors-in-variables bias, discussed above. As seen in Table 16.1, the *PHYPOP* and *RAD* coefficients are remarkably stable. All the others perform at least as poorly as in the micro-regressions. One should note that, although R^2 is higher, the parameter estimates are determined with far less precision than in the micro-regressions.[1]

(2) *Supply Equations*

Tables 16.2–16.4 present the results of the supply equations. Variants containing the predicted wage (identified by circumflexes over the wage variables) differ substantially from those that do not, probably reflecting multicollinearity to a considerable extent. The discussion of the supply equations is therefore limited to the wage and income variables and insignificant coefficients that probably do not reflect multicollinearity. Multicollinearity would have been far less severe if there were fewer variables common to both wage and supply equations. For example, it would have been more desirable to use experience for the wage and age for the supply equations if this were possible.

The wage coefficients of the weeks and hours equations suggest quite different responses for the two types of decisions. The supply curve for weeks bends backward far above the mean weekly wage. When the predicted weekly wage is used, the response is substantially higher than when the actual ratio of earnings to weeks worked in

---

[1] In the state runs, each state is weighted by the sample size.

TABLE 16.2
PHYSICIAN SUPPLY EQUATIONS
(standard errors in parentheses)

Weeks

Variant	SEX	A2	A3	A4	A5	FRN1	FRN2	RACEN	WCL1	WCL2	EARNSAL	Y	YS	C1
I	2·22* (0·76)	−0·062 (0·63)	−1·75† (0·74)	−1·53† (0·71)	−0·28 (0·74)	0·17 (0·50)	0·17 (0·48)	2·62* (0·98)	1·36* (0·42)	4·07* (0·57)	−5·51* (0·75)	−0·000066 (0·000030)	0·000014 (0·000039)	0·93* (0·35)
II	2·49* (0·76)	−0·011 (0·63)	−1·55† (0·74)	−1·43† (0·71)	−0·35 (0·74)	0·28 (0·50)	1·03† (0·48)	2·84* (0·97)	1·53* (0·43)	4·47* (0·57)	−3·75* (0·85)	−0·000066† (0·000030)	0·000003 (0·00003)	0·91* (0·34)
III	−0·78 (0·69)	1·32† (0·63)	1·78* (0·63)	1·64* (0·61)	2·02* (0·71)	−0·11 (0·51)	−1·16* (0·43)	−1·01 (0·89)	−0·65 (0·36)	0·58 (0·39)	0·50 (0·35)	−0·000070† (0·00003)	0·00000008 (0·00003)	0·71* (0·35)

Weeks (cont.)

Variant	SD·C1	C2	SD·C2	MARRD	WAGÊW	WAGÊH^2	YR	PHYPOP	CLM	CONSTANT	
I	−6·11* (1·70)	0·51 (0·30)	−4·64* (1·10)	−0·025 (0·46)	0·019 (0·002)	—	−0·000092 (0·00005)	−0·14† (0·06)	0·00011 (0·00006)	41·11 ‡	$R^2 = 0·12$, $\delta_u = 4·71$, $F = 10·54*$
II	−4·95* (1·72)	0·47 (0·30)	−4·75* (1·10)	0·028 (0·46)	0·029* (0·003)	−0·00001* (0·00000)	−0·000094 (0·00005)	0·12† (0·06)	0·00010 (0·00006)	39·56 ‡	$R^2 = 0·12$, $\delta_u = 4·68$, $F = 10·96*$
	SD·C1	C2	SD·C2	MARRD	WAGEW	WAGEW^2	YR	PHYPOP	CLM	CONSTANT	
III	−6·30* (0·35)	0·62 (0·31)	−4·34* (1·12)	−0·035 (0·47)	0·0024* (0·0009)	$-16 \cdot 10^{-6}$ $(0{\cdot}06 \cdot 10^{-6})$	0·00001 (0·00005)	−0·04 (0·05)	0·00001 (0·00006)	47·64 ‡	$R^2 = 0·08$, $\delta_u = 4·80$, $F = 6·94*$

* Significant at the 1 per cent level.
† Significant at the 5 per cent level.
‡ Computer program used does not give standard error of the constant term. Regression based on 1,800 observations.

Table 16.2—(continued)
PHYSICIAN SUPPLY EQUATIONS
(standard errors in parentheses)

Hours

Variant	SEX	A2	A3	A4	A5	FRN1	FRN2	RACEN	WCL1	WCL2	EARNSAL	Y	YS
I	−13·75* (1·44)	9·83* (1·27)	14·88* (1·30)	12·65* (1·27)	8·66* (1·44)	−1·03 (1·03)	−6·08* (0·89)	−10·82* (1·85)	−7·97* (0·74)	−13·79* (0·85)	13·47 (0·93)	0·000042 (0·00006)	−0·00011 (0·00007)
II	−12·03* (1·46)	9·57* (1·26)	14·03* (1·30)	11·87* (1·26)	7·75* (1·43)	−0·59 (1·02)	−4·87* (0·91)	−8·67* (1·87)	−6·91* (0·76)	−12·25* (0·89)	14·58* (0·95)	−0·000039 (0·00006)	−0·000094 (0·000065)
III	−6·74* (1·48)	9·99* (1·35)	9·71* (1·36)	7·55* (1·32)	5·27* (1·52)	0·72 (1·09)	−2·10† (0·93)	−3·65 (1·93)	−3·96* (0·76)	−0·0004 (0·0001)	2·16* (0·74)	0·00000 (0·00007)	−0·00016† (0·00007)

Hours (cont.)

Variant	C1	SD·C1	C2	SD·C2	MARRD	WAĜEH	WAĜEH²	YR	PHYPOP	CLM	CONSTANT	
I	−0·30 (0·71)	1·38 (3·52)	0·25 (0·62)	−0·95 (2·29)	−1·02 (0·96)	−2·38* (0·12)	—	0·00023† (0·00011)	−0·57* (0·11)	−0·00027 (0·00012)	70·49 —‡	$R^2 = 0.32$ $\delta_u = 9.72$ $F = 37.23*$
II	−0·20 (0·71)	1·50 (3·49)	0·10 (0·62)	−3·00 (2·27)	−1·04 (0·95)	−1·01* (0·27)	−0·74* (0·13)	0·00021 (0·00011)	−0·55* (0·11)	−0·00025† (0·00012)	65·38 —‡	$R^2 = 0.33$ $\delta_u = 9.63$ $F = 37.68*$
						WAGEH	WAGEH²					
III	0·50 (0·76)	−1·74 (3·75)	0·87 (0·67)	−6·88* (2·43)	−1·39 (1·02)	−0·31* (0·05)	−0·00089 (0·00054)	−0·00003 (0·00012)	−0·35* (0·11)	−0·00013 (0·00013)	57·32 —‡	$R^2 = 0.22$ $\delta_u = 10.37$ $F = 21.86$

* Significant at the 1 per cent level.
† Significant at the 5 per cent level.
‡ Computer program used does not give standard error of the constant term. Regressions based on 1,800 observations.

1959 is used. For hours, the supply curve appears to bend backward throughout. The negative coefficient of the squared hourly wage term implies that the supply response becomes even more negative as the hourly wage increases. As with weeks, the measured response is lower when the actual wage is used. These differences in responses for weeks and hours are not startling. The data given in the introduction suggest a larger percentage decrease in hours per week than in weeks per year during the 1960s, a period when physician compensation, irrespective of how it is computed, rose rapidly.

One reason for the positive response to the weekly wage may be that physicians expand effort in direct response to patient needs, especially in response to patients in emergency situations. Physicians living in areas where there are few or no other physicians may be reluctant to take long vacations. As Table 16.1 shows, where there are relatively few physicians, the weekly wage is higher. The predicted wage in the supply of physician weeks equation may be picking up a 'need' effect in addition to a positive wage-incentive effect. Even if this is the case, it is reassuring from the vantage point of policy that physicians work harder, at least in the weeks dimension, in response to demand pressures. The hourly wage does not reflect these patient pressures resulting from a low physician/population ratio as directly.

TABLE 16.3

WAGE AND INCOME COEFFICIENTS WITH
NON-EMPLOYMENT INCOME SQUARED
(standard errors in parentheses)

Weeks	Y	YS	Y^2	$WA\hat{G}EW$	$WA\hat{G}EW^2$
Variant I	-0.000144†	0.000014	$0.2.10^{-8}$	0.019^*	–
	(0.000058)	(0.00003)	$(0.2.10^{-8})$	(0.00002)	
Variant II	-0.000138†	-0.0000036	$0.3.10^{-8}$	0.029^*	-0.00001
	(0.000058)	(0.000032)	$(0.2.10^{-8})$	(0.003)	(0.00000)
Hours	Y	YS	Y^2	$WA\hat{G}EH$	$WA\hat{G}EH^2$
Variant I	-0.00010	-0.00011	$0.2.10^{-8}$	-2.38^*	–
	(0.00012)	(0.00006)	$(0.4.10^{-8})$	(0.12)	
Variant II	(0.00012)	(0.000094)	$0.1.10^{-8}$	-1.01^*	-0.074^*
	(0.00012)	(0.000065)	$(0.4.10^{-8})$	(0.27)	(0.103)

* Significant at the 1 per cent level.
† Significant at the 5 per cent level.

One could state with greater confidence that the hours supply curve is backward-bending if the non-employment income (Y) coefficient were strongly negative. However, it is not. From Table 16.2, it is apparent that a $10,000 increase in Y would reduce weeks by 0.66 per year and hours by around 0.4 per week. A Y^2 term has been added to some variants of both supply equations. Wage and income parameter estimates with Y^2 included are given in Table 16.3. Coefficients of both Y^2 terms are positive, but insignificant. Estimates of the Y parameter in both weeks and hours equations approximately double when the Y^2 term is included, but they are still small. Apparently, the income effect diminishes as non-employment income increases. With both wage and income parameters, one may calculate the pure substitution elasticity (ϵ^s), calculated according to a formula given as part of Table 16.4's heading. ϵ^s is calculated at the mean of observations. For weeks, the substitution estimates range from 0·19 to 0·24. For hours, the implied substitution elasticity is negative, a result contradictory to the underlying economic theory. As is evident from Table 16.4, a much larger income effect would be needed for ϵ^s to be positive.

TABLE 16.4

SUPPLY ELASTICITIES

Weeks

Table	Variant	$\dfrac{dWEEKS}{dWA\hat{G}EW}\cdot\dfrac{\overline{WA\hat{G}EW}}{\overline{WEEKS}}$	$-\overline{WA\hat{G}EW}\cdot\dfrac{\partial WEEKS}{\partial Y}$	$=\epsilon^s$
16.2	I	0·166	$-(-0\cdot029)$	$=0\cdot195$
16.3	II	0·178	$-(-0\cdot029)$	$=0\cdot207$
16.3	I	0·166	$-(-0\cdot058)$	$=0\cdot224$
16.3	II	0·178	$-(-0\cdot056)$	$=0\cdot234$

Hours

Table	Variant	$\dfrac{dHOURS}{dWA\hat{G}EH}\cdot\dfrac{\overline{WA\hat{G}EH}}{\overline{HOURS}}$	$-\overline{WA\hat{G}EH}\cdot\dfrac{\partial HOURS}{\partial Y}$	$=\epsilon^s$
16.2	I	$-0\cdot358$	$-(-000034)$	$=\epsilon^s<0$
16.2	II	$-0\cdot235$	$-(-0\cdot00031)$	$=\epsilon^s<0$
16·3	II	$-0\cdot358$	$-(-0\cdot00076)$	$=\epsilon^s<0$
16.3	II	$-0\cdot235$	$-(-0\cdot00074)$	$=\epsilon^s<0$

Numerous reasons for the negative ϵ^s exist; space does not permit one to explore them all here. The large percentage of physicians reporting a zero Y makes measurement error and resulting bias toward zero a definite possibility. Moreover, measured non-employment income may be dominated by its transitory component, which would give a bias in the same direction. Greenberg and Kosters (1970) indicate that several studies employing a similar methodology have found a small, negative or even positive non-employment coefficient and have therefore calculated negative ϵ^s's. The authors attribute the result to a positive bias in the non-employment income coefficient, reflecting an omitted variable, difference in preferences for asset accumulation. They control for differences in asset preferences by including a taste variable in the hours equation, the difference between a person's actual and his predicted assets. Assets are predicted on the basis of the person's age and wage. With the control variable included, the non-employment income coefficient is more negative, and a positive ϵ^s is computed. A weakness in the Greenberg–Kosters approach is that the control variable is an indirect measure of non-employment income; its coefficient in their hours equations is positive. It is, then, not appropriate to consider only the non-employment and not the control parameter estimate as a measure of the 'pure' income effect. A more direct taste measure is needed.

The wage-rate parameter estimates in the Tables 16.2 and 16.3 hours equation also appear too strongly negative. Though negative total wage effects have been found in studies of male labour supply, the wage parameter estimates in these tables are more negative.[1] Part

TABLE 16.5

PHYSICIAN SUPPLY: REDUCED-FORM PARAMETERS

Variable	Weeks	Hours
SEX	−4·61	−0·69
A2	6·38	1·95
A3	6·26	1·83
A4	4·68	1·64
A5	3·26	1·89
FRN1	−0·53	0·019
FRN2	−2·03	−0·61
RACEN	−1·78	−1·03
WCL1	−3·90	−0·25
WCL2	−8·04	1·01
EARNSAL	−0·31	0·39
Y	−0·000042	−0·000066
YS	−0·00011	0·00014
C1	−0·30	0·93
SD·C1	1·38	−6·11
C2	0·25	0·51
SD·C2	−1·95	−4·64
MARRD	−1·02	−0·025
YR	0·00023	−0·00009
PHYPOP	−0·213	−0·073
CLM	−0·00027	0·00011
PT	−19·80	−0·31
M1	4·83	−2·13
M2	−4·09	−1·74
M3	6·66	−3·00
MEDY	−0·0013	0·00032
AGLT5	0·26	−0·17
AGT65	0·10	0·088
SURINPOP	0·018	−0·014
MEDINPOP	−0·038	0·013
RAD	−1·24	0·42
CONSTANT	72.42	50·38

[1] See, for example, Kosters (1966), Greenberg and Kosters (1970) and Rea (1971).

of the explanation may be that the wage parameter estimate picks up time spent investing in human capital on the part of physicians in an early stage of their careers, a period when wages are low. The reduced-form parameter estimates for hours in Table 16.5, showing *A*2 physicians with the longest work-week, support this view. According to the best available evidence, the negative coefficient on the wage variable does not reflect the identification problem discussed in section II. The small impact of hours on wages, calculated from Reinhardt's results, implies an even more negative wage coefficient.

The parameter estimate for spouse earnings (*YS*) is positive in the weeks and negative in the hours equation. Although its *t*-value is very low, the positive sign in the former probably arises because vacations are more difficult to schedule when both husband and wife are employed. The parameter estimate of *YS* in the hours equation implies that a $10,000 increase in spouse income would result in around a one-hour reduction in hours worked. Only a very small percentage of spouses (less than 2 per cent) earned as much as $10,000 in 1959.[1]

All variables to the right of *YS* in Table 16.2, with the exception of the wage variables and *PHYPOP*, do not appear in the wage equation and, thus, should not be as subject to multicollinearity arising from the instrumental variables method. The *C*1 and *C*2 variables have an effect on weeks but not on hours. *SD·C*1 and *SD·C*2 are significant in the weeks but not in the hours equation. *SEX* is highly collinear with the *SD* variables. Sums of *SEX* and *SD·C*1 and *SEX* and *SD·C*2 coefficients, however, are negative and significantly different from zero at the 5 and 10 per cent levels, respectively, in the weeks equation. In the hours, both sums are also negative and significant at the 1 per cent level. The married dummy (*MARRD*) does not enter significantly into either equation. *YR*, reference income, enters negatively in the weeks but positively in the hours equation. The expected sign was positive. Degree days enters positively in weeks and negatively in hours. A positive sign had been anticipated.

(3) *Reduced-Form Parameters*

Considering the wage equations used to obtain predicted wages for the supply equations as structural equations, reduced-form equations for weeks and hours have been calculated. Reduced-form parameters, shown in Table 16.5, are based on Variants I of weeks and hours equations from Table 16.2. The impact of *SEX* is negative on both

---

[1] Previous research on general labor supply relationships shows the cross-substitution effect of the wife's wage on husband labor force participation to be positive and the husband's wage to have a negative impact on wife labor force participation. See Ashenfelter and Heckman (1971) and Cain (1966).

weeks and hours. This variable should be viewed in conjunction with $SD \cdot C1$ and $SD \cdot C2$, which measure the effects of physician mothers with children. With the exception of $SD \cdot C1$ in the hours equation, all these parameter estimates are negative. As indicated above, there are very few physician mothers with children under age two in the sample. The $SD \cdot C$ coefficients may in fact understate the negative sex effect, since physicians who reported no weeks worked during 1959 and/or hours in the March 1960 reference week have been excluded from the sample; some of these non-labor-force participants are likely to be women with small children. In sum, the evidence indicates less market work for the female physician.

With the exception of the $A5$ parameter estimate for weeks, the A parameters reveal monotonically decreasing participation in market work. Withdrawal from market work after age 64 is rather substantial. A geographical area served by a large proportion of older physicians will have a substantially lower effective supply than one that does not, holding other factors constant.

The $FRN1$, $FRN2$ and $RACEN$ coefficients are negative, with one exception. Given its low significance in all the structural equations, $FRN1$ should be considered to have no impact on supply. Both $FRN2$ and $RACEN$ are associated with less work, but the effects shown in Table 16.5 are not very large. On weeks, the $WCL1$ and $WCL2$ parameter estimates vary in sign. On hours, the two are substantially negative, reaffirming evidence from other sources that employed physicians have shorter work-weeks. The $EARNSAL$ coefficient, positive in the weeks and negative in the hours equation, is small in both cases. Reduced-form parameter estimates of the Y through YR variables and of the CLM variable are identical to the structural estimates. The impact of part-time (PT), not surprisingly, is negative. The migration variables have a negative impact on weeks and a positive impact on hours. These results reinforce the interpretation that human capital accumulation, as reflected in hours worked per week, is important in the initial stages of practice formation. Also, the results lend support to the interpretation that patient load pressures are partly responsible for the positive effect of the weekly wage on weeks worked. The physician with less to do takes longer vacations.

Among the area variables, the most interesting is the physician/population ratio ($PHYPOP$). $PHYPOP$ exerts a negative impact on both weeks and hours. According to the Table 16.5 estimates, an increase in $PHYPOP$ by 5 physicians to 10,000 population would reduce mean weeks worked by 0·35 qnd mean hours per week by one. Since increasing the number of physicians in the community reduces the level of effort of the individual physician, increasing the number of physicians in the area will not augment the effective supply of physician services proportionately to the increase in the physician stock.

(4) *Total Effect of a Change in the Hourly Wage on Effective Supply*

Since the weekly and hourly wages have positive and negative impacts on effective physician supply, it is of some interest to know the extent to which the positive weeks effect offsets the negative hours effect when the hourly wage rises. For self-employed male physicians between the ages of 30 and 64, an increase in the hourly wage from $8·58, the mean for this group, to $9·58 would reduce hours worked per year by 48·6, or less than the equivalent of a work-week. Thus, the net withdrawal, even if the above wage parameter estimates are accepted as valid, is not substantial.

V. CONCLUSIONS, POLICY IMPLICATIONS AND FUTURE RESEARCH DIRECTIONS

Even though the preceding results do not suggest it (probably because the insurance measures are crude), more widespread health insurance coverage in the United States has probably increased physicians' earnings. The above estimates indicate, however, that the pure income effect on physician supply is small. Further research, in particular to determine the extent of measurement errors, should be conducted. Other research by the author, on physicians in residency programs, indicates that the income effect on hours spent moonlighting is somewhat higher than the income effect represented by the coefficients of non-employment income in this study.[1] But the residents' non-employment coefficient is also small, about the same as the effect of spouse earnings on physician hours. Since the income measure in the resident study includes spouse earnings, it is perhaps more comparable to the spouse earnings than to the non-employment income coefficient. Analysis of nurse hours of work with the 1960 Census Public Use Sample, using the same definition of non-employment income, shows a substantially higher income effect, especially for single nurses.[2] The higher coefficient for nurses suggests that non-employment income is not generally poorly measured by the Census Bureau in general, but rather that more errors appear in this income component of the self-employed.

Through price control and reimbursement policies associated with government health insurance, the United States government is increasingly a setter of medical care prices. To the extent that prices are reflected in wages, it would appear that low prices would increase

[1] Sloan (forthcoming).   [2] Sloan and Blair (1972).

the effective supply of the existing stock of physicians, which is also a conclusion of the Feldstein (1970) physician supply study.[1] The estimate of the income effect, however, is inconsistent with a backward-bending supply curve and the total wage effect, especially when weeks as well as hours are taken into account, is small.

The output of medical schools has grown in recent years. This trend affects the age distribution of physicians as well as the aggregate physician/population ratio. This study indicates that young physicians work longer, but that the physician/population ratio exerts a negative impact on supply. Future research should investigate the components of physician hours of work to ascertain whether the distribution of hours of work by age is reflected in patient care or primarily in differences in time devoted to human capital investments.

No single data base is completely adequate. Unfortunately, such variables as physician health status, which according to research by Luft (1972) is an important determinant of male work patterns in general, are not available for 1960. Information on disability is available in the Public Use Sample for 1970. A future study based on 1970 data will include this variable.

REFERENCES

Ashenfelter, O., and Heckman, J. (1971), 'The Estimation of Income and Substitution Effects in a Model of Family Labor Supply', paper presented at the Winter Meeting of the Econometric Society (Dec 1971).
Brown, D. M., and Lapan, H. E. (1972), 'The Rising Price of Physicians' Services: A Comment', *Review of Economics and Statistics*, LIV, 1, pp. 101–5.
Brown, M. G. (mimeo), 'Experience and Earnings of Male Physicians: Some Empirical Findings'.
Cain, G. C. (1966), *Married Women in the Labor Force* (Univ. of Chicago Press).
Carnegie Commission on Higher Education (1970), *Higher Education and the Nation's Health: Policies for Medical and Dental Education* (New York: McGraw-Hill).
Center for Health Services Research and Development, American Medical Association (1971), *Reference Data on the Profile of Medical Practice* (Chicago: American Medical Association).
—— (1972), *Reference Data on the Profile of Medical Practice* (Chicago: American Medical Association).
Feldstein, M. S. (1970), 'The Rising Price of Physicians' Services', *Review of Economics and Statistics*, LIV, 1, pp. 105–7.
—— (1972), 'The Rising Price of Physicians' Services: A Reply', *Review of Economics and Statistics*, LIV, 1, pp. 105–7.
Greenberg, D. H., and Kosters, M. (1970), *Income Guarantees and the Working Poor: The Effect of Income Maintenance Programs on the Hours of Work of*

---

[1] See also a critique of the Feldstein study, Brown and Lapan (1972), and Feldstein's rejoinder (1972). Feldstein does not measure the impact of non-employment income on supply.

Male Family Heads (Santa Monica, Calif.: RAND Corporation) (R–579–OEO).

Horowitz, I. (1970), *Decision-Making and the Theory of the Firm* (New York: Holt, Rinehart & Winston).

Kosters, M. (1966), *Income and Substitution Effects in a Family Labor Supply Model* (Santa Monica, Calif.: RAND Corporation) (P–3339).

Kraft, A. (1970), 'The Labor Supply of Nonwhite Married Women', unpublished Ph.D. dissertation (State Univ. of New York at Buffalo).

Leuthold, J. (1968), 'An Empirical Study of Formula Income Transfers and the Work Decision of the Poor', *Journal of Human Resources*, III, 3, pp. 312–23.

Luft, H. S. (1972), 'Components of the Impact of Disability on Earnings', paper presented at the Health Economics Research Organization Session, Toronto (Dec 1972).

Maurizi, A. (1969), *Economic Essays on the Dental Profession* (Iowa City: College of Business Administration, Univ. of Iowa).

National Advisory Commission on Health Manpower (1967), *Report*, vol. I (Washington, D.C.: U.S. Government Printing Office).

Peterson, O., Andrews, L.P., Spain, R. S., and Greenberg, B. G. (1956), *An Analytical Study of North Carolina General Practice, 1953–1954* (Evanston, Ill.: Association of American Medical Colleges).

Rea, S. A., (1971), 'The Supply of Labor and Incentive Effects of Income Maintenance Programs', unpublished Ph.D. dissertation (Harvard Univ.).

Reinhardt, U. E. (1970), 'An Economic Analysis of Physicians' Practices', unpublished Ph.D. dissertation (Yale Univ.).

—— (1972), 'A Production Function for Physician Services', *Review of Economics and Statistics*, LIV, 1, pp. 55–66.

Scitovsky, T. (1943), 'A Note on Profit Maximization and its Implications', *Review of Economic Studies*, XI, 1, pp. 57–60.

Sloan, F. A. (forthcoming), *Supply Responses of Young Physicians: An Analysis of Physicians in Residency Programs* (Santa Monica, Calif.: RAND Corporation) (R–1131–OEO).

—— and Blair, R. D. (1972), 'The Impact of Wage Incentives on the Effective Supply of Nurses', paper presented at the Health Economics Research Organization Session, Toronto (Dec 1972).

Theodore, C. N., and Sutter, G. (1967), 'A Report on the First Periodic Survey of Physicians', *Journal of the American Medical Association*, CCII (Nov) 516–24.

Yett, D. E., Drabek, L., Kimbell, L., and Intriligator, M. (1970), *The Development of a Micro-Simulation Model of Health Manpower Demand and Supply*, vol. I (Washington, D.C.: Bureau of Health Manpower Education, National Institutes of Health–U.S. Government Printing Office).

17 Modeling the Delivery of Medical Services

Judith Lave, Lester Lave and Samuel Leinhardt

CARNEGIE-MELLON UNIVERSITY, PITTSBURG

A three-type model of health care delivery is constructed, in which individuals seek care at a primary care station and may be referred to a clinic or a hospital. The probability of seeking care depends on symptom level. (The demands for medical care depends on cost, ease of access, perception of the efficacy of care, and symptom level; the first three are represented by shifts in the probability of seeking care in the model.) Each provider has efficacy and referral matrices; individuals decide whether to pursue care. The model is simulated to investigate the cost–health status trade-offs. The outcome measure is used to investigate the efficacy of social policies, such as increasing access to the system. The cost–health status frontier is insensitive to a wide range of schemes for weighting symptom levels. The underlying health status of the population is much more important than the quality of medical care in determining the health status.

I. INTRODUCTION

Medical care delivery in the United States is fraught with severe problems. While there is disagreement about the exact nature and extent of these problems, there is general agreement that the high cost of care and its inconsistent availability contribute to adverse health levels. To remedy this situation, the government has initiated several programs which intervene in the market for medical resources. However, because those programs have had unforeseen systemic effects, they have often exacerbated, rather than relieved, the difficulties.

While conscious of the dangers of analyzing whole systems (especially when there are data and conceptual problems), we attempt to develop an analytical model of health care delivery. Our objective is to construct a model general enough to encompass an entire local delivery system and specific enough to permit assessing the consequences of changes in the system. We consider both inputs and outcomes, judging each experiment in a series of simulations in terms of total cost, physician time consumed and alterations in the health status of the serviced population.

We begin by focussing on the factors which influence the demand for medical services and the characteristics of the supply of these services (particularly ambulatory care). These demand and supply considerations provide the foundation for an idealized system for delivery of medical services. We identify three functional units represented in the model by primary care stations, clinics and hospitals. We propose a series of outcome measures which reflect the health status of the population. The model is sufficiently complicated that its implications cannot be derived analytically. We present a simulation of the model to explore its properties. Finally, we summarize the results of the simulation and consider future directions for this research.

II. THE DEMAND FOR MEDICAL CARE

The basic assumption behind our analysis is that individuals make their own decisions as to whether, when and where to seek medical care. This is not to deny the influence of medical personnel and laymen; it simply states that it is the individual who decides to seek or defer care. Government policy can affect these decisions only by manipulating some of the variables which influence demand.[1]

Demand for medical services is a function of three interrelated variables, as shown in equation (1):

$$M = M(HS, A, P) \tag{1}$$

where M is the quantity of medical services demanded, HS is the individual's underlying health status or objective need for medical care, A is the individual's perception of the need for and the efficacy of medical care and P is the price of medical care to the consumer. The price consists not only of the payment to the provider, but also of access costs, time costs of treatment, as well as psychological cost.[2] We assume that the higher the price, the less care will be demanded and the longer people will delay seeking care. When we discuss the medical care delivery system, we shall explore the implications of reducing access constraints and, thereby, the likelihood of increasing the demands on the system.

---

[1] An obvious exception would be mandatory smallpox vaccinations. Arrow [1] gives a good discussion of some economic reasons for government intervention into the medical care market.

[2] For a full discussion of these variables, see J. Lave and Leinhardt [11].

III. THE SUPPLY OF MEDICAL SERVICES

Medical care can be provided on either an inpatient or ambulatory basis. Many medical problems can be treated in either setting. The major difference between the two is that inpatient care is more expensive in the sense that the cost of identical treatment will be much greater.

Let us briefly review the current research that is relevant to modeling medical care delivery systems. Researchers have considered the question of economies of scale in different types of ambulatory care facilities,[1] have experimented with a classification scheme for ambulatory medical patients with respect to the skill required for treatment and the emergency nature of the case,[2] and have undertaken task analyses of different medical specialties.[3] While definitive results have not yet been obtained, the following observations seem reasonable:

1. The major proportion of patient visits does not require specialized resources. This finding suggests that a primary care component, staffed and equipped at an elementary level, may improve efficiency without compromising effectiveness.
2. There is no consistent evidence that economies of scale exist in the production of ambulatory medical services. In fact, there is some evidence that inefficiency increases with size.
3. The cost per case in a particular ambulatory setting is a function of the average complexity of cases treated, the stand-by capabilities of the setting and the level of inefficiency. While this hypothesis has not been tested for ambulatory care, it has been validated for inpatient hospital care.[4] This suggests that medical care delivery might be improved by stratifying facilities and equipping primary care stations to service medical problems specific to the local population.

IV. THE CONCEPT OF HEALTH STATUS

The health status of a population is a crucial factor affecting its demand for medical care. If all access costs are held constant, the

[1] Joseph Newhouse and colleagues at the RAND Corporation, Richard Bailey at Berkeley and Melvin Reder at Stanford have been studying this problem.

[2] Professor Gavett and his colleagues at the University of Rochester School of Management have been working on this problem.

[3] Most of the work appeared in *Pediatrics*. The study by Yankauer *et al.* [18] will probably be a classic.

[4] See Lave, Lave and Silverman [10].

demand for medical care should be directly related to the incidence
of disease.

One might characterize the health status of a population in a
number of ways, each emphasizing a different viewpoint.[1] A
physician might characterize health status in terms of morbidity
and mortality. Thus, one might determine the mortality rate and
the prevalence of certain diseases. The emphasis here would be on
the objective incidence of pathology. Another approach, such as that
typified in the United States National Health Survey, would be to
characterize the disability levels of the population. A third approach,
somewhat similar to the second, would characterize health status
by the distribution of the severity of symptoms in individuals when

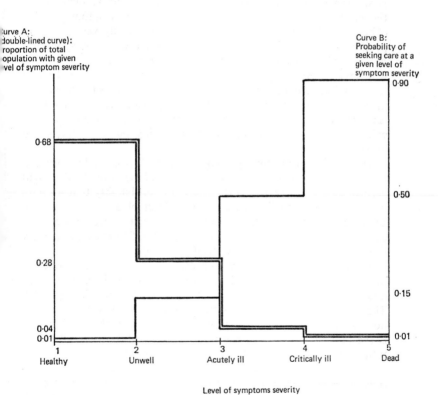

FIG. 17.1   Graphs of the health status and illness behavior for a hypothetical population

[1] For a recent review of the literature on health status, see Hennes [6].

they were surveyed or when they presented themselves for treatment. All three approaches are related and there is a (not necessarily unique) translation among them. We are interested in the process through which an individual decides to seek medical care; thus, the severity of symptoms is likely to be the most relevant health status indicator for our purposes.[1]

We assume that each individual has a level of symptom severity. Using a scale from 1 (no symptoms) to 5 (death), the proportion of the population in each severity level could be tabulated and the information represented in a graph, such as that in Fig. 17.1 (curve A). The horizontal axis describes the level of severity of the symptoms (where 2 might be a mild headache or stomach upset and 4 hemmorrhaging from a principal artery); the left vertical axis is the proportion of the population with a given symptom severity. (The curve demonstrates our belief – an empirically verifiable proposition – that a high proportion will either have no symptoms or very mild ones and that a small proportion of the population will have severe symptoms.) The curve shows that 68 per cent of the population is healthy, 28 per cent unwell, 3·6 per cent acutely ill, 0·4 per cent critically ill, and that the mortality rate is 1·4 per cent. (In any population, the proportions in each symptom class will depend upon a host of factors, including pollution levels and nutrition.[2])

The more severe the symptoms, other factors held constant, the more likely it is that medical care will be sought. The right vertical axis of curve B in Fig. 17.1 is the probability that an individual will seek medical care, given a level of symptom severity. Thus, the curve shows that 1 per cent of healthy people seek care each week, as do 15 per cent of unwell people, 50 per cent of acutely ill people and 90 per cent of critically ill people.

These two distributions can be used to forecast the number of patients in each symptom class who will visit a clinic, physician's office or other institution for primary care, as shown in Fig. 17.2. The distribution of patients is the product of curves A and B. The horizontal axis of Fig. 17.2 is symptom severity, the vertical axis is the number of visits to a primary care institution (or any institution servicing the population) per 1,000 people per week. Individuals with symptom severity (unwell) make the greatest percentage of visits (42·0 per cent). Relatively few people who present themselves have no symptoms (6·8 per cent) or are critically ill (3·6 per cent). Minor symptoms alone, though frequent, are not

---

[1] See Wyler *et al.* [16, 17].

[2] See, for example, Stewart [15], Auster *et al.* [2] and L. Lave and Seskin [12].

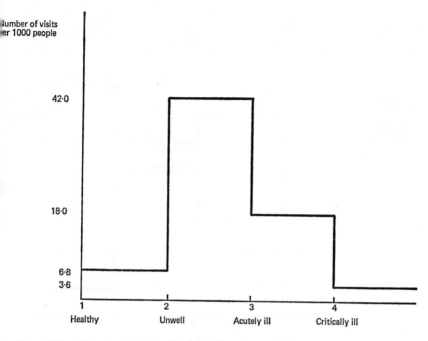

FIG. 17.2 Hypothetical distribution of patient visits at a primary care institution, given cost of obtaining medical care

strongly motivating, and critical symptoms, though strongly motivating, are rare.[1]

Successful medical treatment requires a compliant patient. It is not possible to treat all individuals needing care, but only those seeking care. Steps can be taken to induce more people to seek care so that more people who genuinely need care seek it, but this usually means that many who do not need care will also seek it. The number of individuals seeking care can be increased by manipulating demand variables such as the price of care, the availability of information about care or symptoms, the proximity of care, or attitudes towards the institutions providing care. A decrease in the cost of care will

---

[1] This conclusion is in accord with available evidence on physician visits. For example, Silver [14] estimates that about 71 per cent of pediatric visits could be managed by a trained pediatric nurse practitioner and about 80 per cent by a child health associate. (This equates symptom severity with case complexity.) In a study of H.I.P. patient visits, 36 per cent of physician visits were for acute upper respiratory infection, influenza–grippe and acute bronchitis (Denson [4]).

increase the overall level of demand (i.e. many more patients with all levels of symptom severity will seek care) and will change the symptom distribution of patients presenting themselves for treatment, as shown in Fig. 17.3. Since we expect that the role of factors

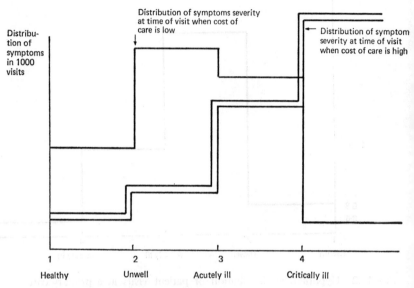

FIG. 17.3 Hypothetical distribution of symptom severity at time of patient visits for different costs of obtaining care

other than symptom severity becomes greater with decreasing symptom severity, we argue that a reduction in cost will have little effect on the behavior of individuals with critically severe symptoms, but will have a significant effect on those people with less severe symptoms.[1]

One measure of the health status of a population is its distribution across the five symptom levels.[2] A survey could be used to estimate this distribution. A more direct method would be to examine the distribution of symptoms appearing in a primary care center. If most patients are in health status 1 or 2 (and the mortality

[1] To give an extreme example, if a town's sole doctor moves away, then people will more likely wait until they are 'really sick' before visiting the doctor in the next town.

[2] A survey could observe (a) the incidence of patient-perceived symptom levels, (b) physician-perceived morbidity levels, and (c) the relationship between (a) and (b). While we focus on measure (a), we sometimes conceive of it as the direct measure of patient perception and sometimes as an indirect measure of physician-perceived morbidity.

rate is low) this implies that access costs are small. If most patients are in health status 3 or 4, the access constraints are severe.

V. A MODEL OF HEALTH CARE DELIVERY

We proceed to sketch a model which embodies the ideas we have been discussing and which isolates the essential parts of a delivery system. In this idealized system, medical care is provided in one of three settings: ambulatory care via a primary care station (P.C.S.), or a clinic (C), or inpatient care via a hospital (H). The primary care station acts as a screen (since patients use it as a referral point) for the other components of the system and provides the primary care that makes up the bulk of personal health services. The P.C.S. has a small and unspecialized staff and a local orientation. It is a traditional physician's office, or a radical store-front, or part of the service of an elaborate clinic. Depending on the population served, it could be staffed by a physician (full or part time), a medical team, a specially trained nurse or a physician's assistant. It is an extension of the clinic and hospital into the community. All three are assumed to be coordinated so as to exploit their relative advantages.

Except for minor changes, the primary care stations, the clinics and hospitals constituting this system are traditional ones, serving the roles they were originally designed to serve, but from which they currently have deviated. For example, in the clinic, only referred patients requiring some special medical skills or equipment are treated; in the hospital, only patients requiring treatment as inpatients are serviced. These institutions need not be spatially separate; the clinic could be within the hospital (as an outpatient department) and could contain one primary care station. It is evident that more primary care stations are needed than referral institutions (clinics and hospitals).

Since the primary care stations offer only elementary medical care and need only limited quarters, the cost of a primary care visit should be less than the cost of a clinic visit. Clearly, a visit to the clinic should cost less than an inpatient day in the hospital.[1] Current estimates would put the cost of a primary care visit at $10, the cost of a clinic visit at $40 and the cost of a hospital stay at $800.

To summarize, the model characterizes health in terms of the

---

[1] For simplicity, we assume that each of the institutions is used to capacity and so the cost of seeing an extra patient equals the average cost per patient. Note that many current clinics and hospitals have so much excess capacity that the cost of treating an extra patient is a small proportion of the average cost per patient.

distribution of symptoms in the population. Medical care is delivered in a primary care station, clinic or hospital. The individual is assumed to make the decision to seek care, depending on his current symptoms; the worse his symptoms, the higher the probability that he will seek care.

A complete model of health care is specified with the addition of a few more concepts. The first is the underlying health status of the population. How rapidly do individuals become better or worse in the absence of medical care? We assume that this function can be represented by a set of probabilities giving the chance that, for example, an individual in health status 3 will get better (go to health status 1 or 2), stay the same, or get worse (go to health status 4 or 5). The second concept is that of the efficacy of the medical care system. This efficacy might be thought of in terms of the probability of improving the health status of a patient, as well as the probability of having to refer a patient to another component for treatment. The final concept is that of the willingness of the patient to comply with a referral (as a surrogate for complying with the treatment regime). We assume that this will depend on the individual's symptoms and the component to which he is referred.

In this model, demand is embodied in the probability of seeking care vector and the compliance matrices. Demand was written as a complicated function of three factors in equation (1). In our model, most of these factors are held constant and, therefore, the function reduces to a single variable, the symptom level of the individual. Thus, the *PSC* and *COMP* are functions only of a symptom level (and place referred). However, the stochastic nature of the formulation implies that other (unmeasured) factors influence demand.

We believe that the essential aspects of any medical care delivery system are present in this model. The differences between existing systems might be represented as differences in staffing (for example, a physician's office versus an emergency room as the primary care station) or in the ambulatory care sector (for example, a two-tier system when the primary care station and clinic are merged, versus a three-tier system when they are separate). There is much to be gained, conceptually, from specifying this model in detail and attempting to determine the probabilities, patient flows and resources required. In addition, the model can be used to contrast the health status distribution, cost and resource requirements of proposed systems for delivering care. If the model is completely specified (assumptions regarding underlying health status, probabilities of seeking care, staffing and efficacy of the three kinds of medical care delivery institutions, number of delivery institutions and compliance probabilities), the implied health status distribution, cost and resource requirements for any health care system can be calculated.

This model was programmed in SIMULA for the Univac 1108 and a simulation run.

VI. THE BASIC CASE OF THE SIMULATION MODEL

The matrices for the basic case are shown in Appendix A. Their interpretation and the functional interrelationships in the model are illustrated by tracing the flow of an individual through the system. The hypothetical population consists of 1,000 people, whose initial health status is described by the 'starting health status of the population'.[1] (Note that the solution to the model is independent of the starting health status, and, therefore, this distribution is arbitrary.[2]) An individual's decision to seek care is described by the 'probability of seeking care' (or *PSC*) vector. Thus, one healthy person in 100 seeks care during a week (or 48 of 100 seek care during a year), 15 unwell people in 100 seek care, etc. The number of people who actually seek care during a week is the product of the starting health status and *PSC* vectors (thus, $682 \times 0 \cdot 01 = 6 \cdot 82$ healthy people seek care during the first week). These figures are illustrated in Figs. 17.1 and 17.2.

Those people who do not seek care are subjected to the underlying factors affecting health, as characterized by the *NATURALEV* matrix. According to this matrix, in the absence of receiving any medical care, someone who is healthy this week has a $0 \cdot 90979$ chance of being healthy next week, a $0 \cdot 08$ chance of being unwell, a $0 \cdot 01$ chance of being acutely ill, a $0 \cdot 0002$ chance of being critically ill and a $0 \cdot 00001$ chance of dying. Similarly, a person in any one of the other health states has the specified probabilities of getting better, remaining the same or getting worse. (Note that deceased individuals remain deceased with probability 1.)

The people who do seek care are treated at the primary care station (P.C.S.). From there they may be discharged, asked to return, or referred to the clinic (C) or hospital (H), depending on their initial symptom level (as shown in the *TRP* matrix). For example, 97 per cent of initially healthy patients are discharged, as are $0 \cdot 90$ per cent of initially unwell patients, $0 \cdot 50$ per cent of initially acutely ill patients and $0 \cdot 20$ per cent of initially critically ill patients.

Depending on the initial health status and the place to which the patient is referred, four matrices describe the health status of the patient after this phase of treatment: *TRPD* for discharge, *TRPP*

---

[1] To simplify computation, whenever someone dies, someone is assumed to be born in the hospital with symptom level 'unwell'.

[2] The current structure does not ascribe any value to preventive care, since healthy patients cannot be improved, and since the probabilities of changing symptom level do not show any benefit from preventive visits. We plan to modify the model to reflect preventive care by having patients who have sought care have a higher probability of remaining in their discharge symptom classification.

for referral to the P.C.S., *TRPC* for referral to the C, and *TRPH* for referral to the H. Thus, 95 per cent of the patients who were healthy when they went to the P.C.S. and who were discharged are now healthy, while 5 per cent of them have become unwell.

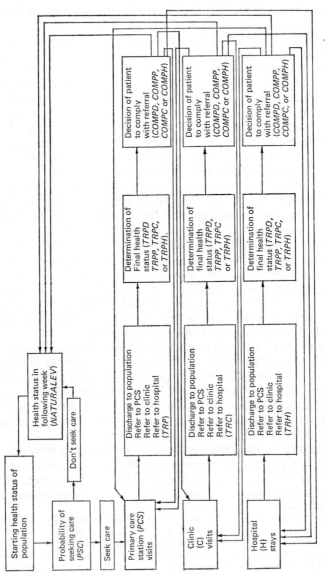

Fig. 17.4 Flow diagram of simulation model

Having received care and been referred to the community, P.C.S., C or H, the individual must decide whether to comply. The *COMPD*, *COMPP*, *COMPC* and *COMPH* matrices describe the compliance behavior of patients depending on health status and place of referral. Thus, someone who is discharged with symptom level 'healthy' leaves the system with probability 0·97 and chooses to seek care at another primary station with probability 0·03, i.e. 3 per cent are non-compliant.

The model can also be illustrated by the flow chart shown in Fig. 17.4. Given an initial health status, the probability of seeking care is used to determine whether a visit is made to the primary care station (if not, the individual's health status for the following week is determined by the *NATURALEV* matrix). From the P.C.S. he is referred to the population (discharged), to the P.C.S., to the clinic or to the hospital (as determined by the *TRP*). The final health status is determined by the initial health status and the place of referral (*COMPD*, *COMPP*, *COMPC* or *COMPH*). If one or more weeks intervene between discharge and the next appointment, the *NATURALEV* probabilities modify the individual's health status. The pattern of referrals from the clinic and hospital are the same, although referral probabilities differ (*TRC* and *TRH*, respectively).

VII. OUTCOMES IN THE MODEL

The health status distribution of the population in each period is one measure of 'outcomes' in the model. Others are the associated cost, number of physician hours required and hospital costs as a proportion of total costs. The physician indices are calculated on the basis of $10 and $\frac{1}{4}$ hour of M.D. time per P.C.S. visit, $40 and $\frac{3}{4}$ hour of M.D. time per clinic visit, and $800 and 12 hours of M.D. time per hospital stay.

Since it is clumsy and somewhat confusing to work with five indices of health status (the proportion of the population which is healthy, unwell, acutely ill, critically ill, and the mortality rate), we used a set of weights to transform the health status vector into a scalar. The first weighting scheme assigns a zero to health state 1 (healthy) and a one to the other health states (0,1,1,1,1). The second, third and fourth give progressively larger weights to the worse health states: (1,2,3,4,5), (1,2,4,8,16), (1,10,100,1,000,10,000). The fifth assigns a positive weight only to the mortality rate (0,0,0,0,1). For each index, the lower the index, the better the general health status of the population.

The five sets of weights differ in the relative weights they give to each health state. For example, scheme 1, which considers only people in the health category, exemplifies the goal of 'complete mental, physical and social well-being'. The second through fourth indicate that death is worse than critical illness, which is worse than acute illness, which is worse than being unwell, which is worse than being healthy. Finally, scheme 5 considers only the mortality rate. These five schemes cover the most commonly discussed goals for a health care system.

VIII. SIMULATIONS RUN

The model relates the health of a population to the cost of achieving it, given certain system parameters. Here we consider the effects which changes in these parameters have on output of the system. We motivate our discussion by showing how the parameter changes can be related to real-world policy measures.

The first set of parameter changes investigated were the probability of seeking care. Demand would increase with an increase in health insurance coverage, an improvement in the transportation system, a decrease in the monetary cost of seeking care, an increase in the perceived efficacy of medical care and an increase in the warmth and general attitudes of the providers of medical care. The first set of simulations to study the effect of changes in the health care system focused on changing the components of the *PSC* matrix.

The second set were the efficacy with which the medical care is rendered. Improved medical knowledge, better-trained personnel and improved specialization should increase the quality of medical care (increase the probability of a successful encounter) and change the *TRP* matrix.

The third were changes in compliance behavior. The introduction of health care expediters, educational programs and provision of transportation to health care facilities are examples of factors that can generate improvements in compliance.

The fourth were changes in the underlying health status of the population. Changes in the occupation mix, personal habits, air pollution levels and life-style, for example, will affect the general level of health, the *NATURALEV* matrix. In Appendix B we summarize the characteristics of the situation.

IX. RESULTS

In Table 12.1 we present the various output measures for 27 simulations. The distribution of the population across the four health states is given in columns (1)–(4); the monthly mortality rate is in column (5). The next three columns present the numbers of visits

TABLE 17.1

Case No.	Health study distribution					Visit distribution			Costs			Health status index			
	(1) Healthy	(2) Unwell	(3) Acutely ill	(4) Critical	(5) Deceased (health index E)	P.C.S.	Clinic	Hospital	Total cost	M.D. time	% hospital cost/total cost	A	B	C	D
1	680·9	279·6	35·9	2·8	1·2	311·9	13·0	5·6	8,119·99	180·93	55·172	319·59	1,365·24	1,425·82	22,092·74
2	558·4	397·5	40·4	3·2	1·4	120·2	8·2	4·7	5,265·00	102·25	70·909	442·46	1,494·20	1,562·34	25,381·53
3	629·1	327·8	38·9	3·3	1·2	228·1	10·5	5·6	7,208·66	151·52	62·517	371·32	1,421·12	1,487·13	23,633·78
4	745·7	217·8	33·1	2·8	1·0	436·4	13·4	6·2	9,833·66	229·53	50·168	254·76	1,297·04	1,352·68	19,314·79
5	794·4	172·3	30·0	2·9	0·9	564·8	15·8	6·3	11,320·99	275·73	44·519	206·06	1,244·98	1,206·32	17,302·98
6	785·6	179·0	32·1	2·9	1·0	764·3	16·7	8·0	14,684·32	362·98	43·402	214·90	1,256·20	1,310·73	18,648·59
7	567·6	402·6	26·7	2·7	1·0	133·9	10·0	4·7	5,525·33	108·92	68·533	432·97	1,468·49	1,516·55	19,652·80
8	664·2	274·7	53·2	7·5	1·7	290·8	11·8	5·6	7,858·66	172·96	57·007	336·93	1,411·13	1,512·37	32,827·55
9	682·2	279·2	35·5	2·6	1·0	301·9	11·1	4·9	7,356·66	167·37	52·923	318·17	1,362·09	1,418·52	19,309·44
10	685·0	275·4	35·6	3·5	1·1	332·8	14·0	6·1	8,793·00	195·00	55·802	315·58	1,361·95	1,423·33	21,299·31
11	676·4	281·4	38·4	3·1	1·5	347·5	39·5	13·3	15,669·66	304·68	67·732	324·37	1,374·13	1,441·27	25,394·05
12	683·8	276·0	36·7	3·0	1·1	335·9	24·6	6·1	9,250·66	204·03	53·041	316·84	1,363·63	1,424·89	21,505·68
13	683·1	277·8	35·5	3·1	1·3	322·5	14·0	4·8	7,599·33	175·21	50·180	317·74	1,364·15	1,426·24	22,922·49
14	678·8	281·9	35·8	2·9	1·1	303·0	10·5	5·2	7,608·99	171·26	54·572	321·66	1,366·88	1,425·85	20,530·38
15	679·3	280·0	37·5	2·7	0·8	314·1	9·2	5·4	7,802·33	176·00	55·026	321·00	1,366·67	1,424·10	18,259·29
16	758·7	219·9	20·0	1·2	0·6	229·1	6·7	2·8	4,824·33	115·37	46·984	241·71	1,266·35	1,297·98	12,298·77
17	588·6	351·3	54·1	5·4	1·8	411·7	18·5	8·7	11,815·32	255·47	58·907	412·61	1,484·15	1,579·54	32,722·73
18	835·3	143·7	19·3	1·3	0·7	686·3	12·3	5·3	11,619·99	301·96	36·718	164·97	1,189·17	1,221·00	12,168·99
19	746·8	217·0	32·6	2·9	1·2	457·8	15·1	6·8	10,650·33	245·96	51·329	253·79	1,296·48	1,354·25	21,332·64
20	734·4	212·8	47·1	5·1	1·6	852·6	21·1	10·1	17,450·32	421·24	46·303	266·62	1,329·65	1,414·57	28,506·02
21	627·2	330·1	38·8	3·2	1·1	210·9	8·8	3·7	5,393·33	120·89	54·388	373·18	1,422·15	1,486·08	22,149·00
22	683·3	276·9	36·3	3·1	1·1	314·9	14·2	4·0	6,944·66	164·03	46·463	317·48	1,364·15	1,245·21	21,327·07
23	744·9	219·3	32·9	2·5	1·1	467·7	17·3	5·4	9,688·66	233·66	44·588	255·78	1,297·58	1,352·37	19,553·21
24	785·2	179·1	32·6	2·8	0·9	792·5	21·0	6·1	13,671·99	353·53	35·888	215·36	1,256·81	1,310·49	17,554·75
25	438·7	339·1	132·6	86·3	3·8									2,398·5	
26	625·8	282·5	62·4	29·3	1·5									1,698·8	
27	215·0	344·9	206·2	226·6	7·0									3,654·4	

each month to the primary care station, the clinic and the hospital. In columns (9)–(11) various measures of resource use are given: total cost, monthly M.D. hours needed, and hospital costs as a proportion of total medical costs. Finally, the five health indices are given. (Note that the last index is merely the mortality rate, health status E.) The characteristics of the separate runs are given in Appendix B. We shall discuss only two of the output measures: health index C (whose weights are 1,2,4,8 and 16) and the total costs of the system. The qualitative results are unchanged if any of the other health indices are read.

(1) *Changing the Probability of Seeking Care*
In the first eight cases we study the effect of changing the probability of seeking care *ceteris paribus*. In the first six cases the probability of seeking care changes for only the first two health states, healthy and unwell. The extremes are represented by case 2, which sets both these probabilities to 0, and case 6, which sets them at 0·1 and 0·5 respectively. In cases 7 and 8 additional changes in the probabilities of seeking care for health states are made. In Fig. 17.5 the resulting health status index is plotted against total cost. The points are labeled by case number and can be thought of as approaching an efficiency frontier in which the trade-offs between health status and cost are shown.

A number of interesting results are obtained. For example, case 5 dominates case 6. Despite the fact that the *PSC* is lower for case 5, the resulting overall health status is higher and the total costs lower. This result arose because we assumed that the health status of a 'healthy' person cannot be improved: at best, he is not affected; at worst, his health status is lowered. Such a structure is not peculiar to our model. A healthy person seeking medical care in the real world cannot be made better off; however, he can be exposed to infectious disease, he may receive badly performed tests, or may react adversely to unneeded medication.[1]

The locus of points for cases 1 through 5 indicates that there is a trade-off of $23 per month for each point improvement in the health index. Thus, for $23 per month, one person moves (on net) from a state of unwell to one of healthy; for $132 one person moves from being acutely ill to healthy; for $322 one person moves from being critically ill to being healthy; and for $345 the death rate is

---

[1] The current structure does not ascribe any value to preventive care, since healthy patients cannot be improved, and since the probabilities of changing symptom level do not show any benefit from preventive visits. We plan to modify the model to reflect preventive care by having patients who have sought care have a higher probability of remaining in their discharge symptom classification.

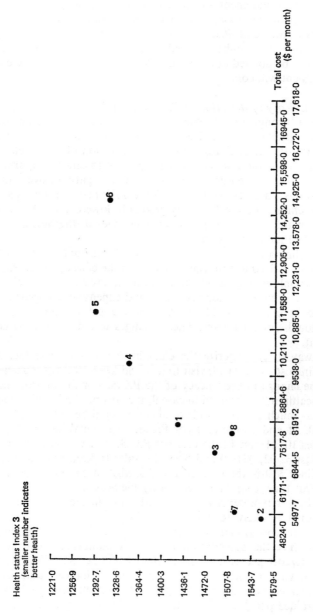

FIG. 17.5   Outcomes of simulation cases 1–8: health status index 3 versus cost

lower by one death per month with the additional person being healthy. This statement of trade-offs is not strictly accurate. A comparison of cases 2 and 5, for example, indicates that the additional expenditure of $6,055 reduced the death rate by only 0·5 per month while the number of healthy persons increased by 236. It should also be pointed out that one cannot choose *a priori* where the improvement will come.

(2) *The Efficacy of the Primary Care Station*
In cases 9 through 12, the efficacy of the P.C.S. is varied. The outcomes are graphed in Fig. 17.6. In case 9 the *TRP* matrix is changed so that the P.C.S. discharges a higher proportion of its patients to the community, and refers a lower proportion to other components. The result is a marked decrease in cost and a slight improvement in health status. In cases 10, 11 and 12 the *TRP* matrix is changed so that the efficacy of the P.C.S. is gradually lowered. Lowering the efficacy of the P.C.S. results in slight changes in the health index and marked increase in cost.

These simulation results assume, throughout, that the cost of a P.C.S. visit is fixed at $10. Improvement in the efficacy of the P.C.S. can occur only by increasing physician time, having more specialists present, or using more sophisticated (and expensive) equipment. A decrease in efficacy could result from the substitution of para-professionals for physicians. These changes would change the cost of a visit.

One way to characterize the changing costs is to calculate the change in cost for a P.C.S. visit that would keep total cost constant, given the change in the efficacy of the P.C.S. For the improvement in the health index obtained in case 9, the cost per P.C.S. visit could rise by as much as $2·52 while total costs would be unchanged. For cases 10, 11 and 12 the cost per P.C.S. visit would be unchanged. For cases 10, 11 and 12 the cost per P.C.S. visit would have to fall by at least $2·02, $21·70 and $3·36 in order to keep total cost constant. Since $10 is the cost of a P.C.S. visit, it cannot be reduced by $21·70; thus, case 11 is necessarily inefficient. Case 12 is interesting since it represents a greater reduction in the efficacy of the P.C.S. than is likely to result from the substitution of a highly trained paraprofessional, such as a nurse practitioner or physician's assistant. Yet the substitution of such a paraprofessional could reduce the cost per visit by more than $3·36 (a reduction of 33·6 per cent). Thus, comparisons of cases 1 and 12 indicate that under some circumstances it may be practical and efficient to have a highly trained paraprofessional take over the primary care role.

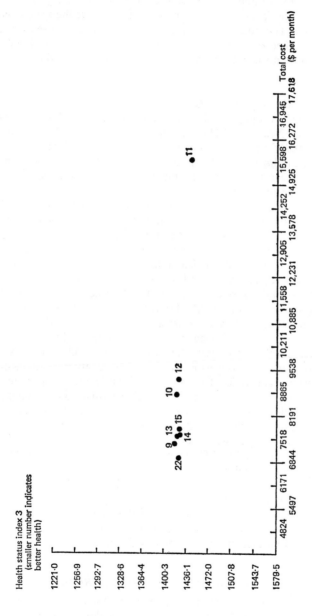

FIG. 17.6 Outcomes of simulation cases 9–15 and 22; health status index 3 versus cost

(3) *The Role of Compliance in Keeping Appointments*
Cases 13, 14, 15 and 22 explore the effects of changing the probabilities that patients will keep appointments or leave the system when
discharged. The outcomes are graphed in Fig. 17.6. These cases are
interesting because large changes in the compliance probabilities
have almost no effect on health status and only a slight effect on
cost.

(4) *The Underlying Health Level*
What would be the general health status of the population if there
were no medical care? The answer is given in case 25, where the
NATURALEV matrix in the basic case is powered to determine
what the equilibrium health status would be without medical intervention. The resulting health status distribution is lowered significantly. For example, the health index number of 2,398·5 is far
worse than that of any of the previous cases where some medical
care was provided. In comparing the resulting health status distribution to the basic case, the greatest differences appear in health
states 3 and 4 and in the mortality rate. Thus, the model reflects the
assumption that initial medical intervention is most successful in
dealing with severe disease and in lowering the mortality rate.

   Cases 26 and 27 reflect the effects of respectively raising and
lowering the underlying health of the community. The *NATURALEV*
in case 26 reflects a lower propensity to get ill, while that in case
27 reflects a greater propensity. The resulting health indices are
extremely sensitive to these changes, with the index for case 26
being comparable to the worst cases examined above with medical
intervention. The index for case 27 reflects a greater propensity.
The resulting health indices are extremely sensitive to these changes,
with the index for case 26 being comparable to the worst cases
examined above with medical intervention. The index for case 27
is almost three times as large (as bad) as the index for the basic
case. Again, the major differences occur in the mortality rate and
in health states 3 and 4.

(5) *Compound Experiments*
In cases 16 through 24 we have varied two or more parameters
simultaneously to study the compound effects. The outcomes are
graphed in Fig. 17.7 and all the outcomes are shown in Fig. 17.8.

X. SUMMARY AND CONCLUSION

We have described a technique for modeling the delivery of medical
care which describes the various trade-offs available in the system. A

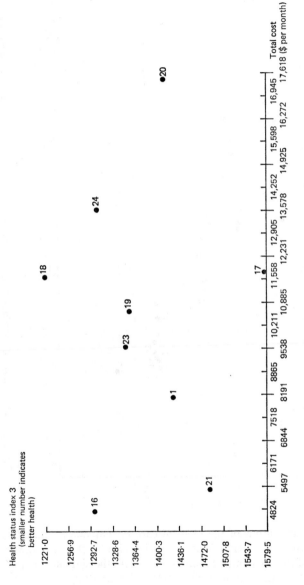

FIG. 17.7 Outcomes of simulation cases 16–21 and 23–24: health status index 3 versus cost

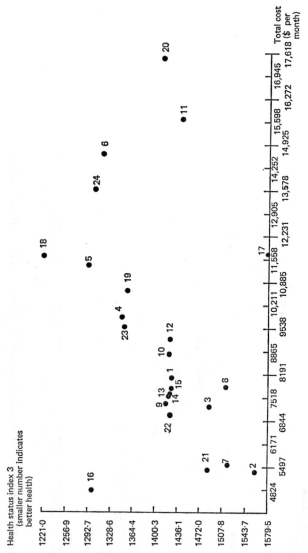

Fig. 17.8 Outcomes of simulations of combined cases: health status index 3 versus cost

measure of output of the medical care system was proposed as the distribution of individuals across various health states. A simulation model of this system was then built. Within the simulation model we found the equilibrium health states, the resulting cost, physician time, and the proportion of total cost spent on hospital care. Finally, we characterized the health state by a health index in which weights were given to the various health states to get a scalar index.

The simulation model was used to trace the implications of changes in the probabilities of seeking care, in the efficacy of the primary care station, in the population's compliance behavior and in their underlying health status. Changes in the *PSC* were used to derive an efficiency frontier relating improvements in health to the cost of care. When parameters of the system were within a reasonable range, the various outcomes indicated that the most important differences occurred in the trade-offs between the first two symptom classes, rather than in the more serious illnesses or the death rate. Changing the efficacy of the P.C.S. at a given cost per visit had little effect on the health index, but a significant effect on cost. Changing compliance probabilities had little effect on outcomes. Finally, changes in the underlying health levels had major effects on outcomes and appeared to be the most important parameters in the determination of cost and health status. A number of different indices of health status were calculated, using a variety of different weighting schemes. Little effect was noticed. The qualitative conclusions remain unchanged if physician time, rather than monetary costs, is used as the cost measure.

We believe we have demonstrated that our approach is feasible. We intend to proceed to explore our model more thoroughly and to proceed with a more careful estimation of its parameters. Work in progress includes the consideration of a two-tier system; allowance for chronic conditions; inclusion of a changing population base; recognition of extra-system care; and chronic non-compliance. Our objectives are to develop a general method for analyzing the delivery of medical care as a system.

REFERENCES

[1] Arrow, Kenneth J., 'Uncertainty and the Welfare Economics of Medical Care', *American Economic Review* (Dec 1963).
[2] Auster, Richard, Leveson, Irving and Sarachek, Deborah, 'The Production of Health: An Exploratory Study', *Journal of Human Resources* (Fall 1969).
[3] Bashshur, R., Shannon, G. and Metznev, C., 'Some Ecological Differentials in the Use of Medical Services', *Health Services Research* (Spring 1971).
[4] Denson, P. M. *et al.*, 'Medical Care Plans as a Source of Morbidity Data', *Millbank Memorial Fund Quarterly* (Jan 1960).
[5] Feldstein, Martin, 'The Rising Price of Physicians' Services', *Review of Economics and Statistics* (May 1970).
[6] Hennes, James D., 'The Measurement of Health', *Medical Care Review* (Dec 1972).

[7] Kaplan, Robert S. and Leinhardt, Samuel, 'Determinants of Physician Office Location', *Medical Care* (May–June 1973).

[8] Lave, Judith R. and Lave, Lester B., 'Medical Care and its Delivery: An Economic Appraisal', *Law and Contemporary Problems* (Spring 1970).

[9] ——, —— and Morton, Thomas E., 'The Physician's Assistant: Exploration of the Concept', *Hospitals, J.A.H.A.*, 1 June 1971.

[10] ——, —— and Silverman, Lester P., 'Hospital Cost Estimation Controlling for Case Mix', *Applied Economics* (Sep 1972).

[11] —— and Leinhardt, Samuel, 'The Delivery of Ambulatory Care to the Poor: A Literature Review', *Management Science* (Dec 1972).

[12] Lave, Lester B. and Seskin, Eugene P., 'Air Pollution and Human Health', *Science*, 21 Aug 1970.

[13] Leinhardt, Samuel, 'Ambulatory Care for the Poor in Pittsburgh, Part II: An Inventory of Primary Care Facilities', Working Paper, Carnegie-Mellon Univ. (Nov 1970).

[14] Silver, Henry K., 'New Patterns of Personnel for Children's Services: A Blueprint for Child Health Care for the Next Decade', paper presented at the 38th Annual Meeting of the American Academy of Pediatrics, Chicago, 18 Oct 1969.

[15] Stewart, Charles T., 'Allocation of Resources to Health', *Journal of Human Resources* (Winter 1971).

[16] Wyler, Allen R., Masuda, Minoru and Holmes, Thomas H., 'Seriousness of Illness Rating Scale', *Journal of Psychosomatic Research*, XI (1968).

[17] ——, —— and ——, 'The Seriousness of Illness Rating Scale: Reproducibility', *Journal of Psychosomatic Medicine*, XIV (1970).

[18] Yankauer, A., Connelley, J. P. and Feldman, P., 'Pediatric Practice in the United States', *Pediatrics*, Supplement (Feb 1970).

APPENDIX A

PARAMETERS FOR BASIC MODEL: CASE 1

Starting Health Status of the Population

Healthy	Unwell	Acutely ill	Critically ill	Deceased
682	277	37	4	0

PSC: Probability of Seeking Care

Healthy	Unwell	Acutely ill	Critically ill	Deceased
0·01	0·15	0·50	0·90	0

TRP: Referral Matrix for the Primary Care Station

	P.C.S. 1	Clinic 1	Hospital 1	Community
Healthy	0·015000	0·010000	0·005000	0·970000
Unwell	0·050000	0·040000	0·010000	0·900000
Acutely ill	0·360000	0·110000	0·030000	0·500000
Critical	0·360000	0·340000	0·100000	0·200000
Deceased	0·000000	0·000000	0·000000	0·000000

TRC: Referral Matrix for the Clinic

	P.C.S. 1	Clinic 1	Hospital 1	Community
Healthy	0·050000	0·040000	0·010000	0·900000
Unwell	0·100000	0·080000	0·020000	0·800000
Acutely ill	0·200000	0·100000	0·050000	0·650000
Critical	0·150000	0·300000	0·150000	0·400000
Deceased	0·000000	0·000000	0·000000	0·000000

TRH: Referral Matrix for the Hospital

	P.C.S. 1	Clinic 1	Hospital 1	Community
Healthy	0·150000	0·030000	0·020000	0·800000
Unwell	0·200000	0·050000	0·050000	0·700000
Acutely ill	0·200000	0·100000	0·100000	0·600000
Critical	0·200000	0·150000	0·150000	0·500000
Deceased	0·000000	0·000000	0·000000	0·000000

TRPD: Symptom Determination after Treatment for a Patient Discharged from System

	Healthy	Unwell	Acutely ill	Critical	Deceased
Healthy	0.950000	0·050000	0·000000	0·000000	0·000000
Unwell	0·600000	0·350000	0·050000	0·000000	0·000000
Acutely ill	0·300000	0·600000	0·099000	0·000000	0·001000
Critical	0·200000	0·650000	0·140000	0·000000	0·010000
Deceased	0·000000	0·000000	0·000000	0·000000	1·000000

TRPP: Symptom Determination after Treatment for a Patient Told to Report to P.C.S.

	Healthy	Unwell	Acutely ill	Critical	Deceased
Healthy	0·900000	0·090000	0·010000	0·000000	0·000000
Unwell	0·500000	0·400000	0·100000	0·000000	0·000000
Acutely ill	0·200000	0·500000	0·298000	0·000000	0·002000
Critical	0·100000	0·550000	0·335000	0·000000	0·015000
Deceased	0·000000	0·000000	0·000000	0·000000	1·000000

TRPC: Symptom Determination after Treatment for a Patient Told to Report to Clinic

	Healthy	Unwell	Acutely ill	Critical	Deceased
Healthy	0·850000	0·100000	0·040000	0·010000	0·000000
Unwell	0·400000	0·350000	0·200000	0·048000	0·002000
Acutely ill	0·150000	0·500000	0·250000	0·092000	0·008000
Critical	0·030000	0·550000	0·290000	0·105000	0·025000
Deceased	0·000000	0·000000	0·000000	0·000000	1.000000

TRPH: Symptom Determination after Treatment for a Patient Told to Report to Hospital

	Healthy	Unwell	Acutely ill	Critical	Deceased
Healthy	0·800000	0·110000	0·070000	0·019000	0·001000
Unwell	0·350000	0·350000	0·250000	0·045000	0·005000
Acutely ill	0·120000	0·440000	0·280000	0·142000	0·018000
Critical	0·010000	0·460000	0·290000	0·165000	0·075000
Deceased	0·000000	0·000000	0·000000	0·000000	1·000000

COMPD: The Probability Distribution that a Person
Discharged from the System Will Obey

	P.C.S. 1	Clinic 1	Hospital 1	Community
Healthy	0·030000	0·000000	0·000000	0·970000
Unwell	0·080000	0·000000	0·000000	0·920000
Acutely ill	0·200000	0·000000	0·000000	0·800000
Critical	0·500000	0·000000	0·000000	0·500000
Deceased	0·000000	0·000000	0·000000	0·000000

COMPP: The Probability Distribution that a Person
Told to Report to the P.C.S. Will Do So

	P.C.S. 1	Clinic 1	Hospital 1	Community
Healthy	0·500000	0·000000	0·000000	0·500000
Unwell	0·650000	0·000000	0·000000	0·350000
Acutely ill	0·800000	0·000000	0·000000	0·200000
Critical	0·950000	0·000000	0·000000	0·050000
Deceased	0·000000	0·000000	0·000000	0·000000

COMPC: The Probability Distribution that a Person
Told to Report to the Clinic Will Do So

	P.C.S. 1	Clinic 1	Hospital 1	Community
Healthy	0·050000	0·450000	0·000000	0·500000
Unwell	0·100000	0·555000	0·000000	0·350000
Acutely ill	0·180000	0·670000	0·000000	0·150000
Critical	0·200000	0·750000	0·000000	0·050000
Deceased	0·000000	0·000000	0·000000	0·000000

COMPH: The Probability Distribution that a Person
Told to Report to the Hospital Will Do So

	P.C.S. 1	Clinic 1	Hospital 1	Community
Healthy	0·250000	0·000000	0·600000	0·150000
Unwell	0·200000	0·000000	0·700000	0·100000
Acutely ill	0·150000	0·000000	0·800000	0·050000
Critical	0·080000	0·000000	0·900000	0·020000
Deceased	0·000000	0·000000	0·000000	0·000000

NATURALEV: The Underlying Health Status
Transition Probabilities

	Healthy	Unwell	Acutely ill	Critical	Deceased
Healthy	0·909790	0·080000	0·010000	0·000200	0·000010
Unwell	0·100000	0·849300	0·050000	0·000600	0·000100
Acutely ill	0·040000	0·090000	0·799000	0·070000	0·001000
Critical	0·001000	0·020000	0·060000	0·889000	0·030000
Deceased	0·000000	0·000000	0·000000	0·000000	1·000000

APPENDIX B

CHARACTERIZATION OF SIMULATION RUNS

Case   1: Matrices shown in Appendix A; $PSC = (0.01, 0.15, 0.5, 0.9)$.
  2: $PSC = (0, 0, 0.5, 0.9)$.
  3: $PSC = (0.005, 0.075, 0.5, 0.9)$.
  4: $PSC = (0.02, 0.3, 0.5, 0.9)$.
  5: $PSC = (0.04, 0.5, 0.5, 0.9)$.
  6: $PSC = (0.1, 0.5, 0.5, 0.9)$.
  7: $PSC = (0, 0, 0.9, 0.9)$.
  8: $PSC = (0.01, 0.15, 0.25, 0.45)$.

  9: *TRP* improvement (P.C.S. more efficacious); 0.98 as compared to 0.97.
 10: *TRP* decrement compared to basic model; 0.94 compared to 0.97.
 11: *TRP* decrement compared to case 10; 0.80 compared to 0.94.
 12: *TRP* decrement compared to case 10; 0.90 compared to 0.94.

 13: Compliance to referrals: seek care more often than basic model.
 14: Compliance to referrals: seek care less often than basic model.
 15: Compliance to referrals: *COMPD* = basic, *COMPP* better than 14, *COMPC* and *COMPH* worse than 14.

 16: Underlying health status improved relative to basic model (0.92379 v. 0.90979).
 17: Underlying health status worse than basic model (0.895790 v. 0.90979).

 18: Combination of cases 6 and 16.
 19: Combination of cases 4 and 10.
 20. Combination of cases 6 and 17.
 21: Combination of cases, 3, 9 and 14.
 22. Compliance to referrals: case 14 except *COMPD* = basic.
 23: Combination of cases 4, 10 and 22.
 24: Combination of cases 6, 10 and 22.

 25: No medical intervention, *NATURALEV* of basic model.
 26: No medical intervention, *NATURALEV* improved (as in case 16).
 27: No medical intervention, *NATURALEV* worsened (as in case 17).

Summary Record of Discussion

This session took up the papers by Dr Davis on hospital cost determinants, by Professor Sloan on physicians' labor supply functions, and by Professors J. Lave and L. Lave and Leinhardt on a simulation model of the health care system.

A. Dr Davis's paper

Professor J. Lave, introducing Dr Davis's paper, mentioned the great number of rival theories which had been used to explain the rapid rise in American hospital costs. Some of these have stressed supply-side factors: technical improvements, inelastic supply of facilities, non-medical factor costs. Others have stressed the increased demand for hospital services and its price inelasticity. In addition, there are case-mix theories which are difficult to classify on a demand-supply basis. Dr Davis's paper is an ambitious attempt to judge between these theories or, rather, to combine them in a quantitative way. She has concluded that increased demand was responsible for about 45 per cent of the rise in costs, changes in the case-mix for about 17 per cent, and the rising factor costs for the bulk of the remainder.

Professor J. Lave's criticisms were primarily econometric and secondarily data-related. On the econometric side, she felt that the Davis data (for hospitals, i.e. firms) had not been well aggregated to apply to the entire hospital industry. She felt that the case-mix should have been included as an endogenous variable, instead of being exogenous as in the Davis paper. She found no independent supply model in the paper, inasmuch as some supply factors are demand-induced; for example, the length of the patient's mean stay in the hospital is both a demand and an input factor, and residuals of hospital stay about their mean are correlated with other independent variables. While Dr Davis used a reduced form, and fitted it statistically, Professor J. Lave doubted that this was legitimate, since the structural models were incomplete.

As regards the data on which Dr Davis had relied, Professor J. Lave pointed out that while the supply data are for individual hospitals, the demand data are aggregated. Hospitals vary so widely among themselves that the combination was, in her opinion, risky. Also, the data cover periods both before and after the inauguration of the Medicare and Medicaid programs. Since, as discussed already in Dr Friedman's paper, these programs altered the demand structure considerably, the pre-Medicare and post-Medicare data should have been analyzed separately.

Nevertheless, most of the signs in the Davis equations are as expected. The exceptions relate to the mean stay variable already mentioned.[1] Professor J. Lave did not understand why either increased population density or increased insurance coverage should lead to increased mean hospital stay. She noted that within a given hospital a number of empirical studies have shown that length of stay, for any given cause, is not affected

[1] *Dr Davis* replied in a postscript that the mean stay variable had both the predicted sign and size.

by the presence of an insurance plan. Perhaps there has been some confounding with case-mix variables, and perhaps some aspects of physician behavior may be involved.

Dr Davis replied that she had originally planned to separate pre- from post-Medicare data, but length constraints prevented reporting these results. A separate paper finds that what is important was increased insurance coverage in any form, and that insurance coverage had, indeed been one of her independent variables.[1] She also agreed that she would have preferred to have either direct data or good surrogates on the case-mix variable, but did not feel that her dependent variables were greatly dependent upon the case-mix.

Mme. Sandier, speaking from French experience, said that rising hospital bills were a major problem in the French health care system, amounting to 40 per cent of the total, and rising by 9 per cent per annum in real terms, while hosital days per case were rising only by 2 per cent. The physical volume of tests and similar procedures – X-rays, for example – is growing faster than the mean stay.

While claiming no competence to criticize the econometrics of the Davis model or of production functions in general, Mme Sandier doubted the feasibility of much labor–capital substitution in hospitals. She also said that wages and salaries were rising there in money terms at approximately the same rate as in the French economy generally.

Professor Emi said that it was important, at least in Japan, to distinguish between hospital costs associated with admitted patients and with outpatient care. The ratio between admitted patients and outpatients is important, and perhaps should have been included in the Davis model. Influence on hospital costs might also, at least in Japan, be exercised by the physicians' fee structure, another omitted variable.

Professor Evans, from his knowledge of Dr Davis's data base, believed that outpatient costs had not been included. He wondered, however, how teaching costs had been handled in the teaching costs included in the Davis sample. He also wondered whether the sample included only voluntary hospitals, or whether the proprietary hospitals (covered in Professor Rosett's paper) had been represented. Finally, he felt that Medicare had caused a major shift in hospital cost functions by increasing the proportion of aged patients. *Dr Davis* indicated that a dummy variable for teaching hospitals had been included in the model and the sample restricted to voluntary hospitals. The proportion of Medicare patients was included in some specifications, but found to be insignificant.

Dr Phelps deplored the stress on the (unavailable) case-mix variable, which might itself be only an artefact whose effects are covered by other variables already available.

Dr Davis argued that number of admissions is a preferable output measure if some adjustment for case-mix is made. Certainly, the number of days spent in the hospital is a poor measure, if people simply remain in the hospital longer and convalesce there instead of at home. She also

---

[1] See 'Hospital Costs and the Medicare Program', *Social Security Bulletin* (Aug 1973).

added that a number of area-wide studies have found that insurance affected the demand for hospital care in a similar fashion.

Professor Fuchs associated the growth of hospital insurance primarily with the growth of the mean length of stay. He also said that labor expenditures have, until recently, increased faster than non-labor expenditures in hospitals, but that this was no longer true in countries he knew about. He wondered about the Japanese case.

In *Mr Kaser's* view, the main issue relative to rising hospital costs is the way technical improvements are to be paid for, and hospital facilities kept up to date. He felt that physicians tried to accomplish this by payments out of hospital receipts; hence hospital costs were rising. He went on to ask Dr Davis whether the rising number of hospital physicians might not be a factor in rising hospital costs. (Dr Davis's data had not included material on this point.)

Professor Liefmann-Keil, returning to a point she had made previously, said that the decreasing size of households was a factor in rising hospital costs, especially when combined with the increasing age of the population. (In West Germany, 25 per cent of the population lives in one-person households.) As a result, there is increasing demand for hospitals to supply services formerly supplied by family members. At the same time, hospital wages were formerly governed by relief standards, but now are more competitive with the regular labor market. As an additional factor, Professor Liefmann-Keil mentioned the tendency for teaching hospitals to seek out interesting patients and keep them hospitalized longer, sometimes at high cost.

To close discussion of her paper, *Dr Davis* replied particularly to Professors J. Lave and Liefmann-Keil. Population density variables lead systematically to longer hospital stays; in rural areas, many are admitted but few stay for long periods. (*Professor J. Lave* repeated her previous view that this may be a case-mix problem.) Many of Professor Liefmann-Keil's points were, in Dr Davis's opinion, valid. The type of patient household should, somehow, be included. Just as in Germany, tight labor markets had raised hospital labor costs somewhat disproportionately in the United States in the late 1960s. The influence of physicians in raising hospital costs needed also to be recognized explicitly.

B. *Professor Sloan's paper*

The assignment of introducing and discussing the Sloan paper had been allocated originally to Professor Feldstein, who was prevented by illness from attending the conference. *Dr Friedman* had volunteered to take over Professor Feldstein's assignment at short notice.

Professor Sloan's study of physician allocation of time between work and leisure was, said Dr Friedman, decidedly superior to previous studies because it was less aggregative, and because it was based more closely upon the standard economic model of the labor–leisure choice of a self-employed individual. (This individual is a demander of cooperant inputs, and a supplier of his own time under conditions of diminishing returns in terms of utility.)

Is the supply of physicians' hours backward-bending? That is to say, do increases in physicians' hourly wages from professional practice reduce the time they devote to this practice when the substitution effect is offset by an income effect? Professor Sloan has made separate estimates for hours per week and weeks per year, and also included such other variables as age, sex, amenities of life and ethical responsibilities, either directly or by proxy. An overall net effect appears to be that each $1 increase in the professional hourly wage of American physicians will lead, on average, to some 49 hours less work per year. To this extent, the supply of physicians' hours is indeed, backward-bending.

To some extent, Dr Friedman continued, there was a bias in Sloan's estimates because average and not marginal income data were relied upon. He was surprised at Professor Sloan's finding the sex variable unimportant, but the Sloan sample had included few female physicians. Professor Sloan's results indicated that younger doctors worked more than older ones; Dr Friedman wondered whether time spent on research and on keeping up with new knowledge had been taken into account.

He would also have expected salaried physicians to work fewer hours than the self-employed, but this distinction does not appear in Professor Sloan's results. Extraneous (non-employment) income also has the 'wrong' sign in Professor Sloan's equations, increasing hours where the economist would have expected the opposite result. It may also be important to estimate the effect of group practice, where it existed, upon physicians' labor–leisure choices. In general, Dr Friedman felt, the most essential and surprising aspect of Professor Sloan's results is that it was apparently the higher return per unit of labor time, not higher income as such, which reduced physicians' supply of effort.

Responding to these comments, *Professor Sloan* said that it would be interesting, if possible, to disaggregate his results further and study, separately, special types of physicians' labor supply. He mentioned, particularly, seeing 'disagreeable' patients. He also would like to see some allowance made for the 'demand creation' effects mentioned in the Evans paper; nothing of the sort had been included in his own paper. On the distinction between marginal as distinguished from average income from additional hours of professional practice, Professor Sloan agreed that it might well be as important in practice as in academic theory, but said he had found no data whatever on marginal incomes. As for the sex variable, he said that it was confounded with the family-sized variable, which had, indeed, appeared in his supply equations.

Professor J. Lave asked the first question from the floor, inquiring whether the physicians in Professor Sloan's sample varied widely among themselves in hours per week or weeks per year. The reply was that the standard deviation of hours per week was 5 or 6, but that the great majority of the physicians in the sample reported themselves as working between 48 and 52 weeks per year.

M. Foulon suggested that the data might show an upward bias, in that they sometimes came from physicians' wives, who were worried about their husbands' working too hard, neglecting their health and domestic responsibilities, etc. *Professor Sloan* referred, on the other hand, to the

American Medical Association claim that most published estimates of physicians' hours of work were too low.

Professor Robinson noted the limitation of Professor Sloan's study to American data. He wondered what international comparisons might show. In a public system like the British, he suspected that there might be some bimodality, with one group of physicians working very hard and another doing relatively little. *Mr Cooper* replied that the average general practitioner in the British system worked 42 or 43 hours per week, and commented further on the difficulty of defining 'work' in medical practice.

Professor Evans wondered about the anomalous effect of outside income. He suspected that many physicians underestimate and underreport such income, reducing it as far as possible by 'expenses of practice' to minimize their income-tax liabilities. There followed some discussion of the importance and details of physicians' tax avoidance (and tax evasion) practices on the American scene, with Professor Evans feeling that these were more important in distorting reported data than did Professor Sloan.

Professor Liefmann-Keil suggested that even more disaggregation of the data might be in order. For example, the flexibility of both hours and weeks on the job are greater for the self-employed than for the salaried physician. The patient mix may also be important; some specialties involved more irregular hours than others, or interfered to a great extent with scheduled vacations, and, in addition some sorts of patients may be more disagreeable than others. In regard to physicians' non-wage income, finally, physicians' behavior may vary with the source of such income. Income related to one's practice indirectly, such as the proceeds from drug sales, may have different effects than income from stock dividends upon the physician's labor–leisure choice.

Dr Bell commented upon Professor Sloan's treatment of the sex variable. Instead of using a dummy variable in a pooled regression, Dr Bell believed, Professor Sloan should perhaps have worked with separate samples of men and women physicians.

M. Foulon thought that some French data might provide interesting comparisons with Professor Sloan's American data. For France, he felt that ten or a dozen variables were important. The average French general practitioner, he said, works 55 hours a week, as against 48 for the specialist. In addition to the general practitioner/specialist distinction, he continued, a number of other distinctions were important. One should distinguish between time actually working and time 'on call'. As for age, there seemed to be an 'inverse U-shaped relation', with the younger and older men working less than those in their middle years. Family size, sex, physician density, amount of postgraduate training, type of practice (individual, group, salaried). outside interests and the amount and nature of non-professional income sources were all important. Some anomalies were found here too. For example, the apparent importance of the physician density variable may reflect a special situation in the South of France, where many older physicians congregate in partial retirement.

To close the discussion of his paper, *Professor Sloan* recognized the presence of errors in measurement in some of the variables in his equations. Replying more specifically to Dr Davis, he agreed that separate regressions might have been run excluding the women in his sample, as an alternative to his use of a sex dummy. He repeated, however, that the number of women in his sample was too small to permit a significant separate study of the female physicians based on his data.

C. *Professors L. Lave, J. Lave and Leinhardt's paper*[1]

Professor Intriligator was the formal discussant of this joint paper. He found in it two major innovations. One was the use of a specific objective function: medical care was to be provided to attain a target health level, and the cost estimated accordingly. The second was the reliance upon a simulation model. In this simulation, health states are ranked subjectively (by the patient himself) from 1 through 5. The health care system was depicted as a three-stage screen, with separate time and money costs at each stage. Cost estimates are based upon probabilities of moving from one health status to another in a Markov chain, making allowance for possible non-compliance with referral from one stage of the health system to another.

Using arbitrary, but plausible data with a hypothetical population, Professors Lave, Lave and Leinhardt concluded tentatively that improvement in the underlying health status of the population (at the outset) was probably the most important single factor in reducing the cost of reaching a target health care level, while increases in the efficacies of various stages of the health system were more important than increases in the probability of referral from one stage to the next.

Professor Intriligator then criticized the paper on several grounds. (1) He felt that 'cost' was really a transfer payment to the health system from some other elements in society, and that the attained level of health was more closely related to the distribution of benefits and burdens than to their total amount. (2) He felt that the state of health is difficult to measure, and that such societal measures as we have are influenced by distributional factors. He found the present paper's subjectivism inconsistent with previous comments by the Laves at this Conference. (3) He wondered about the numbers and probabilities in the paper. Was the model presented as potentially operational or merely as a 'think piece'? Also, probabilities were presented in an either–or manner. A patient would either move from one stage of the health-care system to another or he would not, but in the real world a great deal depends upon *how much* treatment and of *what sort* he receives at each stage. (This, in turn depends upon the patient's age, sex, social class, insurance status, etc.) Professor Intriligator admitted feeling that the econometric model developed by himself and his associates had been more successful in capturing these aspects of the health care system. (4) The authors claimed that the health care system was too complex for formal modeling, and that it

[1] This paper appears in a slightly revised version, differing from the original only in small details. The revisions do not appear to have affected the trenchancy of the comments.

required treatment by simulation methods, but he (Professor Intriligator) was able to reduce their model to a pair of fairly conventional linear programming problems closely related to each other.[1]

Replying particularly to the critical portions of the Intriligator introduction, *Professor L. Lave* felt that Professor Intriligator had suggested both simplifications and complications, but that on balance, the Lave–Lave–Leinhardt model remained richer than the alternative linear programming formulation suggsted by Professor Intriligator. (The differential complications, however, did not really matter.) He and his associates believe that their model *is* essentially operational, in the sense that all essential inputs can be estimated; admittedly, the health status estimates are subjective only. Moreover, it would appear that the simulation model is robust, in that fairly substantial changes in the input variables do not seem to change the outcomes greatly, Professor J. Lave added that the probabilities in the model take account of demand as well as supply aspects of the medical care system.

Professor Bronfenbrenner seized upon the last point. Demand as a quantity entered the model, but not demand functions (quantity demanded as related to prices, incomes, etc.). He doubted, on methodological grounds, the validity of simulation models purporting to explain economic behavior without reference to economic variables, in the manner of the current 'doomsday' simulations made under the auspices of the Club of Rome.

Professor Leinhardt answered the charge that the model had neglected distinctions between different qualities of health care. He pointed out that people's access to the system is rationed and that patients cannot always have the type they want. If they cannot have the type they want, they may refuse compliance with referral to that particular stage of the health care system. This is one interpretation of the 'compliance' variable which enters into the model's transition probabilities.

Professor Williams raised the question: whose view of a patient's health status is relevant, his own subjective view or the physician's objective one? At the initial stages of contact of the individual with the health system, the paper's subjective view is probably right, Health as an end-product, however, may be quite another matter. It is up to the physician to determine whether a prospective patient will be accepted at all or discharged from a hospital. The point is especially important if the physician has an incentive to induce people to reapply for higher and higher stages of care.

Professor Emi asked two questions. (1) What, if any, is the role of medical associations in governing access and discharge to the health care system, or the definition of health status variables? (2) Has there been any allowance for regionalism and inter-regional differences at any point in the global simulation model presented here?

Professor L. Lave replied (to Professor Wiliams primarily) that filtering of health care applicants by suppliers is largely ineffective, as compared

[1] The Intriligator reformulation of the Lave–Lave–Leinhardt model is omitted here.

to filtering by patients themselves. Everything is determined by the patient, he believed, citing a Detroit study that some 60 per cent of prescriptions were never filled. As for Professor Emi's query about regions and regionalism, the system was a macro-system operating within any area determined by geography. It might be a country or a city. Professor Lave went on to suggest that, since the most effective means of reducing health costs is improving the initial state of health, there should be more stress on preventive medicine, pollution control, reduction of smoking and similar measures.

M. Foulon and *M, Dupuy* found the simulation model too hypothetical for practical use in decision-making. The concept of 'health status' they found too subjective and variable for statistical estimation, although M. Dupuy admits the importance of the individual's perception of his own health status. Both men agree that it is better to drop such notions as 'health stock' and 'health status' in favor of readily available indicators.

Mr Kaser agreed generally with Professor Williams, despite the reply by Professor L. Lave. He introduced into the discussion the notion of 'trade-off' between the importance of subjective and objective estimates of health, and wondered whether it could be treated as a constant. He himself thought it was highly variable, depending on the patient's initial position and the speed with which it might be changing. In rebuttal, *Professor Leinhardt* stressed again that the patient's subjective views determined compliance with whatever might be recommended by the health care system. *Professor Intriligator* felt that the notion of health status was useful only for society; for individuals, reliance exclusively on either subjective of objective measures is dangerous. His own solution would be to use transition probabilities (of movement from one health care subsector to another) without reference to any measures of health status whatever.

Professor Lévy felt that application of the paper's simulation model might result, in practice, in underestimation of the demand for preventive medicine, and in concentration upon the curative aspects of the medical profession's work. This is because, in health status 1–2 (the 'healthier' states, in the simulation model), any individual experiences so slight a demand for health care assistance, except for occasional and perfunctory supervision and inspection. *Professor Williams* replied that, in a British context, the patient's self-perceived medical state is not the governing factor in his use of the physician's services. Even the healthy man wants counseling, reassurance and information from a physician whom he trusts. (Is the average general practitioner very effective at this point? Not in Britain, according to *Mr Cooper*.) More important than one's health status in determining one's use of medical services are one's ingrained habits, including, particularly, persistence.

Dr Grossman stated that subjective health measures of health status have statistical validity. They are correlated highly with objective measures. They are also associated with such variables as hospitalization and disability. Also Dr Grossman continued, we should not forget the psychosomatic side of medicine. It often happens that a psychological malaise at time t is reflected in (or causes) a physical ailment at time $t + n$.

Closing the session, *Professor L. Lave* agreed particularly with Dr Grossman's support of the subjectivist position. Physicians themselves take the same view, as regards people's demand for periodic physical check-ups. If by objective health status we mean clinical morbidity, it makes no great difference in statistical work whether we use subjective or objective health status measures. Investigations of motivation (to seek medical assistance) have related it to health status as a highly important variable. Both in the real world and in the simulation model, healthy people do, in fact, seek care – primarily, however, for preventive reasons. This may not be adequate, but it is certainly better than nothing at all.

18 Measuring the Effectiveness of Health Care Systems[1]

Alan Williams

UNIVERSITY OF YORK

Much economic analysis of health care systems employs measures of effectiveness which relate to workload or provision rather than to the health status of the individual. A conceptually correct measure is sketched out, and it is argued that such a measure is operationally feasible, though it requires careful analytical treatment, and a clearly specified division of responsibility between various research disciplines, administrators and policy-makers, all of whom would be involved in generating and processing the relevant information. It is also argued that some effort should be devoted to wide-ranging, routine, longitudinal monitoring of individual health states as a source of such information, and a brief account is given of a proposed field trial, relating to the care of the elderly in Britain, designed to demonstrate the possibility and usefulness of this approach.

I. THE PROBLEM AND ITS SETTING

In my mind's eye I have an image of a health care system whose sole function is to ensure that the community it serves derives the maximum net benefit from its existence. The community it serves (its 'clients') comprise sick people and those who suffer pain, grief anxiety, etc., because of that sickness, both now and contingently in the future. It does not include, as such, those whose livelihood depends upon providing the inputs which the health care system requires, except in so far as they are 'clients' in the meaning given above. Moreover, this community wishes its health care system to be run in a manner which reflects the values of the community,

[1] In this paper I have drawn heavily on the work of three colleagues, Anthony Culyer, Robert Lavers and Kenneth Wright, who should be credited with joint responsibility for its more solid parts. The actual edifice is mine, so if it seems a bit shaky, blame the bricklayer, not the brickmakers. I should also acknowledge the stimulus provided for this work by the support given to various parts of it by the Department of Health and Social Security, the Institute of Municipal Treasurers and Accountants, the Nuffield Provincial Hospitals Trust and the Social Science Research Council.

despite the fact that the health care system is so large and complex that a great deal of decentralization of resource allocation decisions is necessary. The basic problem I wish to examine is 'how can we measure the "efficiency" of such a system?' or, put in more everyday language, 'How can we tell whether that health care system is serving the community as well as it could?'

The simple-minded economist's formulation of this problem would be to establish production functions for the various health-affecting activities which the system might embrace and from these estimate marginal social costs, then elicit the preference function of the community for the outputs of the system, and optimize (i.e. maximize the difference between total social benefits and total social costs). At this level of abstraction, this way of formulating the problem might be assigned to that class of economic propositions labelled 'true but unhelpful', but because it is both true *and* fundamental, it is nevertheless a useful reference point for the discussion.[1]

In practice, we have difficulty implementing it as an operational research strategy for several reasons:

(*a*) Production functions are ill-defined, owing to our ignorance of the physiological, psychological and sociological influences affecting the efficacy of therapeutic or supportive activities.[2]

(*b*) In costing the inputs into these activities we are often unclear at a conceptual level as to the proper realm of discourse (i.e. over what range of considerations we are suboptimizing in an imperfect world), and even when we are clear on that score, the data at our disposal are frequently inadequate (drawing heavily on financial data from large public agencies and from the well-organized markets which happen to exist, with rather poor data on true opportunity costs, especially as felt by the clients themselves).[3]

[1] This framework is developed further as a means of disentangling notions of 'need', 'trade-off', etc., in Appendix A of A. J. Culyer, R. J. Lavers and Alan Williams, 'Health Indicators', in Andrew Shonfield and Stella Shaw (eds.), *Social Indicators and Social Policy* (London: Heinemann, for the Social Science Research Council, 1972).

[2] A particularly pungent exponent of this view is A. L. Cochrane, *Effectiveness and Efficiency: Random Reflections on Health Services* (Nuffield Provincial Hospitals Trust, 1972).

[3] For instance, the simple notion that the client's time is also valuable is slowly gaining explicit recognition in 'scheduling' and 'location' studies in the health care system. It does not always spill over as fully as it should into comparisons of institutional versus domiciliary care, however, with some odd effects on policy choices. See, for instance, R. Wager, *The Care of the Elderly* (London: Institute of Municipal Treasurers and Accountants, 1972).

(c) The community's preference function is a will-o'-the-wisp, because we are not sure that the community actually has one, or even has a set of concepts and a language in which to discuss what is involved in developing one, not to mention much idea as to who should play what role in that process.

In this paper I shall not discuss the difficulties arising under (a), though we shall have to take note of them. The agenda of business to discuss under (b) is long and fascinating, and is the area of health studies where the economist's role is pre-eminent. But my interests lie in area (c), because I think it is here that the most appalling weaknesses of current studies into the efficiency of health care systems (by economists and others) are manifest,[1] and although it is not, strictly speaking, 'economics', there appears to be some reluctance by other professional groups to plunge into the difficult territory of devising 'output' measures for health care systems which are going to serve the economists' purposes in answering the basic question posed earlier.[2]

I begin, therefore, by setting out (in section II) certain desiderata which I think any such 'output' measures should fulfil, before going on (in section III) to outline a strategy for devising such measures. Section IV reports briefly on some work I am currently directing which forms part of this strategy, and in section V I offer some observations on why I think economists need to devote more of their time, energy and skill to this kind of work.

II. DESIDERATA

Ideally, we seek an estimate of the benefits of health-affecting activities measured in monetary units commensurate with the relevant cost estimates. Before setting out the schemes by which such measures might be evolved, two cautionary disclaimers are in order: (a) using monetary units as a measure of value does not imply

---

[1] It even defeated the ingenious M. S. Feldstein (*Economic Analysis for Health Service Efficiency*, Amsterdam: North-Holland, 1967), who was forced to accept the convention that 'a hospital's outputs are measured as the numbers of cases treated in each of several categories' (p. 169), and among his list of ways of improving the model is included the tentative hope that one day 'it may be possible to relate selected measures of population health to the care being received' (p. 286).

[2] Which is not to claim that no one else is active in this field. Besides the work cited later, note should be taken of D. F. Sullivan, *Conceptual Problems in Developing an Index of Health* (Washington, D.C.: Office of Health Statistics Analysis, Departments of Health Education and Welfare, 1965), and S. Fanshel and J. W. Bush, 'A Health Status Index and its Application to Health Status Outcomes', *Operational Research*, XVIII, 6 (1970).

accepting any particular *mode of valuation* and, more specifically, it does not imply acceptance of market values, and still less of a 'cash flow' approach to the evaluation of health care systems; (*b*) in order to purge the subsequent discussion of any risk of misunderstanding on that score, I am going to use the convention that all the so-called 'economic' benefits (like getting people back to work more quickly, saving costs which would fall on other services, etc.) are treated as *negative costs* and offset against the items on the input side.[1] Thus, only 'humanitarian' benefits are considered here.

One other important preliminary matter needs to be made clear, and that is that, because it is the client's state which is our central interest, the measures we are seeking must be to do with the client's state. I apologize if that seems too trite and banal to be worth mentioning, but it is not as trivial as it seems at first sight. In this context, it is not only important to distinguish between indicators of state of health (like mortality and morbidity measures, days of restricted activity, etc.) and provision indicators (hospital beds per thousand population, doctors per thousand, etc.).[2] But it is also important not to be led into believing that numbers of cases, episodes of treatment, hospital bed-days occupied, are true 'output' measures, even though they refer to clients, because they are concerned with throughput or workload, not to 'output' in terms of amelioration of an individual's state of health compared with what it would otherwise have been. A still more tempting trap for the unwary is set by measures of 'need', such as nursing dependency scales, which indicate the quantity and quality of care required by a patient. Although these measures are closely associated with client state in terms of social functioning, they specify *inputs* needed, which is precisely what we must avoid prejudging.[3]

Moreover, it is the community's valuations of that state which are relevant. This may or may not coincide with the individual's own valuations of his own state, or indeed with any particular individual's valuations of any other client's state. I am going to duck

---

[1] This obviously leaves the calculation of 'net benefits' unaffected, but means that we might have to think of some activities as having negative *net* costs if, for instance, the 'economic' benefits outweighed the costs. Such cases I do not regard as very interesting from our standpoint, since all such activities should obviously be pursued in a rational society, as the 'humanitarian' benefits are free goods. The interesting cases are those where the humanitarian benefits can be obtained only by the sacrifice of other good things (i.e. where their costs are positive).

[2] See, for instance, Culyer, Lavers and Williams, op. cit., for a fuller discussion of the shortcomings of some of the existing work based on these approaches.

[3] This distinction is clearly drawn in V. Carstairs and M. Morrison, *The Elderly in Residential Care* (Scottish Home and Health Department, 1971).

the very large and difficult set of intellectual philosophical problems which surround the processes by which 'community' values emerge. I shall merely refer to a 'dialogue' between the parties, without investigating the power and influence relationships at work therein. What I shall do, instead, is indicate the proper *professional* roles of the various parties, and try to provide them with a communication system which reduces the area of ignorance and risks of confusion in the conduct of that dialogue. As an 'efficiency' analyst I would be reluctant, in principle, to attempt more, and enormously self-satisfied if I achieved anything significant even in that apparently limited task.

This measure of benefits should also be capable of wide application and not specific to particular conditions, or to the inputs of particular services; otherwise it will be of severely restricted value. This means that it has to refer to a context in which the client's state can be assessed in a fairly general manner, and it leads, inexorably, to an approach based on the general *social* functioning of the client, i.e. his or her ability to conduct the essentials of everyday living free of pain. This goes well beyond measurement of blood pressure, pulse rate, etc., and also beyond the identification of conditions (e.g. pneumonia, pregnancy, arthritis), and even beyond the noting of physical disabilities (missing index finger, blind in one eye, loss of one leg below the knee), because it rests on the question: 'To what extent is this individual unable to carry out painlessly the activities which the community would expect individuals of that age and sex normally to be able to carry out?'

The final desideratum is that the measure should be capable of being made operational, which implies that it must be capable of routine application and use, which in turn implies that it must not make inordinate intellectual demands, nor intolerable demands in time and energy, upon those responsible for collecting and processing the information. Although high-powered research and development work may be required to test it out in the initial phase, it should be designed to run on low-powered inputs in the long run.

III. A SOLUTION IN PRINCIPLE

The basic elements in the proposed scheme are:

(*a*) a set of descriptive categories concerned with the client's state in terms of pain-free social functioning;

(*b*) a relative evaluation process that converts these states into index points;

(*c*) an absolute valuation of points in money terms.

In this section the general properties of each element will be described, before presenting a brief account of some empirical work designed to help us with element (*a*).

If we are to build up an index of health (or, in this case, of ill-health), we need to measure both intensity and duration. 'Intensity' is here interpreted as having two dimensions, 'pain' and 'restriction of activity'. The first step would be, therefore, to experiment with simple standardized descriptions of painfulness and of the extent to which activity is restricted, to see if there is any consensus among medical personnel as to how painful and how restricting particular conditions are, using these descriptive categories. The initial descriptive stage may be represented as in Fig. 18.1 below.

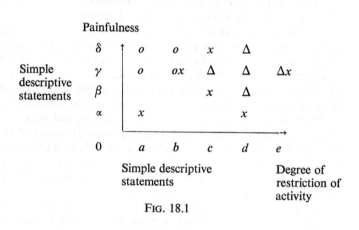

FIG. 18.1

α, β, γ and δ are simple descriptive statements concerned with painfulness (such as 'mildly uncomfortable', 'very comfortable', 'extremely painful', etc.). *a*, *b*, *c*, *d* and *e* are simple descriptive statements concerned with restriction of activity (such as light work only, confined to house and immediate vicinity, confined to house, confined to bedroom, confined to bed, etc.). The symbols *o*, *x* and Δ each refer to different medical conditions. Each *o* plotted on Fig. 18.1 represents a different expert's assessment of the most appropriate description of the effect of that condition (e.g. one says, *a*, δ, another says *a*, γ, another says *b*, δ, and yet another *b*, γ). Similarly, each *x* and each Δ represent corresponding judgments by various experts of the most appropriate descriptions of each of those conditions. If there is any consistency in these judgments (as there is to *o* and Δ in the example in Appendix B), some 'norm' will be indicated as the standard description for that condition; where no consensus exists (as with *x* in the example) it is likely that the condition under study needs to be more closely specified.

However, supposing that we had each condition clearly ascribed to a pain category (α, β, γ, etc.) and a restricted-activity category (*a*, *b*, *c*, etc.), we should now need to establish the trade-off between them (e.g. is the combination *γa* better or worse than the combination *βc*?). This pairwise comparison is, essentially, a *social* judgment and should be recognized as such, but may have to be made in practice by medical people. This first evaluative step is set out diagrammatically in Fig. 18.2, where the lines are embryonic indifference curves, and it is desirable to be as 'close' to zero as possible.

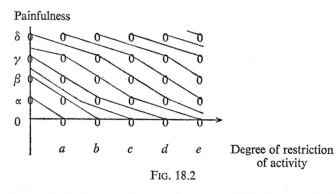

FIG. 18.2

In the example shown, the combinations (β, 0), (α, *a*) and (0, *b*) are equivalent to each other, but better than (γ, 0) and (0, *c*) which are equivalent to each other). Those, in turn, are better than the next group of equivalents (β, *a*), (α, *b*) and (0, *d*), and so on.

Despite the fact that describing the intensity of pain is notoriously difficult, and that interpersonal comparisons are bound to be rather arbitrary, medical personnel can and do make such comparisons between stages and classes of condition, and such comparisons already have to be assimilated into judgments about 'acceptable' degrees of physical disability and pain at the diagnostic and therapeutic level when determining courses of treatment. It is, therefore, suggested that it should be possible to move to the second (partial evaluative) stage and construct, say, a 10-point scale of intensity of ill-health along the following lines:

0 = normal
1 = able to carry out normal activities, but with some pain or discomfort
2 = restricted to light activities only, but with little pain or discomfort

  3–7 = various intermediate categories reflecting various degrees of pain and/or restriction of activity
    8 = conscious, but in great pain and activity severely restricted
    9 = unconscious
  10 = dead

Since it is intended to use these numbers as *weights*, and not simply as *rankings*, it is important to stress that society's judgments concerning the relative importance of avoiding one state rather than another are represented by the actual numbers attached to each respectively, e.g. state 2 is *twice as bad* as state 1, and state 10 is ten times as bad. This implication must not be shirked, and it must be regarded as a statement about *health policy* (and is to be made by whoever is entrusted with that responsibility, e.g. the politicians), and not a technical statement about *medical condition*.[1] In terms of Fig. 18.2, this would be represented by attaching index numbers to each of the contour lines.

As to duration, this will be based on the outcome of scientific investigations, cast in statistical terms. For instance, recovery from a particular disease will follow one time path (incorporating both intensity and duration) in 90 per cent of the cases, another in a further 9 per cent, and yet another in the remaining 1 per cent. Chronic cases where no (or little) improvement in intensity is to be expected will have a duration equal to the life expectancy of that class of individual, and the duration of the 'gain' from postponing death where successful treatment is possible will be similarly measured. A 'successful' treatment is *not only* one which reduces intensity and duration but could also be one that reduces intensity without affecting duration, or vice versa; or even that increases one at the expense of the other, provided the net outcome is to *reduce* the index number (a product of intensity *and* duration). The important sources of information here are the medical statisticians, since it is purely empirical information that is required at this stage in the process.

Fig. 18.3 illustrates how this would work for any particular condition. The diagram starts at a point of time, 0, when the condition in question is diagnosed. In the illustrative example the first two weeks are spent in further observation, decision as to appropriate treatment, and waiting for therapeutic facilities to become available. The prognosis without treatment (or with the best treatment other than that under consideration) is represented by the broken line, and may be described as a steady deterioration from

    [1] M. Magdelaine, A. A. Mizrahi and G. Rösch, 'Un Indicateur de la morbidité appliqué aux données d'une enquête sur la consommation médicale', *Consommation*, no. 2 (1967), in their work on a similar indicator, fail to make this clear.

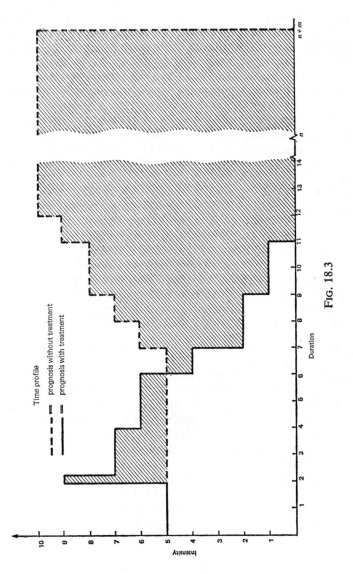

FIG. 18.3

approximately week 7 until death in week 12. This would be the standard prediction for this class of case. The average expectation of life for a person of that age/sex, etc., is represented as $n+m$, which may be rather large if necessary (e.g. 50 years). The prognosis with treatment is represented by the solid line, and may be described as two weeks of severe restriction of activity (in the pre-operative, operative and immediate post-operative phases), plus possibly considerable pain, with a steady improvement in condition during the ensuing three weeks, a convalescent phase from weeks 7 to 9, and a further two weeks taking it easy in the normal environment, after which the patient is completely normal (as far as this condition is concerned).

The index *score* (representing the 'effectiveness' of this treatment) would be the area lightly cross-hatched *minus* the area heavily cross-hatched, obviously including in the former the interval omitted in the horizontal scale as drawn. This particular example would, obviously, be a highly effective treatment if applied to people with long life expectancy, and less so the shorter life expectancy. Both the time profiles used would be derived from statistical analyses of clinical results, or on experimental data if the former were lacking. It is up to the medical statistician to provide these key data. A further sophistication which could be introduced, if necessary, would be to apply a discounting factor which would give less weight to future states of health compared with present states, and, hence, reflect the greater weight which people seem to attach to the 'here and now' rather than to more distant prospects.

Certain features of this sytem are noteworthy:

(a) It enables preventive as well as therapeutic activities to be incorporated.

(b) Although much more difficult in practice, in principle it can embrace mental illness.

(c) It treats one week of suffering at any particular intensity level as being equally undesirable irrespective of the identity of the patient. Other distributional assumptions are possible in principle, but would make the analysis much more complicated.[1]

(d) It relates only to patients, and does not include infectivity, or the pain and suffering caused to others by the patient's condition. Neither of these shortcomings are insuperable in principle, but as a practical matter they will be difficult to overcome in the near future.

(e) The *satisfaction* felt by patients themselves (or their friends and relatives) is not regarded as an independent consideration in this formulation, and to do so would raise such enormous

---

[1] This is a particular manifestation of a more general problem in compiling social indicators, which is that we may not wish to count each individual on a one-for-one basis when certain people register poor readings on many different indicators, e.g. health, education, crime, poverty.

difficulties for any health indicator that the matter is mentioned here only so that it is not lost sight of.

The primary purpose of such an indicator is to facilitate cost-effectiveness studies, by providing a quantification of the purely humanitarian benefits to be used in conjunction with economic costs (and benefits) in order to improve the effectiveness of health services in the face of severe resource limitations. But it could also generate, as a by-product, improved indicators of the state of (ill) health of a community if used as part of the basic information matrix in a national survey of the state of health of the community.[1] If successful, this would fill an important gap in our present knowledge, for it would include cases where people had not presented themselves for treatment, or where those giving treatment were unaware of the patient's condition between episodes of treatment.

This leaves us with the final step, which is attaching money values to index points. There are various ways of approaching this thorny issue. The one least likely to raise strong emotional objections is simply to calculate the *implied* values placed on marginal points by exisiting allocations of resources,[2] and to argue that if there are discrepancies, and the relative points values are right, then resources should be shifted from activities yielding high cost points at the margin to those where marginal points are relatively cheap. A more direct method has been used in the field of crime, by getting respondents of vaiious kinds to say how serious they thought one crime was relative to another, from which an index of crime seriousness was constructed.[3] Once people get used to this kind of discourse, one could then pose the question: 'Are these marginal points values of the right order of magnitude relative to other things?' It might

[1] For a brief description and methodological critique of such surveys, see Forrest E. Linder, 'National Health Interview Surveys', in W.H.O., *Trends in the Study of Morbidity and Mortality*, Public Health Papers No. 27 (Geneva, 1965). It may be that the 'General Household Survey' will become a suitable vehicle for such an investigation in the U.K.; see C. A. Moser, 'Some General Developments in Social Statistics', *Social Trends*, no. 1 (London: H.M.S.O., 1970) pp. 7–11.

[2] e.g. John Hawgood and Richard Morley, 'Inverse Linear Programming as a Means of Estimating Librarians' Benefit Criteria' (Durham Univ., 1969); subsequently applied to health services by A. M. D. Porter, 'Planning Maternity Care', unpublished M.Phil. thesis (Univ. of Durham).

[3] See T. Sellin and M. E. Wolfgang, *The Measurement of Delinquency* (New York: Wiley, 1964), and M. L. Chambers (Univ. of Lancaster), 'Construction of a Utility Function for a Police Force', paper presented to an R.E.S. Specialist Conference on Decision Analysis, Lancaster (Jan 1973). This has been carried a stage further to derive an actual tariff of money values by D. C. Shoup and S. L. Mehay, *Program Budgeting for Urban Police Services* (Institute of Government and Public Affairs, Univ. of California at Los Angeles, 1971).

be possible to help inform such judgments better by pointing out the kinds of awards which the community regards as fair if someone is moved from health state to health state for a given duration through no fault of his own,[1] and compare this with the sums the community seems willing to devote to preventing similar changes from happening by the provision of health care. Before long, we may even reach a stage when some bold politician[2] will have the nerve to put the issue to his constituents in these terms, e.g. 'If elected, my policy will be based on a 5 per cent increase in the value of a health point' (i.e. 'I think we ought to be prepared to devote an extra 5 per cent of the community's resources to improving health by one unit at the margins'). This 'price' thus becomes a 'cut-off' point for decentralized resource allocation decisions in health care systems, and one which will force decision-makers to pay regard both to medical effectiveness (expected points score) and social valuations (as indicated by the 'price' of a point).

IV. WHERE SHOULD WE START?

I am not so crazy as to imagine that by this time next year (or even in ten years time) we could have the provision of health care rationalized in this way, even if all the parties whose cooperation is necessary were sold on the idea, so we need to face the problem of research priorities and testing during the developmental learning phase. I am convinced that the major stumbling-block at present is the absence of any widely used standardized descriptive categories of social functioning,[3] and without these we cannot get off first base,

---

[1] Some preliminary analysis of this kind has been done for the U.K. by Rachel Rosser and Vincent Watts, 'The Measurement of Hospital Output', paper presented to the O.R. Society Conference, Lancaster (Sep 1971). It is likely that more will be undertaken as a result of an S.S.R.C.-financed project on 'The Cost of Human Impairment' under D. S. Lees at Nottingham University, and the recent setting-up of a Royal Commission on Civil Liability and Compensation for Personal Injury.

[2] So far we have at least reached the stage where the Minister responsible for road investment is willing to publicize the sum he uses in investment appraisals as the value of avoiding fatal accidents: in 1968 it was £8,800, of which £3,800 represented tangible costs (including loss of output) and £5,000 an allowance for 'warm-blooded' costs (pain, grief, suffering, etc.). See *Annual Reports of the Road Research Laboratory* (London: H.M.S.O.).

[3] There are plenty of special-purpose ones, many of which do not even get into the literature. A few of the published ones which seem capable of wider application are: Jessie Garrard and A. E. Bennett, 'A Validated Interview Schedule for Use in Population Surveys of Chronic Disease and Disability', *British Journal of Preventive and Social Medicine*, xxv (1971); E. M. Gruenberg and S. Brandon, 'Measurement of the Incidence of Chronic Severe Social Breakdown', *Millbank Memorial Fund Quarterly*, xliv (1966); M. Hamilton, 'A Rating Scale

so I have become a major advocate (and a minor organizer) of *longitudinal* surveys[1] of clients, these surveys needing to be broad in coverage both as regards the clients' conditions and the health care agencies treating them.

For tactical reasons, the care of the elderly has been selected as the test area, covering hospitals, general practitioners, welfare homes, domiciliary support, etc., in both urban and rural areas of England and Wales. In order not to try to clear too many hurdles at once, no index is being calculated, so we are operating at the level of Fig. 18.1 above. This does not, however, preclude individual agencies from supplying their own relative valuations of client states if they wish, and it will give them a set of categories across which they can sensibly do so. Nor does it preclude statistical analysis of the results designed to see what transitions from state to state are associated (*ceteris paribus*) with the various treatment modes, so that one can begin to build up the basis for prognoses along the lines of Fig. 18.3, though in several (incommensurable) dimensions rather than in the common currency of 'health points'.

In our study, client state has three dimensions (physical mobility, capacity for self-care and mental state), each of which is ranked on a four-point scale, so that there are 4^3 ($=64$) logically possible different states. Clients are to reassessed at three-monthly intervals, so that (if we add the state 'dead' to those already mentioned) it will be possible to compile a 64×65 matrix of 'transitions', which can be repeated (and combined) at three-month intervals to give three-month, six-month, nine-month, twelve-month, etc., transitions. The fundamental research task will be to try to identify (from a sizeable package of background information on clients, which is also being collected at each assessment) what statistically significant associations exist between the different transitions experienced by people starting in the same state and the different treatment modes provided by the health care system. But a more immediately important operational payoff may well be the focusing of routine records on

for Depression', *Journal of Neurology and Psychiatry*, XXIII (1960); A. I. Harris, *Handicapped and Impaired in Great Britain* (London: H.M.S.O., 1971); B. Isaacs and F. A. Walkley, 'The Assessment of the Mental State of Elderly Hospital Patients Using a Simple Questionnaire', *American Journal of Psychiatry*, CXX (1963); S. Katz *et al.*, 'Studies of Illness in the Aged: The Index of Independence in Activities of Daily Living', *Journal of the American Medical Association*, CLXXXV (1963); J. Tunstall, *Old and Alone* (London: Routledge & Kegan Paul, 1966).

[1] These are not unusual in the field of child care, but much rarer elsewhere. See W. D. Wall and H. L. Williams, *Longitudinal Studies and the Social Sciences*, S.S.R.C. Reviews of Current Research (London: Heinemann, 1972).

client states and a more general dissemination and testing of category systems of this kind (see appendix for a brief outline of the contents of schedule to be used).

This project will be at the pilot stage (with some 500 test observations) during 1973 and, if no fatal flaws emerge, will run on a fairly large scale (10,000 or so observations) during 1974 and 1975. But it will still be but a beginning in the task ahead, because it still will not include any agreed set of index weights across client states (still less their evaluation in money terms), nor will it provide detailed knowledge of production functions but only broad indicators of the relative effectiveness for one client group of whole packages of care, and it is not concerned with the measurement of costs. However, it is focused on the appropriate primal element in the problem, and is the first stage of a carefully mapped escape route from the intellectually imprisoning confines of the measures of workload and throughput (and even input) which too often are pressed into service as measures of the effectiveness of health care systems.

V. CONCLUDING OBSERVATIONS

No one step in this 'escape route' seems infeasible, though when viewed *in toto* the whole programme may appear a daunting task. Fortunately, economists need not (and, indeed, should not) play a central role in every phase of the work, though I think it would be extremely valuable if the work undertaken by others were well informed as to the data requirements and underlying philosophy of the economists' optimizing models of health care systems, and it may well be that this can only be achieved by having economists involved in an advisory way with work which they (and others) may not regard as their own particular specialty.

I am fortified in this view by the great dangers I see in the opposite course (which is that economists concentrate entirely on the estimation of costs and 'economic benefits'), because this, unfortunately, taints us with the stigma of a 'commercial' or 'G.N.P.'-oriented approach to health care systems,[1] and while I should be the last to deny that G.N.P. considerations are relevant, I should not wish anyone to think that I believed them to be predominant. It seems, therefore, to be extremely important that we demonstrate our practical concern for health service effectiveness in broader terms than these, and the plan of work set out in this paper is designed to do precisely that.

[1] See, for instance, A. H. Packer, 'Applying Cost Effectiveness Concepts to the Community Health System', *Operations Research*, xvi, 2 (1968) 227–53.

APPENDIX

OUTLINE CONTENTS OF ASSESSMENT SCHEDULE AND BACKGROUND INFORMATION CONCERNING CARE OF THE ELDERLY

A. ASSESSMENT SCHEDULE

The assessment schedule has three divisions concerned with mobility, capacity for self-care and mental state. The factors considered in each of the divisions are as follows:

(1) *Mobility*
- (*a*) Ability to get in and out of bed and/or chair.
- (*b*) Ability to negotiate a level surface.
- (*c*) Ability to climb stairs.
- (*d*) Ability to walk outdoors.

(2) *Capacity for Self-Care*
- (*a*) Ability to feed self.
- (*b*) Ability to dress self.
- (*c*) Ability to wash self.
- (*d*) Ability to make a hot drink.
- (*e*) Ability to cook a meal.
- (*f*) Ability to light a fire.
- (*g*) Ability to shop.
- (*h*) Whether or not continent.

(3) *Mental State*
- (*a*) Intellectual processes – memory, orientation of person and place.
- (*b*) Loneliness and desolation.
- (*c*) Depression.
- (*d*) Boredom.
- (*e*) Motivation towards independence.
- (*f*) Anxiety.
- (*g*) Anti-social or self-harming behaviour.

Care has to be taken in this division to distinguish general feelings of mood from pathological mental disorders which are to be recorded in the background information.

B. BACKGROUND INFORMATION

(1) *Personal and Socio-economic Status*
- (*a*) Age.
- (*b*) Sex.
- (*c*) Marital status.
- (*d*) Occupation or previous occupation of self or spouse.
- (*e*) Income.

(2) *Domestic Environment*
    (*a*) Type of house.
    (*b*) Facilities, e.g. hot water, location of toilet, bath, etc.⎫
    (*c*) Shared or sole use of accommodation.   ⎬ for people
    (*d*) Warden or other people officially in attendance.   living in
    (*e*) Presence of alarm system.   ⎭ community
    (*f*) Residential or nursing home:
        public or private
        type of home
        facilities available
    (*g*) Hospital ward:
        general, medical or surgical
        geriatric – assessment or
        rehabilitative
        – continuing care
        psychiatric.

(3) *Medical Condition*
Based on broad systematic classes, e.g.
Injuries or diseases of:
    Cardiovascular system
    Locomotor system
    Central nervous system.

(4) *Social Contacts*
    (*a*) Visits received from
        relatives
        friends and neighbours
        tradesmen, etc.
    (*b*) Visits made to
        relatives
        friends and neighbours.
    (*c*) Casual visits to
        social clubs
        shops
        church, etc.
    (*d*) Other 'non-face-to-face' contacts, e.g.
        telephone calls
        letters.
    (*e*) Interest in current affairs – newspapers, radio, TV.
    (*f*) Use of spare time.

(5) *Use of Services*
Use of local authority, hospital, general practitioners, etc., and
voluntary services.

19 Health Indicators and Health Systems Analysis

Émile Lévy

UNIVERSITÉ DE PARIS–DAUPHINE

The main points raised in this paper are:
The solution proposed by a number of authors, i.e. a final result indicator expressed as a scale with several degrees, is not practical in the short run.
It is not adequate to data at hand, and it presents the risk that useful information might be lost.
The health state is a very complex phenomenon. Even a superficial system analysis indicates that it presents four aspects:
(a) the vulnerability aspect (exposure to risk factors like disease);
(b) the morbidity aspect, itself being divided into several expressions depending on the agent (subjective, diagnostic or objective morbidity);
(c) the protection aspect (by medical services and social insurance);
(d) the result aspect (physical and mental validity, duration of life).
The problem remains that the information we possess is expressive, in the best case, of only one of these aspects.
Now, it is just as dangerous to highlight one of these to express the health status as it is to aggregate all of them because of weighting problems revealed.
The solution suggested here is a linked set of data on these four aspects, which has to be reordered in relation to each specific problem (priorities, choice of techniques, etc.).

I. INTRODUCTION

The problem of the formulation of a set of social indicators, in the sense of indicators of well-being, has been raised vigorously in all advanced societies for several years now. This undertaking is strongly encouraged by all international organizations (the U.N.,

O.E.C.D., the European Communities, etc.), for the subject of health always figures prominently among the themes of research on social indicators. That is, although the list of social preoccupations varies, in part, depending on the period or the country involved, preoccupation with the state of health itself is a constant that nobody would dream of questioning. One might even say that health indicators are often taken as a preferred example of social indicators.

At least two reasons may be given for this exemplary situation: on the one hand, the field of health has the obvious advantage of being able to derive its support from a special system of production and distribution of care; on the other, the data regarding life expectancy at birth and, to a lesser degree, mortality rates (particularly infant mortality rates) have seemed, for a long time, to acquire the rank of synthetic 'indicators' of the state of public health.

Nevertheless, as the specialists realize, the situation in this area is far from being favorable as one might think.

In fact, it seems clear that the data on mortality in advanced societies are far from expressing the totality of health problems – especially since the improvements in life expectancy have become slight, or even non-existent, and since certain types of morbidity (the chronic degenerative kind) play an ever-increasing role here.

On the other hand, the relationships between the state of health and the system for producing and distributing care are rather obscure, and the 'product' of this system is also hardly, or poorly, defined in terms of final results. Hence, a certain degree of confusion reigns at the level of the indicators proposed or utilized by planners, where, along with the above-mentioned factors, there can be found the indiscriminate admixture of the number of doctors per patient, the number of beds per patient, per capita medical expenditures, etc.

We should like, therefore, to devote ourselves, in this paper, to greater lucidity in the search for health indicators, following upon several others who have preceded us[1] and whose papers will be discussed. The ideas contained in this paper are based on research done a year ago for the French Commissariat Général du Plan, and the French situation is, obviously, our point of reference.

II. SOME PRELIMINARY CONSIDERATIONS

Before discussing the principles of this research, it is not at all

[1] In particular, see the list of papers cited by B. Morando, 'De Certains Travaux Relatifs aux Indicateurs de Santé', *Bulletin de l'INSERM*, no. 2 (1968) and the majority of references which follow in our text.

pointless to recall the four types of questions that are asked in advance of any investigation of health indicators.

(1) *Indicators of Health, or Indicators of the State of Health?*

Actually, the terminology is ambiguous with respect to what one is studying. Sometimes it seems certain that one wants to express the real 'state' of health of a population, in terms of a final result, and of an abstraction of the factors that determine or explain it; at other times, it seems that one is particularly anxious to assign preeminence to the indicators of the effectiveness of the system for producing and distributing care; and at still other times, it seems that any quantitative data, whether physical or financial, relating to the area of health, might be considered as an indicator of health in the broad and vague sense of the term.

In the first instance, one is dealing with indicators of health; in the second, one is dealing with indicators of the functioning of the health system.

If we can assert, when faced with this choice, that we must place greater emphasis on the indicators of the *state* of health, one of our main methodological hypotheses has to derive from the fact that we cannot neglect, *a priori*, the indicators of the system, to the extent that they might throw light on the significance of the indicators of the state.

(2) *Indicators of Health for Whom?*

The interested groups are at least three in number: public opinion, administrators and planners, and the doctors themselves. And it seems probable that the needs of each are not all the same.

It has been maintained[1] that it was necessary to seek a synthetic indicator that was simple and obvious for the sake of public opinion and for the needs of political debate; to throw light upon the course of social progress and to bring out the actions of society which accompany economic growth or reflect upon it in the long run, from that point of view.

And it is true that one finds it especially difficult to discuss health, and that statistics generally put out by the press or by politicians are numerous, confused, and hard for the average citizen to decipher.

It is also true that administrators and planners need indicators which go beyond the simple instrument panel that makes it possible to trace the evolution of the state of public health. For their purposes, useful indicators are those which allow them to reintegrate

---

[1] R. E. Bickner, 'Measurements and Indices of Health', in *Methodology of Identifying, Measuring and Evaluating Outcomes of Health Service Programs, Systems and Subsystems*, Conference Series, H.E.W., P.H.S., H.S.M.H.A.

health within its social context, to identify the impact of the system of production and distribution of care, to clarify the choices and, ultimately, to evolve sanitary planning which goes beyond medical and charitable institutions.

As for the doctors, they, in particular, need indicators for measuring the effectiveness of their activity. That is, the scale of analysis should also vary, since, for the latter, the need for measurement of effectiveness occurs at the level of their specific actions, and they also need to clarify the choice which they make among alternative therapies for a given ailment. Therefore, much more refined indicators than those intended for planners are required for doctors.

But from the fact that the needs for indicators differ it would be impossible to deduce that:

(*a*) the problem of formulating a synthetic indicator of the state of health is of no interest to planners or the medical profession: or

(*b*) that the global indicator and specific indicators must be entirely independent of each other. On the contrary, it would be more satisfactory if there existed an interconnection among them, even if it were particularly difficult to conceive of.

(3) *Why Health Indicators?*

One aspect of this problem was just touched upon, when we mentioned the types of special needs of the three categories of users.

But even if one were to limit the problem of needs to those of the planner, it is still not so easy to clarify the goals one strives for in the search for a health indicator.

One could be dealing with an apparently modest goal, that of *recognizing* a past and/or present situation. This is the case when one poses questions like those in the draft American Social Report:[1] how far have we come in the state of public health? And, in the light of this objective, one could ask whether life expectancy, mortality rates, morbidity rates, etc., correctly express the phenomenon under study in its entirety and in its evolution. It is the perspective of an 'instrument panel' to which we have already alluded, and which harmonizes, naturally, with the desire for worthwhile settings which function as alarm signals or 'blinking' lights.

At an even higher level of exigencies, one might wish to establish indicators that would allow us not only to recognize a situation or watch an evolution, but even to *grasp* its reasons, the factors in it, and to measure their respective impacts. This presupposes a more

---

[1] *Towards a Social Report* (Washington, D.C.: U.S. Department of Health, Education and Welfare, 1969).

advanced effort at analysis, in order to unravel the maze of complex interrelations.

At the most ambitious level, one finds the orientation which consists of seeking a system of indicators to serve as a basis for *making decisions*, as in a model for simulation, for example, which permits one, over a period of time, to predict consequences of a decision, or of a set of proposed measures, on the state of health of a population.

But one must admit that it is unrealistic to place oneself at this level of ambition in the area of health economy. For it is obvious that those sectors in which one has available an adequate amount of information (notably epidemiological information) and a correct understanding of the relationships in order to formulate such models are relatively few in number. It is only for a few pathologies that we know the natural history and the effectiveness of various possible techniques for diagnosis, treatment or prevention. And we fear that it will be a long time yet before we will be able to extend this type of study to all phenomena of illness and health.

There is always a great temptation to aim for a coherent set of indicators that would have a descriptive, explicative, prospective and decision-making value, all at the same time. And certainly, all these objectives are related. But, from an operational standpoint, it remains no less necessary to distinguish among them, lest one risk missing them altogether. Even from the planner's point of view alone, in which I decided to place myself here, the myth of a system of health indicators 'good for everything' seems dangerous and inadequate. But these are not the same indicators that would be useful for determining objectives or priorities, for formulating programs of action (and then for checking the adequacy of the means to the ends) and for ultimately evaluating the result of these actions. Considerations of economic and social costs of illnesses and financial indicators, in particular, do not play the same role at all these levels.

(4) *Health Indicators – How?*

The problem we should like to raise here is common to all research on social indicators. One always finds a distinction between two types of approaches: an 'ascendant' and statistical-empirical one that consists in starting with existing information, screening it with respect to established criteria,[1] and retaining those data that have the desired degree of significance to express, directly or indirectly, the state of a public's health; and a 'descendant' one, that starts out

---

[1] For example, cf. a note by the Commissariat Général du Plan Français, 27 July 1969, which defines several criteria: sensitivity, fidelity, unequivocal meaning, and synthetic nature of social indicators.

by defining the phenomenon to be measured *a priori* (say, a scale of states of health), then seeks out the types of information it needs for this purpose, and eventually recommends the adoption of systems for collecting new information, if it has found gaps in its earlier results.

In the first case, which lies within a short-term operational perspective, one will satisfy oneself with expressing some data deemed to be significant within the scope of a coherent scheme that is to serve as a 'reading frame' for a complex social reality. In the second case, the approach starts out by being prejudiced in the direction of the theoretical level, and can hope to end up with an integrated system of quantified information only after a moderate or a long period of time.

Actually, these two approaches are always used in conjunction, and the satisfactory solution is one that aims to make the combination work. But it is apparent that the proportions of them have differed markedly in studies undertaken in recent years.

At the conclusion of these preliminary considerations, at least one essential conclusion imposes itself on those investigating the matter of health indicators, namely: quantitative information regarding health becomes 'indicators' only when one has defined the question or questions one is actually asking oneself. The notion of an indicator is always a relative one, always necessarily finalized, and meaningful only within a specific frame of reference and with regard to one specific function.

III. THE CRITICAL RESULTS OF PREVIOUS WORK ON HEALTH INDICATORS

It is certainly impossible to take account of all the studies that have been made on this problem; one can select only a few that illustrate certain of the methodological choices presented above and collect the results of these choices.

Particularly in regard to the last methodological option, one distinguishes two great series of studies: the empirical-statistical, on the one hand, and on the other, the *a priori* searches for indicators of the level of health.

(1) *Empirical-Statistical Attempts*

The property common to all such attempts has to do with the fact that one is attempting to make optimum use of existing information to express the health phenomena that characterize a population. Under this common constraint, the approaches differ, depending on whether one intends simply to interrelate these data or to combine them.

(i) *Interrelation of the data within an over-all format.* A significant piece of research using this approach is that of Delors in his paper on social indicators,[1] oriented towards the second theme, protection of health.

After a general presentation of this theme, wherein he mainly defines the different aspects of morbidity, he distinguishes the problem of measuring the level of health from that of establishing the characteristics of the health system.

Regarding the former problem, he uses three indicators to state it: life expectancy at birth as a synthetic indicator; infant mortality rates as being 'directly linked with the technical effectiveness of care'; and the main causes of death as expressing the structure of morbidity and, thus, the level of development of society.

Regarding the latter problem, he characterizes it by classical indicators which he terms 'measures': the number of hospital beds, the number of visits (to the hospital or the doctor), total per capita density of doctors and paramedics, etc.[2]

As he notes, aside from the fact that certain data might be contested in the appraisals to which they give rise (infant mortality and causes of death, in particular), the effort at interrelating these data is rather slight and the format underlying the list of indicators is rather well worn. Generally speaking, the connection between 'measuring' indicators and 'result' indicators is not certain, and one is usually dealing with a simple juxtaposition. This line-up of numerical data is not fruitless, however, for it is nonetheless, the first attempt from which a certain picture emerges, however nebulous and difficult it may be to interpret the French medical situation and its recent evolution.

(ii) *Assembling the data in a synthetic indicator.* I shall be referring in this section, to three illustrations of this process: Chiang's studies,[3] those by the Division of Indian Health, U.S Department of Health,[4] and the Olson Report.[5]

More directly centered on the problem of measuring the result and thus, the state of health, these studies have all chosen time as the common denominator of the data which they assemble.

[1] J. Delors, *Les Indicateurs Sociaux* (Paris: Éditions SEDEIS, 1971).

[2] Ibid., pp. 27–43.

[3] C. L. Chiang, 'An Index of Health: Mathematical Models', N.C.H.S., 2nd series, no. 5 (1965).

[4] Division of Indian Health, 'Principles of Program Packaging in the Division of Indian Health' (Silver Springs, Md., 15 Jan 1966).

[5] *Towards a Social Report*, op. cit.

For Chiang it is a matter of expressing per annum, say, the time lost by the population owing to morbidity and mortality, in order to deduce the mean period of health.

In the Olson Report, the famous indicator – life expectancy, excluding confinement to bed – is based on a line of thinking very similar to the above, since he is dealing with an estimate of life expectancy in good health, the latter being defined by the fact of not being in bed (or deceased).

Finally, we have the *Q* indicator of the Division of Indian Health, which is really a method for determining priorities; it is expressed for each ailment in terms of the total number of days lost because of sickness, according to the type of care received and the mortality ratio, taking into account the varying figures for productivity according to age level.

In each case the following objections may be raised:

(*a*) that health cannot be reduced simply to the absence of sickness or of death;

(*b*) that the phenomena taken as a criterion for sickness are debatable (time in bed, reduced activity, etc.);

(*c*) that the weighted coefficients are either non-existent or entirely arbitrary:

(*d*) that the respective impact of socio-economic conditions and of the system of production and distribution of care does not appear there.

(2) '*A priori' Searches for Indicators of the Level of Health*. The dominant idea in the second group is the rejection of diagnostic categories, or rather, the desire to go beyond counting maladies as a basis for the health indicator, Rather, one will discuss manifestations or consequences – both at the level of the individual and at the level of society – of different ailments, instead of an account of the ailments themselves. Thus, there appears here the idea of a scale, to be formulated and tested, of different levels of health at which different groups of the population are found.

But sometimes the indicator is one-dimensional, while at others it is two- or three-dimensional.

(i) *The one-dimensional indicator*. Most of the attempts belonging to this group are characterized by:

(*a*) The notion that the only *common denominator* of the state of health that goes beyond the notions of morbidity and mortality other than time is the *level of validity*. Whether one expresses this in terms of 'functional sufficiency', as Sanders has done,[1] or as capacity or incapacity, as Sullivan has done,[2] or even as 'independence in everyday life', as Katz *et al.* have have done,[3] it is still the same principle one is dealing with; that is, that the scale of different levels of validity could be expressive of the global state of health of individuals and of groups.

(*b*) The second characteristic of these propositions is that in the two first cases, at least after the methodological principles of these indicators have been posed, no calculation over an extended base has resulted.

In other words, aside from any intrinsic difficulty in establishing the indicator based on this concept, one might seriously doubt whether in most countries credible statistical elements exist that might permit one to calculate it. And if reference is made to data on absenteeism in business or to working days compensated because of illness, provided such exist,[4] it seems likely that what one might be measuring with such data would be mostly a reflection of specific institutions (social security) or of relationships between individuals and their work, rather than the state of their health itself. Thus, only direct surveys of samples of individuals, which are a major task, would permit one first to test and then to calculate this indicator regularly. Moreover, this indicator would remain quite normative (what are the normal functions of an individual at a given age?) and, despite its 'unifying' quality, it could not express all aspects of the state of health. Furthermore, this is the reason why indicators have been proposed that take account of several dimensions.

(ii) *The multi-dimensional indicator.* In recent years, three studies have been made in France, Great Britain and the United States, in directions that definitely converge.

CREDOC (Centre de Recherches et de Documentation sur la Consommation) has elaborated a so-called indicator of morbidity on the basis of its studies of medical consumption[5] in three dimen-

---

[1] B. S. Sanders, 'Measuring Community Health Levels', *American Journal of Public Health*, LIV, 7 (1964).

[2] D. F. Sullivan, 'Conceptual Problems in Developing an Index of Health', *Vital and Health Statistics*, 2nd Series, no. 17 (May 1966).

[3] S. Katz *et al.*, 'Studies of Illness in the Aged', *Journal of the American Medical Association*, CLXXXV (1963).

[4] Which is not the case, particularly in France, where workdays lost owing to sickness and paid for by social security are not broken down by causes.

[5] M. Magdelaine, A. A. Mizrahi and G. Rösch, 'Un Indicateur de la Morbiditié Appliqué aux Données d'une Enquête sur la Consommation Médicale', *Consommation*, no. 3 (1967); auf *Enquête Pilote 1965–66 sur les Soins Médicaux*, fasc. 4: 'Un Indicateur de Morbidité: Analyse des Risques Vitaux et d'Incapacité (CREDOC, 1971).

sions, and then in two. In its first version, this involved combining the following into a six-degree (level) scale:

(a) invalidism, or consequences of the pathological state on living conditions (inconvenience, confinement to bed, work stoppage);

(b) risk of dying;

(c) duration of the illness (or its pattern of development).

All these dimensions are expressed in terms of prognose for the future made on the last day of the survey, and the synthesis of this is done in six degrees of morbidity.

In the second version, CREDOC's indicator combines only two dimensions:

(a) the vital risk (calculated in five classes of ratios from no negative prognosis to a surely bad prognosis);

(b) the risk of incapacitation (calculated in eight classes of ratios, from no incapacity to permanent confinement in bed or a grave condition).

A doctor was the one who, on the basis of the totality of information and the list of afflictions, placed each person in the appropriate class. These two dimensions, then, remain distinct, and the classification serves mainly to establish proportional connections among them, with the number of ailments or the evolution of treatments or distributions as related to geography, age, etc.

In the same spirit, Culyer, Lavers and Williams in a recent article,[1] recommended a two-dimensional health indicator, these dimensions being intensity and duration of illness, with intensity having two components, namely the degree of suffering and the degree of restriction from activity. Te express intensity, the authors propose to establish, on the basis of expert judgments, some kind of indifference curves connecting the two components; these curves would be equivalent to a scale of intensity of illness in a certain number of degrees (ten, for example).

As for the duration, it would be a matter of expressing this for each ailment as a function of observations by the medical profession.

In these two dimensions, the indicator could serve as a basis for cost-effectiveness studies (by comparing a profile of the evolution of the illness under a given treatment with the profile of spontaneous evolution), well as expressing the state of public health based on data collected in surveys of health carried out directly among the population.

[1] A. J. Culyer, R. S. Lavers and A. Williams, 'Social Indicators: Health', *Social Trends*, no. 2 (1971).

Finally, in the case of Fanshel and Bush,[1] if the concept of activity versus inactivity appears to be essential for establishing an eleven-degree scale of states to which values are attributed, their classification actually integrates the notions of inconvenience or isolation (confinement to bed, hospitalization, etc). Moreover, the notion of gravity of illness is taken into account through the medium of prognosis, which draws its support from the preceding health indicator to give it a dynamic dimension (in terms of probabilities of passage of the indicator from one level to another). As with the preceding authors, it would thus be possible for each group in the population to compare the effective course of life in terms of passage along various levels until death at a given age, to an ideal profile that would place this life at the highest level throughout its duration (standard).

Beyond these suggestions, the authors are primarily concerned with showing that it is possible to balance the different states of activity in order to obtain a synthetic indicator, whether by economic criteria or by sociological or medical criteria, and, in the final analysis, by the method of dual comparisons.

As for valorization of the indicator, this can be done either in terms of equivalence (of states) in time (days or years of life), or in terms of equivalence in the number of persons (x persons in state A equivalent to y persons in state B).

Aside from the differences that characterize these attempts (like the place reserved for the prognostic aspect, or the fact of proceeding, or not proceeding, to an aggregation (combination), the proposals for multi-dimensional indicators made in this spirit elicit two fundamental remarks:

(*a*) They have the undeniable advantage of *setting the problem in its true form:* that is, as a level of health in terms of a final 'output', and to this extent they start out on the right track.

They also have the advantage of recognizing several dimensions of the state of health: some collective, others individual; some in terms of levels, and others in terms of duration. Finally, although they are based upon the different categories of traditional nosology, they try, undeniably, to avoid the negative view of health (diseases) in order to evolve towards a more positive conception, closer to the O.M.S.'s definition (even though they are more oriented towards expressing physical health than mental health).

(*b*) But in most cases, these indicators turn out to be difficult to compute on the basis of existing information. That is, they

[1] S. Fanshel and J. W. Bush, 'A Health Status Index and its Application to Health Services Outcomes', *Operations Research*, XVIII, 6 (1970).

are set in a long-term perspective of research and of the establishment of new data.

In this perspective one might then ask if, instead of aiming for a synthetic indicator like those that have been proposed to us, one might not expect some partial measure or other, obtained from individuals during preventive examinations, might turn out to be a good 'indicator', in the sense that it might express the level of health better than some precise phenomenon (such as height, weight or some other dimension).

For the aggregative logic inherent in the preceding indicators, provided that they can be expressed numerically, leads to an expression of the level of health that would neither be clearly perceptible to the population itself, not very useful for throwing light upon particular decisions for planners or administrators. Just what would be meant by an indicator that moved from 7·8 to 7·9 for a given age class, if not that things seem to be improving?

(3) *Summary*
In the final analysis, the information that can be derived from all the recent experiments in the search for health indicators is the following:

(*a*) If the desire for an immediate operational opening surpasses the other considerations, the figures proposed as indicators are not very satisfactory. Either they do not express the entire phenomenon under investigation (the state of health), when one is dealing with synthetic indicators, or else, in the case of a battery of indicators, the interrelationships among the latter cannot be grasped.

(*b*) But if, on the contrary, the research is preceded by a conceptual and analytical approach, as in the last cases aforesaid, the conclusions arrive at a dead-end – at least for the moment – at the numerical level.

Thus, it is definitely the proportion between modeling efforts and systematic analysis of the problem, on the one hand, and the desire to arrive quickly at statements of numerical indicators for the entire population, on the other hand, which seems to be the heart of the problem.

IV. METHODOLOGICAL SUGGESTIONS FOR ESTABLISHING HEALTH INDICATORS
The perspective in which we have chosen to situate ourselves lies at the crossroads of the methodological axes that have just been

defined. With an operational approach to the effort to make optimal use of existing information, it must take account of the constraints implicit in the conception of this information and in its scope; but in the hope of reaching our goal as quickly as possible – namely, an understanding of the state of public health – we shall sort out and interrelate the data retained from an effort at modeling. That is to say, our approach is characterized by the detour we are imposing on ourselves, from an anlysis of the system of health, to arrive at the indicators. Without this detour, hopefully a 'productive' one, the state of the question runs the risk of being closed in by the dilemma mentioned.

Three essential principles, which will be quickly developed, arise from this starting-point.

(1) *To Start with a Health System Analysis*
This analysis may be more or less ambitious, but even if it is still rather rudimentary, it must clearly distinguish among the different coherent subsets of variables that characterize it in order to find the most important interrelationships.

(i) *The breakdown into three subsystems.* If, by a health system, one means quite a vast body of data and variables – ranging from the socio-economic of biological characteristics of individuals to the mechanisms for financing health expenses, passing through morbidity and mortality, doctors, hospitals, medical research, etc. – it is useful to break this body of data up into three subsystems, each governed by its own logic. This breakdown is justified by an observation that was made in regard to the French situation, in particular, namely, that we are in an area where it is not the same individual who feels the need, makes the (therapeutic) decision, and finances it. Thus, all three – the patient, the doctor and the disbursing body – are concerned with health, but from different points of view and very different possibilities for action.

    (*a*) *A first subsystem*, then, is made up of different 'states' of health through which individuals pass as a function of genetic factors (cultural level, habitat, social-professional category, way of life, etc.), and interventions by (or recourse to) medical institutions. Let us call this the circuit of 'states'. This is the one primarily concerned with the search for indicators of the state of health.

    (*b*) *A second subsystem* is made up of the apparatus for production and distribution of care. Its functional logic is, therefore, that of any productive system. In integrating a certain number of factors of production into specific enterprises, it is subject to certain constraints and its actions are motivated by certain incentives. Its missions, which are numerous, but which it can fulfill only to unequal degrees, are all linked up with the same finality, which is the improvement of the level of health; but the structures and functioning of this apparatus have the effect of letting it pursue its goal only with more or less success.

(c) *A third subsystem* is composed of different mechanisms for financing health expenses, mechanisms which are heterogenous to the extent that some of them are ascribable to the laws of the market, while others originate from a more or less extensive collective community of interests.

The collective taking-charge of medical liability through the intermediary of social institutions (health insurance, mutual insurance, etc.) and the correlative fact that many prices in the health sector are 'political' prices have a specific impact both on the structures and the functioning of those offering services (subsystem 2) and on the behavior of recourse to care and the medical situation of those making the demand (subsystem 1).

Next to more profound analysis of the first subsystem, then, it is the study of its interrelations with the other two that seems essential (see Fig. 19.1).

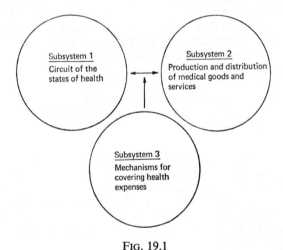

FIG. 19.1

(ii) *Thorough analysis of subsystem 1.* One question antecedes any effort at thoroughly analyzing this subsystem. That is the question of the choice which has been formulated in terms of a *positive or negative conception* of the state of health.[1] In fact, the possibility of this being expressed by illness or non-illness is being challenged more and more and efforts are being made to advocate a so-called 'positive' conception of health in accordance with the definition by the O.M.S. Moreover, many attempts at finding synthetic indicators which were cited above go along with this line of thought.

But aside from the fact that one is obliged to note the lack of data and the difficulty in collecting them in order to reverse the perspectives and to characterize states of more or less good health, the choice we are faced with thus runs the risk of depriving us of everything we might know, however imperfectly, concerning the malady.

Actually, the problem of constructing indicators is a different one; it consists in the choice between an expression of the medical state of a population *in terms of cases* and *in terms of individuals*. What the proponents of the so-called positive system appeal for is that, really, the individual remains the privileged unit of measurement, and that he does not find himself mutilated in an expression in terms of cases (of illnesses).

The point of contention, thus, is the possibility of taking counts (for all aspects that characterize the state of health: risk factors, illnesses, invalidism, etc.) that respect the individual unit, whereas most of the numerical data are taken in different, non-summable counting units. This requirement will most certainly have to be taken into consideration in the future; it leads us once again, to call for special efforts in new studies of the longitudinal type, using representative samples of the population.

But while we are waiting for national governments to decide to set up such means of investigation, what can we do?

It seems realistic not to deprive ourselves of available information on sickness, and to admit – at least provisionally – the notion of morbidity as the keystone to analysis and measurement of states of health.

Thus, if one agree with the line of demarcation of the existence of an illness to characterize these states, the main problem that presents itself in the search for indicators is that of *the different expressions of morbidity*.

For morbidity can be conceived of as the codage worked out by an individual, or by an institution, of a set of data relating to an individual 'state of health'.

Depending on the characteristics of the 'encoder', his aptitudes and his dominant concerns, one arrives at different parlances (cf. Fig. 19.2).

[1] B. Cazes, 'Les Préoccupations Sociales dans le Domaine de la Santé', Essai de classement, Division des Affaires Sociales de l'O.C.D.E. (Jan. 1972).

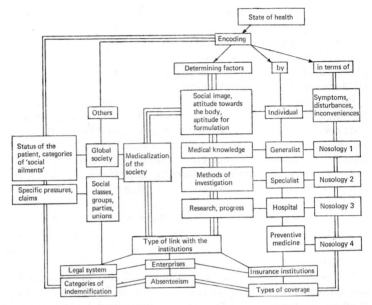

FIG. 19.2   Different approaches to morbidity

The 'diagnostic' is the *encoding* realized by a medical institution. This diagnostic is extracted from a general *typology* of all *possible* diagnostics corresponding with the practice of the institution under study (nosology).

Starting from the general nosology corresponding with the medical knowledge of the moment, as well as the level of development of the technical means for investigation, each medical institution utilizes a *partial nosology* for its own purposes. This nosology corresponds both with the level of medical knowledge of the personnel using it, with the level of the available means of investigation (technical and non-technical) and with the nature of the health problems that the insitution in question is supposed to treat.

The diagnostic achieved by a medical institution (the G.P., the specialist, the hospital center, etc.) is, thus, only one of the elements of the indefinite set of *possible discourses on the state of health*. In our society it has been invested with the prestige surrounding a scientific discourse. Nevertheless, depending on the medical institution that offers it, this discourse will have a more or less scientific and more or less prestigious aspect. One of the essential elements that will mark the more or less 'scientific', or 'objective', aspect of such a discourse is the fact that, like any measure, it is tainted with a certain amount of error due to the experimentation itself. To conduct a measurement is to disturb in some way the phenomenon being measured. Yet all medical discourse and diagnosis operates within a context where knowledge is not being sought for its own sake, and, thus, where the precautions taken to ensure elementary conditions of objectivity of measurement are not brought together.

On the contrary, and paradoxically, the closer one gets to the very conditions of objectivity of measurement, the more one tends to eliminate the subject himself, to negate him as a 'person' or 'totality' possessing his own discourse and perception; and extreme objectivity – that of an autopsy – even goes so far as to deny life to the other person.

Thus, the very problematics of medical discourse is connected with this ambivalent situation in which two irreducible discourses confront each other with the doctor–patient relationship, which cannot be mutually denied without annihilating the relationship itself.

In the case of *epidemiological inquiries*, the dimension we have just evoted – that of a therapeutic relationship linked with a certain socio-economic context – disappears. Here, knowledge is sought for its own sake, and the gathering of data is surrounded by a set of precautions directed towards ensuring scientific validity. But even here, this is done at the price of considerable *reduction* of the pathology to the level of symptoms taken on the subject under standardized conditions. The subject exists only as a support for these symptoms; the epidemiology is almost analytic and reductionistic, in the image of the dominant scientific method of the 'natural' sciences.

Within the framework of the social science survey based on the analysis of morbidity, the subject and its discussion are, on the other hand, taken as a whole. But the representation of the illness, the faculty of devoting attention to one's body, the possibility of formulating signs and symptoms – all are inextricably bound up with smatterings of technical discussions which one has memorized in the course of successive passages through the health system, and with recollections of information popularized by the media. The result is a strange discourse that one might translate, in certain cases, in terms of felt or expressed morbidity.

Finally, one may thus distinguish three dimensions or aspects of morbidity, which can hardly be reconciled:

(a) the morbidity which an individual feels;
(b) the morbidity diagnosed by the medical profession when one has recourse to its care;
(c) the morbidity objectivized via systematic examinations or epidemiological inquiries.

On the basis of the preceding hypotheses, a *circuit of states of health* can be formulated which brings out the passage of individuals through these states, not only in a process of evolution, but also by juxtaposition or association (multiple afflictions, for example). This formulation, thus, grants privileges to one stage – that of illness – while differentiating the various situations in which an individual may find himself in regard to it; but it also retains the factor of risk upstream, and that of death downstream, stabilization with or without *sequelae* (aftermaths), and healing. And to these states are connected all possible types of intervention by the apparatus of production of medical care (cf. Fig. 19.3). From the standpoint of

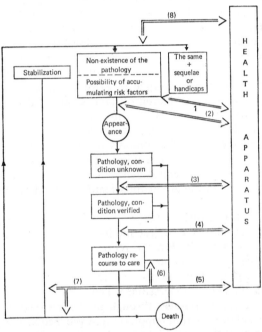

FIG. 19.3 (1) Limitation of the possibility of accumulating risk factors by certain consumptions (certain types of consumption). (2) Prevention. (3 and 4) Screening. (5, 6 and 7) Principal recourse to the health apparatus with a view to cure. (8) Limitation of the risks with regard to *sequelae* and handicaps; correction of these harmful consequences

such a diagram, the level of health of a population at a given moment appears as the result of a series of passages or non-passages from one level to another in the circuit. But this is precisely where the problems begin. In this way, the death of a sick person might ameliorate the state of health of a population; the appearance of an illness would have the same consequence as its failure to disappear, and the failure of it to appear would amount to its being cured. Actually, in defining the state as the consequence of all these fluxes, one is, supposedly, already aware of the operation of all these factors.

One last particular must be brought out concerning this diagram. At all the levels which it distinguishes, and in all the processes of passage, there actually intervene a great many exogenous (to this circuit) factors: genetic and socio-economic factors. But, for these innumerable factors and connections, medical socio-economics or epidemiology provide only partial clarification. The latter, particularly, prevents us from 'endogenizing' more than a few of these aspects in the form of 'risk factors' of illnesses. But the fact that we have kept only this notion in our diagram certainly does not mean that we deny a role to all those which we did not include, at all points on the circuit.

(iii) *Relationships with the two other subsystems.* In the search for health indicators, the apparatus for the production and distribution of care (subsystem 2) and the mechanisms for financing (subsystem 3) interest us only to the extent that their influence on it, and especially the quantity of data they provide us with, yield us information on the state of public health.

Yet although this influence is considered obvious just because it is there and is the justification for the existence of these two subsystems, its measurement is made only very imperfectly, and that is because of their own logic of functioning.

The functional logic of subsystem 2 is, as we have already said, that of a productive system. Since it is made up of enterprises that differ broadly in size and productive functions, from private offices up to university hospitals and the pharmaceutical industry, with a whole series of intermediate forms along the way, it combines the factors of production (doctors, paramedical personnel, equipment, chemical and pharmaceutical products, etc.) to make it possible to obtain goods and medical services. Thus, the offer seems to us to be an offer of actions (by doctors, dentists, laboratories, etc.), of days of hospitalization, and of medical goods.

The logic of such a system, while liberal medicine continues to penetrate it even in its attenuated form, whether it relies upon profit-making or status-seeking incentives, leads to a certain number of known consequences; the multiplication of acts and days of hospitalization, the more rapid development of technical acts, the channeling of progress towards innovations with material supports,[1]

[1] C. Lefaure, 'L'Innovation et le Progrès Technique dans le Secteur de la Santé: Approche Économique', D.Sc. Econ. thesis (Paris, 1972).

etc. It also leads to a preference for certain types of actions (diagnosis, treatment) over and above others (prevention, tracing). Certain health needs will find researchers, doctors and specific institutions ready to meet them, whereas others will have to remain unmet for quite a while, since they are unable to mobilize the essential incentives of the system. Finally, the medical system has obviously not quite felt the need to prove its own efficiency in terms of results in the state of health in order to pursue its activity.

As a result, it is not surprising that, up to the present, we do not have a system for observation that would permit us to measure these results on the scale of a population, and that the sole 'output' of this system which we were measuring in the National Accounts of Health[1] should be this body of actions, days, etc., which tells us nothing about the evolution of the state of health that derives from it.

At the very most, we can be experts, in France, for example, at diagnoses referred to by actions, days of hospitalization, or medicine.

The operation of the mechanisms for financing health expenses, especially the collective mechanisms (social security, mutuals, assistance), has its effect on:

(a) individuals, in their behavior of resorting to its assistance (care);
(b) the structures and function of subsystem 2 and, thereby, on health activities that concern individuals.

With regard to the first type of activity, one should distinguish between two aspects – that of the type, and that of the level, of protection.

We are rather ill-informed on the first aspect, but the studies we were able to carry out in this area seem to show that the type of protection (social insurance, mutuals, private insurance, or assistance from the state) appears to play a relatively slight role in behavior, since the other variables that influence them have the effect of unifying this behavior independently of the mechanism for financing to which the appeal is made. But this does not mean that these collective mechanisms, as a whole, have not improved people's reliance on care.

As for the level of protection, its influence is hardly more clearly discernible. Nevertheless, it seems that with the aid of specific regulations (which, say, in France exempt the insured person from being charged for certain diseases or, especially, for certain types of hospital care) or of specific institutions (medical-social centers), a

---

[1] Cf. 'Méthodologie des Comptes Nationaux de la Santé', *Économie et Santé*, no. 2 (Paris: Ministère de la Santé et de la Sécurité Sociale, 1972); and CREDOC, *Comptes Nationaux de la Santé: Évaluation de la Consommation Médicale 1966, 1967, 1969.*

person can be more or less encouraged, depending on the case, to have recourse to care and prevention.

But it is primarily the second type of action – on the structure of care units – that is important. Because of subsidies accorded to certain investments and, especially, because of tariffing different actions, days of hospitalization, and pharmaceutical products, the agencies concerned with social security are able to favor certain of these actions and products, and, thus, favor certain of these enterprises to the detriment of others. In this way, restraints have been placed on false teeth or house calls, while private hospitalization has been encouraged to a relative degree.

Whatever the consequences of these actions, one must recall that the structure of the collective financing mechanisms only transfers the state of power relationships among social groups (the state, employers, workers, health personnel), and that, for a given situation of balance in these relationships, the proper logic of this system consists in ensuring the financing of care while checking the growth of expenses – in other words, that it be provided by the imperative of financial equilibrium.

And this imperative impels subsystem 3, just as if it does subsystem 2, which it finances, to measure its results in terms of actions, days, etc., and of expenses correlated with its products, rather than in terms of improvements in states of health brought about with their aid. Thus, it is logical, though regrettable, that collective organizations for financing expenses provide us with so little information on our problem.

(2) *From descriptors of the System to Health Indicators*

With the preceding analyses in mind, one might think that the quantitative information that allows us to describe the structures and function of the health system as a whole would be rather considerable, though incomplete on some points. These data will be called descriptors, though only a certain number of them can be kept for throwing light upon the medical situation in a country.

(i) *In reference to subsystem 1*, which is still the one most involved with indicators of the state of health, a small number of data available for France deserve out attention.

Above morbidity. Only environmental variables retained in the form of risk factors of one or several affections can regularly be taken into consideration. This is the case for the consumption of tobacco, alcohol, fats or sugars, and certain others. The difficulty consists in the fact that although the epidemiological studies show clearly the relationship of a simple factor or of multiple factors in the case of a pathological condition, they do not permit us to show

Risk factors   *Diseases*

   R_1 Tobacco

   R_2 Alcohol consumption M_1

   .   Age

   .   Working conditions M_2

   .   Obesity   .

   R_j (One pathological condition may constitute a risk factor .

        for another: diabetes–ischemia.)   .

                                                  M_k

Etiological studies

  (*a*) Simple factor:

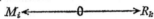

$$M_i \longleftarrow \quad 0 \quad \longrightarrow R_k$$

  (*b*) Multiple factors:

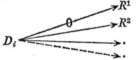

                              R^1 Methods:

                 0   R^2 descriptive

        D_i model

  (*c*) Synthetic analysis of certain factors:

                        synthetic indicator of health:

        $R_i \longrightarrow$ mortality, life expectancy

  (*d*) Global systemic analysis

           R_1 M_1

           R_2 M_2

            .   .   Not realized

            .   .

            .   .

           R_j M_k

Fig. 19.4. The connection between risk factors and maladies

the interplay of several factors on several such conditions (cf. Fig. 19.4).

It is no less true that retention of the statistical series concerning certain of these factors in a set of health indicators would be indispensable, according to the possibilities and countries involved. Thus, in France, the factor of alcoholism should certainly be one of these indicators, if one goes by certain statistical analyses.[1]

[1] L. Lebart, 'Analyse Statistique Régionale des Consommations Médicales', mimeo (CREDOC, 1969), and idem, 'Recherches sur le Coût de Protection de la Vie Humaine dans le Domaine Médical', mimeo (CREDOC, 1970).

At the level of morbidity. We provide some light on the nature of the *morbidity experienced* in non-periodical surveys both of the psychosociological type[1] and of the epidemiological type, always based on limited, non-representative populations. But the indicators which they provide could hardly have any value as indicators.

In dealing with *morbidity diagnosed* by the medical profession, we find ourselves in an area of more codified information which is, thus, easier to follow in time.[2]

In this way, in France, we have statistics on hospital morbidity that will be extended progressively to include all hospitals (excepting those in the private sector), and a survey of private offices based on a panel of 1,600 doctors per annum.[3] But all these data have to do with diagnoses made in a doctor's office or a hospital, and, thus, do not really reflect incident or prevalent morbidity.

Although their value as data might be limited to diagnoses when care is available and their technical imperfections might still be certain, these series of data can be utilized in a battery of indicators of the state of health.

As for *objective morbidity*, it is not objective, unless it be through specific epidemiologic surveys[4] with no follow-up or systematic examinations on non-representative samples, since only volunteers offer themselves and preventive medicine still does not know how to interpret them correctly.

But on the occasion of surveys of consumption it was possible[5] to measure the divergence between incident and prevalent morbidity over a six-month period and the type of morbidity that meant recourse to a doctor, a specialist or a hospital. Such surveys could, thus, be a report of more extensive information on morbidity, and, thus, indicators.

At the level of mortality. It seems that the most homogeneous data (with respect to the preceding) and that which is most useful in a system of indicators are the statistics of the causes of death by age group reported annually;[6] so much so, that in many studies they are

---

[1] C. Herzlich, *Santé et Maladie: Analyse d'une Représentation Sociale* (Paris: Mouton, 1969).

[2] For example, cf. Framingham's surveys on cardiovascular ailments.

[3] A survey by Idrem-Dorema, published up to 1968, in the *Bulletin de Statistiques Sociales*, séric Santé, by the Ministère des Affaires Sociales.

[4] In particular, cf. the survey called 'Soissons: Recherches sur les Besoins de Santé d'une Population', *Bulletin de l'INSERM* no. 3 (1969).

[5] C. Guillot, A. A. Mizrahi and G. Rosch, 'La Morbidité d'une Population et ses Relations avec les Recours aux Soins Médicaux', *Rev. Epidém. Méd. Soc. et Santé*, XIX, 4 (1971).

[6] INSERM, *Statistique des Causes Médicales de Décès* (annually), obtainable from 3 rue Léon Bonnat, Paris 16e.

still practically the only ones retained as indicators of the level of health.

(ii) As for the data linked with subsystems 2 and 3, the results of the analysis we have presented indicate that their informative power regarding the state of health is rather feeble.

In the case of the variables in the offering of medical care, global factorial analyses have already been made based on the causes of death, on medical consumption, on the number of doctors and hospital beds; and various socio-economic variables in the French departments[1] show only that the first preponderant factor, which explains 38 per cent of the total dispersion, is the standard of living as seen from the medical angle (medical equipment and personnel, health, longevity). They also show that it is impossible to compute the connection for a given age group between the mortality rate and the level of medical consumption, for this relationship, in the case of the French departments, is marginal, as compared with the disparities (in mortality) as a result of alcoholism.

So the physical or financial data turn out to be of little help. The same holds for data on individuals who are the object of special protection and on indemnified (compensated) work stoppages (time off from work).

The detailed report made by the French agencies of social security about those benefited by the government for illnesses of long duration (which prevents any financial charges being required from these individuals reflects more closely the evolution of an institution and its changes in regulations than it does the evolution of the most gravely ill patients. As for periods of indemnified time off, these are not even sorted out by cause, as we have already said. Their significance would remain obscure in the light of the multiplicity of factors that could become involved there.

In conclusion, when one follows the train of thought we have used for the French case, it appears that:

1. In the present state of the statistical information which we have, one should not look for a miraculous indicator, a 'trick' indicator. The difficulties encountered, both at the level of comprehending the phenomena and at the level of evaluating them, make the formulation of a good synthetic indicator premature.
2. If the approach uncovered by those who seek such an indicator at the level of the consequences of illness (degrees of validity) or by those who would promote a 'positive' conception of illness seems interesting, it still does not seem possible to

[1] Lebart, op. cit.

ignore the traditional categories, i.e. the nomenclature of illnesses, and, thus, avoid thinking in terms of cases rather than of individuals.

3. We must, therefore, start out by establishing a 'battery' of indicators in the absence of any unique indicator; this battery of indicators would be characterized by three dimensions:

   (*a*) *indicators of vulnerability* of the population, made up of series having to do with the major risk factors and their distribution in the population (by age, sex, etc);

   (*b*) *indicators of morbidity* which, in the present state of affairs, can be formulated only by diagnoses made by city or hospital doctors, even if one might raise the objection that here one is measuring the level of medicalization, rather than the level of health;[1]

   (*c*) *indicators of mortality*, derived from the statistics on causes of death.

These three types of indicators must be interrelated, yet remain distinct from each other. The two latter have the advantage of being based on an identical nomenclature, with their combined development in time thus lending itself more readily to interpretation. On the other hand, the combination of the first one with the other two turns out to be more delicate, except when the risk factors have to do with a quite specific ailment.

From this starting-point one must look for all possible combinations of indicators for each large group of ailments that are defined by the former, and evaluate their significance (for example, the three series of indicators increasing in parallel, or two of them increasing and one decreasing, etc.).

4. It is urgent to recommend to national governments, agencies of social security, and the medical profession, to allow the necessary means for developing data that go beyond diagnoses and to allow us to evaluate both the result of medical actions and, in a general way, the longitudinal surveys of representative samples of the population or of patients.

[1] D. Defert, 'Réflexions sur l'Appréciation des Niveaux de Santé: Préalable Méthodologique', *Bulletin de l'INSERM*, xxii, 6 (1967).

20 The Quality of Hospital Services: An Analysis of Geographic Variation and Intertemporal Change[1]

Martin S. Feldstein

HARVARD UNIVERSITY

In studying the operation of any nation's health care system, it is useful to have an economic measure of the quality of care that is provided at different times and places. This paper discusses the conceptual problems of defining an aggregate quality index and develops the formulae required to make this operation. A price index for hospitals' non-labor inputs is constructed, using weights based on the 1963 United States input–output study. The substantial and persistent variation in the overall price of inputs is then analyzed with a cross-section of time-series data. The same sample is then used to examine the intertemporal change and geographic variation in the quality of hospital services.

I. INTRODUCTION

Economists are generally accustomed to discussing the prices and quantities of goods and services while saying rather little about their quality. At a formal level, different qualities of the same product may be treated as a set of different products. As a substantive matter, however, the determinants of product quality and the dynamics of product change are significant problems that have been unduly neglected.

For health services, in particular, the quality of care is an important issue to which economists have given too little attention. This has been particularly true in empirical research.[2] In studying the operation of any nation's health care system, it is useful to have an economic measure of the quality of care that is provided at different

---

[1] I am grateful to Virginia Ambrosini and Bernard Friedman for assistance with the calculations; to the Harvard Economic Research Project and the Office of Business Economics, U.S. Department of Commerce, for providing unpublished data; and to the National Center for Health Services Research and Development for financial support.

[2] The quality of health services has been discussed in a number of studies, including Arrow (1963), Feldstein (1967, 1971a, 1973a), Grossman (1972), Newhouse (1970), Pauly and Redisch (1971) and Reder (1969), but none of these incorporates a quality measure into an empirical analysis.

times and places. As I shall explain, such a measure is important, not only for monitoring the general performance of the health care system, but also for analyzing the demand for care, forecasting the effects of changes in the method of financing, and assessing the welfare implications of policies that would alter the expenditure on health services.

A good measure depends on its purpose. For a regulatory agency charged with evaluating the quality of care being provided, or for a cost–benefit analyst who is examining the desirability of a particular program, the only suitable measure of quality is an assessment of the effects of care on the health of the relevant population. The current study is less ambitious. I want a measure that will be useful for rather *aggregative* analyses of the quality of hospital services. I shall consider a measure to be useful if it permits us to assess the extent and change of geographic variation in the quality of care, and if it can be used as an index of quality in an econometric model of the health care sector. I have no doubt that the measure presented in this paper is a crude one, but I believe that, by the standards that I have defined, it is also a useful one. I hope that, by directing attention to this issue and providing an operational measure of quality, I shall succeed in encouraging others to deal with this important subject.

The next section will discuss the conceptual problems of defining an aggregate quality index and will develop the formulae required to make this operational. A key variable used in calculating the quality measure is a price index for hospitals' non-labor inputs. Such an index was constructed using input weights based on the 1963 United States input–output study; the method and results are described in section III. Section IV analyzes the substantial and persistent geographic variation in the overall price of inputs. Section V then examines the intertemporal change and geographic variations in the quality of hospital services. A final section indicates a number of directions for future research.

II. THE MEASUREMENT OF QUALITY

My original interest in developing an aggregate quality measure was motivated by work that I was doing on the demand for hospital services (Feldstein, 1971*b*). Using a pooled cross-section sample of time series for each of the individual states of the United States for 1958 through 1967, I estimated equations relating the demand for hospital admissions and for mean durations of stay per case to the price of care net of insurance and to other explanatory variables including income, population density and the availability of physicians. The dependent variables were adjusted for interstate differences in the demographic composition of the population. A typical equation could be summarized as:

$$ADM_{it} = k_0 \ NP_{it}^{\alpha} \ e^{\gamma_0 t} \ (\pi_j X_{jit})^{\beta_j} \ U_{it} \qquad (1)$$

where ADM_{it} is the demographically adjusted admission rate, NP_{it} is the price net of insurance and deflated by the consumer price index, t is a time trend, the X_{jit} are other explanatory variables, and U_{it} is a disturbance term. The subscripts i and t refer to the state and the year. The equation was estimated by a consistent instrumental variable procedure after a logarithmic transformation. The time trend reflects both technical progress and the changing popular attitudes about hospital care.

The specification of equation (1) implicitly assumes that other variations in quality, through time or between states, do not affect demand. I accepted this as a basis for analysis on the assumption that patients were not likely to be able to discern and respond to actual variations in the quality of services provided. Nevertheless, I was concerned about the lack of specific testing of this assumption. Moreover, when I later analyzed the role of the physician in the demand for hospital services,[1] I recognized that the patient may often act as he would if he had the expertise to perceive quality differences. If a more appropriate specification includes the quality of care, Q_{it}, i.e.

$$ADM_{it} = k_0 \ NP_{it}^{\alpha} \ e^{\gamma_0 t} \ (\pi_j X_{jit})^{\beta_j} \ Q_{it}^{\eta} \ U_{it} \qquad (2)$$

the omission of Q_{it} leads to incorrect inferences about the other demand parameters and, perhaps, about the qualitative behavior and efficiency of the health care system in general. If quality and price are positively correlated,[2] the price elasticity estimated in equation (1) would be biased toward zero.[3]

More generally, my analysis of hospital cost inflation (Feldstein, 1971*a*, 1971*b*) rested largely on changes in the quality or 'style' of hospital care. In *The Rising Cost of Hospital Care*, I developed a theoretical model of quality change in a context in which individual demand for care does reflect the quality of services. To test this model and to integrate it with the earlier empirical work, an operational

[1] The theory of a 'generalized agency relation' between the patient and his physician is developed in Feldstein (1973*b*).

[2] While a strong correlation might be assumed to exist, the correlation would actually be attenuated by differences in local costs and, more important, by the use of price net of insurance. This point is discussed again in section v.

[3] This actually depends on a positive partial correlation between quality and price, given all the other variables in the equation.

measure of the quality of hospital services in each state is needed. Finally, the analysis of the welfare economics of health insurance depends on the effect of quality on demand. More specifically, the welfare gain or loss that results from changes in the level of health insurance depends on the effect of changes in the resource input per patient-day on the quantity of care demanded at each price (Feldstein, 1973*a*).

The constant elasticity specification of equation (2) suggests a simple 'constant elasticity' model of the relation of quality to resource inputs:

$$Q_{it} = k_1 e^{\gamma_1 t} R_{it}^{\rho} \tag{3}$$

where R_{it} is a measure of the resource inputs per patient-day. The constant k_1 is an arbitrary choice of units, but γ_1 and ρ are unknown parameters. If this relation is substituted into equation (2), it is clear that the parameters k_1 and γ_1 are not identified. The constant term of equation (2) becomes $k_0 k_1^{\eta}$ and the time term becomes $\gamma_0 + \gamma_1 \eta$. Similarly, the coefficient of R_{it} is $\rho\eta$. The estimation therefore provides neither the parameters of the quality function (equation (3)) nor the elasticity of demand with respect to quality (η). Nevertheless, this estimate of equation (2) may provide all the information that is required for practical analysis. Note first that the estimated price elasticity of demand (α) would no longer be biased by the omission of Q_{it}. Moreover, the analysis of hospital cost inflation and the welfare economics of insurance depend only on the effect of additional resource inputs on the demand for care, i.e. on the combined parameter $\rho\eta$.[1]

The simple specification of equation (3) implies strong assumptions. The technical progress that occurs with time is neutral in that it raises the quality in the same proportion at all levels of resource inputs.[2] The efficiency with which resources are turned into the quality of service is assumed constant, or is subsumed into the time term. For this reason, the specification is more useful for the analysis of a large group of hospitals than for comparing individual hospitals. No distinction is made among the different types of quality increase that may be produced with additional resource inputs. In my earlier

---

[1] Equation (3) specifies a non-stochastic relation. Introducing a multiplicative random error poses no special problem. Since R_{it} must be treated as an endogenous variable in estimating equation (2), some form of instrumental variable procedure will be used. This is sufficient to permit consistent estimation even if Q_{it} contains an unobserved random error.

[2] See Feldstein (1971*a*, chap. 4) for an analysis of non-neutral technical change in this context. Even such neutral technical progress can be either 'cost-increasing' or 'cost-reducing', depending on preferences and market structure.

analysis of hospital cost inflation (1971*b*), I assumed that a relation like equation (3) exists between inputs and *quality as perceived by the providers*, i.e. quality in terms of the providers' preferences. For demand analysis, the relevant aspect is quality as perceived by the patients and their physicians. More generally, hospitals may differ in the way in which they allocate additional resource inputs per patient-day to increase the several different dimensions of the 'quality' of service: the efficacy of treatment, the intensity of treatment (i.e. reduction in duration of stay with given overall efficacy), the level of patient amenities, and the extent of facilities and services that appeal primarily to the providers. The particular mix of the quality facets that is chosen will depend on the market conditions faced by each hospital. In short, using resource inputs to measure quality is only a first approximation that will be more suitable for some purposes than for others.

The resource input per patient-day (R_{it}) can be measured as the ratio of an index of average cost per patient-day ($JACPPD_{it}$) to an index of hospital input prices ($PRIN_{it}$):

$$R_{it} = \frac{JACPPD_{it}}{PRIN_{it}}. \tag{4}$$

Data on average cost per patient-day are published annually for individual hospitals and as state averages.[1] The index of average cost per patient ($JACPPD_{it}$) is defined as the ratio of average cost per patient-day in state *i* and year *t* ($ACPPD_{it}$) to the national average in a base year:

$$JACPPD_{it} = \frac{ACPPD_{it}}{ACPPD_{a0}}. \tag{5}$$

The subscript *a* denotes a national average and the subscript 0 denotes the base year. Note that equation (5) implies that the national average of *JACPPD* in the base year is 1. No index of input prices ($PRIN_{it}$) exists on a state or even on a national basis. An important aspect of the current study has been the development of such an index. This input price index is also scaled so that it has a national average of 1 in the base year.

Two types of inputs may be distinguished. Labor inputs are purchased in a relatively local market. Substantial interstate differences

---

[1] See, e.g., American Hospital Association (1967). The data used in the current study refer only to non-federal short-term general and other special hospitals. They specifically exclude mental hospitals and other long-stay facilities. The definition of cost also excludes capital costs; this is likely to result in an underestimate of costs by only about 10 per cent, but may also introduce some differential bias between observations.

in wage rates can therefore persist. It is important to have a separate wage index value for every state and year. Non-labor inputs are generally available in a national market. A single price index for non-labor inputs is therefore sufficient.[1]

The basic input price index to be used in the current study is a Laspeyres index of wages and non-labor inputs:

$$PRIN_{it} = \frac{w_{it} N_{a0} + \pi_t J_{a0}}{w_{a0} N_{a0} + \pi_0 J_{a0}} \tag{6}$$

where w_{it} is an index of hospital wages for state i;

π_t is national price index for non-labor inputs;

N_{a0} is the national average quantity of labor inputs in the base year;

J_{a0} is the national average quantity of non-labor inputs in the base year.

The average hospital wage in state i and year t is measured by the ratio of total hospital payroll to the number of full-time equivalent employees.[2] This procedure fails to make specific allowance for local differences or changes in the job mix or quality of employees. This is probably not a serious deficiency. A previous analysis showed no evidence of substantial overall change in the average job level of hospital employees in the decade 1956–66 (Feldstein, 1971*a*, pp. 57–8). The job mix and quality of employees may, however, differ across states. Further disaggregation of the labor input would be desirable. The average payroll per full-time equivalent employee was then converted to an index number with a national average of 1 in 1958. A corresponding measure of the quantity of labor inputs in each state and year was defined by dividing the payroll costs per patient-day by the wage index. N_{a0} is the national average of these quantities for the base year, 1963.[3]

The national price index for non-labor costs (π_t) is defined as a weighted average of the separate price indices for all the products

[1] A national price index for hospital inputs was previously developed in National Advisory Commission on Health Manpower (1967), Taylor (1969) and Feldstein (1971*a*). No geographical disaggregation was attempted. More important, each of these studies used the general wholesale price index to measure the price of hospital non-labor costs.

[2] The data, published by the American Hospital Association, exclude most physicians.

[3] The wage and non-labor price indices, w_{it} and Π_t, are *scaled* to be 1 in 1958, the first year for which data is analyzed in the current study. This choice of scale obviously does not affect the analysis. The *weights* in the index number of equation (6) are the 1963 national quantities. The choice of a base year does, of course, affect the behavior of the index. 1963 was chosen because of the availability of the detailed input–output data that will be discussed in the next section. This base year is also conveniently in the middle of the current period of analysis.

purchased by the hospitals. The construction of this index is the subject of the next section. There is obviously no physical measure of the average base year quantity of non-labor inputs (J_{a0}). Instead, J_{a0} is defined by analogy with N_{a0} as the ratio of non-labor costs to the price index of non-labor inputs, i.e.

$$J_{a0} = \frac{ACPPD_{a0} - w_{a0}N_{a0}}{\pi_0}. \tag{7}$$

The resource input measure (R_{it}), defined by equations (4) through (7), reflects variation among states and through time. Although this is important for monitoring the extent and change in the inequality of resource use, it may be inappropriate for demand analysis. The demand for hospital care may respond to changes in the quality of services that are produced locally, but may not reflect interstate differences in the quality of care. Stated somewhat differently, patients may perceive and respond to the *relative* quality of services but may not know, be able to judge or respond to the *absolute* level of the quality of services. An increase in the quality of services in a particular market may increase the demand for those services, but the initial level of services may not affect the initial level of demand. To explore the implications of this hypothesis requires a resource input index that reflects changes through time but not across states. This could be accomplished by dividing each value of R_{it} by R_{i0}, the value of R_{it} in the base year. An alternative and more appropriate index would permit the weights on w_{it} and π_t to differ among states. To do so it is only necessary to replace N_{a0}, J_{a0} and w_{a0} in equations (6) and (7) by N_{i0}, J_{i0} and w_{i0}. The state-specific indices constructed in this way will be denoted RS_{it}. Note that they will all be equal to 1 in the base year. All interstate variance in other years will reflect differences in the rates of change of resource inputs.

III. INPUT–OUTPUT TECHNOLOGY AND A PRICE INDEX FOR HOSPITAL NON-LABOR INPUTS

This section describes the construction of a new price index for hospital non-labor inputs based on technological information developed for input–output analysis and on detailed price indices provided by the Office of Business Economics of the U.S. Department of Commerce and by the Bureau of Labor Statistics of the U.S. Department of Labor. The new index will also be compared with the general wholesale price index that has previously been used as a proxy for non-labor hospital costs.

The hospital non-labor price index is defined by the equation:

$$\pi_t = \sum_k a_{k0} q_{kt} \tag{8}$$

where a_{k0} is the quantity of input k used by hospitals in the base year; q_{kt} is the value of the price index in year t for inputs of type k. This price index is scaled so that $q_{k, 1958} = 1$ for all k.

The 1963 United States input-output table of order 367 contains information on the purchases of the hospital industry (industry number 77·02) from each of the other industries.[1] These data were then aggregated to the two-digit I.S.P. level,[2] since price indices are generally not available on a more detailed basis. 35 of 86 two-digit industries are sources of hospital inputs. These are listed with their 1963 sales to the hospital industry in Table 20.1. 12 of the 35 industries supplied extremely small quantities, less that $6 million each in 1963 and, collectively, less than 1·5 per cent of total hospital non-labor purchases. These small industries were therefore ignored in constructing the price index. Deflating the remaining 23 values of sales to 1958 dollars (by the individual price indices described below) provided the values of the a_{k0}'s required by equation (8).

The 23 price indices for the industries (the q_{kt}'s) were derived from several sources. The Office of Business Economics (O.B.E.) of the U.S. Department of Commerce provided unpublished time series of implicit deflators for the value of production of each two-digit I.S.P. *manufacturing* industry. This relates to industries 13 through 64 inclusive. The published O.B.E. composite index of construction costs[3] was used for industry 12, maintenance and repair construction. The wholesale price index (W.P.I.) component for processed foods was used for the purchases of agricultural products (industry 2) and the W.P.I. component for producers' finished goods was used for industries 81 and 82.[4] The remaining industries are classified as services in the I.S.P. system. Because there are no wholesale price indices for the purchases of services by business firms, components of the consumer price index were used for these industries.[5] Although a more

---

[1] The input–output table and a discussion of methods is published in U.S. Department of Commerce (1969). The hospital industry (77·02) corresponds to S.I.C. industry 8061. It includes all forms of hospitals (but not convalescent homes, rest homes, etc.), and is therefore broader than the average cost per patient-day data that exclude long-term institutions.

[2] Note that the two-digit input–output industry (I.S.P.) level is *not* the same as the two-digit S.I.C. (Standard Industrial Classification). For an analysis of the S.I.C. categories corresponding to I.S.P. industries, see *Survey of Current Business* (Sep 1965) p. 33.

[3] See U.S. Department of Commerce, *Business Statistics*, 1967 ed., p. 51.

[4] These are treated as 'dummy' industries in the construction of the input–output table. They are best considered as a residual for otherwise unallocated purchases.

[5] More specifically, the following C.P.I. components were used: I.S.P.66, non-durables less food and apparel; I.S.P.68, fuel and utilities; I.S.P.71, rent; I.S.P.75, transportation services; for the remaining six industries, 'other services'.

TABLE 20.1

COMPONENTS OF A PRICE INDEX FOR
HOSPITAL NON-LABOR INPUTS

Source industry Number	Industry title	Hospital purchases in 1963 ($m)
1	Livestock and livestock products	5·0
2	Other agricultural products	29·9
7	Coal mining	4·2
12	Maintenance and repair construction	143·3
14	Food and kindred products	218·2
19	Miscellaneous fabricated textile products	12·8
24	Paper and allied products, except containers and boxes	21·7
26	Paperboard containers and boxes	4·2
27	Chemicals and selected chemical products	23·0
29	Drugs, cleaning and toilet preparations	317·1
31	Petroleum refining and related industries	19·4
32	Rubber and miscellaneous plastics products	27·4
35	Glass and glass products	1·8
36	Stone and clay products	2·4
41	Screw machine products, bolts, nuts, etc., and metal stampings	0·8
55	Electric lighting and wiring equipment	0·1
58	Miscellaneous electrical machinery, equipment and supplies	0·5
59	Motor vehicles and equipment	0·6
62	Professional, scientific and controlling instruments and supplies	95·9
63	Optical, ophthalmic and photographic equipment and supplies	50·0
64	Miscellaneous manufacturing	3·2
65	Transportation and warehousing	42·8
66	Communications, except radio and television broadcasting	50·1
68	Electric, gas, water and sanitary services	192·4
69	Wholesale and retail trade	187·5
70	Finance and insurance	44·3
71	Real estate and rental	450·3
72	Hotels and lodging places; personal and repair services, except automoblie repair	58·0
73	Business services	91·9
75	Automobile repair and services	20·0
77	Medical, educational services and non-profit organizations	5·1
78	Federal government enterprises	32·3
79	State and local government enterprises	5·3
81	Business travel, entertainment and gifts	159·1
82	Office supplies	25·6

detailed matching of price indices with the specific categories of hospital inputs might be pursued, it is unlikely that the extra work would repay the effort.

Table 20.2 presents the price index for hospital non-labor costs derived according to equation (8) and the corresponding annual values of the wholesale price index. From 1958 through 1967, hospital non-labor costs rose 13·1 per cent, compared with 5·7 per cent for the wholesale price index and 15·5 per cent for the consumer price index.

TABLE 20.2

PRICE INDEX FOR HOSPITAL NON-LABOR COSTS

Year	Hospital non-labor price index (π_t)	Wholesale price index[a] (WPI_t)	Consumer price index[a] (CPI_t)
1958	1·000	1·000	1·000
1959	1·009	1·002	1·007
1960	1·023	1·003	1·024
1961	1·034	0·999	1·035
1962	1·044	1·002	1·047
1963	1·052	0·999	1·060
1964	1·064	1·001	1·073
1965	1·081	1·021	1·091
1966	1·109	1·055	1·123
1967	1·131	1·057	1·155

[a] The published W.P.I. and C.P.I. indices have 1967 = 100; they have been rescaled for convenience in comparison with π_t. The numbers in the table have also been rounded.

The wholesale price index is not a very satisfactory measure of the price of hospital non-labor inputs. It substantially understates the overall rise in hospital non-labor prices. Although the correlation between the two series is 0·88, this is largely due to the common trend. This is shown by equation (9):

$$\pi_t = 0·34 + 0·57\ WPI_t + 0·0106\ TIME \quad R^2 = 0·993. \qquad (9)$$
$$\quad\ (0·08) \qquad\ (0·0006)$$

the relative standard errors imply that the partial correlation of π_t and *TIME* is substantially greater than the partial correlation of π_t and WPI_t.

The consumer price index is actually a better proxy for the hospital non-labor price index during the period 1958–67. The simple correlation between CPI_t and π_t is 0·999, and a regression analogous to equation (9) shows that the coefficient of CPI_t (0·90, s.e. 0·07) is much more important than the coefficient of *TIME* (0·001, s.e. 0·001). It would, of course, be necessary to compare substantially longer series of π_t and CPI_t before deciding whether the consumer price index could generally be used as a proxy for hospital non-labor input prices.

IV. GEOGRAPHIC VARIATION IN INPUT PRICES

Before examining the variation and change in the quality of services, it is worthwhile looking briefly at the behaviour of input costs. The input price index ($PRIN_{it}$) defined by equation (6) has been evaluated for each state and year. Table 20.3 summarizes the distribution among states for each of the years from 1958 through 1967; the index is scaled so that the average value of $PRIN_{it}$ for 1963 is equal to 1·0.

TABLE 20.3

GEOGRAPHIC VARIATION IN INPUT PRICES

Input price index ($PRIN_{it}$)

Year	National average	Standard deviation	Coefficient of variation	Maximum	Minimum
(1)	(2)	(3)	(4)	(5)	(6)
1958	0·851	0·061	0·072	1·012	0·756
1959	0·884	0·066	0·075	1·044	0·771
1960	0·914	0·075	0·082	1·092	0·788
1961	0·937	0·074	0·079	1·122	0·807
1962	0·963	0·078	0·080	1·156	0·837
1963	1·000	0·106	0·106	1·433	0·843
1964	1·023	0·089	0·087	1·241	0·881
1965	1·061	0·088	0·083	1·272	0·934
1966	1·079	0·087	0·081	1·292	0·938
1967	1·150	0·096	0·083	1·396	1·009

The average input price rose 35 per cent, from 0·85 in 1958 to 1·15 in 1967. If this is compared with the 13 per cent increase in the price of non-labor inputs (shown in Table 20.2), it is clear that average wages have risen very much faster than the price of non-labor inputs. The 35 per cent increase in the price of inputs can also be compared with the 85 per cent rise in average cost per patient-day during the same period. The higher cost of inputs can, by itself, account for only two-fifths of the higher cost per patient-day.

The variation in input prices among the states is quite significant. The average input price in the highest-cost state (column (5)) has generally been about 35 to 40 per cent higher than the average price in the lowest-cost state (column (6)). This range reflects a symmetric distribution with a coefficient of variation of about 0·08, as shown in column (4). It is clear that there has been no tendency for the relative inequality of input prices to increase or decrease during the decade.

The average increase in input prices during the decade was approximately as large as the 1958 interstate range of input prices. Moreover, the rate of price increase varied rather substantially, from 26 per cent in Wyoming to 50 per cent in New York. Despite this relatively rapid and varied increase and the importance of the local wage component, the specific interstate pattern of input prices has remained quite stable. The correlation between $PRIN_{it}$ in 1958 and 1967 is 0·91. The relation between the two sets of prices is also very close to proportional. Equation (10) shows that the elasticity of $PRIN_{i,\ 1967}$ with respect to $PRIN_{i,\ 1958}$ is approximately 1:

$$\log PRIN_{i,\ 1967} = 0\cdot110 + 1\cdot055 \log PRIN_{i,\ 1958} \quad R^2 = 0\cdot83. \tag{10}$$
$$(0.070)$$

This equation indicates that there has been no tendency for lower input prices to 'catch up' with the national average or for states with higher input prices to be brought back into line. This is also shown by the absence of a significant correlation between the relative increase in the input price ($PRIN_{i,\ 1967}/PRIN_{i,\ 1958}$) and the input price level in 1958; the actual correlation (0·12) is positive and insignificant.

The persistence of substantial interstate variation in input prices and the stability of the pattern of differentials reflect the general absence of a single national market for labor and, more specifically, the special characteristics of the labor market for hospital employees. The preponderance of low-skilled workers and the substantial number of married women both weaken the tendency for wages to equalize across areas. But this is just the supply side of the labor market. A full explanation of the interstate differences in wages and of their variation through time also requires an analysis of hospitals' demand for labor services and their wage policies. Although an attempt to explain these changes lies beyond the scope of the current paper,[1] the stable interstate variations indicate that a cross-section of states should be a useful data base for developing such an analysis.

The pattern of input prices implies that residents of different states must pay quite different prices to purchase the same level of quality.[2] The effect of this on the choice of quality level will be considered in the next section. It does imply that any federal program of health care or health insurance that tries to provide the same quality of services in all states will distribute quite unequal dollar benefits. Similarly,

---

[1] See Altman (1971) and Benham (1971) for interesting attempts to develop econometric models of the labor market for hospital nurses. In Feldstein (1971a) I discuss why the non-profit nature of the hospital may make the usual supply and demand analysis inadequate for explaining the wages of hospital employees.

[2] It is worth reemphasizing the caveat that some of the wage differentials may actually reflect quality differences in personnel.

a program that provides the same dollar benefits per patient-day will distribute quite unequal real benefits.[1]

V. GEOGRAPHIC VARIATION AND INTERTEMPORAL CHANGE IN QUALITY

The index of resource use per patient-day (R_{it}) has been evaluated using the definition of equations (4) through (7). To emphasize the relation between resource use and quality discussed in section II, I shall refer to R_{it} in the following analysis as an index of quality. A comparison with the definition in equation (3) shows that this ignores the role of time and implies that quality increases proportionately with resource inputs ($\rho = 1$). Ignoring time has no effect on relative interstate variation, but does understate the amount of quality increase during the decade. If quality is a convex function of resource inputs ($\rho < 1$), the following analysis overstates the relative variation in hospital quality. The general qualitative conclusions, particularly about the stability of that variation and of its geographic pattern, would be unaffected.

TABLE 20.4

GEOGRAPHIC VARIATION IN HOSPITAL QUALITY

			Hospital quality index (R_{it})		
Year	National average	Standard deviation	Coefficient of variation	Maximum	Minimum
(1)	(2)	(3)	(3)	(5)	(6)
1958	0·868	0·075	0·086	0·706	1·052
1959	0·888	0·078	0·088	0·693	1·033
1960	0·912	0·087	0·095	0·729	1·075
1961	0·967	0·086	0·089	0·770	0·123
1962	0·982	0·092	0·094	0·790	1·167
1963	1·000	0·102	0·102	0·743	1·204
1964	1·037	0·093	0·090	0·840	1·233
1965	1·078	0·096	0·089	0·867	1·292
1966	1·139	0·103	0·090	0·952	1·355
1967	1·185	0·123	0·104	0·966	1·454

Table 20·4 summarizes the interstate distribution of quality for each year in the decade. The interstate variation is substantial and persistent. The coefficient of variation remains between 8·5 and 10·5 per cent and indicates no clear trend in relative inequality. The quality index is generally 50 per cent higher in the maximum state than in the minimum. The pattern of quality differences also remained

[1] The persistent interstate differences in wages may also have an important implication for any possible future national wage policy for the health industry. Any attempt to set national wages would conflict with the natural forces that have led to the current differentials. The result might be shortages in some areas and excess supply in others.

relatively stable from the beginning to the end of the decade; the correlation of $R_{i,\ 1967}$ and $R_{i,\ 1958}$ is 0·81.

Although the rate of quality increase for some states did depart substantially from the mean – the increases ranged from 17 per cent to 57 per cent with a mean of 37 per cent – there was no overall tendency for the low-quality states to move upward more rapidly. The elasticity between the quality levels at the beginning and end of the decade is approximately 1:[1]

$$\log R_{i,\ 1967} = 0·305 + 0·966 \log \bar{R}_{i,\ 1958} \quad R^2 = 0·653. \tag{10}$$
$$(0·105)$$

This is also confirmed by the low and insignificant correlation of the growth of quality ($R_{i,\ 1967}/R_{i,\ 1958}$) and its 1958 level: $r = 0·045$.

The persistence and stability of the pattern of quality differences requires further explanation. A simple hypothesis is that quality is high where the price of quality is low, i.e. that there is an inverse relation between R_{it} and $PRIN_{it}$ across states for each year. Data for 1967 clearly contradict this. The correlation between $R_{i,\ 1967}$ and $PRIN_{i,\ 1967}$ is actually positive and significant ($r = +0·71$).[2] One possible explanation of this is that the input price index is higher in states where other factors that increase the quality of care are also above average. Equation (11) relates the logarithm of quality to the logarithm of real per capita income (*INC*), a measure of insurance coverage (*INS*)[3] and the input price index.[4]

$$\log R_{it} = -3·83 - 0·175 \log (INC) + 0·043 \log INS \tag{11}$$
$$(0·132) \qquad\qquad (0·071)$$
$$+ 1·24 \log PRIN_{it} \quad \bar{R}^2_{1967} = 0·52.$$
$$(0·25)$$

Neither of the two demand variables is significant, while the price elasticity is large and with the wrong sign. Similar results are obtained for other years.[5]

[1] Note that this equation also yields the elasticity of $Q_{i,\ 1967}$ with respect to $Q_{i,\ 1958}$. This elasticity is independent of the value of ρ and, of course, of the time term: $\log Q_{it} = \log k_1 + \rho_1 t + \rho \log R_{it}$. The first two terms are constants while ρ multiplies both the dependent and independent variables.

[2] Note that the usual errors-in-variables problem would tend to bias the coefficient toward zero. Moreover, since R_{it} is defined as the ratio of a cost index to $PRIN_{it}$, errors of measurement in $PRIN_{it}$ would be expected to introduce a negative bias.

[3] *INS* is defined as the proportion of hospital charges paid directly by patients; see Feldstein (1971*b*, pp. 859–61).

[4] Note that the use of log R_{it} rather than log Q_{it} changes the scale of the coefficients but not their relative magnitudes or *t*-statistics.

[5] The simple correlation of quality and income is, however, positive; the 1967 elasticity is 0·30 (s.e. = 0·08).

The implication of equation (11) is clear. The local price of hospital inputs is not exogenous but is jointly determined with the quality and quantity of hospital care. The forces that raise the local quality of care also increase the price of hospital inputs. This may operate through the usual forces of supply and demand for hospital labor. States with higher quality per day are also likely to have more patient-days per capita. Both factors raise the demand for hospital personnel and therefore the local wage. Moreover, because of the special non-profit character of the hospital, the positive correlation of wages and hospital quality may also reflect a deliberate 'philanthropic' wage policy on the part of hospitals. Hospitals that are insulated from the usual competitive market pressures may choose to use their discretionary market power to raise both the quality of services and the wages of hospital employees.[1]

The emphasis on geographic differences in the quality of hospital services should not obscure the fact that the rapid growth of individual quality levels is at least as significant as the inequalities that exist at any time. The state with the lowest quality level in 1965 had already achieved the national average of 1958. Since this measure ignores the effect of the passage of time on scientific progress and general innovation, it understates the extent to which changes in the absolute level of quality may dominate relative differences. In assessing the overall performance of the health care sector, it is important to remember that dynamic adjustments may be more important than static inequality or inefficiency.

To conclude this section, I shall return to the issue of the role of quality in the demand for care and, more specifically, to the problem of the bias in the estimated price elasticity when a measure of quality is not included in the demand equation. The discussion of section II showed that the price elasticity of demand would be biased toward zero if there is a positive partial correlation between the logarithm of the net price variable (NP_{it}) and the logarithm of the resource input variable (R_{it}).[2] The parameter ρ that relates resource input to quality affects the magnitude of the bias but not its existence or sign. Although a full analysis of this question lies beyond the scope of the current paper, it is interesting to examine the simple correlation

---

[1] A model of the hospital choosing the quality of services is presented in Feldstein (1971*b*). The notion of a 'philanthropic wage policy' is developed in chap. 5 of Feldstein (1971*a*). I am currently extending the econometric model to examine the question of 'philanthropic wage policy'.

[2] If the equation is estimated by two-stage least squares or some other instrumental variable procedure, the bias is more complicated and depends on the correlation of the omitted variable with the instruments. If the first stage has a low residual variance, this will not differ appreciably from the ordinary least squares bias.

between price and quality. Since the demand equation is specified to be linear in the logarithms of the variables, I shall consider the correlation between the logarithms of price and the logarithms of the quality or resource input variable.

For the entire ten-year sample, the correlation between $\log R_{it}$ and the logarithm of the real price per patient-day[1] is, as would be expected, very high: $r = +0.943$. The correlation is almost the same when attention is limited to a single year; for 1967 it is $+0.940$. It should be emphasized that the price variable in these correlations is the gross price charged by the hospital and not the price net of insurance that is actually paid by the patient. The correlation of resource input and net price is substantially lower: 0.633 for the entire period and 0.607 for 1967. Finally, if we assume that demand depends only on the *within*-state changes in quality and not on the differences among states, we must look at the relation between $\log (NP_{it})$ and $\log (RS_{it})$.[2] For the entire decade, this correlation is only 0.327. All these correlations suggest that omitting a measure of quality from the demand equation is likely to result in a downward bias of the estimated price elasticity. Since only simple correlations have been examined and the problem of simultaneity has been ignored, this must be regarded as a plausible hypothesis and a reason for more work rather than as a definite conclusion.

VI. QUESTIONS FOR FUTURE RESEARCH

The previous sections have already indicated several research problems that are suggested by the current study. These include the role of quality in the demand for care and the extent of 'philanthropic' wage-setting in non-profit hospitals. Closely related is the question of how input prices affect the level of quality and the rate of product innovation.

The period since 1967 has seen an extremely rapid increase in hospital costs. It would be valuable to extend the current study to more recent years. Of particular interest would be the effect of the very substantial growth of federal health care funds for the poor and the aged on the interstate distribution of quality.

An international comparison of the extent of interregional variation in the quality of services would shed light on the effect of health sector organization and financing on the equality of care. I suspect that such differences in quality variation between national health

---

[1] The price variable is defined as the average cost per patient-day deflated by the annual consumer price index.

[2] Recall that RS_{it} is constructed so that it equals 1.0 in every state in 1963 and therefore only reflects intertemporal change. See section II for more detail.

services, like the British, and private non-profit systems, like that in the United States, are relatively small. It would be of further interest to examine the relation in different national settings between local quality and variables such as income and urbanization.

Finally, a quite different economic measure of quality should be examined and related to the current analysis. Hedonic quality indices assess quality by the market's willingness to pay for attributes of a product (see Griliches, 1971). If the agency relationship between patients and physicians is relatively complete,[1] a hedonic quality index (with adjustment for insurance) would be an appropriate normative measure of quality. The relation between the hedonic index and the current real input measure of quality could be investigated. Such an analysis would help us to understand the way in which the local market structure affects how hospitals allocate additional resource inputs between the services and facilities valued by patients and those valued by the providers.

The quality of care and the process of product change are central to any analysis of the health care sector. Although the measurement problems here are potentially enormous, quite simple measures may be useful in a number of areas of aggregate analysis. I hope that the current study will encourage further work on this important subject.

[1] See Feldstein (1973b) for a discussion of a complete and incomplete agency model of the physician's role in the demand for hospital care.

REFERENCES

Altman, S. H., *Present and Future Supply of Registered Nurses* (Washington, D.C.: U.S. Government Printing Office, 1971).

American Hospital Association, *Hospitals, Journal of the American Hospital Association: Guide Issue* (1967).

Arrow, Kenneth J., 'Uncertainty and the Welfare Economics of Medical Care', *American Economic Review*, LIII (Dec 1963) 941–73.

Benham, Lee, 'The Labor Market for Registered Nurses: A Three-Equation Model', *Review of Economics and Statistics*, LIII, 3 (Aug 1971) 246–52.

Feldstein, M. S., *Economic Analysis for Health Services Efficiency: Econometric Studies of the British National Health Service* (Amsterdam: North-Holland, 1967).

——, *The Rising Cost of Hospital Care* (Washington, D.C.: Information Resources Press, 1971a).

——, 'Hospital Cost Inflation: A Study of Nonprofit Price Dymanics', *American Economic Review*, LXI, 5 (Dec 1971) 853–72 (1971b).

——, 'The Welfare Loss of Excess Health Insurance', *Journal of Political Economy* (1973a).

——, 'Econometric Approaches to Health Economics', in M. Intriligator and D. Kendrick (eds.), *Frontiers of Quantitative Economics*, vol. II: (Amsterdam, North-Holland, 1973b).

Griliches, Z. (ed.), *Price Indexes and Quality Change* (Cambridge, Mass.: Harvard Univ. Press, 1971).

Grossman, M., *The Demand for Health: A Theoretical and Empirical Investigation* (New York: National Bureau of Economic Research, 1972).

National Advisory Commission on Health Manpower, *Report*, 2 vols. (Washington, D.C.: U.S. Government Printing Office, 1967).

Newhouse, J. P., 'Toward a Theory of Nonprofit Institutions: An Economic Model of a Hospital', *American Economic Review*, LX, 1 (Mar 1970) 64–74.

Pauly, M., and Redisch, M., 'The Not-for-Profit Hospital as a Physicians' Cooperative', unpublished paper (1971).

Reder, M. W., 'Some Problems in the Measurement of Productivity in the Medical Care Industry', in V. Fuchs (ed.), *Production and Productivity in the Service Industries*, vol. XXXIV of *Studies in Income and Wealth* (New York: Columbia Univ. Press, 1969).

Taylor, V. D., *The Price of Hospital Care* (Santa Monica, Calif.: RAND Corporation, May 1969).

U.S. Department of Commerce, *Input–Output Structure of the U.S. Economy*, 1963, vol. I (Washington, D.C.: U.S. Department of Commerce, Office of Business Economics, 1969).

Summary Record of Discussion

The three papers presented at this session advocated rival approaches to the problem of measuring the effectiveness of health care. Because of the absence of one of the authors (Professor Feldstein), due to illness, the format of the session differed from that of most of the earlier ones. The three papers were presented in order, together with prepared discussions; these presentations were followed by open discussion.

The papers in question were by Professor Feldstein on measuring the quality of hospital services in particular, by Professor Lévy on health indicators in the analysis of the health care system, and by Professor Williams on measuring the effectiveness of health care in general.

Mr Culyer presented and discussed Professor Feldstein's paper. The Feldstein proposal, he said, was to measure the quality of hospital *output* in terms of the quality of hospital *inputs*. Quality indexes were computed separately for labor and non-labor inputs, deflated respectively by indices of wage rates and of capital-goods prices. When cost per case rose above the costs of inputs, as it has, the differential may be taken as an indicator of quality improvement.

Mr Culyer criticized this approach as misguided 'ingenuity', primarily on the ground that the quality of health output was not in practice, related very closely to the quantity of health inputs as estimated by the Feldstein method. Not being himself an econometrician, Mr Culyer limited his criticism to conceptual aspects.

The main reason for Mr Culyer's skepticism about Professor Feldstein's use of input quantity as surrogate for output quality was that, in his own opinion, it was not a good surrogate in practice. The quality of output was related not only to the quantity of inputs, but to the quality of transformation of inputs and outputs, i.e. to choice of technique.

Mr Culyer gave several illustrations of problems which concerned him. Two were: Is long bed rest, whatever its quantity, really related to the quality of health care in tuberculosis. Is surgery, whatever its quality, really as necessary in pediatric tonsillectomy as we have assumed, or is a non-surgical approach to tonsillitis preferable? There was abundant evidence that choice of techniques in treatment was not related to cost, nor was the effectiveness of alternative treatments in terms of their outcomes (quality) systematically related to cost.

In Mr Culyer's view, the entire production function approach (to the measurement of health quantity and quality) is questionable, since a definition of quality in terms of inputs deprives us of the opportunity of testing the *hypothesis* that inputs and quality vary together, but to test the hypothesis, one would need to measure final outcomes. There is no short-cut to the direct measurement of health output, and British experience has convinced him (Mr Culyer) that such direct measurement is possible. Professor Feldstein's indices of input quality avoid the problem rather than solving it. The patient's subjective feeling, Mr Culyer added (referring to the Lave–Lave–Leinhardt paper), is also important, but by no means the whole story. What he himself hopes for is separate measurements and predictions of the utilization of health facilities (related to subjective feelings) and of objective health quality.

Professor Williams then introduced and discussed Professor Lévy's paper. Professor Lévy's position is that no one set of indicators can serve all purposes, and that the optimal research strategy would make use of existing statistics to the maximum possible extent. These include 'upstream' indicators of vulnerability (such as alcohol and tobacco consumption), 'alongside' indicators of morbidity (as felt subjectively, as diagnosed initially, and as reflected *ex post* in published data), and 'downstream' indicators of mortality and life expectancy. All these indicators should, somehow, be interrelated within the system, but Professor Williams did not believe that the Lévy paper handled the interrelation problem satisfactorily.

Although himself an advocate of an alternative position, Professor Williams looked with sympathy and encouragement on Professor Lévy's efforts, provided one realizes that the data are unreliable, that the unreliability is communicated to consumers of the data, and that no strong policy recommendations are based upon such data.

Even for the short term, however, Professor Williams prefers his own approach to continued work with what he called 'the present garbage'. For the long run, he felt the Lave–Lave–Leinhardt approach might be more productive. As for the 'upstream–downstream' distinction stressed in the Lévy paper, he felt that this would be helpful only in the long run. He also expressed the view that longitudinal (time series) studies of medical-economic statistics were basic, and suggested that Professor Lévy concentrate on these, rather than on inter-country or inter-system comparisons.

Discussion then passed to Professor Williams's own paper, which was introduced and discussed by *M. Dupuy*. M. Dupuy praised this paper for considering the interests of consumers (patients) and for minimizing confusion between inputs, outputs and throughputs. In particular, it was preferable, in his (M. Dupuy's) opinion, to cost–benefit analysis, which was related too closely to conventional economics.

The Williams system, as M. Dupuy understands it, operates in three stages. First, two-dimensional severity indexes for particular conditions may be constructed, the two dimensions being pain to the patient and restriction of activity. Second, the estimate (by physicians) of indifference curves in this (ordinal) restriction of activity–pain space. Third, transferring the results to a cardinal scale by policy-makers in the health area. In addition, the use of 'human capital' notions may be helpful in placing monetary values upon shifts in the various indifference curves.

This strategy, said M. Dupuy, is far from optimal, particularly in its reliance on physicians in the second stage. Professor Williams assumes, in M. Dupuy's opinion, a closer connection between the patient's state of health and his satisfaction level than exists in practice. Moreover, he does not take into consideration the fact that the doctor's appreciation on the patient's state of health is not merely a technical application, but is dependent upon the doctor's social value, which may greatly differ from the patient's own value. In a sense, the Williams indicators are throughputs and not outputs, because the final outcome, the patient's well-being, is dependent upon the patient's psycho-social background, and is variable both over time and with the socio-cultural environment. In some cultures, and in some classes, more concern for physical ailments is legitimized than in other cultures and classes. Our standards of comfort vary, depending on whether we are on camping trips or living in our own houses. Compulsory wearing of safety belts in automobiles and compulsory physical examinations may lower subjective feelings of well-being, even though the objective results are as desired by those who propose such requirements.[1]

If we ever obtain an adequate indicator of the final outcome of health activities, said M. Dupuy, it will be by collaboration of economists, sociologists and psychologists. This interdisciplinary collaboration may not provide quantitative results in short order, but this is not (at least not to M. Dupuy) a *sine qua non* condition. What is really important, in M. Dupuy's opinion, is to try to understand what really concerns people. Otherwise, there is a great danger of imposing an extrinsic rationality on the health system.

Dr Christiansen opened discussion from the floor by sympathizing with both the Williams and the Lévy approaches, and expressing the view that usable cost–benefit analysis was a matter of the distant future. The main thrust of his interpellation, however, was to expand the Dupuy critique of the Williams paper. Professor Williams's two-dimensional analysis might well be adequate for problems of geriatrics and of surgery, but he (Dr Christiansen) was puzzled as to its applicability to conditions like the contagious diseases, secondary syphilis, the anemias, or early pneumonia. In Dr Christiansen's opinion, several more dimensions are needed for intensity indexes, or for any attempts to combine such micro-indexes to measure the health status of an individual or a population. Also, the question of time (until health is restored) should be considered more carefully, especially when we are dealing with the early stages of chronic conditions, or with 'health euphoria', where the easy way out may be to leave the condition untreated and maximize short-term benefits to all concerned.

Dr Friedman expressed concern for the ideological implications of the discussion.[2] Some of the objective health measures advocated at the Conference, he feared, might involve too great delegation of power to decision-makers and away from individuals (patients) themselves.

Professor Fuchs wished that more attention had been paid throughout to the problems of mental illness, which are of increasing importance

---

[1] To illustrate his differences with both the Williams and the Lave–Lave–Leinhardt papers, M. Dupuy prepared a diagram which was made available to Conference participants but is not reproduced here.

[2] He also inquired, relative to the Dupuy diagram (not reproduced here), whether one could fit educational campaigns (changing persons' subjective viewpoints on health matters) into such a presentation.

in the developed countries. He felt that they were being relegated to 'another conference', despite the thin and tenuous line between mental and physical ailments suggested by the term 'psychosomatic'. He also wondered how the health care system should deal with the insane person who believed himself well and/or everyone else 'sick'.

Professor Intriligator hoped, eventually, for a more direct and immediate approach to the health quality problem than is involved in Professor Williams's paper. He also would like more technical detail than had been made available in that paper.

Professor J. Lave felt that there was a great deal of overlapping between the Lévy and Williams papers (presented at this session) and the paper of which she had been co-author. The problem of seeking care (in the Lave–Lave–Leinhardt scheme) is, indeed, related closely to the psycho-social complex of elements dealt with by Professors Lévy and Williams, and M. Dupuy. On the other hand, Professor Lave felt that the current group of papers were ignoring the problem of cost, which is important, especially for patients in relatively good health. Concern for cost has been the rationale for nominal charges, less to shift the cost to the patient than to discourage marginal calls upon the health care system's limited capacity. She also felt that discussion of 'health status' and 'health care quality' in the large was too aggregative. What is important is not an aggregate health status indicator, but the specific individual decisions about treatment of specific ailments.

Professor Evans (and also *Mr Kaser*) disagreed with Professor J. Lave on the usefulness of health charges. In Canada, said Professor Evans, only the doctors complain about 'overuse' of the health care system by the relatively healthy. Nominal charges would have little or no effect on the total demand for health services. Granted, the poor would use them less, but the rich might well use them more, because of any possible reduction in waiting time. *Professor L. Lave* felt that the cost problem included time as well as money. In fact, the main cost of health care is patient's time lost. When, as he said, doctors believed that 80 per cent of cases do not really need professional care, charges would save the time of the 20 per cent of patients who do need such care.

At this point the Conference adjourned for a mid-morning intermission with the understanding that Professor Williams should present an 'intermediate view' of the health quality problem as he saw it, with special reference to his own scheme, immediately afterwards.

Professor Williams proposed to omit ideological positions and avoid controversy. For somewhat the same reasons, he felt it might be better to drop the distinction between 'objective' and 'subjective' measures of health states. A better distinction, in his opinion, was between 'other-perceived' and 'self-perceived' states.

The question of breadth versus narrowness of definition was more substantial. We are dealing with matters of community interest, to be decided, if at all, in a collective fashion. We want tools which policy-makers can use, but with which the electorate can be satisfied. In a similar fashion, some measure of social control over the medical profession is desired, but it should not be direct or arbitrary. These considerations point in principle, perhaps, to a wider definition, including specifically psychological considerations of the sort mentioned by M. Dupuy and Professor Fuchs. But this is at present too difficult to be operational. It is desirable that any index should not require the services of too highly trained people. It is also desirable to rely somewhat upon the views of physicians, if only because the health care system must also rely on their professional judgment, sometimes overriding that of the patient himself. In his own system, the weight of medical view is expressed in the aggregation system for his proposed health indicator. It may be too large or too small a weight – this is a matter for policy judgment – but in any case, the patient may have his day, if not in court, in the polling place.

Following the Williams 'intermediate view', *Professor Perlman* shifted the discussion to health indicators and the Lévy paper. He said (and *Mr Kaser* agreed) that the indicator problem is an interdisciplinary one, which cannot be settled by economists alone. In addition to psychology and sociology, contributions are required from medicine, epidemiology, statistics and law. But at the same time, these other disciplines are likewise at sea, and await the contributions of economists. There will be a major conference on health indicators in 1975 for European countries, and meanwhile the World Health Organization is being kept informed (at its own request) of the proceedings here. Only its tight budget kept W.H.O. from sending an observer or participant to Tokyo for this conference.

M. Foulon turned the discussion back to the sixth session, by discussing the role of the patient's own conception of his health state. He thought that the patient's subjective conception is important, but perhaps different from his health stock or status as objectively determined. (The second, for example, may be additive as between individuals, while the first is not.) Correlation between the two is difficult. Each may be useful for its own purposes: objective and quantitative indices for production functions, and qualitative ones for judging self-perceived welfare levels. Similar problems also arise when one is dealing with education. *Professor J. Lave* expressed herself in general agreement, adding that it was perhaps possible to combine self-perceptions and other-perceptions for decision-making purposes and objecting to 'polarization' between the two. Returning also to her disagreement (before the intermission) with Professor Evans and Mr Kaser, Professor Lave thought that the difference was primarily statistical, and related to the *probability* that the health care system might be bogged down with minor ailments in the presence of health insurance or the British N.H.S.

Dr Kleiman addressed himself to the Williams indifference curve scheme. He agreed that one should start with indifference curves, but we should, at the same time, realize that the present set of preferences revealed by such curves are not given by God. Rather, they result from experience with existing transformations of health inputs into health outputs, and from the existing cost structure. When and how these functions should be changed remains a policy problem. Moreover, Dr Kleiman continued, health is a public good, to which inter-dependent utility functions apply. Conventional economic analysis requires considerable modification to work well in such cases.

At the same time, Dr Kleiman characterized as 'abdication of responsibility' the tendency of several other participants to leave problems of social choice to the electorate or to the politicians. The general public is volatile and not dispassionate. It is affected, for example, by epidemics in the recent past or by the short-term future, which tend to warp electoral judgments.[1]

Mr Cooper said that Professor Williams had relegated more responsibility both to physicians and to the electorate than he need have. We should not confuse want and need; the latter can be assessed by outsiders, and there is little disagreement about it. In the same way, according to Mr Cooper, the Professors Lave and Professor Leinhardt underestimate the importance of need in their transition probabilities. There has also been, again in Mr Cooper's view, too much concern with the burden of minor illnesses on the health care system, and not enough with the 'iceberg of illness' which remains undiagnosed and untreated. (This iceberg is not considered in the Williams scheme either, as far as Mr Cooper could see.)

Dr Friedman agreed with the other speakers as to the importance, in a planned system of health care, of having simple and readily available measures of health care and effectiveness. But such systems tend, he feared, to forget the opportunity costs of improving the system's performance, which involve the allocation of resources between health care and the remainder of the economy. He (Dr Friedman) was also concerned lest patient preferences be forgotten. He saw a basic problem in structuring incentives in a planned system in such a way that patient preferences are revealed and taken into account. Accordingly, he thought that education and information were important governmental activities in any health care system. Finally, he thought that, however much they could be improved upon, such conventional measures as mortality rates and life expectancies remained useful measures of a health care system's success.

Professor Robinson thought that the problems of evidence (of a health care system's success) and evaluation (in financial terms) had best be separated. He wondered whether the evaluation problems, in particular, might not best be studied in the armed services, because the evidence problems are less serious there. For many decisions of resource allocation in particular, the evaluation problem is the main one. It is complex, and involves comparing a multiplicity of health states as well as weighting or adding up effects on different individuals. However, these problems are handled – however badly – by the courts, in connection with damage suits involving particularly accidents, and the results are translated into monetary terms. Could not health economists utilize this experience as well? *Professor J. Lave* replied that work was, indeed, in progress along the lines that Professor Robinson had suggested.

[1] As if to bear out Dr Kleiman's statement on this point, Tokyo had a smallpox scare the week after the Conference adjourned, on the basis of one case – a Japanese who had just returned from Bangladesh.

At this point, *Professor Levy* presented certain conclusions of his own, and also his view of the Williams proposal. His five principal conclusions to date were: (1) 'Final result' indicators were not practical; his own solution, involving a multiplicity of indicators, was, admittedly, 'second best'. (2) The health status of any individual is also complex, involving his exposure to risk, his degree of morbidity (subjective, diagnostic and objective), his protective resources (including the financial), and also the prospective effects of whatever ailments he might have. (3) Use of any single simple indicator loses a great deal of information; the final result of its use is to high-light one aspect of our information at the expense of all the rest. (4) The multiplicity of different diseases and different risks makes the problem more complex and more delicate. (5) Health status indicators are, to some extent, variable with the problem being studied, and are also subject to 'technique priority', meaning that changes in statistical technique may change their relative feasibilities.

On the Williams proposal, in particular, Professor Levy saw no close relation between the subdivision of the health system and the single, overall Williams indicator; in fact, there may be an inconsistency involved. He thought that a general overall decision-making model was unrealistic and overly aggregative. He also believed that one's vulnerability to disease depended upon one's health status as well as the reverse; this aspect of the problem had been generally ignored thus far.

Mr Pole agreed that the Williams proposal might be improved by greater attention to what he (Mr Pole) called 'chicken–egg situations' of simultaneous causation in opposite directions, but he thought it best to discuss the proposal primarily in terms of its technical efficacy. In reply, *Professor Fuchs* felt that economists should avoid getting themselves involved in technological problems where doctors know so much more. Economists should limit themselves to studying the behavior of physicians, planners, patients, etc., both positively and normatively.

Dr Christiansen wondered whether Professor Williams had answered his earlier doubt about the validity of the Williams measures of intensity, i.e. whether the judgments involved were such that physicians agreed upon the outcome. To this direct question, *Professor Williams* answered that he had found his measures valid in an aggregative sense, meaning most of the time. Additivity, however, Professor Williams continued is another problem which involves political judgment. He (Professor Williams) is an egalitarian, and would weight all people's illnesses equally. But he has not proposed that economists – egalitarian or not – make such evaluations themselves.

Professor Intriligator agreed with Professor Fuchs that behavior should be studied, and felt that the Feldstein model shoud be interpreted as judging health quality by market behavior, rather than as using inputs as surrogates for output. He thought that the Williams paper proposed to equate quality with effectiveness. This, he thought, might be misleading if, for example, 'quality' involved a longer waiting period.

Dr Friedman also approved of the emphasis upon behavior. He said that economists focus on value-neutral conditions for the correct answers to social questions. If for whatever reason, redistribution of income or wealth is desired from the health care system, it is certainly legitimate to inquire whether or not it is being achieved, and also what the side-effects may be. To this, *Professor Kleiman* added that economists always made value judgments, and that they should admit doing so.

Mr Pole said that economists had the duty to insert the problem of resource allocation into discussions which, without them, tended to assume an economy of abundance. Also, they should judge the efficiency of such allocation. For this purpose, it is desirable to use production functions so that marginal productivities can be estimated.

M. Foulon commented, with special reference to morbidity indicators, that some part of morbidity was always hidden by errors of patients and doctors. This was particularly true in psychosomatic cases, as other participants had indicated. He also added that any measure of health care effectiveness was difficult in the presence of simultaneous and related illnesses, as in geriatric practice, where a treatment effective for one condition may exacerbate another.

The task of a final summary was left to *Professor Williams*. He began by discussing the economist's role: providing a framework for interdisciplinary dialogue, as well as securing usable information. (As an example, he agreed with Mr Pole that production functions were, in principle, as applicable in medicine as in industry.) He went on to claim that economic expertise may relate to non-market behavior – planning, politics, etc. – despite some of the derogation of 'conventional economics' at this conference. He felt that he was agreeing with both Drs Kleiman and Friedman on the necessity of making normative judgments and labeling them as such. To say, merely, 'study behavior' may dodge a number of the most important issues at hand.

Relative to Professor Robinson's suggestion to study what the courts are doing to evaluate health and life, Professor Williams pointed out that lawyers and judges would like to have more and better economic data; it is a case of 'the blind leading the blind'. But to return to the main theme, Professor Williams repeated, the main role of the economist was to provide a framework for interdisciplinary dialogue. The Williams proposal, concluded its author, was one such framework which could be applied operationally.

21 Smoking and the Economics of Government Intervention[1]

Anthony B. Atkinson
UNIVERSITY OF ESSEX

If the existence of a relationship between smoking and disease is accepted, the question arises of the desirability of government intervention to reduce tobacco consumption. This paper is concerned with the economic aspects of this question and, in particular, with the development of an underlying theoretical framework. The model of individual smoking behavior is based on utility maximization, but also allows for imperfect knowledge and habit formation. The welfare economic implications are then explored, and related to various estimates of the 'cost' of smoking. The paper also considers the choice between taxation and health education as means of reducing smoking, and brings out the point that more information about the health risks of smoking is not necessarily socially desirable.

I. INTRODUCTION

A recent review of the evidence concerning the relationship between smoking and the incidence of cancer stated that 'it is now clear that smoking plays a significant role in the production of most cancers of the upper digestive tract, the respiratory tract, and the bladder' (Doll in [1], p. 10). More generally, the prospective studies of Doll and Hill [4], Hammond and Horn [3] and others have shown a substantially higher mortality rate from all conditions. A selection of the evidence from the Hammond and Horn study is presented in Table 21.1 and Fig. 21.1. How far this excess mortality can be attributed to smoking has been the subject of controversy, but in the case of the specific conditions mentioned by Doll, the relationship appears to be well established. In the case of lung cancer, the excess mortality is very substantial (see Table 21.2).

[1] This paper grew out of a joint project on the economic consequences of smoking between the M.R.C./D.H.S.S. Epidemiology and Medical Care Unit, Northwick Park Hospital, and the Department of Economics, University of Essex. Many of the ideas arose from discussions with Joy Skegg, who is the Senior Research Officer working on the project, and I am grateful to C. C. von Weizsäcker and C. J. Bliss for their comments.

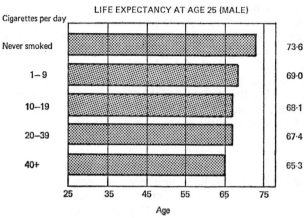

FIG. 21.1   Life expectancy at age 25 (male)

TABLE 21.1

MORTALITY RATIO (NON-SMOKERS = 1.00),
UNITED STATES

Lifetime smoking history	Men aged 45–54	Men aged 65–74
Pipe only	0·96	1·06
Cigar only	1·17	1·05
Cigarettes only	2·20	1·58
Cigarette and other	1·88	1·36

Source: Hammond in [1], Table 1.

TABLE 21·2

MORTALITY RATIO FOR LUNG CANCER
(NON-SMOKERS = 1·00)

Study	Current cigarette smokers	Current pipe/cigar smokers
British doctors	16·9	4·6
U.S. veterans	12·1	1·7
U.S. 9 counties	10·0	–
Canadian veterans	11·7	–

Source: Doll in [1], Table 1.

If the existence of a relationship between smoking and the incidence of disease is accepted, we should then consider the desirability of government intervention to reduce tobacco consumption, and the form which this intervention should take. It is with the economic aspects of these questions that this paper is concerned. Section II reviews the empirical studies which have been made of the costs of smoking in Britain, and suggests that the underlying welfare economic framework has not been adequately considered. As a first attempt to remedy this deficiency, a theoretical analysis of the case for intervention (by taxation or by health education) is presented in sections III and IV. This analysis is based on a highly stylized model of smoking behaviour,[1] but the starkness of the assumptions made may serve to demonstrate the need for further research, and this need is discussed in the final section of the paper.

II. ESTIMATES OF THE 'COST' OF SMOKING

A number of estimates have been made in recent years for the 'cost' of smoking in Britain, including those by Peston (in [1]), the Royal College of Physicians [2] and the Department of Health and Social Security.[2] The use of inverted commas is justified on the grounds that these studies appear to view cost in a rather different light, and it is with these differences that this section is primarily concerned.

The most straightforward approach – and one commonly adopted by doctors – is to view the problem as parallel to that of vaccination against, say, polio. For the expenditure on vaccination (health education to publicize risk involved in smoking) there is a return in reduced health costs, reduced sickness absence, the value of the lives saved, etc. It is this approach which appears to be the basis of the estimate of a total cost of £150 million made by Preston, which is made up of the following items:

	£m
Treatment cost	50
Lost production as a result of sickness	290
Cost of premature death	150
Fires	20

The analogy with vaccination is not, however, valid, since campaigns against smoking may impose costs on those giving up smoking (or, indeed, on those continuing) which have no parallel in the case of vaccination. A much more natural approach for an economist is that based on the divergence between social and private benefits and costs. In the extreme case where smokers are assumed to possess full information about the health risk, and where there are no habit effects, the argument for intervention would have to be based on the costs

---

[1] Some readers may conclude that only a non-smoker could put forward such a model!

[2] Estimates have been made for other countries (see, for example, [5]), but these are not discussed here.

imposed on others, e.g. health costs and the net tax contribution.[1] It would be possible to interpret the Department of Health and Social Security figures as being concerned with these divergencies, and they estimate that a 100 per cent reduction in smoking would lead, in the long run, to the following reduction costs imposed on others:

	£m
Health costs	– 12½
Social security payments	– 60
Taxes paid	+210

(The net *increase* in health costs arises from the fact that the savings on smoking-related disease are offset by the higher subsequent health costs for survivors.)

The approach just considered meets with resistance from the medical profession, but it has the merit of treating smoking in the same way as other activities in which individuals voluntarily assume risks, such as, for example, skiing. It would not be suggested that the social desirability of the latter should be assessed simply in terms of the working hours lost and the health costs, without any reference to the consumption benefits from skiing, and if smoking is to be treated differently, then an argument has to be made to this effect. At the same time, the extreme form of the approach outlined above is clearly not a realistic basis for policy-making, and allowance has to be made for imperfect information, for the addictive nature of tobacco, and for the social forces influencing its consumption. In the following sections, an attempt is made to incorporate these factors, and to see under what assumptions different approaches to the measurement of the costs of smoking would be valid. The analysis is also concerned with the relative merits of two main forms of intervention: publicity concerning the health hazard, and taxation. The advocates of increased government intervention tend to assume that these two approaches are perfect substitutes, but it is far from clear that this is necessarily so.

III. THE INDIVIDUAL SMOKING DECISION

(1) *The Basic Assumptions*

(i) A person plans his consumption of cigarettes C_t in period t and his consumption of other goods X_t subject to the budget constraint.

$$X_t + p_t C_t = E_t$$

[1] In this case, no allowance would be made for the risk to the smoker. As it is put by Mishan [6]: 'If smoking tobacco causes 20,000 deaths a year, no subtracting from the benefits, on account of this risk, need be entered, inasmuch as smokers are already aware that the tobacco habit is unhealthy.'

432   *The Economics of Health and Medical Care*

where E_t is exogenous and p_t denotes the price of cigarettes (inclusive of tax).

(ii) A person maximizes the expected utility derived from consumption over the remainder of his lifetime: i.e. at time V,

$$\max W_V = \overset{t=T}{\underset{t=V}{\Sigma}} U[X_t, C_t, Z_t]F_t$$

where F_t is the probability of his being alive in period t, Z_t is a variable reflecting past consumption (the effect of habit) and U is a concave function.[1] It is assumed that $U \geqslant 0$ for the relevant E_t.

(iii) The survival rate F_t depends on the death rates from smoking-related diseases δ_t^s and other causes δ_t (exogenous):

$$F_t\_F_{t-1} = -(\delta_t^s + \delta_t)F_{t-1}.$$

The deaths from smoking related diseases are assumed to be a function of age and current cigarette consumption. This assumption is not fully consistent with the evidence of Doll, which suggests that past consumption is also important, but may be a reasonable first approximation.

(iv) The person is covered by a state health service which is financed by a uniform tax (unrelated to the incidence of illness).

On the basis of the four assumptions described above, it is possible to characterize the utility-maximizing behaviour of the individual. In order to simplify the analysis we shall, however, add the following extra assumptions:

(v) The person lives for only two periods ($t = 1, 2$) and $E_1 = E_2 = E$.

(vi) The survival rates are given by

$$F_1 = e^{-A_1^* C_1}, \ F_2 = e^{-A_2^* C_2} G_2$$

where G_2 is the survival rate for a non-smoker, and it is assumed that $A_1^*(1 + G_2) < A_2^*$.[2]

(2) *Smoking Behaviour: No Habit Formation and Perfect Knowledge*

We consider, first, the case where U does not depend on Z_t and where the person has perfect knowledge of the relationship between smoking and mortality.

At the beginning of period 1, he maximizes

---

[1] The cardinal nature of U is clearly important. It should be noted that other formulations of the individual's objective function may be more attractive, e.g. maximizing the expected average flow of utility.

[2] Empirically, it appears that for constant C, $F = e^{-pct^5}$ where t denotes number of years smoking (Pike and Doll [7]), so that this assumption does not appear unreasonable.

$$W_1 = U(C_1)e^{-A_1^* C_1} + U(C_2)e^{-(A_1^* C_1 + A_2^* C_2)} \, G_2$$

where $U(C)$ denotes $U(E - pC, C)$. If he survives to consume in period 2, he chooses C_2 to maximize

$$W_2 = U(C_2)e^{-A_2^* C_2} G_2$$

so that his plan is intertemporally consistent (i.e. he carries out at the beginning of period 2 his consumption planned at the beginning of period 1). The first-order conditions for maximization are

$$\frac{\partial W_1}{\partial C_2} = e^{-A_1^* C_1}[U'(C_1) - A_1^*\{U(C_1) + U(C_2)e^{-A_2^* C_2}G_2\}] \leq 0 \qquad (1)$$

with equality if $C_1 > 0$ (and $C_1 = 0$ if $\partial W/\partial C_1 < 0$),

$$\frac{\partial W}{\partial C_2} = G_2\, e^{-(A_1^* C_1 + A^* C_2)}\, [U_1(C_2) - A_2^*\, U(C_2)]^1 \leq 0 \qquad (2)$$

with equality if $C_2 > 0$ (and $C_2 = 0$ if $\partial W/\partial C_2 < 0$).

We may characterize the solution in terms of the value of $U^1(0)/U(0)$:

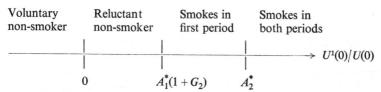

| Voluntary non-smoker | Reluctant non-smoker | Smokes in first period | Smokes in both periods |

$$0 \qquad\qquad A_1^*(1 + G_2) \qquad\qquad A_2^*$$

'Voluntary' non-smokers are those who would not choose to do so even if there were no health risk ($U^1(0) < 0$). For those people with $U^1(0) > 0$, we have either $C_1 = C_2 = 0$ ('reluctant' non-smokers), or $C_1 > 0$, $C_2 = 0$ or $C_1 > 0$, $C_2 > 0$ (as shown in Fig. 21.2).

(3) *Imperfect Knowledge*
Suppose that the individual believes the risk to be determined by A_1 and A_2. If $A_2 < A_2^*$ (the true value), it is clear that the number of smokers is higher. Moreover, for a person who previously was ignorant of the health risk, knowledge that $A_2 > 0$ will lead him to cut down the amount smoked (from $\bar{C}$ in Fig. 21.2). At the same time, it is not necessarily true that increasing knowledge of the risk leads to reduced consumption. If A_2 increases, then C_2 falls; but if A_1 is constant while A_2 increases, then C_1 rises. A person in period 1 knows that expected utility in period 2 is lower, and therefore there is less incentive to cut down in period 1.

These results show that the spread of information about the health

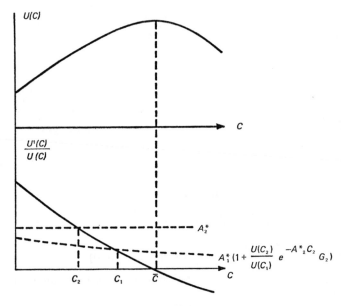

FIG. 21.2

hazard reduces the number of smokers, but may increase consumption among young continuing smokers where the publicity is directed particularly at the risks in later life (as with lung cancer).

It may also be noted that increased knowledge about the health risks may reduce the responsiveness of consumption to price change. If

$$U = C^\alpha(E - pC)^{1-\alpha} \quad (0 < \alpha < 1)$$

the elasticity of demand in period $2(\epsilon_2)$ is given by

$$\frac{1}{\epsilon_2} = 1 + \frac{A_2C_2(1 - \alpha)}{(1 - A_2C_2)(\alpha - A_2C_2)}.$$

On the assumption that $A_2C_2 < \alpha$, the elasticity falls as A rises above zero: e.g. if $AC = 0.05$ and $\alpha = 0.10$, the elasticity would be halved.

(4) Habit Formation

The introduction of habit via the dependence of utility in the second period on C_1 is straightforward. On the assumption that $\partial v/\partial z < 0$, the person, must allow, in period 1, for the reduction in the later utility as he becomes habituated to tobacco consumption. If the person behaves myopically, and ignores this interdependence, then he will later 'regret' his earlier decision and may (depending on the form of U) raise his planned consumption C_2.

This formulation of the habit-forming effect of tobacco is similar to that put forward by Preston [9], Pollack [10] and von Weizsäcker [11], but it may not fully capture its addictive nature. Peston, for example, referred in the case of tobacco to the 'widespread evidence of large numbers of people who recognize its dangers and would like to give up, but are unable to do so'. Moreover, it can be argued that the habit may be transmitted to others (e.g. across generations). These considerations may be incorporated by supposing that individuals inherit a level of consumption C_0, that there are substantial costs of adjustment involved in reducing this level, and – in an extreme form – that the consumer is intrinsically indifferent about the allocation of his expenditure,[1] i.e.

$$W = U[E, g(C_1/C_0)] \, e^{-A_1 C_1} + U[E, g(C_2/C_1)]e^{-A_1 C_1 + A_2 C_2)} \, G_2$$

where g represents the cost of adjustment, having a shape similar to that shown in Fig. 3, and $\partial U/\partial g < 0$. With suitable modifications, the analysis can be carried out as before.

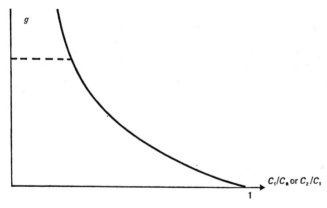

FIG. 21.3   Note: there is assumed to be discontinuity at zero

(5) *Relationship with Empirical Demand Studies*
An analysis of the demand for tobacco in Britain in the period 1951–1970 suggests the following conclusions [8]:

[1] Although the model would clearly be valid only within a limited range of variation in p. This formulation has some similarity with the model of Becker [12].

(a) The price elasticity is low, in line with earlier studies. It is around 0·4 for women and is not significantly different from zero for men.

(b) The spread of information about the health risks following the report of the Royal College of Physicians in 1962 led to no reduction in the consumption of cigarettes by women, but a fall of around 10 per cent in the case of men (although this tended to disappear over time).

The second of these findings could be explained by the fact that women smokers tend to be younger, and – as shown above – increased knowledge about the risk at older ages may lead younger people to increase their smoking. Alternatively, it could be explained by the health education campaign having been less successful in reaching women. This would be consistent with the difference in price elasticities, since we have seen that increased awareness of risk may lower the price responsiveness.

IV. THE WELFARE ECONOMICS OF GOVERNMENT INTERVENTION

On the assumption that social welfare can be regarded as a sum of individual utilities, we can distinguish between changes affecting the welfare of the smoker and those representing transfers between the smoker and others. In the latter category come health costs (with a national health service), the excess of consumption over production (benefits received less taxes paid and savings), the emotional burden borne by relatives and other externalities. This corresponds to the kind of method used to value lives by Weisbrod [13] and others, and the theoretical issues involved are not considered further here.

If we focus on the effect on the welfare of the individual smoker, the relevant component of the social welfare function W^* coincides with the individual lifetime utility W where $A_1 = A_i^*$ and there are no habit effects. In that case there is no divergence between private and social decisions. With this extreme case as a bench-mark, we may consider the effect of more reasonable assumptions.

Suppose first that $A_i < A_i^*$ but that there are no habit effects. In such a case, the social welfare function could take (at least) two forms:

I. $W_I^* = U(C_1)\, e^{-A_1^* C_1} + U(C_2)\, e^{-(A_1^* C_1 + A_2^* C_2)} G_2$

or

II. $W_{II}^* = U(C_1)\, e^{-A_1 C_1} + U(C_2)\, e^{-(A_1^* C_1 + A_2 C_2)} G_2.$

The rationale of I is that social welfare depends on individual one-period utilities defined *ex post* (i.e. an individual not surviving to consume is supposed to have zero utility). In this case, the individual's expectations with respect to his survival are not relevant. In case II, on the other hand, the social welfare depends on individual one-period utilities defined *ex ante*, so that the survival rates expected by the individual (e^{-AC}) are relevant. The product $U(C_i)\,e^{-A_iC_i}$ represents individual expected utility, and this is summed across the survivors at the beginning of each period to give social welfare W_{II}^*.

In the case where $A_i = 0$, the individual chooses $C(P)$ determined by $U^1(C) = 0$. If there is a value p^1 such that $(Cp^1) = 0$, we can calculate the associated change in welfare on criterion I from increasing p to p^1.[1]

$$\Delta W_I^* = U(0)(1 + G_2) - U(\bar{C})\,e^{-A_1^*\bar{C}}(1 + e^{-A_2^*\bar{C}}\,G_2)$$

$$= U(0)(1 + G_2)(1 - e^{-A_1^*\bar{C}}) + U(0)\,G_2\,e^{-A_1^*\bar{C}}(1 - e^{-A_2^*\bar{C}})$$

$$- [U(\bar{C}) - U(0)]\,e^{-A_1^*\bar{C}}(1 + e^{-A_2^*\bar{C}}\,G_2).$$

Since $1 - e^{-A^*\bar{C}}$ is the death rate, the first two terms represent the value of the lives lost as a result of smoking-related disease, where this value equals $U(0)$ times the life expectancy of non-smokers. The final term represents the loss of utility (if $U(\bar{C}) > U(0)$) to surviving smokers from being forced to give up smoking. If we were to take criterion II, then

$$\Delta W_{II}^* = U(0)\,G_2(1 - e^{-A_1^*C_1}) - [U(\bar{C}) - U(0)](1 + e^{-A_1^*\bar{C}}\,G_2)$$

which is clearly smaller than ΔW_I^*. This reflects the fact that the improvement in their survival prospects will not be recognized by those who are unaware of the risk in any case.

Let us now suppose that the change in smoking is brought about by health education, rather than by taxation: i.e. A_i is increased from 0 to A_i^*. If this is sufficient to ensure that the person does not smoke, then the change in welfare over the initial state is identical to that given before for both criteria. the At same time, the change in W_{II}^* may be decomposed into:

$$\Delta W_{II}^* = \Delta W_I^* - U(\bar{C})[1 - e^{-A_1^*\bar{C}}] - U(\bar{C})\,G_2e^{-A_1^*\bar{C}}(1 - e^{-A_2^*\bar{C}}).$$

The last two terms represent the change in welfare brought about by the individual perceiving the true value of A_i^*; the effect of health education is to change the evaluation of any given state under W_{II}^*. This brings out the differences between W_I^* and W_{II}^*. The former does

---

[1] Where the revenue is handed back in a lump-sum form.

not allow for the cost imposed on individuals through their awareness of the risks they are running – or, in the case of taxation, that they do not perceive the improvement in their survival prospects.

If we now turn to the model incorporating the effects of habit, as represented by the cost of adjustment, we can see that the value of g may depend on the method by which the reduction in smoking is brought about. If it involves individual response to health education campaigns, then there would undoubtedly be costs associated with giving up and, as a consequence, $U(0) < U(\bar{C})$. If there were to be (effective) prohibition, the psychic costs of the will-power involved might be avoided, but there would still be personal withdrawal costs. It seems unlikely that – in this model of habit formation at least – $U(0) \geq U(\bar{C})$ for those who are currently smokers, and we cannot on these grounds ignore the last term in ΔW_I^*.

Choice between Taxation and Health Education
Let us suppose that the government wishes to reduce the consumption by a representative smoker to a certain level $C_2 = \hat{C}$ in the second period of his life, and that it has a choice between achieving this through an increase in p and through increasing A. If we assume for convenience that U has the simple form

$$U = (C + \gamma)^\alpha (E - pC)^{1-\alpha}$$

the first-order conditions give

$$\frac{\alpha}{\hat{C} + \gamma} - \frac{p(1 - \alpha)}{E - p\hat{C}} = A_2.$$

On the assumption that there are values of p and A satisfying this condition (and $A \leq A^*$), then the trade-off between them is given by

$$\frac{dA_2}{dp}\bigg|_{C \text{ constant}} = -\frac{(1 - \alpha)E}{E - p\hat{C})^2}.$$

On criterion I, we can see that

$$\frac{dW_I^*}{dP}\bigg|_{C \text{ constant}} = \frac{\partial U}{\partial p} e^{-A_2^* C}.$$

If the revenue is handed back in lump-sum form, then $\partial U/\partial p = 0$ and the level of welfare is unchanged. On the other hand, with criterion II,

$$\frac{dW_{II}^*}{dp}\bigg|_{C \text{ constant}} = \frac{\partial U}{\partial p} e^{-A_2\hat{C}} - \hat{C} \ W_{II}^* \frac{\partial A_2}{\partial p}$$

which will be positive (for $\hat{C} > 0$), so that tax measures are clearly preferable in this case. If we further assume that the costs of health education exceed those of tax collection (as certainly seems reasonable at the margin), the case for tax measures is even stronger.

This analysis brings out the important point that more information about the health risks of smoking is not necessarily socially desirable (even if it can be disseminated costlessly). There is a tendency for economists to believe that more information is always desirable (although doctors have, of course, always been aware that this is not so). Under criterion II, for example, we have

$$\frac{\partial W^*}{\partial A_1} = \frac{\partial W^*}{\partial C_1} \frac{\partial C_1}{\partial A_1} - C_1 \, U(C_1)e^{-A_1 C_1} + \frac{\partial W^*}{\partial C_2} \frac{\partial C_2}{\partial A_1}$$

$$\frac{\partial W^*}{\partial A_2} = \frac{\partial W^*}{\partial C_1} \frac{\partial C_1}{\partial A_2} - C_2 G_2 \, U(C_2)e^{-(A_1^* + A_2)C_2} + \frac{\partial W^*}{\partial C_2} \frac{\partial C_2}{\partial A_2}.$$

From the conditions for individual maximization of W (interior solution) $\partial W^*/\partial C_2 = 0$, so that the last term vanishes and

$$\frac{\partial W^*}{\partial C_1} = \frac{\partial W}{\partial C_1} + U(C_2)e^{-A_1 C_1} [A_1 e^{-A_1 C_1} - A_1^* e^{-A_1^* C_1}]$$

which is negative if $A_1^* C_1 < 1$ and approaches zero as $A_1 \to A_1^*$. It is clear, therefore, that if there are people who would continue to smoke even if they are fully aware of the health risk,[1] then there is a point beyond which further information is not desirable even if it can be provided at no cost.

V. IMPLICATIONS FOR FUTURE RESEARCH

In section II, I suggested that there were two approaches to the measurement of the cost of smoking, and from the analysis of sections III and IV it can be seen that they represent two polar cases:

	Individual knowledge of health risks	*Habit formation*
Pure divergence approach	Perfect knowledge by individual	No habit formation
'Vaccination' model	Individual perception of risk not relevant	Allocation explained solely by habit, no costs of adjustment

The progression from one to the other can be seen as follows. With perfect information and no habit effects, it is only the costs imposed on others which are relevant, and in broad terms these can be

---

[1] In this case, the only term in $\partial W/\partial A_1$ and $\partial W/\partial A_2$ which is relevant is the middle one, and this is negative.

measured by the loss of net production (present value of contribution to production minus consumption) and the health costs. An approximate estimate of the costs in this form in 1971 is that they would amount to £200 million.

If we now assume that people are unaware of the health risks and that the correct criterion of social welfare is W_I^*, then we have to add the elements under ΔW_I^*.

(i) plus the intrinsic value of the lives lost,
(ii) minus the costs to smokers from giving up.

If, following conventional practice, item (i) is approximated by the value of consumption plus an allowance for 'the value of life as such' (Peston), the total cost equals that calculated on the vaccination approach (approximately £500 million in 1971) minus item (ii). This latter item can be neglected only if we assume that the addictive nature of tobacco is such that individuals are, in fact, indifferent about the allocation of their expenditure and if the elimination of smoking could be achieved with no personal adjustment costs. If this is not the case, then the true costs under criterion I would be less than those calculated on the vaccination model. Some idea of the difference is provided by the fact that there are over 20 million smokers, so that if the cost to each of giving up smoking were only £5 per annum, then the cost is reduced by £100 million. To reduce the total cost to that obtained on the pure divergence approach would require a cost per smoker of only £19 per year. Moreover, we have seen that criterion II, which takes into account the individual's perception of risk in evaluating different outcomes, would lead to a still lower estimate.

The main purpose of this paper has been to argue that the 'cost' of smoking is far from being a straightforward issue, and that it raises a number of difficult questions in addition to those, such as the valuation of human lives, which usually arise with cost–benefit analysis in the health field. These questions include the determinants of smoking behaviour and the correct formulation of the social welfare function;[1] and there are other important issues not discussed here, such as the redistributional consequences of measures to reduce smoking.[2] I hope that this paper will stimulate work to provide better answers than those given here.

[1] For a discussion of this question in the context of the rather similar problem of decisions about family size, see Mirrlees [14].
[2] Between 1958 and 1971, the proportion smoking cigarettes among social class I (professional, etc.) fell from 54 per cent to 37 per cent, whereas the proportion for social class V (unskilled) fell only from 61 per cent to 59 per cent.

REFERENCES

[1] Richardson, R. G. (ed.), *The Second World Conference on Smoking and Health* (London: Pitman, 1972).

[2] Royal College of Physicians, *Smoking and Health Now* (London: Pitman, 1971).

[3] Hammond, E. C., and Horn, D., 'Smoking and Death Rates', *Journal of the American Medical Association* (1958).

[4] Doll, R., and Hill, A. B., 'Mortality in Relation to Smoking: Ten Years' Observation of British Doctors', *British Medical Journal* (1964).

[5] 'The Estimated Cost of Certain Identifiable Consequences of Cigarette Smoking upon Health, Longevity and Property in Canada in 1966', mimeo.

[6] Mishan, E. J., *Cost–Benefit Analysis* (London: Allen & Unwin, 1971).

[7] Pike, M. C., and Doll, R., 'Age at Onset of Lung Cancer', *Lancet*, 27 Mar 1965.

[8] Atkinson, A. B., and Skegg, J. L., 'Anti-Smoking Publicity and the Demand for Tobacco in the U.K.', *Manchester School* (1973) (forthcoming).

[9] Peston, M., 'Changing Utility Functions', in M. Shubik (ed.), *Essays in Mathematical Economics* (Princeton Univ. Press, 1967).

[10] Pollak, R. A., 'Habit formation and Dynamic Demand Functions', *Journal of Political Economy* (Aug 1970).

[11] von Weizsäcker, C. C., 'Notes on Endogenous Change of Tastes', *Journal of Economic Theory* (Dec 1971).

[12] Becker, G., 'The Economics of Irrational Behaviour', *Journal of Political Economy* (1961).

[13] Weisbrod, B., *Economics of Public Health* (Philadelphia: Univ. of Pennsylvania Press, 1961).

[14] Mirrlees, J. A., 'Population Policy and the Taxation of Family Size', *Journal of Public Economics* (1972).

22 Allied Health Personnel in Physicians' Offices: An Econometric Approach[1]

Michael D. Intriligator
and Barbara H. Kehrer
UNIVERSITY OF SOUTHERN CALIFORNIA − AMERICAN
MEDICAL ASSOCIATION, CHICAGO

This paper develops a simultaneous equation model of allied health personnel employed in physicians' offices, which include nursing, technical and secretarial-clerical workers. The first three equations explain weekly hours demanded of each of the three types of allied health personnel as functions of the degree of delegation of tasks; own wage; visits; own capital; and, for nurses, the technician wage and, for technicians, the nurse wage. The fourth equation explains degree of delegation as a function of employment of all three types of allied health personnel, nurse rooms, technician rooms, malpractice insurance premiums, and percentages of low- and middle-income patients. The model was estimated separately for four specialties, general family practice, internal medicine, obstetrics–gynecology and pediatrics, using, data for solo practice physicians obtained from the Seventh Periodic Survey of Physicians, conducted by the American Medical Association in 1972. Estimated parameters of the model and implied elasticities of demand for allied health personnel are reported.

I. INTRODUCTION

The purpose of this paper is to study the employment and utilization of allied health personnel employed in physicians' offices. A simultaneous equations model is developed to take account of complex interrelationships between the demand for various aides and several factors affecting their utilization. The model is specified in section II, estimated parameter values for alternative categories of practice

[1] The paper reports on research in progress on Contract No. HSM 110–70–354 from the National Center for Health Services Research and Development, U.S. Department of Health, Education and Welfare. The authors wish to acknowledge useful suggestions and comments from colleagues at both the University of Southern California and the American Medical Association. We are especially grateful to Bud S. Schnierle, of the A.M.A., for computational assistance.

are presented in section III, and conclusions are presented in section IV.

II. SPECIFICATION OF THE MODEL

The four endogenous variables of the model are:

N = weekly hours worked by nursing personnel
T = weekly hours worked by technical personnel
S = weekly hours worked by secretarial-clerical personnel
D = the degree of delegation of tasks to allied health personnel.[1]

These variables, each referring to a particular medical practice, are the jointly dependent variables explained by the interaction of endogenous and exogenous variables in the model.

Exogenous variables of the model, variables determined by mechanisms lying outside the scope of the model, and which affect the endogenous variables but are not affected by them, are:

w_N = hourly product wage of nursing personnel (relative to the price of an official office visit)
w_T = hourly product wage of technical personnel (relative to the price of an initial office visit)
w_S = hourly product wage of secretarial-clerical personnel (relative to the price of an initial office visit)
V = total patient visits produced
K_N = capital stock available for nursing services
K_T = capital stock available for technicians' services
K_S = capital stock available for secretarial-clerical services
M = annual malpractice insurance premiums paid
Y_p = percentage of patients with low incomes
Y_m = percentage of patients with middle incomes.

All variables refer to a particular practice.

In most demand–supply models, including models of factor price and quantity are taken as endogenous variables. Here, quantities, in particular weekly hours worked by allied health personnel, are taken as endogenous, with prices, in particular wages, taken as exogenous. This assumption of exogenously determined wages reflects the institutional character of the physicians' offices. The wages paid by physicians depend primarily on wages paid by larger institutions. Wages of nurses and technicians are based largely on wages paid by hospitals, while wages of secretarial-clerical personnel are based largely on prevailing wage rates in general business.[2]

---

[1] A detailed discussion of the definitions of the variables used is provided in the appendix to this paper.

[2] With respect to nurses, see Donald E. Yett, 'Causes and Consequences of Salary Differentials in Nursing', *Inquiry*, VII (Mar 1970) 78–99.

Wages are product wages – money wages divided by the price of an initial office visit – to be consistent with price theory which stipulates that, for cost minimization, such prices are the important variables affecting employment decisions. Patient visits, numbers of rooms and malpractice insurance premiums are also taken as exogenous, since they can be considered policy variables from the standpoint of the physician. The other exogenous variables of the model – the percentage of patients who have low incomes and the percentage of patients with middle incomes – may influence delegation and employment of aides, but are clearly not affected in turn by them.

The first three equations of the model relate to the demand for each category of allied health personnel. Symbolically, using signs to indicate expected signs of partial derivatives:

$$N = N(D; w_N, w_T, V, K_N) \tag{1}$$
$$ + \quad - \quad + \quad +$$
$$T = T(D; w_N, w_T, V, K_T) \tag{2}$$
$$ + \quad + \quad - \quad + \quad +$$
$$S = S(D; w_S, V, K_S). \tag{3}$$
$$ + \quad - \quad + \quad +$$

These equations relate to the derived demand for allied health personnel since, wages being treated as exogenous, the number of weekly hours worked by allied health personnel is demand-determined. These equations can be interpreted as labor requirements equations under the assumption of given number of visits and capital stock.

An increase in the degree of delegation, which refers here to delegation of health services tasks (e.g. taking blood pressure, immunizations), is espected to increase the demand for all three types of allied health personnel, *ceteris paribus*. An increase in a practice's propensity to delegate health-related tasks will tend to increase its demand for nursing and technical personnel to perform those tasks. With respect to secretarial personnel, the more a practice delegates health services tasks to nursing and technical personnel, the less time will the latter be able to spend on secretarial and clerical functions and, hence, the greater will be the demand for secretarial personnel, *ceteris paribus*.

According to classical theory, an increase in own wages will reduce demand, while an increase in wages of other factors may increase demand (where the factors are substitutes) or decrease demand (where factors are complements). Thus, in all three equations the sign for the own wage is expected to be negative. The signs of the technician wage in the nurse equation and the nurse wage in the technician equation are expected to be positive to reflect substitutability between the two factors. Secretarial-clerical personnel are not expected to exhibit significant substitutability or complementarity with either nurses or technicians and, hence, only the own wage is included in equation (3).[1]

Inclusion of number of patient visits scales the functions and captures the effects of simple ratio staffing patterns dictating, for example, a certain number of nurses for a certain number of patient visits. Capital stock specific to each type of allied health personnel, measured by number of rooms, is, presumably, a complementary factor of production, judging from the fact that one reason physicians give for not hiring additional allied health personnel is that office space is limited.[2]

The fourth equation of the model relates to the degree of delegation of health services tasks to allied personnel in the practice. Symbolically:

$$D = D(N, T, S; K_N, K_T, M, Y_p, Y_m).$$
$$\quad\; + \;\; + \;\; + \;\; + \quad\; + \quad - \;\; \pm \;\; + \tag{4}$$

The signs of the coefficient of all three allied health personnel variables are expected to be positive. Presumably, the more nursing or technician hours are available to the practice, the more tasks may be delegated, and, hence, the greater degree of delegation. As suggested above, secretaries may relieve nurses and technicians of clerical duties and, therefore, promote the delegation of nursing and technical functions.[3] Increased numbers of nursing and technical rooms may, other things being equal, increase delegation, with physically larger practices delegating more, simply because space is available for delegation.

Increased malpractice insurance premiums are expected to reduce the degree of delegation in a medical practice. Higher malpractice premiums are assumed to reflect both a greater probability that a

[1] This approach was suggested by the results of earlier work in estimating a preliminary version of the model. (Michael D. Intriligator and Barbara H. Kehrer, 'A Simultaneous Equations Model of Ancillary Personnel Employed in Physicians' Offices', paper presented at the winter meetings of the Econometric Society, Toronto, 29 Dec 1972.)

[2] Alfred Yankauer, John P. Connelly and Jacob J. Feldman, 'Pediatric Practice in the United States, with Special Attention to Utilization of Allied Health Worker Services', *Pediatrics*, xlv(2) (Mar 1970) 543.

[3] In the course of discussion during the Conference, Professor Williams pointed out that inclusion of S in the delegation equation is inconsistent with our exclusion of W_S from the nurse and technician equations and the exclusion of W_N and W_T from the secretary equation. We should have indicated that the decision regarding which wage variables were included in each of the first three equations was influenced by our expectations regarding *relative* degrees of substitutability and the desire to avoid problems of multicollinearity (simple correlation coefficients between each pair of wage variables are greater than 0·7 in all four specialities).

physician will be used for malpractice[1] and larger settlements for malpractice suits. At the same time, greater delegation of health services tasks tends to increase the risk of a malpractice suit.[2] It is expected that, the greater the risk of a malpractice suit already confronting a practice, the less willing the physician will be to incur greater risk by delegating health service tasks to allied health personnel. Hence, the sign of the coefficient of malpractice insurance premiums is expected to be negative.

Patient resistance to delegation may be related to patient income. It has been suggested that middle-income patients are most receptive to delegation. In contrast, high-income patients who may feel they are paying to be seen by a physician may insist upon treatment by the physician himself, while low-income patients may feel they are receiving second-class service if they are treated by aides.[3] At the same time, low-income patients are likely to have less power than other patients to have their preferences implemented. To test these conjectures about the effect of patient income on the degree of delegation in a practice, the percentage of patients with low incomes (less than $5,000 per year) and the percentage of patients with middle incomes (between $5,000 and $15,000 per year) are included as explanatory variables in equation (4). The expected sign of the coefficient of Y_m is positive, reflecting greater acceptance of delegation by middle-income people, while the sign of the coefficient of Y_p may be either negative or positive, reflecting, respectively, greater resistance or lack of power to have one's preferences implemented on the part of low-income patients.

Mean values for all variables in the model are given in Table 22.1.

III. ESTIMATION OF THE MODEL

Estimates of the simultaneous equations model described by equations (1)–(4) were obtained by utilizing data collected in the American Medical Association's Seventh Periodic Survey of Physicians[4] and applying the technique of two-stage least squares. The model was estimated separately for four alternative specialities:

[1] The size of malpractice insurance premiums paid tends to be positively related to the riskiness of the physician's specialty and the propensity of patients to sue in the community in which the practice is located.

[2] Richard P. Bergen, 'Liability for Use of Paramedical Personnel', *Connecticut Medicine*, xxxv (Feb 1971) 78–80.

[3] See Louis R. Pondy, Bobby H. Dampier, Thomas R. Rice and Andria Knapp, 'A Study of Patient Acceptance of the Physician's Assistant', G.S.B.A. Paper No. 27 (Durham, N.C.: Graduate School of Business Administration, Duke Univ., Feb 1970).

[4] These data are described in the appendix.

TABLE 22.1

MEAN VALUES OF VARIABLES USED IN THE MODEL
(standard deviations in parentheses)

Variable	Specialty			
	General/family practice	Internal medicine	Pediatrics	Obstetrics–gynecology
N	28·856	14·920	37·611	28·536
	(28·197)	(25·286)	(29·881)	(29·200)
T	8·386	12·225	9·722	4·680
	(19·524)	(23·218)	(21·419)	(15·143)
S	40·546	36·835	38·494	41·070
	(29·486)	(25·730)	(22·660)	(27·948)
D	25·018	20·195	19·393	18·000
	(25·276)	(21·604)	(23·072)	(20·107)
w_N	0·384	0·209	0·309	0·226
	(0·142)	(0·103)	(0·091)	(0·105)
w_T	0·396	0·218	0·341	0·225
	(0·139)	(0·109)	(0·113)	(0·090)
w_S	0·333	0·182	0·269	0·175
	(0·144)	(0·093)	(0·084)	(0·068)
V	178·395	119·242	175·028	126·560
	(91·261)	(58·576)	(58·775)	(56·574)
K_N	3·118	2·408	3·472	2·400
	(1·609)	(1·000)	(1·424)	(0·808)
K_T	1·200	1·150	0·806	0·800
	(0·905)	(0·923)	(0·577)	(0·700)
K_S	2·386	2·117	2·306	2·260
	(0·892)	(0·758)	(1·037)	(0·944)
M	1,247·009	701·583	474·500	2,204·340
	(6,731·406)	(808·329)	(526·126)	(1,576·312)
Y_P	27·114	15·342	22·111	12·780
	(23·874)	(15·235)	(19·917)	(13·811)
Y_m	60·091	61·233	0·667	72·220
	(23·439)	(20·503)	(18·036)	(17·717)
Number of cases	220	120	36	50

general/family practice (220 cases), internal medicine (120 cases) pediatrics (36 cases) and obstetrics–gynecology (50 cases). Only solo practice physicians are included in the study.[1]

The model may be summarized as follows:

$$Y_i = \sum_{j-1}^{4} \beta_{ij} Y_j + \sum_{k-1}^{11} \gamma_{ik} Z_k, \ i = 1, \ldots, 4,$$

where i refers to each of the four equations in the model, Y_j refers to the four endogenous variables, Z_k refers to the eleven exogenous

[1] Solo physicians are defined as those who devoted more than 50 per cent of their medical practice time to solo practice in 1970. We intend, in later work, to estimate the model by type of practice; in particular, to compare results for group and solo practice physicians.

variables,[1] and the β_{ij} and γ_{ik} are slope coefficients some of which are preassigned a value of zero.

Elasticities may be calculated at the mean values by scaling. For example,

$$\gamma'_{ik} = (\bar{Z}_k / \bar{Y}_i) \cdot (\partial Y_i / \partial Z_k) = (\bar{Z}_k / \bar{Y}_i) \cdot \gamma_{ik}$$

where γ'_{ik} is the elasticity of variable Y_i with respect to variable Z_k, barred symbols representing mean values of these variables.

Estimated coefficients of the model are reported for general/family practice physicians in Table 22.2, for specialists in internal medicine in Table 22.3, for pediatricians in Table 22.4, and for specialists in obstetrics–gynecology in Table 22.5. The remainder of this section discusses these results. This analysis will not include a general discussion of signs and significance of coefficients since the tables speak for themselves. Instead, the focus will be on in-interpreting the results.

In the estimated equation for nurses, summarized by the first column in Table 22.2, the most significant variables are number of patient visits per week and nurse wages. The value of the visits coefficient (0·0632) can be interpreted more readily in terms of its reciprocal, 15·82, which gives the number of additional patient visits which, for given wages, capital (examining rooms) and extent of delegation, would lead to using one additional hour of nursing services per week. This number of visits for an added nursing hour may seem high, but it must be recalled that other variables are being held constant and that the same number of visits is generating demand for other types of allied health personnel at the same time. Thus, referring to the secretary equation, it may be seen that 8·66 extra visits (the reciprocal of 0·1154, the coefficient of visits in equation (3)) lead to one additional secretarial hour of service. Combining these two results, an additional 20 visits per week lead to an extra 2·31 secretarial hours *and* an extra 1·26 nursing hours, with the number of rooms in the practice, in particular, held constant. In contrast, statistically significant results for the other specialties reveal that, in internal medicine, 6·26 extra patient visits (the reciprocal of 0·1597) are associated with one extra secretarial hour, while in pediatrics, only 5·22 extra visits result in an extra nurse hour and 6·35 extra visits result in an extra secretarial hour.

The effect of rooms on allied health personnel hours may be analysed by considering the coefficients of the three rooms variables in Table 22.2. Thus, one extra examining room, K_N, increases the number of nurse hours per week by 2·8, one extra laboratory or

---

[1] The additional exogenous variable is the constant value of unity, accounting for a constant term in each equation.

TABLE 22.2

TWO-STAGE LEAST SQUARES ESTIMATES OF THE MODEL FOR SOLO GENERAL/FAMILY PRACTICE
(*t*-statistics in parentheses)

Explanatory variables	N	T	S	D
		Dependent (endogenous) variables		
N				$-0\cdot5442$
				$(-1\cdot24)$
T				$0\cdot7942$
				$(0\cdot43)$
S				$0\cdot6619$
				$(2\cdot19)\dagger$
D	$0\cdot4505$	$0\cdot1945$	$0\cdot3674$	
	$(2\cdot40)\dagger$	$(1\cdot14)$	$(1\cdot95)*$	
w_N	$-62\cdot6386$	$-10\cdot1345$		
	$(-3\cdot18)\ddagger$	$(-0\cdot67)$		
w_T	$25\cdot1381$	$7\cdot4054$		
	$(1\cdot26)$	$(0\cdot48)$		
w_S			$-15\cdot6978$	
			$(-1\cdot29)$	
V	$0\cdot0632$	$0\cdot0051$	$0\cdot1154$	
	$(3\cdot11)\ddagger$	$(0\cdot31)$	$(5\cdot42)\ddagger$	
K_N	$2\cdot7782$			$3\cdot3449$
	$(1\cdot97)\dagger$			$(2\cdot19)\dagger$
K_T		$4\cdot6232$		$2\cdot5416$
		$(2\cdot13)\dagger$		$(0\cdot22)$
K_S			$5\cdot9093$	
			$(2\cdot37)\dagger$	
M				$0\cdot00006$
				$(0\cdot13)$
Y_p				$-0\cdot2589$
				$(-1\cdot41)$
Y_m				$-0\cdot2399$
				$(-1\cdot72)*$
Constant	$11\cdot7629$	$-1\cdot9834$	$1\cdot8770$	$15\cdot0949$
	$(1\cdot81)*$	$(-0\cdot40)$	$(0\cdot26)$	$(1\cdot32)$
R^2	$0\cdot285$	$0\cdot113$	$0\cdot305$	$0\cdot257$

Number of cases = 220.
Second-stage significance levels: $* = 0\cdot90$, $\dagger = 0\cdot95$, $\ddagger = 0\cdot99$.

TABLE 22.3

TWO-STAGE LEAST SQUARES ESTIMATES OF THE MODEL FOR SOLO INTERNAL MEDICINE

(*t*-statistics in parentheses)

Explanatory variables	N	*Dependent (endogenous) variables* T	S	D
N				0·5550
				(1·75)*
T				0·2953
				(0·65)
S				−0·0834
				(−0·37)
D	0·5259	1·1292	−0·0301	
	(0·96)	(1·84)*	(−0·07)	
w_N	−97·6835	147·7747		
	(−1·39)	(2·17)†		
w_T	74·5721	−151·3979		
	(1·24)	(−2·56)†		
w_S			−10·5511	
			(−0·3862)	
V	0·0529	−0·0267	0·1597	
	(0·91)	(−0·47)	(3·21)‡	
K_N	5·0689			−3·5896
	(2·10)†			(−0·83)
K_T		4·1321		0·5932
		(1·36)		(0·16)
K_S			8·4404	
			(2·91)	
M				0·00002
				(0·01)
Y_p				−0·0836
				(−0·49)
Y_m				0·0262
				(−0·16)
Constant	−10·0311	−10·0592	2·4478	22·2100
	(−1·07)	(1·16)	(0·21)	(1·12)
R^2	0·174	0·182	0·178	0·083

Number of cases = 120.
Second-stage significance levels: * = 0·90, † = 0·95, ‡ = 0·99.

TABLE 22.4

TWO-STAGE LEAST SQUARES ESTIMATES OF THE MODEL FOR SOLO PEDIATRICS

(*t*-statistics in parentheses)

Explanatory variables	Dependent (*endogenous*) variables			
	N	T	S	D
N				0·2107
				(0·76)
T				0·0099
				(0·03)
S				0·1036
				(0·27)
D	0·3815	0·2117	0·3454	
	(1·07)	(0·88)	(1·33)	
w_N	−148·4068	86·8071		
	(−2·02)*	(1·60)		
w_T	112·7332	−144·3304		
	(1·86)*	(−3·26)‡		
w_S			−24·4121	
			(−0·49)	
V	0·1915	0·0320	0·1574	
	(2·23)†	(0·52)	(2·19)†	
K_N	−0·4914			4·2578
	(−0·14)			(1·39)
K_T		9·9380		−0·7452
		(1·73)*		(−0·09)
K_S			0·0894	
			(0·02)	
M				0·0131
				(1·42)
Y_p				−0·0347
				(−0·10)
Y_m				0·3105
				(0·93)
Constant	5·8791	14·3303	10·6089	−31·0610
	(0·31)	(0·99)	(0·74)	(−1·05)
R^2	0·346	0·323	0·253	0·304

Number of cases = 36.
Second-stage significance levels: * = 0·90, † = 0·95, ‡ = 0·99.

TABLE 22.5

TWO-STAGE LEAST SQUARES ESTIMATES OF THE MODEL FOR SOLO OBSTETRICS–GYNECOLOGY

(*t*-statistics in parentheses)

Explanatory variables	*N*	*T*	*S*	*D*
N				0·2212 (0·51)
T				0·3458 (0·46)
S				0·6291 (3·01)‡
D	−0·2530 (0·65)	0·0747 (0·28)	0·4444 (0·83)	
w_N	−33·7989 (−0·60)	15·7366 (0·43)		
w_T	29·9848 (0·45)	−61·0370 (−1·43)		
w_S			−85·4494 (−1·46)	
V	0·0806 (0·91)	0·0032 (0·06)		
K_N	10·3885 (2·18)†			−5·9971 (−0·85)
K_T		1·7318 (0·47)		0·1026 (0·02)
K_S			5·9032 (1·08)	
M				−0·0009 (−0·27)
Y_p	+			0·1416 (0·35)
Y_m				0·5181 (1·83)*
Constant	−1·1664 (−0·09)	11·7372 (1·62)	24·9406 (1·77)*	−38·6541 (−1·42)
R^2	0·165	0·094	0·266	0·305

Number of cases = 50.
Second-stage significance levels: * = 0·90, † = 0·95, ‡ = 0·99.

X-ray facility, K_T (which may consist of only a corner of a room), leads to an extra 4·6 technician hours per week, and one extra waiting room or business and administrative office, K_S, leads to an extra 5·9 secretarial hours per week. These numbers may appear low, but this may be the result of holding the number of visits constant. If visits increase with rooms, the number of nursing hours resulting from an additional room will increase. For example, if each additional examining room increases weekly visits by 50, using the estimated coefficient for V, an extra examining room results in approximately 6 additional nursing hours per week.

Statistically significant results for the other specialties indicate that the effects of rooms on demand for allied health personnel hours is generally greater than in general/family practice. In internal medicine, an extra examining room leads to 5·1 extra nurse hours, one additional X-ray or laboratory facility to 4·1 extra technician hours, and one additional waiting room or business and administrative office to 8·4 secretarial hours. In obstetrics–gynecology, an extra examining room results in an extra 10·4 nurse hours.[1]

Turning now to the wage variables in Table 22.2, only the nurse wage in the nurse equation is significant, with the expected negative sign. The reciprocal of this coefficient suggests that an increase in the hourly product wage of nurses is $0·015 would result in a decline of one nurse hour. (In interpreting this product wage coefficient reciprocal, it is useful to note that the mean initial office visit fee in general/family practice is approximately $10; thus, an increase of $0·015 in the hourly product wage would, at the mean, represent an increase of $0·15 in the undeflated hourly money wage.)

All statistically significant estimates for the wage variables in the other specialties have the expected signs. Thus, in internal medicine, an increase of $0·006 in the hourly product wage for nurses leads to an increase of one technician hour, while an increase of $0·006 in the technician hourly product wage leads to a reduction of one technician hour. In pediatrics, an increase in the technician wage of $0·006 leads to a decline of one technician hour.

According to the reported coefficients for variable D in the first three columns in Table 22.2, employment of nurses seems to be the most responsive to degree of delegation, in terms of both the size of the coefficients and their statistical significance.

---

[1] It is worth noting that, in all but one case – the secretary equation for internal medicine – in which the rooms variable coefficient is higher than that for general/family practice, the visits variable is not statistically significant. Thus, some of the 'visits effect' may be included in the rooms coefficient, i.e. there may be some problem of multicollinearity between the rooms and visits variables.

The estimated delegation equations indicate that, in general/ family practice, examining rooms is significant and positive at the 95 per cent level, which is consistent with previous findings that physicians regard inadequate space as a barrier to increased delegation.[1] Number of nurse hours is significant and positive at the 90 per cent level in internal medicine, and number of secretary hours is significant and positive at the 99 per cent level in obstetrics–gynecology, indicating that greater availability of allied health worker services increases delegation. Percentage of patients with middle incomes is significant and negative in general/family practice, but significant and positive in obsterics–gynecology. The latter is consistent with expectations of greater delegation when patients are in the middle-income bracket.

TABLE 22.6

CALCULATED DEMAND ELASTICITIES
FOR ALLIED HEALTH PERSONNEL

Elasticities of demand for	Elasticities with respect to						
	w_N	w_T	w_S	V	K_N	K_T	K_S
	General/family practice						
N	−0·834	0·345	–	0·391	0·300	–	–
T	−0·464	0·350	–	0·108	–	0·662	–
S	–	–	−0·129	0·508	–	–	0·348
	Internal medicine						
N	−1·368	1·089	–	0·423	0·818	–	–
T	2·526	−2·670	–	−0·260	–	0·389	–
S	–	–	−0·052	0·517	–	–	0·485
	Pediatrics						
N	−1·219	1·022	–	0·891	−0·045	–	–
T	2·759	−5·062	–	0·576	–	0·824	–
S	–	–	−0·171	0·716	–	–	0·005
	Obstetrics–gynecology						
N	−0·268	0·236	–	0·357	0·874	–	–
T	0·760	−2·934	–	0·086	–	0·296	–
S	–	–	−0·364	–	–	–	0·325

Table 22.6 reports estimated elasticities obtained by deflating the slope coefficients in Tables 22.2 through 22.5, using mean values of the variables reported in Table 22.1. It is of interest to consider the demand elasticities for allied health personnel with respect to their own wages. For example, in general/family practice, a 10 per cent increase in the price of an initial office visit, which would reduce

---

[1] Yankauer *et al.*, op. cit.

product wages for all allied health personnel by 10 per cent (assuming money hourly wages were held constant), would increase nurse hours by 8·3 per cent, decrease technician hours by 3·5 per cent and increase secretary hours by 1·3 per cent. In internal medicine and pediatrics, both the demand for nurses and the demand for technicians are elastic with respect to the own wage, in contrast to general/family practice. In obstetrics–gynecology, demand for nurses and for secretaries is highly inelastic, while demand for technicians is elastic with respect to the own wage.

Elasticities with respect to visits and with respect to rooms are also reported in Table 22.6. A given percentage increase in visits or rooms generally increases demand for all categories of allied health personnel in all four specialties, but by a smaller percentage than the original increase. In particular, the demand for technicians is quite inelastic with respect to visits in all specialties, while the demand for secretaries is quite inelastic with respect to secretary rooms in all specialties.

IV. CONCLUSION

This paper has reported on a simultaneous equations analysis of physicians' decisions regarding the hiring of allied health personnel and delegation of health services tasks to such personnel. The results of this analysis should be of value, not only to economists concerned with markets for health manpower, but also to public health policy planners concerned with improving the efficiency of delivery of health services in physicians' offices.

APPENDIX

(1) *Source of the Data*
Data on all variables were obtained from the Seventh Periodic Survey of Physicians (P.S.P.) conducted by the American Medical Association in 1972. This large-scale survey obtained responses from over 5,000 physicians in all forms of medical practice and in all specialties.

(2) *Definitions of Variables*
1. *Weekly hours worked by nursing, technical, and secretarial-clerical personnel.* The Seventh P.S.P. requested information on full-time equivalent employment of nine types of allied health personnel during the most recent complete week of practice. Three of these types of aides – registered nurses, licensed practical nurses, and nurses' aides – were aggregated into a nurse group, and three – X-ray technicians and assistants, laboratory technicians and assistants, and medical technicians – were aggregated

into a technician group. The other categories of personnel included in the questionnaire were: secretaries, receptionists, bookkeepers, etc., which constitute the secretarial-clerical category used in this paper; and pharmacists and others, which were not included in this study.

The Seventh P.S.P. also requested respondents to indicate the number of hours per week worked by an average or typical full-time equivalent allied health employee in their offices. The full-time equivalent employment figures for each of the three groups of workers were then multiplied by hours per week to yield total nursing, technician and secretarial-clerical hours worked per week, respectively. In those cases in which the physician did not answer the hours per week question, the mean value of 38 hours per week was used.

It should be noted that a physician may hire less than one full-time worker in any one of the three groups of allied health personnel, either by hiring a part-time worker or by having one person work at more than one type of job. Thus, one half-time employee might work 10 hours per week as a nurse and 10 hours per week as a secretary.

2. *Degree of delegation of tasks to allied health personnel.* The Seventh P.S.P. asked respondents to indicate the percentages of times each of ten specific tasks was performed by an allied health employee. These tasks were: (1) history-taking; (2) blood pressure; (3) well-child examination; (4) cast application or removal; (5) minor sutures; (6) skin preparation for minor surgery; (7) immunizations; (8) taking E.K.G.s; (9) chest X-ray; and (10) instruction of patients (exercises, diet, medication routine, etc.). These tasks were selected for inclusion in the P.S.P. questionnaire because, in some practices, they are performed only by the physician, while in others they are sometimes or always performed by an allied health worker supervised by a physician.

A single measure of the degree of delegation was obtained for each practice by forming an average of the percentage of time responses for those tasks which were considered relevant to the specialty of the physician These are as follows:

General/family practice: taking blood pressure, cast application or removal, skin preparation for minor surgery, immunizations, E.K.G.s, X-rays and instruction of patients.

Internal medicine: taking blood pressure, immunizations, E.K.G.s, X-rays and instruction of patients.

Pediatrics: taking blood pressure, skin preparation for minor surgery, immunizations, E.K.G.s, X-rays and instruction of patients.

Obstetrics–gynecology: taking blood pressure, immunization, X-rays and instruction of patients.

The criteria which were used to determine whether a given task was relevant for the delegation measure for a given specialty were: whether the mean response to the question by physicians in the specialty was greater than 5 per cent and whether more than half the physicians in the specialty gave valid responses to the question. Two exceptions were made, however. First, taking X-rays was included in the OBG index, even though fewer than half the OBG specialists answered the question, in order to include a task in the OBG index of delegation that is often done by a technician. Second, taking histories qualified for all four indexes according to both criteria, but it was not included because histories may be self-taken by the patient, and we are interested in delegation from physician to allied health workers. Finally, it is interesting to note that, on the basis of the first criterion, well-child examinations were not included in the delegation index for pediatrics. The reason for this is that, although about two-thirds of the pediatricians responded to this question, its mean was only 3·1 per cent, indicating that, by and large, pediatricians do not delegate well-child examinations to allied health personnel.

3. *Hourly product wages.* Total weekly expenditures on each category of allied health personnel were divided by the number of hours worked by all persons in that category to yield the average hourly money wage (including fringe benefits) for that category of personnel within the practice. This money wage was then divided by the usual, or customary, fee for an initial office visit. Seventh P.S.P. returns provided the expenditure, employment and price data. (When physicians failed to respond to the fee question, the mean initial office visit fee for the specialty and census division in which the practice was located was used instead. Where allied health personnel were employed but the physician did not give information on salaries, these were recoded with the mean salaries for the particular types of allied health personnel in the census division in which the practice was located.)

Where physicians employed no nurses or no technicians or no secretaries, it was necessary to assign a wage to the practice, since a wage rate of zero would clearly be inappropriate. In the case of zero secretaries, the wage used was the mean value of the salaries paid to secretaries in the census division in which the practice was located, divided by the price of an initial office visit. In the case of zero nurses (or zero technicians), a weighted salary measure was created in which the mean values of the salaries of each of the three component types of personnel were weighted according to the relative probability of each type of worker being hired first in the group.

4. *Practice capital stock.* Respondents to the Seventh P.S.P. were asked to indicate how many rooms of the following types comprised their working environment: waiting rooms, examining rooms, laboratory facilities, X-ray facilities, and business and administrative offices. Three capital stock variables were computed on the basis of these questions: (1) capital stock complementary with nursing services, consisting of examining rooms; (2) capital stock complementary with technicians' services, consisting of laboratory facilities and X-ray facilities; and (3) capital stock complementary with secretarial-clerical services, consisting of waiting rooms and business and administrative offices.

5. *Malpractice insurance premiums.* Malpractice insurance premiums paid by the practice were obtained in the Seventh P.S.P. as part of professional expense information for 1970.

6. *Percentage of patients with low and middle incomes.* The Seventh

P.S.P. obtained information on the percentage of patients with low, middle and high incomes (the breaks between these categories being $5,000 and $15,000, respectively), but the model utilizes only the percentage of patients with low and middle incomes.

7. *Patient visits.* Finally, patient visits for the most recent complete practice week (consisting of office visits, hospital visits, nursing home visits and other visits) were obtained directly from the Seventh P.S.P.

23 Econometric Forecasts of Health Services and Health Manpower[1]

Donald E. Yett, Leonard Drabek, Michael D. Intriligator and Larry J. Kimbell

UNIVERSITY OF SOUTHERN CALIFORNIA

This paper presents the Human Resources Research Center (H.R.R.C.) macroeconometric model of the health care systems of the United States and examples of its use in the study of health services and health manpower. This model contains 37 behavioral equations and identities treating both demand and supply factors in the markets for health services and health manpower. The model explains utilization rates and prices of health services, occupancy rates and beds for inpatient institutions, and employment and wages for health manpower. The model is used for structural analysis by studying estimated coefficients and implied elasticities. The paper reports estimated price, income and insurance elasticities of demand for hospital inpatient and outpatient care and for visits to medical specialists and to surgical specialists. The model is also used for policy evaluation via simulating future values of variables of the health care system under alternative assumptions as to policy variables. The paper reports analyses of two types of policy initiatives, the first involving features of various national health insurance plans and the second involving policies designed to increase the total number of physicians.

I. INTRODUCTION

Econometric models of the health care system can play an important role in forecasting and policy evaluation. These models have already been useful as pedagogical devices to remind individuals of the complex interrelationships among the various institutions and markets of the health care system. Recent developments in health economics, however, suggest the possibility of a much wider and more important

[1] Research described in this paper was supported, in part, by the Community Profile Data Center of the U.S. Public Health Service under Contract No. HSM–110–69–1. The authors wish to express their appreciation to Royal A. Crystal, Chief, Community Profile Data Center, and his staff for advice and assistance, and to their colleague, Robert T. Deane, for his help and valuable suggestions throughout the project.

use for econometric models. These developments include: greater availability of both formal models of, and data relevant to, economic aspects of the health care system; a more quantitative approach on the part of health economists; and a demand on the part of health planners, both for more quantitative analyses and for analyses that treat the entire health care system, rather than portions of this system. The uses of econometric models that will undoubtedly receive the most emphasis over the next several years are structural analysis and policy evaluation.

Structural analysis refers to the quantitative analysis of the impacts of endogenous, exogenous and policy variables on relevant variables of the health care system. Structural analysis is conducted by a systematic evaluation of the empirical content of the estimated coefficients of the structural equations of the model. Examples of structural analysis include the determination of elasticities, such as the price elasticity of demand for inpatient and outpatient health care, and the determination of impact multipliers, such as the impact of Medicare expenditures on bed days in hospitals or the impact of insurance benefits on patient visits to physicians.

Policy evaluation refers to the quantitative determination of the impacts of alternative policies on the health care system. There are several approaches to policy evaluation; the one emphasized here is simulation, that is, a determination of future values of variables of the health care system under alternative assumptions as to policy variables. Examples of policy evaluation include the determination of the consequences of national health insurance and of the production of additional physicians for both health services and health manpower.

This paper presents examples of the use of the Human Resources Research Center (H.R.R.C.) macroeconometric model of the health care system of the United States to study health services and health manpower.[1] Section II gives an overview of the model, sections III and IV, respectively, present some structural analyses and policy evaluations using the model, and section V gives our conclusions.

II. THE H.R.R.C. MACROECONOMETRIC MODEL: AN OVERVIEW

The H.R.R.C. macroeconometric model of the health care system of the United States contains 37 behavioral equations and identities to deal with the complex interactions in the health care system. It in-

---

[1] For a discussion of the H.R.R.C. macroeconometric model, see Yett *et al.* (1971a, 1971b, 1972). For other econometric models of the health care system, see M. S. Feldstein (1967, 1971) and P. J. Feldstein and Kelman (1970). A related approach is that of the H.R.R.C. model, discussed by Yett *et al.* (1970, 1972).

cludes both demand and supply factors in the markets for health services and health manpower. While limited to personal health services (excluding mental health, drugs and dental services), the model does explicitly treat various categories of health service institutions and health manpower.[1] The six categories of health services institutions and seven categories of health manpower in the model are:

Health service institutions:
  Voluntary and proprietary short-term hospitals.
  State and local governmental short-term hospitals.
  Skilled nursing homes.
  Outpatient units of non-federal hospitals.
  Offices of medical specialists in private practice.
  Offices of surgical specialists in private practice.

Health manpower
  Medical specialists and general practitioners in private practice.
  Surgical specialists in private practice.
  Physicians employed by hospitals.
  Hospital interns and residents.
  Registered nurses employed by health service institutions.
  Allied health professionals employed by health service institutions.
  All other personnel employed by health service institutions.

The 37 endogenous variables of the H.R.R.C. model include utilization rates and prices of health services, occupancy rates and beds for inpatient institutions, and employment and wages for health manpower. The 35 exogenous variables of the model are either variables determined outside the health care system, such as population and income, or variables representing policy instruments, such as benefits paid under government insurance programs (Medicare and Medicaid) and services provided by federal hospitals.

The equations explaining the demand for health services are conceptually similar across different types of providers. Quantity demanded is measured by an observed utilization rate for the service: bed days for inpatient care and patient visits for outpatient care. Explanatory variables for each of the demand equations include prices, income, insurance and demographic variables. These variables were selected on the basis of previous empirical findings as well as *a priori* theory. For example, demand for inpatient days at short-term voluntary and proprietary hospitals depends on prices of hospital and related services, income, insurance enrollment and benefit variables,

---

[1] See Yett *et al.* (1971*a*, 1971*b*, 1972) for a discssion of the detailed structure of the model. A listing of the variables and the estimated equations of the model is available upon request.

Medicare and Medicaid expenditures, and the proportion of the population aged 65 years and over.

The demand for governmental hospital services is determined in a different way from the demand for private hospital care. Historically, governmental hospitals have treated indigent patients at zero or near-zero price. The demand for patient days at state and local governmental hospitals does not depend on prices, but does depend on income, insurance and demographic variables. Patient days at federal hospitals are treated as exogenous.

Hospital supply of inpatient services is specified in terms of the identity: patient days equals occupancy rate multiplied by number of beds. The model treats the number of beds in any period as predetermined, while occupancy rate can vary, subject to a maximum value. Increases in occupancy, after a lag, result in the construction of additional facilities.

The specification of demand and supply equations for nursing homes is similar to that for short-term voluntary and proprietary hospitals, with demand determined by price, income, and Medicare and Medicaid expenditures, and supply determined by occupancy rate and employees per bed in such institutions.

The two basic sources of outpatient care are hospital-based outpatient units and physicians' offices. The model determines number of hospital outpatient visits on the basis of demand and supply equations similar to those for hospital inpatient units.

Demand for and supply of physicians' services (for both medical and surgical specialists) jointly determine the number and price of visits. Demand for physicians' services depends on price, income, insurance, Medicare and Medicaid, and demographic variables. The supply of physicians' services depends on physician hours, which, in turn, is determined by the stock of physicians. The stock of physicians is adjusted for graduations from medical schools, for immigration of foreign-trained physicians, and for the loss of physicians due to deaths and retirements.

Hospital staff physicians are treated as in perfectly inelastic demand, while interns and residents are a fraction of those from the previous period plus current graduates of medical schools.

The model explicitly treats demand for and supply of nurses, the former depending on the quantity of services produced and the wage, and the latter depending on the wage and the stock of nurses.[1] While allied health professionals are treated similarly, the demand for other health manpower is dependent on the quantity of services produced and an exogenously determined wage.

[1] For detailed analyses of the markets for registered nurses, see Yett (1970) and Deane and Yett (forthcoming).

The model was estimated by ordinary least squares using recent cross-section data for states. The intercept terms for each equation were then adjusted in order to scale the model to fit national data for a given year. The model is a non-linear system of simultaneous equations, and the solution technique employed was the Gauss–Seidel method.[1] It was simulated using time-series data for the period 1960–70 to test this procedure, in particular to evaluate the ability of the model to track the historical period. The simulations closely matched the historical data for this period.

III. STRUCTURAL ANALYSIS USING THE H.R.R.C. MACROECONOMETRIC MODEL

The H.R.R.C. macroeconometric model can be used for structural analysis by studying the estimated coefficients of the model. Consider, for example, the price, income and insurance elasticities of demand shown in Table 23.1.[2] While the demand for hospital services is inelastic with respect to the price of hospital services, it is greater than zero. The prices of related medical services were also included in the first regression equation to test for the existence of interactions between demands for specific services.

Interactions between sectors are represented by the relative price terms. One important implication of the structural coefficient estimates is that outpatient care is a substitute for inpatient care. Thus, the estimates suggest that lower prices for outpatient care enable some patients to avoid hospitalization and others to spend fewer days in the hospital. Since inpatient care is far more costly, such substitution is of clear policy importance. The finding of a positive cross-elasticity with respect to the price of outpatient clinic visits supports this interpretation. Another interesting interaction is observed with respect to the services of medical and surgical specialists. The negative cross-elasticities suggest that increases in the prices of these services reduce the demand for inpatient care because they increase the total bill for a hospital stay.

Table 23.1 also gives estimates of elasticity of demand for outpatient clinic services and visits to private practice medical and surgical specialists. The former exhibited the greatest price sensitivity, with a unitary own-price elasticity and a positive cross-elasticity with respect to the price of inpatient care.

Two of the most important federal programs impacting on the

---

[1] The Gauss–Seidel algorithm has been used in the simulation of econometric models of the nation's economy. It was first applied to this task by Norman (1967).

[2] Since the model was estimated in linear form, the elasticities are computed at mean values.

TABLE 23.1

CALCULATED DEMAND ELASTICITIES FOR SPECIFIC MEDICAL SERVICES[a]

	Price of inpatient hospital care	Price of an outpatient clinic visit	Price of medical specialist care	Price of surgical specialist care	Income	Medicare benefits	Medicaid benefits	Enrollment in private health insurance plans
Patient days at short-term voluntary and proprietary hospitals	−0·31	0·07	−0·39	−0·14	−0·14	0·46*	−0·002	0·35*
Visits to hospital-based outpatient clinics	0·88*	−1·02*	−	−	−	0·44**	−0·05	−0·03
Visits to medical specialists in private practice	−	−	−0·06	−	0·42*	0·35*	0·04*	0·03
Visits to surgical specialists in private practice	−	−	−	−0·29	0·19	0·57*	0·01	0·03

[a] A dash (−) indicates that the variable was not included in the regression equation.

An asterisk (*) implies that the regression coefficient was statistically significant at greater than the 5 per cent level.

United States health care system are Medicare and Medicaid. The former covers persons over age 64, and the latter covers medically indigent individuals, for both inpatient and outpatient services.[1] The fact that these programs are potentially subject to change by policy-makers underscores the importance of studying their impacts on the United States health care system. Table 23.1 summarizes the impacts of these policy variables on demand for services of inpatient and out-patient institutions.

It shows that Medicare expenditures exert a substantial positive influence on the demand for medical services. The coefficients of the Medicare variables are highly significant in each equation. The effect of Medicaid is less pronounced, with the principal impact being on the patient visits to medical specialists. The regression results indicate that Medicaid expenditures for physician services tend to reduce outpatient clinic utilization and increase demand for private practice physicians. These findings are consistent with the program's goal of substituting paid services for charity care to low-income persons.

IV. POLICY EVALUATION USING THE
H.R.R.C. MACROECONOMETRIC MODEL

The basic objective in developing the H.R.R.C. macroeconometric model is to provide policy-makers with a method for anticipating the probable impacts of alternative policy initiatives affecting the health care system. This is accomplished via simulation, in which the model is solved over time under alternative assumptions regarding values of the included policy variables. The impacts of policy initiatives are then analyzed by comparing time paths of relevant health care variables, given the policy change, with their values without the change, the latter representing a 'base run' which postulates that no significant policy initiatives have been adopted. The 'base run' is, thus, a *status quo* simulation which serves as the control solution for comparisons with particular policy change simulations. In simulating years for which historical data are not available, projected values of the exogenous variables are used to generate conditional forecasts for the endogenous variables of the model.

Two types of policy initiatives have been studied, using the H.R.R.C. macroeconometric model. The first type involves features commonly considered for various national health insurance (N.H.I.) plans.[2] The second type involves policies designed to increase the total number of physicians.

---

[1] The total expenditures under these programs in 1970 were \$7·5 billion for Medicare and \$5·8 billion for Medicaid.

[2] See Yett *et al.* (1971*b*).

Features of N.H.I. plans, rather than complete plans, were analyzed because it is much easier to study and understand impacts of specific features than to comprehend the simultaneous, and possibly offsetting, impacts of the multiplicity of features of a complete plan. By identifying these impacts, moreover, one can determine the overall effects of alternative 'composite' plans. The implementation of N.H.I. can be described in terms of the H.R.R.C. econometric model. In the H.R.R.C. model, the initial impact of N.H.I. is to expand health insurance coverage, stimulating consumers to demand greater amounts of patient days and patient visits from health care institutions. This greater demand tends, during the current period, to increase both prices and quantities in the health services markets – with the degree of price inflation being a function of the responsiveness of health services supply.

The number of beds is not influenced within the current period, so an induced change in capacity is not immediately forthcoming. Therefore, the increase in patient days raises occupancy rates at inpatient institutions. Over several periods, the increase in occupancy rates and the higher prices for inpatient services lead providers to augment the number of beds, and, depending on how substantially the supply of beds responds, to ameliorate the rate of price inflation. The increase in demand for patient visits to physicians, and the increase in the prices for these visits, tends to increase the (implicit) demand for physicians; but this does not increase the number of medical and surgical specialists which, for the nation as a whole, is highly inelastic in the short run. Greater amounts of patient days in hospitals and nursing homes, and larger numbers of visits to hospital outpatient clinics and physicians' offices, increase the demand for health manpower which, depending on the availability of such manpower, increases their employment and wages.

Three N.H.I. plan features have been analyzed using the H.R.R.C. macroeconometric model: coverage, coinsurance and capitation.[1] *Coverage* refers to the fraction of the population covered by the plan, and is simulated in the model by increasing the proportion of the population enrolled in health insurance plans to one.[2] *Coinsurance* refers to the percentage of health costs paid by the insured population. The effects of coinsurance were simulated in the model by assuming the level of effective prices entering the demand functions for health services to be 25 per cent of the market price.[3] *Capitation*

---

[1] The results of these N.H.I. simulations can be obtained from the authors.

[2] The estimated values of these variables in the base run were 0·90 for hospital insurance, 0·85 for surgical insurance and 0·75 for regular medical insurance.

[3] The proposed 'National Health Insurance Partnership Act' contains provision for a 25 per cent coinsurance rate. The proposed 'National Health In-

refers to whether the plan involves reimbursement on a capitation or fee-for-services basis, and was simulated by increasing the population covered by capitation reimbursement plans from 6 million in 1970 to 46 million in 1980.[1] The model was then solved under the assumption of reduced utilization rates for these individuals.[2] The three simulations indicated that the dramatic increase in utilization, prices and wages due to full coverage of the population was offset somewhat by coinsurance and, to a lesser degree, by capitation reimbursement. For example, inpatient days provided by short-term private hospitals, which increased by over 200 per cent from 1970 to 1984 in the coverage experiment, was reduced by more than 25 per cent as a result of coinsurance but by less than 10 per cent as a result of capitation reimbursement.

The second type of experiment analyzed the impact of programs designed to increase the supply of physicians. In this simulation experiment, the model was solved under the assumption that medical school graduates would increase from 8,280 in 1970 to 14,487 in 1980.[3] However, owing to the fact that physicians typically receive internship and residency training, an increase in graduates precedes, by three to four years, an increase in the number of practicing physicians. This policy was analyzed by comparing the simulation of its impact relative to the N.H.I. coverage experiment. The results indicated that, at least over the ten years following the policy designed to increase the supply of health manpower, there was no significant effect of this added health manpower on utilization, prices or wages. By 1984 there was no perceptible difference in either inpatient or outpatient utilization as a result of the added manpower. The only perceptible difference was in the price of outpatient visits, which was reduced by less than 3 per cent.[4]

---

surance and Health Services Improvement Act' and the 'Health Care Insurance Act' both call for 20 per cent coinsurance. See Yett *et al.* (1971*b*).

[1] This increase was selected because it constitutes one of the announced goals of the sponsors of the proposed Health Security Act. See Yett *et al.* (1971*b*).

[2] The amount of shift in utilization resulting from capitation is exogenously imposed, based on comparisons of utilization differentials observed for prepaid and fee-for-service practices. Specifically, a 30 per cent reduction in hospital days, a 5 per cent reduction in medical visits to physicians and a 43 per cent reduction in surgical procedures were derived from the findings of previous studies. See Yett *et al.* (1971*b*).

[3] This trend represents a target goal set by the Bureau of Health Manpower Education of the National Institutes of Health. See Yett *et al.* (1971*b*).

[4] Of course, there can be beneficial effects in later years due to increased manpower. For example, each additional physician educated by 1980 is expected to work until about 2015, so six-sevenths of his working life lies beyond the simulation period.

V. CONCLUSIONS

This paper has presented an overview of the H.R.R.C. macroeconometric model – a 37-equation model of the health care system of the United States – and a discussion of two uses of the model – structural analysis and policy evaluation.

Only recently has there developed an appreciation of the enormous potential of econometric models for analyzing the complex nature of the health care sstem aynd for guiding policy decisions affecting it. Each of these uses of the model is of considerable significance.

Structural analysis using an econometric model can be considered a logical step in the development of health economics – a development that started with verbal analyses, proceeded to geometrical analyses, progressed to quantitative analyses of individual sectors of the health care system, and is now beginning to treat quantitatively the complete system. With an estimated econometric model it is possible to perform policy experiments on the model rather than on the 'real world', and therefore to avoid the costly consequences of 'real world' experimentation.

The basic conclusion of this paper is that econometric models of the health care system are feasible, and can be of considerable value to both health economists and health planners. They are capable of forecasting not only the initial impact of a policy initiative, but the secondary and tertiary impacts as well. Studies which deal with only one aspect of the health care system cannot provide this type of policy guidance because they fail to take account of the complex interdependencies in the system.

REFERENCES

Deane, R. T., and Yett, D. E., 'The Development of an Econometric Model of the Market for Nurses', final report on a project supported by U.S. Public Health Service Grant NU 00274, Division of Nursing, Bureau of Health Manpower (forthcoming).

Feldstein, M. S., 'An Aggregate Model of the Health Care Sector', *Medical Care*, v (Nov–Dec 1967) 369–81.

——, 'An Econometric Model of the Medicare System', *Quarterly Journal of Economics*, LXXXV (Feb 1971) 1–20.

Feldstein, P. J., and Kelman, S., 'A Framework for an Econometric Model of the Medical Sector', in H. E. Klarman (ed.), *Empirical Studies in Health Economics* (Baltimore: John Hopkins Press, 1970) pp. 171–90.

Norman, M. R., 'Solving a Nonlinear Econometric Model by the Gauss–Seidel Iterative Method', paper presented at the Econometric Society Meetings (Dec 1967).

U.S. Department of Health, Education and Welfare, *Analysis of Health Insurance Proposals Introduced in the 92nd Congress*, printed for the use of the Committee on Ways and Means (Washington, D.C.: U.S. Government Printing Office, 1971).

U.S. Social Security Administration, Office of Research and Statistics (written by Waldman, Saul, and Peel, Evelyn), 'National Health Insurance: A Comparison of Five Proposals', Research and Statistics, Note No. 12, 23 July 1970.

Yett, Donald E., 'The Chronic Shortage of Nurses: A Public Policy Dilemma', in H. E. Klarman (ed.), *Empirical Studies in Health Economics* (Baltimore: John Hopkins Press, 1970) pp. 357–89.

——, Drabek, L., Intriligator, M. D., and Kimbell, L. J., 'The Development of a Micro-Simulation Model of Health Manpower Demand and Supply', in *Proceedings and Report of Conference on a Health Manpower Simulation Model*, vol. I (Washington, D.C.: U.S. Department of Health, Education and Welfare, 1970) pp. 9–173.

——, ——, —— and ——, 'A Macreconometric Model for Regional Health Planning', *Economic and Business Bulletin*, XXIV (Fall 1971a) 1–21.

——, ——, —— and ——, 'The Use of an Econometric Model to Analyze Selected Features of National Health Insurance Plans', paper presented at a joint session of the Health Economics Research Organization and the American Economic Association, New Orleans, 28 Dec 1971b.

——, ——, —— and ——, 'Health Manpower Planning: An Econometric Approach', *Health Services Research*, VII (Summer 1971) 134–47.

Summary Record of Discussion

This session returned to what may be called the standard format, with three papers discussed in order. These papers were by Professor Atkinson on public regulation of smoking, by Professor Intriligator and Dr Kehrer on physicians' employment of paramedical assistants, and by Messrs Yett, Drabek, Intriligator and Kimbell on econometric forecasts of health services and manpower. Floor discussion, however, treated the last two papers simultaneously.

A. *Professor Atkinson's paper*
Professor Moriguchi's introduction and critique stressed Japanese experience. Tobacco and gunpowder, said Professor Moriguchi, were both brought to Japan by the Portuguese in the sixteenth century. In each case, attempts to ban the import failed and were replaced by taxation.

In Professor Atkinson's two-period model of consumer behavior, the consumer is aware that his behavior at t_1 with regard to smoking will effect his chances of survival to t_2. However, this probability is estimated by smokers subjectively as a, whereas its true objective value is a^*. The government can affect smoking either by taxing tobacco consumption or by reducing the differential $(a–a^*)$ at a cost, by anti-smoking campaigns. The effect of such a campaign may, however, be to raise a_2 while lowering a_1. In that case, the campaign may operate to stimulate smoking among the young in particular, while putting off the risk of death to a further future. Japanese experience appeared to Professor Moriguchi to illustrate precisely this result. Taxation, on the other hand, produces more reduction in smoking for a given expenditure of public funds. This is both because tax collection is relatively cheap and because providing additional information may have the 'wrong' results.

To some extent, however, the Atkinson conclusions depend upon certain prior assumptions. For example, the tobacco tax revenue is supposedly without effect on the total and the direction of public expenditures (other than for tax collection). This conception of public expenditures as lump sums is conventional, but not realistic. Also, the price elasticity of demand for tobacco products is extremely low, especially among the male population. This means that the main effect of taxation may be an income redistribution unfavorable to smokers; Professor Atkinson does not explore the effects of such redistribution. Furthermore, externalities are ignored – particularly, effects on indoor air pollution. Experiments on the size and importance of this effect are under way in Japan. Their results would certainly modify the Atkinson conclusions, and might even change them qualitatively.

Replying to Professor Moriguchi's comments, *Professor Atkinson* pointed out that his paper had originated as an interdisciplinary study with epidemiologists. He agreed, accordingly, that externalities are important, and cited experiments with rats, aimed at their measurement. The issues involved, however, are not peculiar to smoking, and the observed results do not appear so large as to alter his own preference for taxation over education. Women in particular, said Professor Atkinson, are not responsive to health education, while their price elasticity of demand for tobacco is higher than that of men.

Mr Culyer, as a smoker, suggested that the present alternatives to smoking, particularly additional eating and drinking, might have worse effects on mortality than smoking itself. He also wondered whether externalities would be less.

Dr Phelps said that the price elasticity of demand for tobacco products in the United States is currently estimated at about 0·4, and that in addition to suffering higher mortality rates, smokers finance the medical care of ailments related to smoking. This cost is quite high in the United States, although perhaps not in the United Kingdom. (In the United States, lung tumors are treated by high-cost surgery, whereas British practice uses cheaper methods.)

Dr Friedman believed that the sizes of the first-period mortality rates (a_1, a_1^*) may be crucial to the Atkinson model, and that any two-period model makes insufficient allowance for the inevitability of death. He thought a three-panel might not be preferable, and, hence, wondered whether an education campaign might not be more successful if it involved systematic misinformation about the a_1^* – presenting it as higher than its actual value.

Professor Bronfenbrenner wondered whether the model might not be over-aggregative, in that it ignored important differences between heavy and light smokers.

Referring to the externality problem, *Professor L. Lave* felt that tobacco taxes are already high enough to offset such externalities as medical care to non-smokers. He asked for more consideration of other externalities to the non-smoker, whose comfort and, possibly, health were affected by exposure to the smoking of others.

Professor Lévy inquired whether the Atkinson model allowed for the additional medical-sector G.N.P. brought on by smoking, and whether it distinguished adequately between the annual and the total (or lifetime) costs of smoking.

Mr Pole felt that smoking, like surfing (but apparently not unlike skiing), has addictive effects, and that much utility analysis of the tobacco problem ignores these effects. He said that education directed specifically at the top of the income distribution might be more effective than education directed at the masses directly, since the latter tend to imitate upper-class habits. As regards income distribution issues, finally, tobacco taxes already contribute to 'secondary poverty' in Britain, as would appear from family expenditure data. British entry into the E.E.C. promises to reduce this effect.

Dr Kleiman began his intervention by mentioning another type of externality. A (a non-smoker) believes B (a smoker) suffers subjectively from his smoking habit and is sympathetic, even though the facts may be the other way. He wondered whether there may not be a third alternative to taxes and educational campaigns in models like the Atkinson one, namely, expenditures to make it easier to stop smoking. Finally, Dr Kleiman denied that reduced smoking would reduce medical-sector G.N.P., as Professor Levy had feared; medical output would simply be redirected. (*Mr Culyer* could not see why the Kleiman externality provided any reason for coercing B, since – if Dr Kleiman's factual conjecture is correct, A would be deprived by such coercion of the pleasures of sympathy with B.)

Professor L. Lave commented on the wide range of mutually inconsistent judgments in the United States about such problems as smoking, alcohol, drugs, automobile driving (without seat belts), motorcycle riding (without crash helmets), etc. If any sense can be made of this congeries of attitudes, it is that new vices are regarded with less tolerance than old ones. His guess was that smoking would now be banned, if it had not already developed and become the basis for a major industry. *Dr Hartwell* also inquired more specifically about the applicability of the Atkinson analysis to alcohol and psychedelic drugs, and about reactions in the tobacco industry.

Replying to the discussion from the floor, *Professor Atkinson* defended his model as a benchmark, not as a realistic model of smoking behavior. At the same time, he felt the decision process in the model does involve the amount of smoking. The two-period model is merely the simplest one available; addition of a third period would not have been worth the added complications. Professor Atkinson also expressed some doubt as to the significance of the externalities involving non-smokers. He said that a welfare economic judgment, such as he had made, does, and should, include both objective and subjective risks under the alternative methods of smoking control, and should also deduct, in each case, the utility loss to smokers. He also agreed that income distribution effects were important. (So, added *Dr Phelps*, were policy reactions if, for example, tobacco monopoly revenue were eliminated, as in the Japanese case.)

B. *Professor Intriligator and Dr Kehrer's paper*

This paper was introduced and criticized by *Professor Sloan*, who began by saying that the problem (hiring of allied medical personnel by physicians) was one to which economists could make significant contributions. This type of medical investment had not thus far been evaluated, and good data was not yet available.

The Intriligator–Kehrer study specifies the number of hours of allied medical personnel time employed by physicians in separate specialties, and also the amount of delegation of specific tasks. It also involves a large number of exogenous variables: wage rates, physical capital investment in medical practice, and malpractice insurance premium costs.

Professor Sloan, however, missed in the paper any model of doctors' decision-making processes. It was not clear whether they were profit- or gross revenue-maximizers, or, perhaps, simply income target-setters.[1]

Professor Sloan was also concerned that some variables might be misspecified as exogenous. The number of patient visits per period was

---

[1] *Professor Intriligator*, in a postscript, says that this model is descriptive, 'which is consistent with physicians acting as cost-minimizers'.

one such. So was the amount of capital. The wages paid to allied medical employees are a more complex variable. Wage *rates*, he agreed, are exogenous for the individual physician, but the actual wages paid are endogenous, depending on the mix of allied medical employees. Perhaps, Professor Sloan said, wage rates and hours per day might have been treated as separate variables.

Conventional empirical analysis assumes all observations in the neighborhood of equilibrium positions. But in the case of physicians, this may be wrong. Are the doctor's capital stock and his hiring of allied medical labor services what he would like them to be, given all prices and incomes?

Professor Sloan did not think that the amount of delegation belonged in an input demand equation, since delegation is a descriptive, rather than a causal, variable. The same might be true of malpractice insurance. (He did not accept a conventional assumption that the use of more aides increases the likelihood of malpractice suits.)

Turning to the Intriligator–Kehrer data, Professor Sloan noted very high variances within specialties, and wondered about the reasons for their existence. He thought that tests for statistical homogeneity should have been made. He also noted that only 435 replies had been used out of a sample of 5,000 medical doctors, wondered why so many had been excluded, and was concerned about possible response biases.

C. Messrs Yett, Drabek, Intriligator and Kimbell's paper

Professor Leinhardt introduced and criticized the paper, as an application to the health area of the macroeconomic modeling techniques which have been used widely for policy evaluation, and also for short-term forecasting. In fact, Professor Leinhardt thought, there were really two papers here, an analysis of past data and a forecast for the period 1971–6.

The model uses the 'system' perspective, utilizes new data (which permit a wider role for econometricians), and makes policy evaluations by simulating the effects of changes both in exogenous variables and in parameter estimates. In this case, 37 equations are used with 35 exogenous variables. The model is estimated using cross-section data on states. The effects of price and insurance changes are included. The effects of possible changes in capitation taxes, coinsurance rates and medical manpower availability are projected as much as fifteen years into the future.

Professor Leinhardt thought the model was subject to criticism as over-aggregated, and as washing out area interactions at local levels, where the data are better and the relations may be more robust.[1] (The example given by Professor Leinhardt was medical care in rural hospitals.) The estimation procedures are open to criticisms: too many interpolations,[2] not enough actual observations. Also, interaction and demographic terms are omitted[3] – particularly the interactions between sets of

---

[1] *Professor Intriligator*, in a postscript, objected; he added that local data were 'considerably inferior to the statewide data'.

[2] In the same postscript, *Professor Intriligator* thought this point erroneous.

[3] Same postscript reaction as note 2 above.

demographic variables. Forecast values of exogenous variables are used, but this procedure is dangerous since such forecasts are constantly revised. Migration is an important aspect of the health care system's problems, but is omitted. The data dealing specifically with the black population and with particular income classes are also poor, and leave the critic wanting to know more about the significance of the differences indicated. No reduced-form equations are supplied, to relate individual endogenous variables to exogenous ones. In this connection, Professor Leinhardt did not find the paper's appendix particularly helpful.

The only 'evaluation variable' of the study appears to be the demand for health care. Supply is omitted.[1] So are any variables relating to health status or cost–benefit ratios. So are such possible changes within the health care system as family practice and increasing paramedical care. He (Professor Leinhardt) would have liked to see more 'retrospective evaluations' of changes which had already occurred. Because of past changes within the health care system, he feels that past experience is a poor guide for long-term forecasts, and would have liked more direct comparisons of different patterns of change.

Following a brief intermission, the last two papers were discussed together. Dr Kehrer replied to Professor Sloan's comments on the Intriligator–Kehrer paper; Professor Intriligator replied to Professor Leinhardt's comments on the Yett–Drabek–Intriligator–Kimbell paper.

The first point to which *Dr Kehrer* replied related to the size of the Intriligator–Kehrer sample and the possibility of response bias. The actual sample of 9,000 had elicited 5,000 responses, with no obvious bias by specialty or geographic location. The further reduction to 435 had come about because the response of only solo practitioners in only four specialty groups were used and because many solo practitioners had failed to answer certain key questions in the questionnaires they had returned.

Disagreeing with Professor Sloan, Dr Kehrer felt that the underlying model was reasonably clear. It involved minimization of costs, given both the level of output and the other (non-labor) inputs used. Were these other inputs and outputs indeed exogenous, as the model had treated them? Perhaps there is some real difference in outlook between herself and Professor Sloan on this issue of specification, but in any case, further experiments with the data will involve increasing its size to permit more variables to be treated as endogenous.

As to 'delegation', Dr Kehrer saw the 'delegation' equation as representing the physician's demand for delegation. The desire for delegation she saw as a cause or propensity, not as an effect of hiring paramedical personnel.

On malpractice insurance, Dr Kehrer agreed with Professor Sloan that delegation did not seem to increase the likelihood of suits. More important appeared to be the geographic location of the physician's practice and also the nature of his specialty; surgeons were particularly likely to be

---

[1] Same postscript reaction as note 2 above.

sued, and there were also wide differences within the surgical specialties.

Replying to Professor Leinhardt's criticism of the Yett–Drabek–Intriligator–Kimbell model, *Professor Intriligator* pointed out that both his Los Angeles group and the Pittsburgh group, including Professor Leinhardt, were interested in the systems approach to health care economics. Even the difference in degree of aggregation is not so great as Professor Leinhardt had indicated. The model is estimated using state data, and he and his group are already working on state and local data from California and Louisiana. Under construction, also, is a micro-simulation model for individuals, which includes many of the variables he had been criticized for omitting. Admittedly, the data are sometimes based on interpolation rather than observation, but one does the best one can with whatever data are available.

Professor Intriligator thought it a misinterpretation to accuse his group of using demand rather than supply as its evaluation variable. He preferred to think of the evaluation variable as being total health service, without regard to the supply–demand distinction. It was true that his model included no health status variable, but he was somewhat skeptical about this concept. They were, however, considering merging with, or embodying into, his micro-model a sub-model like the one of which Professor Leinhardt had been co-author. As for structural changes, Professor Intriligator felt that these could be allowed for by changing the structural parameters of the model. Finally, he agreed with his critics that long-term forecasts were dangerous, but they are inevitable in making long-range plans, and it is better to do them using a formal model than relying upon intuition alone.

Discussion from the floor tended to fluctuate between the two papers in which Professor Intriligator had an author's role, but to concentrate primarily upon the Yett–Drabek–Intriligator–Kimbell one as the larger and more ambitious of the pair. *Dr Davis* began by wondering whether this paper was self-contained and independent of prior work by the same group. She had commented previously on other papers co-authored by Professor Intriligator, and was disappointed to find her prior suggestions ignored here. For example, she noted that the present model does not allow for substitution between inputs by physicians; it is, in other words, a fixed-proportions model. Also, in at least one case (hospital costs), what is presented as an equation appeared to her to be a mere identity. The simulation results she found misleading in at least two ways: (1) There is no way for the volume of hospital care to rise by so much as the forecasts called for, inasmuch as capacity is lacking. (2) Only about 13 per cent of existing cost are out-of-pocket as far as patients are concerned. Professor Intriligator and his co-authors have disregarded the effect of existing insurance schemes.[1] In fact, the newer capitation and coinsurance schemes have represented, not reductions, but increases in the total price of hospital services. *Professor Evans* agreed with Dr Davis, adding that the Yett–Draber–Intriligator–Kimbell forecasts of the effect of massive health insurance were out of line with the actual results of

[1] *Professor Intriligator*, in a postscript, disagreed; they are *not* neglected.

health insurance in Canada. He added that this model seemed to him to involve too much exogeneity in physicians' behavior.

Dr Phelps (still concerned with the Yett–Drabek–Intriligator–Kimbell paper) was disturbed with the low precision and large variances of certain of the equations. He professed himself also unclear about the detail of the data bases, and wondered whether ordinary least squares or simultaneous equation *estimation* procedures had been used. *Professor Bronfenbrenner* added that the forecasting record of the large macroeconomic models of entire economies, which Professor Intriligator had sought to follow, was not particularly good. In particular, even short-term forecasts had required judgmental adjustments at key points. *Professor Rosett* commented on an important difference in this regard, between this health care model and the short-run forecasting macro-models. In these latter, adjustments have given the appearance of plausibility to what might otherwise have been implausible history. Professor Intriligator and his colleagues have refused to fudge or to make adjustments; as a result, their scenario looks implausible as either history or forecast.

Professor Williams shifted discussion to the Intriligator–Kehrer paper by expressing concern with substitution between types of paramedical personnel and, in particular, its asymmetrical character, which the paper had neglected. (For example, a nurse can be assigned some of the functions of a secretary or receptionist, but not the reverse.) He suggested that such delegation differentiations required more study.

Dr Bell said that some of the hours-per-week figures for some types of paramedical personnel in certain specialties looked unrealistic. If they were derived by dividing wages paid by wage rates, the estimates might be biased by failure to reflect part-time, or overtime work.[1]

Professor Fuchs inquired whether there was any such thing as an optimal mix of paramedical assistants for physicians in any speciality, any more than there was an optimal mix of research and teaching assistants for economists. *Mr Kaser* added that routine and the rule of thumb were particularly strong in physicians' hiring practices, and, moreover, that there might be little obvious need for rationality or optimality in these decisions. In *Professor Sloan's* view, the results of the paramedical personnel labor market may not look efficient on paper, but some doctors are better personnel managers than others, and would be quite right to hire 'too little' assistance. (*Professor Fuchs* concurred.) One would therefore expect, continued Professor Sloan, wide ranges of variance to be washed out and concealed by use of sample means. Even so, retorted *Dr Phelps*, mean-value estimates may be unbiased and interesting.

Professor Uzawa then returned to the Yett–Drabek–Intriligator–Kimbell paper to amplify an econometric criticism which he felt Dr Davis had missed. In estimating demand elasticities for patient days in hospitals, Medicare and Medicaid payments are treated as independent variables. But in another equation, Medicaid payments are treated as functions of

---

[1] *Dr Kehrer* believes this point *obiter dicta*; the paper clearly stated that the number of hours worked by allied health personnel was collected directly in the A.M.A.'s Seventh Periodic Survey of Physicians.

patient days. The combined result is upward bias in the estimate of the elasticity of demand for patient days.

Dr Kehrer limited herself, in her final remarks, to acceptance of the Williams criticisms. *Professor Intriligator* replied, however, to certain of the criticisms of the other model. With reference to the Evans criticism, he expressed the view that many physicians' behavioral decisions were, in fact, exogenous, precisely as he had treated them, and that this exogeneity was reflected in, for example, low elasticities of physician demand for paramedical labor. Replying to Dr Davis, Professor Intriligator said that there had been more revisions of his earlier papers than might be apparent on the surface, and that some of the revisions suggested by Dr Davis in earlier critiques were not really needed. As for a possible overstrain on hospital facilities, he admitted that the entire health care system might have to change somewhat to make it feasible, and that such change might take more time than his model allows. Some of his smaller-scale models were, he said, more explicit on this point. Replying to Professors Bronfenbrenner and Rosett, Professor Intriligator expressed the hope that health care models may develop as rapidly and as usefully as the forecasting macro-models. As for Professor Uzawa's claim (that he had overestimated demand elasticity for patient days in hospitals), Professor Intriligator replied that the two equations which Professor Uzawa had referred to were, in fact, independent of each other, being based on two different populations, and he doubted that significant bias remained in his estimates.

Part Five

Method and Methodology in Understanding the Choice of Health Care Systems

24 On the Social Rationality of Health Policies

Jean-Pierre Dupuy

CENTRE DE RECHERCHE SUR LE BIEN-ÊTRE, PARIS

I. Measuring the output of health activities: (1) Introduction. (2) Health expenditure appears to make only a slight impact on overall technical health indicators. (3) Logical criteria systems other than the maximization of an overall technical health indicator. (4) The implicit rationality of health activities and their non-technical outputs. (5) From technical and non-technical outputs to a rational health policy.

II. The Consumption of Medicines in a System of Private Medical Practice: (1) The facts and the questions they raise. (2) The functions of medicines in the doctor–patient relationship. (3) Psychological obsolescence and the outmoding of medicines. (4) The question of overconsumption of medicines.

I. MEASURING THE OUTPUT OF HEALTH ACTIVITIES[1]

(1) *Introduction*

It was tempting to give this paper a different title, like 'Social Indicators in Health Care', or 'On the Measurement of the Efficiency of Health Care Systems'. But this might have proved confusing at a conference where these subjects are treated in other papers under similar headings, but having naught else in common with the approach here adopted.

Yet the basic problem is the same. In the field of health, as in all other fields of economic and social life, it is one of the economist's tasks to 'allocate scarce resources to alternative uses', to quote a well-known phrase. To do so, he needs a composite indicator of results. Take the case, for instance, of how much resources to allocate to the fight against cancer and to providing the country with artificial kidney machines; nothing meaningful can be said about this without a common measure for aggregating the effects of these two different activities. Once such indicators are available, it remains to

[1] There is a translation problem. Another version is 'How to Find Indicators of the Results of Health Activities'.

assess the efficiency of the various possible activities which it is proposed to combine in proportions to be determined. The efficiency of an activity is defined, quite simply, as the level of performance achieved thereby as measured by the chosen indicator or indicators. The problem of allocating given resources between different activities so as to maximize total performance thus becomes a classical problem of programming. We know that, on certain assumptions (convexity, in particular), this problem can be decentralized at the level of individual activities by attaching a value to the indicator. If the latter, for example, is expressed in terms of the number of human lives saved, we arrive at the familiar concept of the 'value of human life' [1].

It follows that to construct indicators of results is the first thing economists, or planners generally speaking, must do prior to any attempt at rationalization. The idea which it is hoped to develop in this paper can be summarized as follows. The only result indicators habitually used in the field of health are based on mortality and morbidity rates, but while these certainly refer to manifest outputs of the health care system, they do not represent the whole of the aims actually pursued by the agents of that system. In other words, to work out a purportedly rational health care system on the basis of these indicators alone would be tantamount to imposing on it an extrinsic rationality. Would it not, in these circumstances, be better to try to discover the real aims consciously or unconsciously pursued by those who make up the health care system? Surely, it is with reference to these real aims that we should judge the performance of the system and define rational policies, and not with reference to indicators expressing no one's aims.

Most of the literature on the economics of health, whether explanatory or normative in intent, seems to take a highly technical view of medical treatment. Most frequently, we find two implicit assumptions. One is that none but 'technical' effects – a patient's life saved or prolonged, pain relief, improved physical comfort – can follow from health activities, the other that all health activities rest on technical decisions. If, for example, a doctor prescribes drugs for his patients, he is supposed to be guided solely by a technical consideration, namely, the effective achievement of desired technical effects. For the economist, this is obviously a convenient view, since it enables him to apply familiar lines of thought in the field of health care. But to regard a physician, or, more generally speaking, anyone who takes decisions which affect other people's health, as a mere technician suggests a disregarding of an important peculiarity of health care. Contrary to the assumptions of the classical consumption model, in the field of health the person who takes decisions is generally not the same as their beneficiary, and furthermore, under any kind of national health scheme, neither is the same as the person who foots the bill. The preferences of the final 'consumer', the patient, are supposed to be unaffected by the existence of the physician, inasmuch as the latter's sole aim is to apply his technical knowledge to the satisfaction of these preferences. But this view of the doctor–patient relationship seems to owe less to reality than to what psychoanalysts mean by rationalization, namely, the reasons by which an individual, when asked to explain his behaviour, spontaneously justifies it while concealing its true motivation. A mere glance at the psycho-sociological and sociological literature on the subject suggests that in health decisions the purely technical aspect is not the only relevant one, and that the doctor–patient relationship is actually much more complex. It will be shown below that the fact that the person who makes decisions and the person who benefits from them are not the same introduces a new and specific dimension into health problems, and that this alone offers the key to any real understanding of the rationale of behaviour in this field.

(2) *Health Expenditures Appear to Make Only a Slight Impact*
    on Overall Technical Health Indicators

The first reason which throws some doubt (but no more than that) on the assumption that the usual performance indicators – that is, crude mortality and morbidity rates – really do represent the sole aims of the health care system is that the results, as measured by these indicators, are very modest indeed [8].

Take, for instance, the effect of health activities on a crude mortality index like life expectancy. We all know that one of the aspects of health problems which causes concern in industrial countries is the feeling that there seems to be no relation between the rate of increase of resources spent on health care and progress made towards lengthening life expectancy or reducing the death rate.

In France, as in nearly all other industrial countries, medical consumption is increasing faster than most other consumption, even though the rates of increase differ for different components (in France, between 1950 and 1964, the quantitative annual increases per head were 12·4 per cent for medicines, and 6·0 per cent for medical services and hospitalization.

However, this growth of health expenditure is matched by a distinct deceleration of life expectancy gains. An average Frenchman born in 1825 could expect to live 39 years; the figure increased to 47 years in 1900 and to 71 years in 1966. In the countries most advanced in the health field, life expectancy lengthened on the average by four years every decade during the first half of the twentieth century, but during the 1950s the gain declined to one or two years in the leading countries, and since 1960 progress has been slower still [16]. The situation in France is typical in this respect. In forty years, from 1932 to the present day, life expectancy at birth rose from 55 to 68 years for men and from 60 to 75·5 years for women. Until 1960, life expectancy for both men and women increased regularly by some six months every year. Since 1960 the curve has been tending to level out, more markedly so for men than for women. The annual increase in life expectancy for women is now only one month, and for men the figure has been oscillating around 68 years since 1965. The fact of higher male mortality, incidentally, is common to all industrial countries, but seems more pronounced in France than elsewhere.

More precise figures can be found in the mortality tables by age and sex. They reveal striking differences during the last forty years in the decrease of death rates for different age groups: the decrease was very sharp for children, considerable for young people and adults, but less marked for the over-50s, especially men. It can be calculated that during these forty years the fall in infant mortality alone was responsible for 20 to 30 per cent of the rise in life expectancy at birth. At present, this same factor accounts for 33 per cent of female and for 50 per cent of male life expectancy gains.

Around the years 1955–60, the mortality table shows a clear break in mortality trends for all ages above 5. Until 1965, mortality rates fell very rapidly, but now they tend to level out or even to increase; for men between 15 and 24, for instance, the death rate is increasing by 2 per cent annually [4].

Disturbing as they are, these facts obviously do not justify the conclusion that medical expenditure is 'ineffective' in reducing mortality, if only because factors other than medical consumption affect mortality, and affect it adversely. Accidents, nutrition, smoking and the way of life in the broadest sense (including, in France, too much drinking) certainly are exercising mounting influence on health and human life in the rich countries. The pathological pattern, too, is changing under the growing impact of certain types of diseases, like chronic degenerative diseases (metabolic, vascular and respiratory), cancer, mental illness, not to speak of accidents and violent death. The common feature in this apparent diversity of diseases and causes of death is that they are all linked to a complex and interdependent set of factors, the so-called risk factors, which are correlative to the way of life in developed countries.

It would seem, then, that the attainment of a given mortality level requires more and more medical care in order to offset increasing incidental morbidity. If we want to push the analysis further, we must, therefore, explain mortality trends in terms of the separate parts attributable to medical consumption and to the environmental and way-of-life variables. Some studies have been made in this direction, mainly in the United States. The results provide presumptive evidence, inasmuch as, at the average level of the different variables in developed countries, mortality changes in time and space are influenced far more by environmental and way-of-life variables than by medical consumption as such, which seems to make little difference [17]. In France, for instance, a recent study by Lebart showed that departmental differences in mortality rates can be explained for the most part by alcoholism. Once this effect is eliminated, we are left with a very weak negative correlation between mortality and expenditure on medical care [14]. For the United States, a study by Auster, Leveson and Sarachek [2] shows a distinctly adverse effect of the income variable, which, at high values, is assumed to express an unhealthy way of life – a diet that is too rich, cars that are too fast, sedentary and harassing jobs, etc. But there is no need to dwell on this point here, since it is dealt with in the very interesting paper that Professor Fuchs has prepared for this Conference [10].

However, the slight impact of health activities as an indicator of the quantity of life will come as no surprise to those who regard it as the primary task of modern medicine to secure for people a certain 'quality of life'. Just because of the prevailing new pathological pattern, medical activities should in any case have much more sophisticated effects than merely to prolong life expectancy, to wit, they should help patients to live with a minimum of discomfort. Along the same line of thought, it can be argued that doctors will tend to minister not only to the sick, but to the healthy as well (e.g. tranquillizers or aesthetic surgery). What we need for the future, the argument continues, is to establish criteria based on morbidity and on the concept of the 'quality of life', however little statistical information there may be at present to work with.

This certainly seems a very useful approach, provided two conditions are met. Firstly, due allowance must be made for the fact that, unlike mortality, the 'quality of life' cannot so simply be defined in terms of physical characteristics, but that psycho-sociological factors play an important part in it, as we shall see presently. Secondly, this last observation must not be allowed to serve as an excuse for shelving the problem of the measurement of the efficiency of medical care.

Admittedly, morbidity statistics are at present still altogether inadequate, since morbidity to a large extent defies observation. If an individual is ill without realizing it or without seeking help from the medical system, his ailment remains unknown and is not recorded statistically. Morbidity can be observed only it it finds expression in the consumption of medical care. Even then it may be statistically elusive, mainly because the production and distribution centres of medical care are so dispersed – at least in France.

However, this is not the chief obstacle for an economist in charge of allocating scarce resources. To this end he needs overall indicators, as we have seen. Even with perfect factual knowledge of morbidity, he still would have to define a common measure, or at least a common scale, for all types of morbidity.

Such few indicators as have been proposed so far do not seem satisfactory. There is an American suggestion, for example, to use an overall health indicator called 'healthy life expectancy', which is total life expectancy less time spent bedridden or in hospital. But this indicator takes no account of the seriousness of the illness (greater or smaller risk of death), of the degree of disability, of the extent to which the trouble is chronic or otherwise, or of the degree of suffering and hence gives no clue to the value of medical care the sole effect of which is, for example, to improve the patient's comfort.

More recent studies go further in this direction, e.g. some of the reports prepared for this Conference [15, 21]. The fact remains that the hypothesis that the primary aim of health activities in highly industrialized countries is to improve the quality of life is, for the time being, neither proved nor disproved. We simply do not have the necessary data, nor, what is more important, any usable conceptual tools.

In any event, my own view, as stated in the introduction, is that, while it is certainly necessary and useful to try and work out an overall technical health indicator based on mortality and morbidity, such research is nevertheless insufficient in that it neglects a major part of reality, as we shall see in the following section. This neglect, incidentally, may well be the cause of the difficulties encountered.

(3) *Logical Symptoms Other than the Maximization of an Overall Technical Health Indicator*

Let us assume that it has proved possible to work out an indicator of a population's state of health, and that that indicator takes account of the quantity of life and of morbidity, including the physical comfort of patients. At once, we are led to suspect that a health policy designed to achieve, with given resources, maximum performance in terms of such an indicator would be very different from what is actually done now.

To prove the point, the rationale of medical decisions may usefully be compared with the repair and maintenance decisions which would be appropriate if it were a matter of using given resources for obtaining maximum performance from a set of industrial machinery (that is, raising to its highest value an indicator integrating in the machines' life-span the quality of their performance at each moment according to their 'state of health'). We sense intuitively that these two types of resource management have little in common.

This, no doubt, is why a French economist and humanist, Bertrand de Jouvenel, said that 'Whereas an economically rational approach would cause priority to be given to the care of persons whose health can be most improved, a social spirit demands that the most seriously ill should be looked after first' [17]. Without claiming that health decisions entirely obey this 'social spirit', it may be assumed that they are influenced by it and come somewhere between the dictates of economic rationality and those of the social spirit. The demands of the latter, as will readily be appreciated, are contrary to management geared to the maximization of any overall indicator of technical performance.

To return to our example of industrial machinery, it can be shown that there exists an age limit beyond which it is preferable to reduce, or indeed stop, all maintenance and not to repair any breakdown. The resources so saved are more efficiently employed in additional maintenance and more thorough repair during the early years. In more general terms, before any decision is taken regarding the extent of repairs when a machine breaks down, one should ask oneself what will probably happen once the damage is repaired; the decision will depend on how much risk there is that the machine will break down again in the future. Clearly, this type of resource management would universally be considered inadmissible with reference to human health. Nobody would ever be in favour of stopping all care to old people above a certain age. Nobody would ever question the legitimacy of care for the dying. No doctor would ever ask himself whether or not to treat a young man of 20 for bronchial pneumonia, just because at that age there is a high risk of dying in a motor accident. The doctor knows only too well that death is stronger than he, and that one illness is followed by another; nevertheless, he will go on treating each illness as it occurs, and society would not wish it to be otherwise.

A good many other decisions and types of behaviour may well appear inconsistent or irrational to an economist intent on maximizing an indicator of technical performance. Compare, for instance, what I shall call 'immediate or primary' health situations and those 'at one stage removed'.[1] In the first case decisions affecting an individual's health are taken by himself with respect to various aspects of his life (his different consumptions, his choice of career, the

---

[1] Again there is a translation problem. The author refers to 'Health situations in the first, in the second and in the third person . . .'; I (the editor) believe that the expression in the text conveys what the author means.

employment of his leisure, etc.). Persons who are well informed about the health consequences of their choices try to reconcile the conflicting claims of their health and those of other satisfactions, and health is not always the winner (in economic terms: the preordering of preferences is not necessarily lexicographically in favour of health, and there is a finite marginal rate of substitution between the weight assigned to health and to other satisfactions). A person may, for instance, deliberately choose an occupation he knows to be trying for his nerves, but which carries prestige, or he may take risks which give him social status, etc. Achilles, remember, prefered a brief life of glory to a long and unworthy one. Now, if such an individual should find himself in the situation of a patient in relation to the medical system, in other words, if his health becomes someone else's responsibility (we call this a 'health situation at one stage removed'), we find a very different type of behaviour dictated by very different preferences. Lay literature and economic research agree that in such a case health becomes the overridingly important commodity, that 'health has no price' (in other words, health comes first in the order of preferences). Medical consumption does in fact seem to be barely influenced by classical economic variables such as price, income (except at very low income levels) or the degree of social protection [18]. Neither the patient, nor the doctor, nor anyone else would wish less than the utmost to be done to restore the patient's health: if it is technically possible to do so, it must be done whatever the cost.

An economist comparing these two types of situations may well be tempted to bewail the inconsistency of human behaviour and will be reminded of other inconsistencies: the environment is polluted and then has to be cleaned up, holes are dug only to be filled in again, etc.

Yet other things look 'irrational' when one compares health situations at one stage removed with those at two stages removed. The former, it will be recalled, are situations involving a personal relationship between a person (or persons) performing a health activity and the person (or persons) benefiting from it, which implies that both are identified. By a health situation at two stages removed, we mean one where no such relationship exists, because one or both of the pair, decision-maker and beneficiary, are unidentified. Cases in point are preventive action aimed at a statistical population (like, in the case of road safety, getting rid of a black traffic spot), or the effects of better public hygiene on the health of the population, etc. There is obviously no strict line of demarcation between situations of these two types. They overlap. Take, for instance, progress in the fight against cancer, Here we have on the one side a group of research workers hard to identify, and on the other side a statistical population of potential cancer victims; this is very close to a health situation at one remove, in so far as it represents a clearly understood message of comfort from society to itself. Inversely, progress in so-called predictive medicine will increasingly lead doctors to attend to individuals who are not really ill, but who, in the light of some of their physical characteristics (such as weight, height, age, sex, blood pressure, cholesterol level, smoker or non-smoker, etc.) run a calculable risk of falling victim to predictable diseases within a predictable period. This is obviously an intermediary situation between one involving an identified victim of a disease and one involving a statistical population. Health situations at one remove and at two removes are merely the two extreme cases of a whole series of situations along a scale of intensity of personal relations between decision-maker and beneficiary of the decision.

So much for definitions. Now, if the aim is to maximize an indicator of 'technical' performance, health situations at one stage removed would seem to be far too greatly favoured compared with those at two stages removed. In the first case, as we have seen, everything happens as though 'health had no price'. With respect to the second, the economists who invented the concept of value of human life have shown that, whether we like it or not, any given preventive action does involve rejected (unaccepted) expenses – which means an implicit decision not to save certain (statistical) lives. Human life and health do, after all, have a finite price (just as in immediate or primary health situations), and this is responsible for an apparent distortion as between health situations at one stage and at two stages removed.[1] Take the example of safety and of the number of lives that could be saved if part of the resources devoted to the safety of astronauts or to rescuing a climber trapped on a cliff were allocated to the prevention of traffic accidents. The same sort of reasoning applies to health. Morbidity in economically developed countries can be attacked in three different ways: by curative medical intervention, generally at a late stage in an ailment's development process, when acute symptoms or complications occur; or by preventive intervention at the stage of a medical check-up; or by direct action on the risk factors. Some experts think that this last method is much the most effective with reference to a purely technical objective. It certainly would require the organization of health policy to be thoroughly overhauled, and would, for example, involve joint policies in several fields now largely outside the scope of existing health systems, as well as the training of dual-purpose experts who are half doctors and half town-planners. Yet this method is neglected at present to the benefit of preventive

---

[1] In the sense that the marginal (not the average) cost of saving a life is very different in the two situations – very high in the first ('health has no price') and medium in the second.

and, even more so, of curative medicine. It looks like another case of the same type of distortions.

Yet another circumstance is bound to appear irrational to our economist. This is that in different health situations at two stages removed, very different values are implicitly assigned to the technical performance indicator (say, a human life saved). Any transfer of resources from one sector to another should, therefore, at given resources, improve the overall performance of the indicator concerned. Relevant calculations have been made in France, though not in the field of health itself (where calculations are complicated by the fact that the effects of most preventive action are not confined to mortality, so that there is no simple choice between cost and years of life), but in the field of safety. These calculations have led to rather startling estimates: 'Everything happens in France at the moment as though a human life were worth, respectively, $30,000 in a road accident, $100,000 in an accident at work in large public company, and $800,000 in an air crash' [19].

(4) *The Implicit Rationality of Health Activities and their Non-technical Outputs*

'Inconsistent behaviour, irrational decisions'! A little humility would befit the economist, as was suggested in the introduction. Before passing judgment, he would do well to try and understand and explain the behaviour and the decisions concerned. He might find some implicit rationality hidden in them.

Actually, there is an implicit rationality and it can be perceived easily enough if we look for what is common to all the cases mentioned above in which, at given resources, a transfer of resources would result in better performance than we have at present, in terms of a crude mortality–morbidity indicator. Any such transfer would lead to the replacement of a certain number of current health activities by others more effective with reference to the indicator, but of weaker psychological impact. Consider, for example, care for a dying person. This care which can be very expensive, does have technical effects, that is, effects on the mortality and morbidity indicators. But these effects may be minute: the person concerned may live a few days longer, and suffer a little less. Undoubtedly, these expenses, which society fully approves whether or not their technical effects are at all appreciable, play another role as well: they demonstrate to the dying, and even more perhaps to his family and friends, not to speak of the doctor himself, that everything possible is being done for the patient and that he is not alone in his last ordeal. Similar considerations apply to the care for the very sick: the more seriously ill they are, the more the very act of caring for them is reassuring and clear evidence that medicine concerns itself not only with people easy to cure.

Generally speaking, it can be argued that any health activity (and, more broadly, any activity concerned with the safety and preservation of human life) has, simultaneously,[1] technical and non-technical effects. The technical effects are so called because they are directly connected with the physical and technical properties of the means employed, and they consist in a prolongation of life, relief of pain and improvement of the patient's physical comfort. The non-technical effects, on the other hand, are not directly connected with the physical properties of the means employed, but rather with their psychological property of signifying something. Their significance may vary; at the level of generality of this discussion, we have to distinguish two dimensions.[2] Health activities may have, firstly, a reassuring effect by signifying the retreat of illness and death, and secondly, an emotional effect (felt by the doctor, the patient and others) by signifying that the doctor takes responsibility for the patient [12]. There would, of course, be no point in distinguishing technical and non-technical effects if they were proportional, that is, if the patient's sense of security and his feeling of the doctor's taking personal responsibility for him were commensurate with the technical efficiency of the means employed. But this is not so. Health activities may well be equivalent in their technical effects and yet have very different significative powers, or non-technical effects.

Let us consider, for example, the sense of security. Psychologists know very well that situations of equal objective insecurity may be lived through in very different ways, and may generate very different feelings of insecurity and anxiety (e.g. fear when travelling in a car or an aircraft). In the field of health, the sense of insecurity experienced in the face of some symptom of illness may have very little to do with the latter's real gravity. Sociological surveys have shown that some people considered seriously ill from the point of view of medical science remained quite unconcerned, and that others were deeply worried by the most benign symptoms [11], which they regarded as the revealing signs of some constitutional weakness and as a foreboding of the inescapable approach of death. Psycho-sociological factors amplify subjective insecurity to a greater or lesser extent. One of the principal of these factors is attention to the body. This is known to vary considerably according to social categories. The limit beyond which an individual feels his physical condition to be impaired ranges from a cut finger in the case of a coal miner to dental

---

[1] In economics, we would speak of joint outputs.
[2] In the second part of this paper, on the consumption of medicines, these notions will be discussed in more detail.

caries in the case of a young lady. Medical attendance itself seems to increase the attention paid to the body. As Boltanski, a French sociologist, writes: 'The practice of consulting doctors increases the number of known diseases, that is, diseases named and established as such; it also enables morbid symptoms to be classified more accurately and hence causes people to perceive them more readily and to pay more attention to them. The end effect is to raise the subjective chances of illness and, *ipso facto*, medical consumption' [3].

Because the state of health and the degree of anxiety felt are relatively independent of each other, actions with equivalent effects on technical indicators may have very different reassuring effects. Publicity devoted to spearhead advances in medicine (heart transplants, cancer research, etc.) is a good deal more reassuring than the construction of sewers. The same applies to the prescription of drugs as compared with advice regarding the general way of life. It is even possible for a positive effect on a technical health indicator to be associated with an alarming psychological effect. A case in point is a system of compulsory medical screening for the early detection of certain diseases, which 'inevitably has the result of lowering the tolerance level for morbid sensations by creating a new, more reflexive and apprehensive attitude to the body' [3]. The opposite is equally true: to smoke, drink, take drugs or eat too much may be means of making people feel more secure and of fighting off anxiety at the price of impairing the health [12].

Let us now consider the other non-technical output of medical activities, which is connected with the quality of the relationship between the person who makes a decision and its beneficiary, and concerns primarily the latter, but also the former as well as third persons. Here again, equivalent technical outputs may be associated with emotional outputs of widely differing effect. It is certainly more gratifying for the doctor if he can bring a baby back to life in the maternity ward, and will give the mother a much stronger impression that 'something is being done for her', than if he simply attends to prenatal check-ups of expectant mothers. With reference to our definition of health situations, there is a general presumption that the emotional output will be much larger in situations at one stage removed than in those at two stages removed or immediate or primary ones.

The non-proportionality of the technical and non-technical effects of health activities creates a situation of conflict between these effects, in the sense that a non-zero weight attached to one type of effect causes at given resources, part of the performance achieved by the other type of effect to be sacrificed. This conflict would appear in an entirely different light if activities having technical effects were distinct from those having non-technical ones, for then there would be conflict only at the level of the distribution of total resources between the technical and the non-technical sector. To be sure, there exist means specifically applied for non-technical effects and devoid of any direct[1] technical effect; examples are a doctor's bedside manner, the kindness of what he says or the attention with which he listens to what the patient has to say (none of these are free, since they use up that very scarce resource which is the doctor's time). But generally speaking, as we have seen, most medical activities exercise simultaneously both technical effects and, thanks to their significative property, non-technical effects.

At this point we begin to discern a certain internal rationality in medical activities, a certain consistency at least in qualitative terms. Everything comes to pass as if a deliberate balance were struck between the weight assigned, respectively, to non-technical and to technical effects, the former being undoubtedly those which play a central part in the definition of what we called earlier the 'quality of life', the 'comfort' of the patient as well as of the doctor and third persons. If we look again, one by one, at all the activities which we have mentioned and which in the light of short-term economic rationality might appear 'unprofitable', we realize that while these activities certainly have mediocre technical effects, their significative effects are outstandingly strong, and stronger at any rate than those of such other activities as would have to be substituted according to the criterion of technical efficiency. Examples are the care given to those who are seriously ill as against those who can recover easily; treatment of actual disease as against disease existing only in probability; action concerned with identified individuals as against a statistical population; and action in fields where the sense of insecurity is strong as against those where it is weak. Everything in effect happens as though the members of society were assessing the value of the performance achieved by non-technical outputs. We may conclude that even though, at present, the technical marginal efficiency of health activities varies greatly in different cases, there does exist, at least in qualitative terms, a tendency towards equalization of their social marginal efficiency, including non-technical outputs.

Let us return to the apparent inconsistency that in health situations at one stage removed, everything happens as if 'health had no price', whereas it clearly does have a price in all other situations. We now see that this social norm is not the expression of a lexicographic order

---

[1] The word 'direct' must be stressed, because actually psychic and somatic factors are so closely interwoven (witness, e.g., the placebo effect) that good performance in non-technical outputs may in itself generate a positive technical effect.

of preferences between health (in the physical sense of the word) and other satisfactions, in which health comes first, but has to do with the type of performance obtainable by the use of technical means for emotional outputs – in plain words, the quality of the doctor–patient relationship. Take, for instance, a simple case where the significative power of the means employed (the significance being that the doctor assumes responsibility for the patient) is linked to their technical efficiency,[1] which we call x. Designating by the variable X_1 the performance obtained with respect to the state of health in the technical sense of the word (mortality–morbidity indicator), we can write

$$X_1 = X_1(x), \frac{dX_1}{dx} > 0. \tag{1}$$

The relation between x and X_2, X_2 being a variable representing the performance obtained in terms of emotional output, the quality of the doctor–patient relationship, is very different. In this case, x acts as a sign, and the performance on X_2 depends not on the absolute value of this sign but on its relative place in a scale of signs. We have to do not so much with efficiency as with the greatest possible efficiency. In other words, what counts is the gap between what the doctor could do and what he actually does. Let us designate by $\bar{x}$ the maximum efficiency possible at a given state of technology and with a given supply of equipment. We can write

$$X_2 = X_2(x, \bar{x}), \frac{\partial X_2}{\partial x} > 0$$

$$\frac{\partial X_2}{\partial \bar{x}} < 0. \tag{2}$$

This is what is really meant by the norm 'health has no price'. This norm does not purport to establish a lexicographic order of preferences between X_1 and other satisfactions; it does mean that when a doctor takes decisions regarding a patient, decisions which can always be considered as the use of existing techniques and equipment (giving the word 'equipment' a very broad sense, including, e.g., the number of doctors, their training, etc.), any failure on the doctor's part to make the utmost use of existing means would incur strong censure (bad performance X_2) as unwillingness to assist a person in danger. But it must be added that in any event the doctor's

[1] This is in fact a simple case, for in reality the significative characteristics of the means employed may be quite different, e.g. their novelty, their cost, etc. (see the discussion of the consumption of medicines in the second part of this paper).

action is conditioned and limited by prior choices regarding techniques and equipment, $\bar{x}$. Necessarily,

$$x \leq \bar{x}. \tag{3}$$

Choices regarding $\bar{x}$ may be made by conscious decision or not, but they are certainly made, and they are different in nature from decisions concerning the use of means. Unlike the latter, they are concerned not with flesh-and-blood patients, but with statistical populations.[1] They are choices in a health situation at two stages removed, where health has a price. In other words, the level of $\bar{x}$ results from weighing the cost of $\bar{x}$, $c(\bar{x})$, against the value of $pX_1(\bar{x})$ of the technical benefit associated with $\bar{x}$.

In concluding this section, let us return for a moment to our starting-point, namely, the observation that health expenditure seems to have precious little influence on crude technical indicators of the state of health. Small wonder, we can now say, for this is not the result which, implicitly, is desired. We may add that, paradoxically, a health policy which, at given resources, carried out such transfers of resources as are necessary to improve performance in terms of an overall health indicator would be regarded as much less reassuring, and hence less efficient, than present policy, even though on the average people would live longer and would be afflicted by less disease.

(5) *From Technical and Non-technical Outputs to a Rational Health Policy*

Now that we have uncovered the implicit rationality underlying behaviour and decisions in the field of health, can we affirm that all is for the best in the best of all possible worlds? Or on the contrary, must this rationality be judged to be ... 'irrational'? It is time to switch from a strictly explanatory to a more normative point of view.

To begin with, there is a temptation to be resisted. It would be wrong to think that only the technical output of health activities should be taken into account, and that, consequently, there is a case for any transfer of resources likely to improve performance with reference to these indicators alone. In any event, advocates of such a policy would stand little chance of seeing it put into effect, given what we have seen above. But we may ask in the name of what principles

[1] However, there are cases where the choice of safety or health equipment is made in conditions similar to those of the choice of the level of its use when there is an accident. In the case of astronauts, for instance, their safety equipment is designed for a very small and well-identified population. The whole range of intermediary cases is obviously possible.

and what ethic we should be required to assume that people's sense of security and freedom from anxiety, and good personal relations, have no weight at all in comparison with their state of health in the physical sense, whereas individuals themselves patently do attach importance to these factors of their well-being and show it by their behaviour. Such a view would, in plain words, be altogether technocratic. We reject it, and in what follows shall take it for granted that any health policy must be judged by its impact on all outputs, technical and non-technical alike.

A more constructive approach is possible. One suggestion is that the non-proportionality of the technical and non-technical effects of health activities is at the root of this problem of choice, and if such be the case, it is because of distortions which make things appear different from what they really are. It might be useful, then, to try and reduce these distortions and make the non-technical effects of health activities match their technical effects. It is perfectly possible that people are simply misinformed about the real efficiency of various health activities. On the one hand, for example, the press makes much of certain spearhead medical techniques, and this publicity gives people a wrong impression of the real possibilities of curative medicine. On the other hand, there is a deplorable lack of information and studies concerning the impact of the environment and of people's way of life on their health. It is suggested that such distortions might be straightened out by health information campaigns, or, better, by real health instruction for the population at large. And it might be well, too, to take a hard new look at certain power relationships, with particular reference to the power which doctors, such as we know them at present, wield in all matters concerned with health.

Measures along these lines would certainly do much to lessen the conflict between the technical and the non-technical outputs of health activities and thus, at given resources, make it possible to obtain improved performance from the first without detriment to the performance of the second. But there is no hope of removing the conflict completely, for at least two reasons.

The first reason is that, leaving aside the time it would take so to refashion individual attitudes, they could bever be changed radically enough. The psychological impact of bringing a new-born baby back to life, to return to our earlier example, would always remain bigger than that of new regulations increasing the number of prenatal check-ups. In other words, when the difference in the non-technical effects of two activities with equivalent technical effects is connected with a purely physical factor, such as whether the decision-maker and the beneficiary (or beneficiaries) of the decision are, or are not, identified individuals and in each other's presence, then this difference simply cannot be reduced to zero [13]. Do what you will, an optimal policy taking account of all the technical and non-technical outputs of health activities will never resemble the management of a set of industrial machinery.

The second reason is that, even though the non-technical effects are linked with technical ones, it still remains a fact that the relational output X_2 is influenced not by the absolute value of technical efficiency, x, but, as we have seen, by the relative value of x with respect to $\bar{x}$. Choices regarding $\bar{x}$, which are those of prime interest to health planners, thus appear in a very different light according as performance is assessed in terms of X_1 alone, or in terms of X_1 and X_2. Any increase in $\bar{x}$ has nothing but advantages so far as X_1 is concerned, since a higher $\bar{x}$ makes room for higher values of $x \leq \bar{x}$. But to increase $\bar{x}$ has, to some extent, adverse effects of X_2, because the impact of any given x on X_2 diminishes when $\bar{x}$ rises (because of the inequality $\partial X_2/\partial \bar{x} < 0$. This is a psychological cost which is associated with any technical innovation in the medical field, and corresponds to the frustration felt by all the people who cannot benefit from this innovation. Here we have another irreducible source of conflict between technical and non-technical effects.

Let us imagine that appropriate measures have been taken in order to minimize the conflict between technical and non-technical effects. Nevertheless, there will still be some conflict. The problem then is to compare the equilibrium state of the health system with an optimal state, the optimum being defined with reference to the whole set of outputs, both technical and non-technical. We can provide an at least qualitative answer on the evidence of the inequality $\partial X_2/\partial \bar{x} < 0$. This psychological cost, which we shall call the 'psychological obsolescence' of the technical qualities x, may formally be characterized as an externality of psycho-sociological nature, since any decision to vary $\bar{x}$ entails a change in the social utility of a given x. Such a decision therefore also alters the choices based on any x, without, of course, any deal being actually struck. There is clear evidence of an interdependence between two decision levels, x decisions and $\bar{x}$ decisions. It is hardly surprising, therefore, that the equilibrium position can be shown to be distorted with respect to the optimal position. More precisely, at the equilibrium position too many resources are allocated to research and development for new techniques, and not enough to the broader application of existing ones [7]. It follows that, in theory, there is a case for action designed to bring the present situation closer to an optimal situation. The same considerations suggest an explanation for the growth of health expenditure much more satisfactory than those usually advanced at present, which all take account only of technical factors [8]. We shall not dwell on these points here, but refer the reader to the theoretical works quoted as well as to the second part of this paper, which deals with the consumption of medicines.

But our final arguments also suggest another way of improving the present situation, that is, of using given resources to enhance the performance of certain outputs without detriment to that of the others. It follows from what has been said (and this will be seen more clearly in the case of medicines) that to bring technical means to bear on problems of human relations leads to bad performance in terms both of technical and of non-technical outputs (the equilibrium is not optimal). We may ask whether it would not be better to devise specific means for dealing with problems of reassurance and personal relations, and reserve technical means for technical purposes. Such an approach would certainly do much to clarify the situation, but it would equally certainly run counter to strong tendencies in industrial societies, where people regard technical progress as the answer to all their problems, though most of these problems have to do likewise with human relationships or with the anxieties of living. We shall discuss this question in more precise terms in connection with the consumption of medicines.

II. THE CONSUMPTION OF MEDICINES IN A SYSTEM OF PRIVATE MEDICAL PRACTICE

So far, the discussion has kept to a very general level and may have appeared somewhat abstract. It will now be illustrated by an analysis of a specific case, namely, the consumption of medicines in a system of private medical practice (which, in France, means that the patient freely chooses his doctor and on a fee-for-service basis). This is a subject on which an interdisciplinary study was carried out under the auspices of the Centre de Recherche sur le Bieu-être (CEREBE) in Paris (9). The research team, which included economists, psycho-sociologists and sociologists, based its findings on a wide-ranging bibliographical analysis as well as on field observations. Using non-directive techniques, the team interviewed some hundred physicians, patients and executives of pharmaceutical firms, and also observed cases of doctor–patient relationships. The principal results of this study are briefly summarized below.[1]

(1) *The Facts and the Questions They Raise*
It has been argued in the first part of this paper that any attempt at rationalizing a social system should be preceded by an effort to

[1] The text which follows is a summary of an article published in May 1973 in the review *Projet* [5].

understand how it works. In the matter of the consumption of medicines, value judgments are often passed on the basis of a very summary and unsatisfactory analysis of the relevant facts. One of these facts is that drug consumption displays one of the fastest growth rates in the whole health care field (in France, its annual growth in the long period is about 16 to 17 per cent, at current prices); this growth is currently justified, if not explained, on the basis of purely technical considerations, whereas precisely known facts suggest that other factors are involved as well.

There is no gainsaying that the pharmaceutical industry produces a rich harvest of innovations, witness a growth rate of 16 to 17 per cent in the consumption of its products. This growth rate may be considered as the sum of several other growth rates, concerning respectively (1) the number of entries into the medical system (consultations and visits): +6 to 7 per cent annually, not to be discussed further here; (2) the number of products per prescription, of which little is known but which is probably close to zero; (3) the average price of medicines prescribed and purchased in the unit period: probably as high as 10 per cent annually, and thus accounting for more than half the rate of growth of expenditure on drugs. In its turn, the high rate of increase in the price of drugs has two causes: (*a*) Every new drug is more expensive than the one it replaces. This has invariably been so in the past and continues to be so, because a higher price is authorized, if indeed not provoked, by a certain number of institutional factors, such as price control (a fixed price for old products and a range of prices for new ones), or the conditions of eligibility for reimbursement by the social security system. (*b*) The renewal rate of the pharmacopoeia is extremely rapid. Products emerge, replace others which disappear from the market, and after an average life of ten years are in their turn driven out by new products; of the medicines now on the market, 70 per cent are less than fifteen years old, and almost half of the industry's turnover is attributable to products less than five years old.

Innovation, therefore, is an essential factor in the growth of expenditure on drugs. But does innovation necessarily mean technical progress? To begin with, not every 'novelty' is *a priori* as good as another, for the term covers a multitude of very different things. Novelty can mean a genuine scientific discovery which enriches therapeutics by a new class of active molecules, or it can mean an existing drug in altered dosage, form or packaging, or with new instructions for use, and indeed it can mean merely a change of name. Something like 250 new pharmaceutical products are launched on the market every year and replace cheaper ones; it certainly looks as though the overwhelming majority of them must be placed on the lowest rungs of the scale of innovation. The point can be proved by American figures, there being reason to think that the French situation is very similar. Between 1948 and 1966, 7,563 articles were launched on the market in the United States (which means, on average, 420 each year); of the total, 1,785 were new pharmaceutical forms of existing products, and 5,778 were new products. The latter consisted of 676 new therapeutic substances, 3,757 combinations of known substances, and 1,345 products launched by a new manufacturer but identical with products already on the market. As regards the 676 new substances, more than half of them were merely new salts or derivatives of some already known molecule. In all, less than 5 per cent of new drugs launched in the United States during the eighteen years in question can rightly be described as genuine major innovations.

These figures will come as no surprise to anyone who knows what sort of research the manufacturers pursue. Most often it is ultra-empirical research, which consists in synthesizing the greatest possible number of molecules and testing them systematically for their activity. This is a lengthy and very complicated process, and also a very expensive one. As Professor J. M. Pelt says: 'Failing any guideline, chemists and pharmacologists proceed by systematic testing of thousands of molecules, like a locksmith devoting all his efforts to making thousands of keys, each better than the one before, in the hope of opening a lock he does not know. The more complicated the lock, the less are his chances of stumbling by accident upon the right key. One ends up by wondering whether it would not be better to dismantle the lock and then make a key that fits' [20]. And in effect, this kind of haphazard, costly and uncoordinated research is the very opposite of genuine fundamental research, which would start out with the 'biochemical lesion' at the bottom of an illness and then try to find ways of treating it.

In any case, there is reason to think that innovation is really a constraint which pharmaceutical manufacturers impose upon each other, rather than a freely chosen aim which furthers their interests. Every manufacturer knows from experience that if he does not bring out novelties, his products will be driven from the market by his competitors' new products. Every one of them is thus forced to innovate and to go in for the kind of research described above, which certainly has the merit of encouraging innovation, though perhaps of doubtful quality, but does so at the cost of making shockingly poor use of the brainpower at hand. In short, it seems that in the present state of the pharmaceutical industry each single manufacturer acts according to his own best interest, given the behaviour of all the others, but that it would be in the best interest of all manufacturers to break out of this situation and adopt other arrangements better for every one of them, not to mention the interests of pharmaceutical research, public health and the social security system. Economists are familiar with this kind of situation of non-optimal equilibrium. The problem is to discover what type of interdependence is responsible for the gap between equilibrium and optimum.

The facts described above are not open to doubt. But how can they be explained? Why is it that these new products, so many of which apparently merely duplicate existing ones, are commercially so successful as to lead to such a situation? The answer no doubt lies in the market, which in this case is rather peculiar in that it consists of all the doctor–patient pairs. Two opposing kinds of explanation are often put forward. One of them, which, needless to say, is the one upheld by the pharmaceutical industry, is that in the light of the most recent biochemical theories, even the slightest change in an existing molecule may have therapeutical implications. It is, of course, true that in matters, say, of metabolism or sensitivity to a foreign body, individual reactions vary very greatly; hence, it is argued, a great many similar products need to be available so that doctors can adapt the treatment to each individual case. The weakness of this argument is to suppose that doctors are expert enough, and sufficiently competent and immune from non-technical considerations, to be able to make such fine distinctions regarding the pharmacodynamic activity of the drugs they prescribe. As will be seen presently, such an interpretation is invalidated by the facts.

Detractors of the pharmaceutical industry suggest an altogether different explanation. Manufacturers, they suggest, can do what they like with doctors; they swamp them with a flood of publicity material, and make them take all this sales talk about doubtful innovations for pure gold. But doctors are not puppets any more than they are omniscient experts. It can be shown that the success of new drugs can in fact be ascribed to their having considerable social utility for patients and doctors alike. But it is not 'technical' utility in the sense of deriving from the drugs' pharmacodynamic activity; rather, it has to do with the significative function of medicines in the doctor–patient relationship. And this links up with the considerations developed in the first part of this paper.

(2) *The Functions of Medicines in the Doctor–Patient Relationship*
Whatever afflicts patients, whether they have had a road accident or suffer from high blood pressure, have cancer or are neurotic, they turn to a doctor in the hope that he will relieve their pain and cure them, which is a technical problem; but they also want help in their state of anxiety. This need for help derives from the patients' feeling

of insecurity, which, as we have seen, is up to a point independent of the real gravity of the disease concerned. A patient expects from the doctor an attitude and a manner which make it quite plain that he takes genuine responsibility for the case. Depending on their social standing, patients may expect mutual trust and understanding, or fatherly devotion, but in any case a technical, detached attitude is not welcome. However, these expectations are highly ambivalent, since they are likewise concerned with outstanding technical competence.

Patients never tell the doctor in so many words that they need this kind of help. Two kinds of repressive factor come into play. One is the defence mechanisms by which an individual safeguards the unity of his ego by putting the blame on the body and, with it, on the exogenous character of the illness. The second has to do with social conformism. Society, and above all its physicians, certainly takes an extremely narrow view of disease and accepts it as such only if it shows every sign of being a mere temporary deviation independent of the sufferer's will.

When people want help from a doctor, therefore, they express their need in purely somatic terms (or, at best, if they belong to the higher socio-cultural classes, in terms of physical treatment of psychical disabilities). Doctor and patient can then agree that things must be put right. But it must be realized that the technical means which the doctor can bring to bear on the satisfaction of the patient's needs have two functions: they should solve the technical problem involved in the patient's illness, but also should in roundabout ways respond to his need for help by making it plain that the doctor is taking charge.

Among these technical means, the prescription of drugs has the immense advantage of making very little claim on the doctor, psychologically and in terms of his time. One of the essential roles of medicines in the doctor–patient relationship is that they are a sign of the doctor's attention. This is a very widespread phenomenon in our society, and can be observed in all cases when one person takes a consumption decision on behalf of others. An example which at once comes to mind is a mother's decision of what to buy for her children by way of clothes, food, toys, etc. However much the popular saying may assert that a gift itself counts less than the spirit in which it is given, the fact remains that what one gives bears direct witness to the attention one devotes to the recipient. A gift having a social or economic value too remote from what one might normally expect in the light of the resources and means of the donor will meet with disfavour. This sign of attention to others may, incidentally, be addressed as much, if not more, to oneself than to the beneficiary concerned; this is certainly true of a mother's decisions concerning her baby, which is quite incapable of appreciating these decisions in terms of the social values which make up society's image of a good mother. Much the same applies to medicines. It certainly is the doctor's bedside manner, his listening to the patient and giving of himself – in short, the judicious administration of what is sometimes called the 'doctor treatment' – which demonstrates medical comprehension so far as the patient is concerned; but given that the issue is confused by the two parties' underlying agreement on technical means, this demonstration would signify little if it were not materially buttressed by the 'gift' of a prescription. To some extent a prescription means for the doctor himself that he is doing his best for the patient. By prescribing such drugs as he judges to be the most effective, the physician proves to himself that he is sparing no effort on behalf of his patient's health, and thus enables himself to forget that, so far as his personal contribution is concerned, and more particularly his time, he certainly does attribute a finite value to other people's health.

If a patient is to feel that his doctor is taking genuine and full responsibility for his case, evidence of comprehension is not enough. The patient must also have confidence in the doctor's ability to take over technical responsibility as well, that is, in his technical competence. But this, in many cases, seems to be somewhat uncertain, or at least is felt by the doctor to be so. Perhaps the reason is that so many people nowadays require treatment for ill-defined diseases with vague and volatile symptoms, or perhaps it is that medical practice is changing as a result of the introduction of drug treatments whose effects are described in terms of easily observable symptoms and clinical signs, so that physicians themselves need not proceed to an etiological diagnosis. This question need not be discussed here. What is certain is that general practitioners themselves state that a large proportion (between 60 and 90 per cent) of the patients they see suffer from what doctors call psychosomatic or functional disorders. What do doctors mean by these terms? Surely not that these patients are malingerers, that there is nothing organically wrong with them, for every doctor can cite cases of a tumor he eventually diagnosed in a patient long regarded as a 'purely functional case'. No, doctors use the word 'functional' precisely when they are incapable of diagnosing a complaint as precisely as they would wish. It is their way of evading responsibility by declaring the trouble to be of psychic origin.

Be that as it may, once again drugs are the answer, for in this case the prescription signifies the doctor's ability to take appropriate action. 'If I'm telling you to take such and such tablets, it follows that I know what's ailing you', he seems to be saying as he writes out his prescription, and this in itself absolves him from making tests or taking the decision to advise the patient to see a specialist or go to a clinic, which might be taken as a sign of incompetence. One can go even further and assert that the prescription, or rather its length, its cash value, the complicated name of the medicines and their novelty for the patient, conveys to the latter the message that he did well to consult the doctor, that his case needs medical treatment and that he would clearly not have managed to get well by himself. A patient of independent mind will thus feel less sorry not to have relied on self-medication. But the medicine can do still more for the patient. It not merely shows him that the doctor knows what ails him, but communicates to him this 'knowledge' in place of the doctor himself, who would often be hard put to it to make an etiological diagnosis and communicate it to the patient. This essential function of communication falls to the manufacturer's directions for use, which are often drafted with an eye to patients as much as to doctors, but in any case are couched in the language of the drug's therapeutic uses and of the symptoms observed. When the patient buys a medicine and unwraps it at home, he will discover, or find it confirmed, that he suffers, say, from high blood pressure or has some 'hepato-biliary malfunction'.

(3) *Psychological Obsolescence and the Outmoding of Medicines*[1]

So much for the significative functions of medicines with respect to patients and also, perhaps primarily, to doctors.[2] The doctor thus appears in a certain sense as a 'consumer' of drugs, and pharmaceutical manufacturers are in no doubt about it.

Let us now see whether and how knowledge of these significative functions can help us to understand some of the seemingly inconsistent facts mentioned earlier.

A doctor and his patient, as we have seen, come to a sort of tacit agreement on a set of technical steps to be taken, even though in part something quite different is at stake. If, therefore, a drug is to perform well with respect to the non-technical aspects of the doctor's and the patient's satisfaction, it must signify technical efficiency. This meaning may be conveyed, in some cases, by the possibility of side-effects which suggest that the drug may be dangerous, or sometimes

---

[1] To avoid any misinterpretation, it should be made clear that to highlight these significative functions in no way means to deny the real pharmacodynamic activity of drugs, nor the real physical relief they bring. But for a proper understanding of drug consumption, it is necessary to take account not only of the technical effects of medicines, that is, those linked to their pharmacodynamic activity, but also of their significative effects. Clearly, both pharmacodynamic and significative effects are produced by one and the same medicine, whether it be an antibiotic or a tonic, a heart stimulant or a tranquillizer.

[2] Again a translation problem. The idea of 'outmoding' refers to the loss of performance (for instance, of a piece of capital equipment) over the course of time.

by the high price of the drug, but most often simply by its newness, a symbol of progress and hope.

But to the extent that the drug acts as a sign, its performance depends, as we have seen, on the relative position of this sign on a scale. In order to obtain good effects, therefore, it is not enough for the drug to signify efficiency; it must signify the greatest efficiency. Let us take a simple example. All general practitioners and rheumatologists know that aspirin is of effective help in rheumatic diseases. But if today a doctor prescribed such an old, familiar and banal drug, after so many new products have succeeded each other on the market since aspirin was first introduced, patients would feel that the doctor was not paying enough attention to their case, or even that he refused to accept responsibility for it (except if the doctor's reputation is so high as to reassure the patient without any further need to prove medical competence; such a doctor can prescribe aspirin). So far as the doctor is concerned, this would certainly not be the best way of demonstrating his competence and his ability to help. Without such non-technical dimensions in the doctor's and the patient's attitude the whole thing would be incomprehensible; aspirin would be regarded as a reasonably effective drug for the case, and it would be prescribed. But if we do take account of the non-technical effects of drugs, then we realize that their performance in terms of the doctor's and the patient's non-technical objectives diminishes with the appearance on the market of a new drug which is more effective or at least believed to be so. To the extent that novelty alone is taken to signify effectiveness, the mere appearance of a new drug is enough to destroy part of the power of older ones. This is precisely what was meant by the term 'psychological obsolescence' as used in the first part of this paper (the significative characteristic x being the novelty of the product in its therapeutic category, and $\bar{x}$ referring to the latest product introduced on the market).

Evidently, the psychological obsolescence of old drugs encourages their displacement by new ones. So does what we shall call the psychological outmoding of drugs. Medicines 'wear out', in the sense not of any loss of pharmacodynamic activity in the course of time (though this can happen, too), but of an erosion of their significative power. Two reasons for this come to mind, each connected with one of two non-technical functions of drugs. In the first place, a drug has the function of demonstrating the doctor's competence. No physician could go on prescribing the same drug for six years without impairing the collective image of continuous progress in therapeutical science. This component of psychological outmoding is an offspring of psychological obsolescence, for it is precisely the experience that old products become obsolescent which creates, in the mind of doctors and patients alike, the image of technical progress and hence causes psychological outmoding. In the second place, a drug signifies that the doctor is taking charge of a case. All patients need this kind of help, but to the extent that any drug's response to this need is not direct, but roundabout, it is hardly surprising that its significative power is brief, 'that this same flower that smiles today, tomorrow will be dying'. The same happens in all cases when people think consumption will answer a problem of another kind: once acquired, the desired object only too often suddenly proves quite unattractive. If a patient feels misunderstood or neglected, he will transfer his dissatisfaction to the medicine prescribed, and he will think either that it is worthless or else too potent and hence dangerous. Doctors are usually very sensitive to this kind of complaint, and in their turn will be quick to prescribe another drug instead, provided of course there is a supply of new ones to choose from.

Now we can see why the market for pharmaceuticals has such an unquenchable thirst for innovations. Manufacturers must meet this demand, for any who fail to do so would quickly be swept off the market. Innovation is needed to offset the destruction of the older products' performance, yet this very destruction grows with an increase in innovations – a vicious circle which shows up the full absurdity of the system. Nor is this all. Since, in these conditions, technical progress simply is not fast enough to provide enough signs of progress for the needs of doctors and patients, there is room for the appearance and commercial success of spurious novelties and minor innovations. While these may contribute little or nothing from the point of view of pharmacodynamic activity, we can see now that they do renew and revive the significative power of pharmaceutical products. The costs, of course, are high all along the line – from research and development through experiments and tests to sales promotion.

(4) The Question of Overconsumption of Medicines
From the above analysis, the following conclusion may be drawn. On the average, the pharmacodynamic power of drugs grows less fast than the resources used in their production. How much of an average annual rise of, say, 10 per cent in the price of drugs is due to genuine progress, and how much to the effort required for producing signs of progress? There are no serious econometric studies on this subject, and therefore no precise answer is possible. But the facts we have recalled in the first part of this paper regarding the overall efficiency of health expenditure as measured by technical indicators suggest that genuine technical progress accounts for only a small proportion.

Another, corollary, conclusion may be drawn. In a system of

private medical practice, expenditure on drugs actually prescribed by doctors is always much higher than would correspond to the purchase of less expensive drugs of equivalent pharmacodynamic effect. This excess expenditure is attributable to the costs of developing, testing and promoting various spurious novelties, not to speak of forgone productivity gains on products with short market life expectations. The amounts involved must be considerable.

Must we, then, conclude that there is waste, overconsumption? One answer has to be ruled out straightaway as unacceptable, as has already been stated: it cannot be said that drugs which duplicate older ones are devoid of social utility, and most certainly such an assertion may not be made without trying to find out first why such drugs are so successful. Nor, however, can we conclude that the existing situation is the best possible one. Drugs appear to be a distinctly inefficient means of obtaining good results with respect to those essential, though non-physical, aspects of doctor and patient satisfaction which have here been discussed.

We are led to ask the following question. Would it not improve the situation if it were possible to remove the present confusion which causes means designed to meet technical requirements to be used also for dealing with problems of human requirements? The answer is certainly in the affirmative so far as technical performances within the scope of the health care system are concerned. If drugs had none but purely technical effects, psychological obsolescence and outmoding would vanish, and pharmaceutical manufacturers would have no reason to oblige each other to innovate at all costs and would thus be free to devote time and resources to fundamental research. There would be clear gains in the field of biochemical knowledge and of the development of really new products, and gains also with respect to the use made of this knowledge and these products. A doctor trying to find the drug most appropriate for the technical problem involved in treating a patient would no longer be side-tracked by considerations extraneous to this technical problem.

There remain the non-technical aspects of the doctor–patient relationship. Here the problem is to substitute something else for drugs in the functions they now discharge, but discharge so badly. The task will not be easy, and certainly this is not the place even to try and outline a solution. But one thing seems obvious, though there are few to recognize it. To tackle the problem of medicines in France is a matter not so much of altering the conditions of production in the pharmaceutical industry (though this may be a useful stage), as of transforming the rules of the game whose name is medical practice. It will readily be appreciated that a satisfactory solution of the problems discussed in this paper, problems which concern doctors and patients alike, will require radical changes in the conditions of medical training and practice. Medical students will need psychological training, the teaching monopoly of hospitals will have to be abolished, genuinely medical post-university teaching will have to be organized by some agency having no connection with the pharmaceutical industry, the status of the general practitioner will have to be upgraded and the manner of his remuneration revised. These are just a few items in the list of necessary reforms.

REFERENCES

[1] Abraham, C., and Thédié, J., 'Le Prix d'une Vie Humaine dans les Décisions Économiques', *Revue Française de Recherche Opérationnelle*, no. 16 (3rd quarter, 1960).
[2] Auster, R., Leveson, I., and Sarachek, D., 'The Production of Health: An Exploratory Study', *Journal of Human Resources*, IV, 4 (1969).
[3] Boltanski, L., *La Découverte de la Maladie, la Diffusion du Savoir Médical* (Centre de Sociologie Européenne, 1968).
[4] Calot, G., and Lery, A., 'La Baisse de la Mortalité se Ralentit depuis Dix Ans', *Économie et Statistique*, no. 39 (Nov 1972).
[5] Dupuy, J. P., 'Le Médicament dans la Relation Médecin-Malade', *Projet* (May 1973).
[6] ——, 'Innovation et Obsolescence Psychologique: Essai de Formalisation dans le Cadre d'une Économie de Marché', *Cahiers du Séminaire d'Économétrie* (1973).
[7] ——, 'Innovation et Obsolescence Psychologique: Application à la Consommation Médicale', to be published.
[8] ——, 'La Croissance des Dépenses de Santé: Un Phénomène Encore Mal Expliqué', to be published.
[9] ——, Ferry, J., Karsenty, S., and Worms, G., *La Consommation de Médicaments: Approche Psycho-socio-économique*, CEREBE Report (Sep 1971).
[10] Fuchs, V., 'Some Economic Aspects of Mortality in Developed Countries', pp. 174–93 above.
[11] Herzlich, C., *Santé et Maladie: Analyse d'une Représentation Sociale* (Paris–The Hague: Mouton, 1966).
[12] d'Iribarne, P., 'A la Recherche de Politiques Rationnelles de Santé et de Sécurité', *Analyse et Prévision*, VIII, 6 (Dec 1969).
[13] ——, 'Les Aspects "Subjectifs" des Politiques de Sécurité', *Annales des Mines* (July 1972).
[14] Lebart, L., *Recherches sur le Coût de Protection de la Vie Humaine dans le Domaine Médical*, CREDOC Report (June 1970).
[15] Lévy, E., 'Health Indicators and Health Systems Analysis', pp. 377–401 above.
[16] Longone, P., *Population et Sociétés*, no. 11 (Feb 1969).
[17] Ministère d'État Chargé des Affaires Sociales–Ministère de la Santé Publique, Report of the Working Party on 'La Science de la Décision en Matière de Santé' (Mar 1973).
[18] Mizrahi, A. and A., 'Un Modèle des Dépenses Médicales Appliqué aux Données d'une Enquête', *Consommation*, XI, 1 (Jan–Mar 1964).

[19] Morlat, G., 'Un Modèle pour Certaines Décisions Médicales', *Cahiers du Séminaire d'Économétrie*, no. 12 (1970).
[20] Pelt, J. M., *Les Médicaments* (Paris: Seuil, 1970).
[21] Williams, A., 'Measuring the Effectiveness of Health Care Systems', pp. 361–76 in this volume.

25 Choice of Technique[1]

Michael Kaser

ST ANTONY'S COLLEGE, OXFORD

A characteristic of medical care supply is the degree of freedom in choice of technique open to the supplier, normally a physician, within the limits or physical availabilities by place and by time in relation to the patient. In view of the rapidly increasing volume of alternative technologies in general, and of information on a patient's condition in particular cases, the clinical evaluation of therapies (efficacy) is urgently required with respect to resources applied (efficiency) and to the resultant health outcome (effectiveness), Health outcomes are not thereby rendered commensurate and remain, in practice, selected by the physician, whose clinical freedom is nevertheless guided towards a cost minimand suitable for a National Health Service-type system.

I. CONCEPTUAL FRAMEWORK

A significant feature of health economics is the attempt to situate health care services in the frame of analyses appropriate to the production and distribution of manufactures through production to consumption. Ideally, the comparative analysis should be applicable both to market and to directive supply of health services or physical goods and hence suitable for discussion within the context of all forms of health planning.

Culyer (1971) has recently reviewed the areas in which health care has been seen as unassimilable to the conventional approach to an economic good. He characterizes them, on the consumer side, as ignorance, uncertainty regarding incidence of need, a degree of consumer sovereignty which leads to non-optimal allocation; and on the supply side, a use which is a composite of final (consump-

---

[1] Acknowledgment is made of discussion with Dr A. E. Bennett, Director of the Health Services Evaluation Group in the Department of the Regius Professor of Medicine, University of Oxford, to Mr David Pole, Dr G. K. Matthew, Dr John Evans and Mr L. B. Hudson of the Department of Health and Social Security, and to A. Creese, Pembroke College, Oxford. A preliminary version of sections of this paper was presented to the Working Group on Evaluation of Public Health Programmes of the European Office of the World Health Organization, Slunchev Bryag, Bulgaria, 29 Aug–1 Sep 1972.

tion) and derived demand (human capital), externalities rank much higher than they would in the cost schedule of a physical good. In a subsequent paper on the relative efficiency of the United Kingdom National Health Service (N.H.S.), he touched on the distinctive characteristic chosen for examination in this paper. Culyer (1972) asked himself[1] whether 'the N.H.S. type of organization [was] likely to produce a medically optimal allocation of resources' on the assumption that 'medical care is a homogeneous entity expressed in terms of an indicator of "output" per unit of time'. He defines a 'medical ideal' as the maximum care technically capable of being supplied regardless of cost; in the market system, 'no one will pay for care beyond the point at which marginal valuation is equal to marginal cost'. In the N.H.S.-type system, no central decision-maker would 'maximize the technical possibilities' irrespective of opportunity cost. Set also within the institutions of the N.H.S., the present paper suggests that more precision can be introduced by a microeconomic approach.

A characteristic of the supply of medical care which distinguishes it from that of other goods and services is the degree of freedom in choice of technique open to the supplier – essentially the physician alone, but sometimes a team[2] or a medical auxiliary working under the supervision of physicians. In establishing or enlarging any other productive enterprise, the entrepreneur chooses a technology whereby capital and current inputs are to be transformed into demand outputs; in the broad sense of having to conform to the supply of resources available to the physician, the decision to create or extend a hospital or to open and equip a practice sets physical limits to the therapies which the physician can apply. Thus within given physical constraints the physician, in each case confronting him, has as wide a choice of therapies (viz. combinations of scarce resources in the form of knowledgeable and skilled manpower, equipment and materials) as his professional expertise and ethic allow. Such choice of techniques includes the withholding of treatment despite the expressed demand of the patient (or his proxies), testimony to which is the long history of the placebo. Like all personal services, time and place of provision are more significant components of value to the consumer than normally for physical goods. The patient has to reach the medical equipment or be administered the drug within limits imposed by the disorder and its natural course; time and

[1] Culyer documents and assesses a discussion mostly compressed into the last decade; the present writer (Kaser, 1960) was perhaps among the first to identify certain of these distinctions and believes a pursuance of this approach to be among the principal tasks of health economists.

[2] In U.K. hospitals such teams are designated a 'firm', a fair presentation of their decision-making power in the terminology of economics.

capacity constraints combine when competitive demand from other patients involves queueing, a subject to which the attention of health economics had been properly directed.

Many professionals work in similar circumstances of an individual relationship to their clients, but the extent to which they can, in practice, choose within a spectrum of possible services is limited. A comparison may be made with a lawyer's advice in chambers or his pleading in court; the verification of its 'correctness' by the law or the judiciary corresponds to the market's constraint on the decisions on production taken by an entrepreneur or to the check of a state control commission (or similar agency) that the manager of a state-run enterprise is conforming to regulations or directives. To the extent that physicians in private practice or profit-making hospitals are paid for services by patients, something of the same regulation applies to medical care, for if a client is dissatisfied (on the evidence of medical decisions taken), he goes elsewhere; an above-average mortality after treatment induces this response among potential clients. Such response is, however, rarer than among, say, litigants with respect to their lawyers, because physicians are reticent about discussing alternative treatments with the lay public. Medical negligence actions have to be sustained in court with considerable difficulty over evidence, whereas the record of a lawyer's success is obtainable from law reports.

The advances of medical science in recent years have greatly multiplied the volume of information available to the physician in making his choice of technique in each given case; in intensive-care units the reaction of the patient to therapy can be monitored moment by moment. Very little research has yet been done, however, to diminish the heavy personal burden of diagnosis and selection of therapy incumbent on the physician in the light of that information, but brief reference is made below to computer diagnosis.

In the United Kingdom, the fee-for-service basis has largely been eliminated; the institution of the N.H.S., which has so reduced the private sector, has permitted the introduction of health planning of a kind for which objectives need to be formulated and their attainment evaluated ('monitored' in United Kingdom government usage), raising, more acutely, problems of choice of therapy and of its evaluation, whether in technical or in economic measure.

II. THE INSTITUTIONAL FRAMEWORK IN THE UNITED KINGDOM

The recent government plans for the reorganization of the National Health Service in the United Kingdom have stressed one of the original principles of the Service, that it 'should provide full clinical freedom to the doctors working in it' (Department of Health and Social Security, 1970, para. 1). The proposals go on to declare that it is the government's policy 'to set clear objectives and standards and measure performance against them'.[1] The present paper deals with objectives relevant to the health care supplied within the administrative boundary of the Department of Health and Social Security (D.H.S.S.); other objectives may predominate, for example, in programmes of school health (now under the Department of Education and Science, but to be transferred to the N.H.S. in 1974), of occupational health (under the Department for Employment) and of environmental health (under the Department of the Environment). The paper considers neither these nor problems arising in management organization or operations research: the D.H.S.S. has commissioned numerous studies in such applications and has a strong technical staff of its own (see Nuffield Provincial Hospitals Trust, 1971) while local authorities have access to the Local Government Operational Research Unit (see Long and Norton, 1972).

The health care activities operated by the D.H.S.S. extend beyond the traditionally defined sphere of public health, which forms part of the first of three divisions of the N.H.S. The first group is that furnished by local health authorities in maternity and child care, midwifery services, home nursing, health visitors, health centres (from which an increasing number of general practitioners operate[2]), home helps (for the sick and disabled),[3] ambulances, social work, after-care, chiropody, vaccination and immunization, health education and other preventive health services. A second division is that of the local Executive Councils, to which all but the very few general practitioners who elect for an all-private practice are under contract, and which also make available general dental, ophthalmic and pharmaceutical services. The procurement of pharmaceuticals, like that of equipment and supplies for hospitals, is to some extent centrally coordinated by the Supplies Division of the D.H.S.S. and by the decisions of the Dunlop Committee. The third division, of hospital and specialist services, is provided by Regional Hospital Boards, Boards of Governors and Hospital Management Committees. The first division is jointly financed by rates (viz. local taxes levied upon immobile property values) and the central rate-support grant, which is intended to equalize social services nationwide. The two others are funded by general central taxation and the N.H.S.

---

[1] Ibid. The same stress is found in the Department's later documents (1971, 1972).

[2] The majority of G.P.s already work in group practice.

[3] 'Homemakers', in United States usage.

constituent of National Insurance employer and employee contributions, plus, to a small extent, minor payments by patients and income from hospital and other charitable endowments.

An American observer of the N.H.S. was 'impressed with the investigative zeal of the British and the many suggestions to diminish or remove deficiencies. Some problems do not easily yield to corrective action. The most troublesome one arises out of the tripartite system' (Lindsey, 1964, p. 50). The binary split of finance[1] and the tripartite division of service constitute a certain obstacle to evaluation, partly because the costs and the benefits relevant to the N.H.S. may relate to different divisions, and partly because of the sheer complexity of coordination between the agencies concerned (in England alone, 119 Executive Councils, 35 Boards of Governors, 14 Regional Hospital Boards, 299 Hospital Management Committees and 158 local health authorities). This aspect, being strictly institutional, is not treated in this note, but the United Kingdom government plans to unify all three divisions from April 1974 within a single service, defining the functions of the new local authorities (to operate also from that date) 'according to the main skills required to provide them rather than by any categorization of primary user' (Department of Health and Social Security, 1970, para. 31). It has adopted the basic features of the scheme delineated by the previous administration, proposing, as its chief change, the insertion of Regional Health Authorities 'responsible for the general planning of the N.H.S. (including the specialities and, in consultation with the universities, the service facilities to be provided in support of medical teaching and research) in each region; for allocating resources to the area health authorities and for coordinating their activities and monitoring their performance' (Department of Health and Social Security, 1971, para. 11).

III. MACRO-AGGREGATES OF HEALTH OUTCOME

Neither the present Conservative nor the previous Labour government proposed full administrative unification of the health and related personal social services, going no further than the assurance of 'strong and binding links', including matching boundaries.

With unification of most of the health service in prospect, the scope for comparative evaluation of its component services is considerably enhanced: Culyer (1972) concluded 'that an appropriate

---

[1] The administration of British social services abounds in this ordinate notation. McNerney (1971) observes that the N.H.S. has been discussed as a triad but should be a 'quintad', viz. adding school and industrial health; after the standard primary and secondary, tertiary education is financed in a 'binary' fashion (local authorities and the University Grants Committee) and teachers' training is proposed to be operated in 'first, second and third cycles'.

approach to comparative health systems should be based upon their relative efficiency in approaching efficient outcomes and in this task only empirical analysis can establish any relevant conclusions'.

Other contributions to this Conference (notably by Williams) have dealt with the concepts of need and demand which underlie the service which a health care system supplies, and no more than a summary seems required in the present paper in connection with the concept of outcome. Matthew (in Nuffield Provincial Hospitals Trust, 1971) defines the 'need' for medical care as existing when an individual has an illness or disability for which there is an acceptable treatment or care, but this is only translated into 'demand' when the individual considers he has a need and wishes to receive care, that being converted into a 'utilization' of health services when he actually receives care. Culyer, Lavers and Williams (1972) carry this concept to a theoretically quantifiable aggregate in their 'measures of the state-of-health' (S.O.H. indicators), against which should be set 'measures of the need-for-health' (N.F.H. indicators), *either*, as targets – more often as the difference between a target and the current level of the indicator (thereby expressing it in terms of the S.O.H. indicator) – *or* attached to a valuation of the intensity of need made by the 'agent responsible for the decision'. They prefer the latter because the former avoids explicit consideration of the S.O.H. indicator. After discussing various quantifications which appear to them unsatisfactory, they present an S.O.H. indicator which encompasses both medical data and judgments and social judgments, viz. by multiplying the intensity of ill-health (pain and/or disability) on a ten-point scale (from normality to death) by the expected period of duration (until recovery or death). They observe that such a valuation would enable preventive as well as therapeutic actions to be incorporated, and treats any particular intensity level as being equally undesirable, irrespective of the economic or other status of the patient.

The degree to which pain is quantifiable is subject to considerable philosophical and physiological difficulty. Ayer (1963) observes generally that 'no amount of gesturing on my part can direct [observers'] attention to a private sensation of mind, which *ex hypothesi* they cannot observe, assuming further that this sensation has no "natural expression" '. Quinton (1968) writes of 'the mistaken analogy' that lies between "I see a tree" or "I touch this stone" on the one hand and "I feel pain" and "I understand this calculation" on the other'. Young (1971) examines this distinction in the light of the requirements of Wittgenstein (1953), that since private experiences cannot be described by a private language, man applies to himself the rules of language he applies in talking about others: 'Even when we say "it hurts" we are not really describing the pain but we are giving the conventionalized response to the situation. . . . Wittgenstein would say that in the statement "I know I am in pain", the word "know" does not have the same meaning as "I know it is raining" because the former cannot be falsified.' Few measurable physiological reactions can corroborate the sensation of pain. Young finds only the 'flexor reflex' – whereby, say, a limb is withdrawn from a pinprick – and the more complex responses of the cerebral cortex which can be demonstrated experimentally by current through an implanted electrode.

Further obstacles to the quantifications proposed by Culyer, Lavers and Williams are their need to treat death on the disability scale: the dilemma, as Fanshel and Bush (1970) had pointed out when considering an earlier 'health status index', is that death terminates pain, whereas most patients would prefer pain to death. Another difficulty is that the prognosis of the course of a disability could be too uncertain to serve as the multiplier to obtain common units of time in pain.

Sociologists seem to be no better placed than economists to measure social indicators relevant to health outcome, at least so far as Plessas and Fein (1972) have summarized forty-five relevant papers. The need for mensuration in macro-aggregates is as much recognized by those working on the medical as by those on the administrative or economic side: a recent book by one of the leading medical proponents of better evaluation procedures opens with the statement that 'if ever we are to get the optimum results from our national expenditure on the N.H.S. we must finally be able to express the results in the form of the benefit that could be obtained if more money were made available' (Cochrane, 1972).

In developed countries there is scant direct information in mortality or morbidity statistics on health outcome (Roemer, 1971; Deniston and Rosenstock, 1970). Neonatal, stillbirth, perinatal and infantile mortality may well describe more the genetic or socio-economic status of a region than its medical services. Morbidity data for England and Wales show a certain 'disease gradient' (from the best in the South-east to the poorest in the North-west and Wales) which is primarily associated with the differing regional availability of services (see Cooper and Culyer, 1972). Considerable reduction in regional variation of service has been effected since the start of the N.H.S. and will continue (see Department of Health and Social Security, 1970), together with promoting the use of services among immigrant or otherwise less advantaged groups of the population.

Two approaches have been used in the United Kingdom for a quantitative survey of morbidity outside ordinary reporting requirements (infectious disease returns and hospital admissions) or the screening procedures discussed below, viz. the prevalence survey and sickness benefit returns. Bennett *et al.* (1970) used a health-outcome measure (defined as inability to perform, unaided, certain activities essential to daily life) in a two-stage prevalence survey based on questionnaires to a randon sample of a local adult population. Sickness benefit statistics are analysed by the D.H.S.S. (see summary, with a commentary and brief international comparison, in Office of Health Economics, 1971), but are affected as indicators of health outcome by the changing attitude to leisure. The trend in underlying conditions is evident in the decline of, e.g., pulmonary tuberculosis, but the increase in more trivial disabilities may often relate to an excuse to stay away from work rather than to a higher incidence.

IV. MICROECONOMIC RATIONING

At the microeconomic level, the N.H.S. has virtually eliminated commodity pricing from the provision of health care. Cooper (1972) observes that rational economic behaviour would indicate that an individual faced with a zero price will consume that good or service until it yields him no further utility. Although he will be deterred by some positive cost (inconvenience, fares to place of service, leisure or work-time forgone), demand would, in principle, be so high that it might as well be infinity.

In practice, demand for health care will gravitate towards whatever level of provision is actually made by the N.H.S., the aggregate resources of which are determined by a political process. Within that limited aggregate, the N.H.S. largely relies on the clinical freedom of the physician, who chooses the intensity and nature of service among many possible degrees and techniques; an immediate threat to life, viz. at the end of that continuum, would generally be adjudged a need for satisfaction, but serious ethical problems interpose themselves even then. Leaving aside 'unmet need' – arising chiefly from a person's inhibitions to present himself to a physician, but also from the time and place at which a physician is available – the physician rarely declines to take action once the confrontation is made, for the very reason just given on the non-verifiability of pain experience. Cook (1972) has recently expressed the physician's view in the N.H.S. that he is 'accountable only to the patients whom he serves and to his own conscience', implying that clinical freedom is a rationing process which he applies to the resources made available by the N.H.S., or, in practice, to their experience of what the Service has provided in the past. Feldstein (1967) has demonstrated that the appropriation of funds for new hospital beds cannot practically be based on data on admissions and waiting lists (the subject of a paper by Culyer to the present Conference) because physicians respond to an enlargement by extending the cut-off point along their need continuum; a forthcoming study by Cooper and Culyer shows that per capita bed availability fluctuates over an 80 per cent range without obvious detriment on the relatively deprived regions. Indeed, they point out, the fact that the Sheffield Regional Board was less well endowed than the Oxford Board on all thirty-one indicators of provision may only prove that the former is more effective. Morris, Ward and Hendyside (1968) have shown that in hernia cases variation in length of hospital stay was not reflected in hospital efficiency, viz. by noticeable effect on patients. Even in prescribing, where accountability has been introduced by relating records of each physician to regional averages, physicians have never been instructed on 'the best buy', i.e. the trade-off between differences in likely therapeutic effect and cost. The shift in relative spending from manpower to drug therapy is partly a technological trend on an international scale, but the N.H.S. may not, according to Cooper (1972), press pharmaceutical manufacturers sufficiently towards reducing prices, and thereby limits provision of care by other means. But the rationing of prescriptions in the N.H.S. would severely prejudice clinical freedom.[1]

V. MICROECONOMIC EVALUATION

The approach which best combines the physician's and the economist's interests in the optimal allocation of resources in an N.H.S.-type system is comprised in the concept of evaluation, the case for which, in general terms, has recently been agreed by the Office of Health Economics (1972) for the N.H.S., and which is the subject of extensive investigation by W.H.O. on an international basis. By avoiding comparisons of health outcome between the conditions treated, it cannot furnish a maximand for an N.H.S.-type system as a whole, but by rationalizing choice of technique at the micro-level it can minimize costs overall for a given, but not intra-commensurate, health outcome. Cost minimization itself would, of course, be rational only to the extent that opportunity costs are represented. The latter condition is not generally satisfied for the national health services of the centrally planned economies, which set as targets a basket of

[1] In some of the national health services of Eastern Europe, where less weight is accorded that freedom but prescription finance is similar to the British, the prescribing of foreign drugs is restricted (to conserve foreign exchange), and a rationing process in money terms is applied to purchase of foreign medical equipment.

service indicators (again, not intra-commensurate). An alternative open to such economies and usable in market economies where N.H.S.-type costs are poor surrogates for opportunity cost is minimization of time. This would, as a current input-model, ideally be an aggregate of the time involved in restoring (within the limits of available technique) to patients an average state of health specific for age, sex and occupation; the time would be that of patient and of the medical and paramedical personnel and these caring for him. Because it is a microeconomic measure (the only one possible when the physician is the selector of technique), problems arise under institutional care of accounting personnel time spread between numerous patients. As a first approximation the times computed need not be weighted, on the assumption that scarcity differentials would be evened out over a large number of cases for comparison. The first phase for this evaluation is measurement of the 'effect of a particular medical action in altering the natural history of a particular disease for the better . . .'. Cochrane (1972), whose definition this is, considers, but rejects, the term 'efficacious' for this measurement in favour of 'effective'. It is suggested that it may be better to reserve the latter for another phase (see below), and conform to the usage of the World Health Organization (1971) in its report on 'Statistical Indicators for the Planning and Evaluation of Public Health Programmes'. These definitions supplement those of 'effectiveness' and 'efficiency' recommended by that Organization's Regional Office for Europe (1967, 1971), and are as follows: 'Efficacy: the benefit or utility to the individual of the service, treatment regimen, drug, preventive or control measure advocated or applied; effectiveness: the effect of the activity and the end results, outcomes or benefits for the population achieved in relation to the stated objectives; efficiency: the effects or end results achieved in relation to the effort expended in terms of money, resources and time.'

That usage was close to definitions for the second two recommended by the reports of the W.H.O. Regional Office for Europe on evaluating public health and dental health services (World Health Organization Regional Office for Europe, 1967, 1971), while the same Office's Working Group on the Evaluation of Public Health Programmes (meeting in 1972) found that because the terms 'efficacy', 'effectiveness' and 'efficiency' were close enough in meaning to lead to confusion, alignment to a common usage would become general. Health economists would probably find no difficulty in using such terms, a more detailed consideration of which is made below.

Efficacy measures a relationship strictly within the observation of medical science, whereas efficiency specifies the result of a given application of techniques. In accord with the concepts applicable in cost-effectiveness and systems analysis by both health economists (e.g. Ingbar, 1964) and public health specialists (e.g. McNerney 1971), effectiveness coincides with the usage of Culyer, Lavers and Williams (1972), who define 'effectiveness of health-affecting activities (E.H.A.A. indicators)' as the effect of a variation in an input of health care on their S.O.H. indicator during given time periods. They see 'effectiveness' indicators as measuring the technical relationships between 'inputs' and 'outputs'.

Evaluation of a health care system can thus be decomposed into medical actions to which, chiefly by randomized controlled trial (R.C.T.), a degree of efficacy can be ascribed (those actions in preventive medicine being assessed as precluding or inhibiting a disease or disability); a chosen application of such an action by the selected use of personnel and materials (capital assest and current supplies) renders such actions efficient; they may be effective in relation to any objective appropriate to the system. The actions and costs thereof cover not only treatment but also screening, diagnosis, place of treatment and length of stay and, if necessary, rehabilitation (Cochrane, 1972).

VI. EXAMPLES OF APPLICATION

Some form of controlled trial is generally required in order to verify or disprove the claim of efficacy in a particular disorder. As a sophisticated technique, the R.C.T. has had little more than two decades in clinical use if it be dated from Daniels and Hill (1952), and is still far from generally applicable or accurate (see Oldham, 1968). Its use is wholly dependent on the clinician's willingness to apply the experimental therapy in certain instances and to withhold it for a control group. Firstly, it may be unethical for the control group to be deprived of the action in question, so general is the concensus of medical opinion that it would be in the interests of the patient. Cochrane (1972) cites three thereby unavailable for R.C.T., viz. surgery for carcinoma of the lung, cytological tests for the prevention of cervical carcinoma, and dietetic therapy for phenylketonuria. Secondly, because of the rarity of cases for similar reasons, reliable measurement (e.g. the use of renal dialysis in porphyria variegata) may be subject to an incorrect assessment of statistical significance. Thirdly, the result of the action may be measured only subjectively, as notably, in psychiatry. Fourthly, the use of a therapy may be of such proven efficiency and urgency that, while withholding would be unethical, no value is to be gained by trial testing (e.g. insulin for acute juvenile diabetes or vitamin B_{12} for pernicious anaemia).

In the absence of ethical problems, efficacies may be confirmed either with R.C.T.s (e.g. drug therapy of tuberculosis) or without it; an example of the latter case arises when there is good experimental evidence that, in the long term, more good is done to the patient than harm (e.g. dosage of iron in raising haemoglobin levels, of anti-depressants in psychiatry). In some instances, R.C.T.s yield equivocal evidence (e.g. tonsillectomy) or show a negative balance for the patient but which (through lack of conviction or communication) persist in practice – demonstrated, for example, by mortality from ischaemic heart diseases after application of tolbutamide and phenoformin to adult-onset diabetics (see Universities Group Diabetes Program, 1970, and Knatterud *et al.*, 1971).

Most work in the N.H.S. on choice of technique in applying an efficacious action to determine its efficiency has been on length of hospital stay and on place of treatment. The correlation of size of institution should be with efficiency rather than with effectiveness, because the consensus now seems to be to relate the findings to medical and social therapy rather than to the comparative cost of achieving given hospitalization effects.

Logically, the place of treatment must be considered before length of stay, and as a preliminary, the optimum time between occurrence of the phenomenon requiring therapy and medical action. An example much discussed is of the provision of coronary-care ambulances in Belfast, for which a medical team is kept in constant readiness to reach cases of myocardial infarction with appropriate equipment (e.g. a defibrillator) as soon as humanly possible (see Partridge and Geddes, 1967). The evaluation of this technique depends, particularly, on the high mortality in the immediate aftermath of the attack, but the situation is part of the general (and occasionally misplaced) belief of ambulance drivers that every second counts in bringing a road-accident casualty to the admissions door. Ford, in Nuffield Provincial Hospitals Trust (1971), finds considerable shortcomings in their conclusions and believes that 'some other way of tackling the problem of sudden and early deaths must be found if real progress is to be made'. She suggests that identification of special risk would be more fruitful.

Five areas may be cited where efficiency is related to place of treatment. In the first place, treatment at the place of case occurrence is chiefly justified on efficiency grounds in the case of transport or industrial accidents and for the convenience of the patient (e.g. therapy in occupational health schemes where the employee is not sufficiently disabled to be off work or is under prophylaxis). The cost in this case is, like that of the coronary-care ambulance staff and equipment, maintained for occasional rather than systematic use, but the latter may range upward from a first-aid kit. Secondly, treatment at the G.P.s surgery (on which the N.H.S. depends, perhaps, more than does any other country[1]) is 'ultimately related to even wider issues, particularly the uncertainty facing the future of the traditional, service-oriented liberal professions in an age of rapidly advancing technology' (Forsyth, 1966, p. 76); in the more specifically microeconomic evaluation, it involves the long-standing controversy over G.P. efficiency (launched in medical literature by Collings, 1950, countered by Hadfield, 1953, and Taylor, 1954). Research has been fairly extensive as a consequence of the establishment of a Royal College of General Practitioners (R.C.G.P.) in 1952 (which has a research unit in Birmingham to provide expert advice to general practitioners desiring to undertake research of their own) and of a Committee for Research in General Practice by the Medical Research Council (M.R.C.) in 1953. A major contribution to the assessment of efficiency is being made by analysis of records of personal and family health events, of which the Oxford Record Linkage Study is the leading example (see, among numerous other accounts, Wilson, in Nuffield Provincial Hospitals Trust, 1971). The problem of individual professional isolation in, e.g., discussion of choice of technique (Forsyth, 1966) has been much attenuated by practice in health centres or in partnerships and by attachments of G.P.s as clinical assistants in local hospitals (one in every four G.P.s in the N.H.S.). Aggregate time-saving has been assessed in patient appointments to replace the surgery queue and in bringing hospital consultants to health centres under such appointments (see Cochrane, 1972); the place of treatment has also been found relevant to doctor–patient communication, seeming to be freer and fuller in a G.P. surgery than in outpatients' departments of hospitals.

The third locus of treatment, the patient's home (when justified by the information at the disposal of the physician), is a normal feature of the N.H.S. The clinical freedom exercised by G.P.s in the United Kingdom has a certain institutional constraint in the tradition of home visiting and sense of duty of the practitioners, both equally strong. Where these are weaker, there may be, as in the United States, some preference for telephone consultation, with reports on lay-applied tests of temperature, pulse, symptoms, etc., or, as in Eastern Europe, more frequent resort to the polyclinic as the expected place of non-hospitalized treatment. This comparison is being considered in the Conference under 'Alternative Health

---

[1] 96 per cent of the population are registered with a G.P., and the N.H.S. in future 'should be centred on the family doctor team' (Department of Health and Social Security, 1970, para. 1).

Care Systems', but at the micro-level within the N.H.S., the relative efficiency of the home versus the hospital has been examined only rarely, e.g. for ischaemic heart disease (Mather *et al.*, 1971, having shown that a rather higher mortality rate is recorded in hospital coronary-care units than at home). Few comparisons have been made within a fourth group – efficiency in treatment at an outpatient department (which, casualty admissions apart, is normally under the N.H.S. only through a G.P.) and in inpatient care. There are studies on hernia operation (Farquharson, 1955), varicose veins treatment (Weddell, forthcoming, cited in Cochrane, 1972, p. 32), and, amid considerable controversy, outpatient abortion by the suction technique.

The fifth area of evaluation on place of treatment, the hospital, by type and size, has atracted most investigation. N.H.S. policy has shifted away from the very large district hospital, and the advantages of the community hospital are being pilot-tested in a number of areas. Much work has been done on the therapeutic effects of length of stay, making comparisons between countries (Logan *et al.*, 1971), between N.H.S. regions and between hospitals (Lipworth *et al.*, 1963; Heasman and Carstairs, 1971).

With given efficacies, a choice of technique may be more or less efficient on account of diagnosis. The very reliance which diagnosis places on observed correlation gives value to the computer at least as ancillary. In trials of computer diagnosis, the principal adverse discrepancy from diagnoses directly by clinicians seems to have been by failure to record rarer disease symptoms on the computer memory. There is very little to add to the generally known efficiency of immunization procedures, save perhaps to remark that the current evaluation in the N.H.S. of whooping-cough vaccine is being made not on efficiency, but on efficacy.

VII. COST-EFFECTIVENESS

Standard costing procedures are in force throughout the N.H.S. and do not, it would appear, give rise to any special problems in relation to evaluation; the problems, as might be expected, arise in determining effectiveness, i.e. in relation to macro-level objectives rather than, as above, to individual cases. Three examples may be briefly cited: screening, hospital utilization and drug-prescribing practice.

Pole (1968) puts the central economic point on the efficiency of screening: 'If screening costs more than not-screening, what we want to know is whether the extra cost is worth while in terms of extra benefit. This may very well be tbe case, even though the ratio of benefit to cost is greater for the non-screening technique than for screening.' The distinction in McKeown (1968) between screening for research and for public health protection implies different valuations of effectiveness. Calculations of costs saved by early revelation of an abnormal condition appear to show screening to be advantageous in finding bacteriuria in pregnant women, and diabetes and deafness in young children; this would also be the case for carcinoma of the breast and of the cervix, for anaemia due to iron deficiency and for glaucoma, if in each case the efficacy were assured of a treatment, after the condition had been demonstrated. On the other hand, screening costs exceed treatment costs for phenylketonuria, rhesus haemolytic disease and pulmonary tuberculosis (Pole, 1968, 1971). The screening programme for the latter has already been suspended by the N.H.S. Since so much depends on the response rate in a screening programme, it is relevant that R.C.T.s on a screening programme in general practice (circulation of questionnaires on a wide range of symptoms and invitations for examinations by the G.P.) have shown no increased rate of physician consultation to follow screening response (Bennett and Fraser, 1972).

The pioneering work of Feldstein (1967) is well known in assessing the optimal intensity of the utilization of hospital facilities either by increasing rates of bed occupation or by shortening the mean length of stay. More work needs to be done on cost-effectiveness of the regional diversity in these indexes and on marginal changes in the admissions queue, viz. in delays experienced by non-acute cases; the subject is being covered in Culyer's paper to this Conference.

He and Maynard (1970) have drawn attention to the cost-effectiveness of choice between drugs which are addictive or otherwise dangerous and those which are not. The cost to hospitals in time consumed by prescribing, obtaining and using dangerous drugs instead of non-dangerous preparations can be considerable: they put a value of £650,000 on time that could be annually saved by such substitution in N.H.S. hospitals of England and Wales.

A caveat should be made, in conclusion, on intangibles arising from institutional factors which may need to be discounted or added in assessing effectiveness. These, and the valuation of public provision in relation to private preferences, are, of course, common to a broad range of public policy issues.

The two topics most relevant to choice of institution within the N.H.S. are the patient's sense of security and his facility for communication with medical staff. Security is perhaps more important because that has been the prime objective of the N.H.S. since its creation, viz. that the risk of sickness be insured by the entirety of taxpayers and National Insurance contributors:

The health service should be financed by taxes and contributions paid when people are well rather than by charges levied on them when they are sick; the financial burden of sickness should be spread over the whole community. In practice the cost of the service has increased so rapidly that it has not always been possible to maintain this principle, but a 'free' service in this sense . . . encourages preventive medicine and early treatment, relieves the sick of financial anxiety and collects the money when people can afford to pay it. (Department of Health and Social Security, 1971)

It is supplemented by private insurance, essentially to obtain quicker service in private beds in the N.H.S. or in nursing homes in the not-for-profit sector (see Webb, 1962), and a Parliamentary inquiry published in April 1972 concluded that this made no net detraction from the overall N.H.S. service after allowance for the payments made. The availability of a G.P. to give reassurance and to guide the patient through the services provided (see Forsyth, 1966), is, hence, a significant contribution to N.H.S. objectives, by assuring a personal sense of security. Security also requires the continuity of care, viz. tracing the efficiency of passage from one section of the N.H.S. as therapy or prophylaxis requires (Forsyth, 1966).[1]

Certain projects now under way should help towards evaluating the degree of patient socialization in hospital (notably the pilot schemes for community hospitals in comparison with larger units already mentioned) and under rehabilitation. More follow-up studies are probably required during after-care, though part of this aspect of evaluation relates to links with other personal social services not covered by the N.H.S. The problem of communication between patient and physician and among hospital staffs has long been recognized (the latter in its measurable aspect especially since Revans, 1960) and seems to require further evaluation.

A forecast of the degree to which preferences shift towards or away from public provision is implicitly required for health planning, the Conference subject for which this paper is offered. Johansen (1971) summarizes the problem. Although it is possible to 'express how much private consumption the country is willing to forgo per unit of joint expenditure used for the satisfaction of collective wants, . . . is

---

[1] Security, as papers to the Conference on inter-system comparison will doubtless state, is not a prerogative of a N.H.S.-type system. For the U.K., the Institute of Economic Affairs (1965) reports a survey in which respondents were asked to decide whether they would prefer, to the N.H.S., a voucher system to purchase medical care on a fee-for-service basis, following the arguments in Lees (1961) and Jewkes and Jewkes (1963) on the value of market forces in health care provision.

it the preferences which are valid before certain measures we put into operation that are to be considered, or should one also consider possible prognostications as to how people's preferences will change as a result of such measures?' One can extend his answer to many other questions raised in this paper: 'Difficult to solve, even on an entirely abstract and logical plane.'

REFERENCES

Ayer, A. J. (1963), *The Concept of a Person and Other Essays* (London: Macmillan).

Bennett, A. E., *et al.* (1970), *Br. Med. J.*, III 762.

—— and Fraser, I. G. P. (1972), *Int. J. Epid.*, I 55.

Cochrane, A. L. (1972), *Effectiveness and Efficiency: Random Reflections on the Health Services* (London: Nuffield Provincial Hospitals Trust).

Collings, J. S. (1950), *Lancet*, I 555.

Cook, D. R. (1972), *J. Roy. Soc. Hlth.*, XCII 1.

Cooper, M. (1972), 'Rationing Health Care Resources', conference paper (publication forthcoming).

—— and Culyer, A. J. (1971), *Soc. Sci. and Med.*, V 1.

Culyer, A. J. (1971), *Oxford Economic Papers*, XXIII 189.

—— (1972), *Kyklos*, XXV 265.

——, Lavers, R. J., and Williams, A. (1972), 'Health Indicators', in A. Shonfield and S. Shaw, *Social Indicators and Social Policy* (London: Heinemann, for Social Science Research Council); also published in *Social Trends*, II (1971) 31.

—— and Maynard, A. K. (1970), *Med.Care*, VIII 501.

Daniels, M., and Hill, A. B. (1952), *Br. Med. J.*, I 1162.

Deniston, O. L., and Rosenstock, I. M. (1970), *Publ. Hlth. Reports*, LXXXV 835.

Department of Health and Social Security (1970), *The Future Structure of the National Health Service* (London: H.M.S.O.).

—— (1971), *National Health Service Reorganisation*, Departmental Consultative Document (May 1971).

—— (1972), *National Health Service Reorganisation: England* (London, H.M.S.O.).

Fanshel, S., and Bush, J. W. (1970), *Operations Research*, VIII 1021.

Farquharson, E. L. (1955), *Lancet*, II 517.

Feldstein, M. S. (1967), *Economic Analysis for Health Service Efficiency: Econometric Studies of the British Health Service* (Amsterdam: North-Holland).

Forsyth, G. (1966), *Doctors and State Medicine: A Study of the British Health Service* (London: Pitman Medical Publishing Co.).

Hadfield, S. J. (1953), *Br.Med.J.*, II 683.

Heasman, M. A., and Carstairs, V. (1971), *Br. Med. J.*, I 495.

Ingbar, M. L. (1964), 'Economic Analysis as a Tool of Program Evaluation: Costs in a Home Care Program', in Bureau of Public Health Economics and Department of Economics, Univ. of Michigan, *The Economics of Health and Medical Care* (Ann Arbor: Univ. of Michigan Press).

Institute of Economic Affairs (1965), *Choice in Welfare* (London: Institute of Economic Affairs).

Jewkes, J., and Jewkes, S. (1963), *Value for Money in Medicine* (Oxford: Blackwell).

Johansen, L. (1971), *Public Economics* (Amsterdam: North-Holland).

Kaser, M. C. (1960), *International Social Science Journal*, XII 409.

Knatterud, G. L., *et al.* (1971), *J. Am. Med. Ass.*, CCXVII, 6, 777.

Lees, D. S. (1961), *Health through Choice* (London: Institute of Economic Affairs).

Lindsey, A. (1964), 'The British National Health Service: Its Organization and Financing', in Bureau of Public Health Economics and Department of Economics, Univ. of Michigan, *The Economics of Health and Medical Care* (Ann Arbor: Univ. of Michigan Press).

Lipworth, L., *et al.* (1963), *Med. Care*, I 71.

Logan, R. F. L., *et al.* (1971), *Br. Med. J.*, II 519.

Long, J., and Norton, A. (1972), *Setting up the New Authorities* (London: Knight.)

McKeown, T. (1968), 'Validation of Screening Procedures', in Nuffield Provincial Hospitals Trust, *Screening in Medical Care* (London: Oxford Univ. Press, for Nuffield Provincial Hospitals Trust).

McNerney, W. J. (1971), 'Financing and Delivery of Health Services in Britain', in G. McLachlan, *Problems and Progress in Medical Care* (London: Oxford Univ. Press, for Nuffield Provincial Hospitals Trust).

Mather, H. C., *et al.* (1971), *Br. Med. J.*, III 334.

Morris, D., Ward, A., and Hendyside, A. J. (1968), *Lancet*, 681.

Nuffield Provincial Hospitals Trust (1971), *Portfolio for Health: The Role and Programme of the D.H.S.S. in Health Services Research* (London: Oxford Univ. Press, for Nuffield Provincial Hospitals Trust).

Office of Health Economics (1971), *Off Sick* (London: Office of Health Economics).

—— (1972), *Medicine and Society* (London: Office of Health Economics).

Oldham, P. D. (1968), *Measurement in Medicine* (London: English Universities Press).

Partridge, J. F., and Geddes, J. S. (1967), *Lancet*, II 271.

Plessas, D. J., and Fein, R. (1972), *Amer. Inst. of Planners J.* (Jan) 43–51.

Pole, J. D. (1968), 'Economic Aspects of Screening for Disease', in Nuffield Provincial Hospitals Trust, *Screening in Medical Care* (London: Oxford Univ. Press, for Nuffield Provincial Hospitals Trust).

—— (1971), 'Mass Radiography: A Cost–Benefit Approach' in G. McLachlan, *Problems and Progress in Medical Care* (London: Oxford Univ. Press, for Nuffield Provincial Hospitals Trust).

Quinton, A. M. (1968), 'Contemporary British Philosophy', in G. Pitcher, *Wittgenstein: The Philosophical Investigations*, LXX (London: Macmillan).

Revans, R. W. (1960), *Hosp. and Soc. Service J.*, LXX 1293.

Roemer, M. I. (1971), *H.S.M.H.A. Hlth.Reports*, LXXXVI 839.

Taylor, S. (1954), *Good General Practice* (London: Oxford Univ. Press).

Universities Group Diabetes Program (1970), *Diabetes*, XIX, suppl. 2.

Webb, E. F. (1962), 'The Impact of BUPA and Similar Schemes on the Market for Medical Care', in D. Mirfin, *Buying Better Health* (London: Acton Society Trust).

Wittgenstein, L. (1953), *Philosophical Investigations*, trans. G. E. M. Anscombe (Oxford: Blackwell).

World Health Organization (1971), *Statistical Indicators for the Planning and Evaluation of Public Health Programmes*, *W.H.O. Tech. Rep. Ser.*, 472.

World Health Organization Regional Office for Europe (1967), *Methods of Evaluating Public Health Programmes* (EURO 0375).

—— (1971), *Planning and Evaluating Dental Health Services* (EURO 5505).

Young, J. Z. (1971), *An Introduction to the Study of Man* (Oxford: Clarendon Press).

Summary Record of Discussion

Two papers were reserved for this final session. The respective authors were M. Dupuy, on the rationale of health policy in general, and Mr Kaser, on the choice of techniques in medical practice.

A. *M. Dupuy's paper*
Mme Sandier undertook the introduction and formal discussion of the Dupuy paper. M. Dupuy believes that 'technical 'indicators represent obvious but incomplete targets for health services. The measurement of the quality and quantity of medical care output should also involve 'quality of life' variables, which would drastically change our collection of indicators. Indeed, medical decisions are sometimes made on this basis already. (When a decision to seek medical care is made by the potential patient himself, we may speak of decision on the basis of the health of the *first* person. When it is made by a physician in the interests of his patient, it is on the basis of the health of a *second* person. But if, as in an increasing number of cases involving preventive measures particularly, it is made by public agencies for the benefit of the community at large, the decision is made on the basis of the health of *third* persons.) M. Dupuy is concerned that considering only such 'technical' variables as mortality and life expectancy might result in decisions lowering the general quality of life, although conflicts may be minimized with improved information. M. Dupuy feels that what he calls 'technical' indicators should be used for evaluating only the technical results of medical care, but that non-technical indicators should be used to evaluate the 'general' results.

Mme Sandier expressed considerable skepticism about the Dupuy proposals, as she understood them. She felt that the distinction between the technical and the non-technical or general results of health care was difficult to draw, especially where mental illnesses are concerned, and varies also by culture and social class. She did, however, recognize the existence of considerable agreement in some advanced societies.

In her view, furthermore, the non-technical effects of medical care were not so important in practice, or so different from the technical ones, as M. Dupuy had presumed. They were also difficult to measure, and over-stressing them might not be optimal resource use, when so much is left to be done on the technical side. Some of these had best be left to other professions while medicine and medical economics concentrated on what M. Dupuy calls the technical aspects of health.

French studies of medical care and health economics indicate that present procedures are very different from those of even twenty years ago, and that this change is the main reason for the growth of medical expenses. It continues to be true that perhaps one-fourth of the population consumes no medical care at all in any given year, while perhaps one-tenth of the population consumes one-half of the total expenditures. There may be some real waste reflected in these figures, but Mme Sandier pointed particularly to advances in the care of premature births and coronary ailments as examples of the causes for increased cost. She also argued that needs for medical care increase over time. Living standards rise, so that, for example, a victim of tooth decay expects a set of false teeth rather than a life of toothlessness. There is also diminished self-production of health care; purchase from specialists (doctors) has replaced home-made remedies. And at the same time, the rise of other commitments and fixed costs has made many people, paradoxically, less

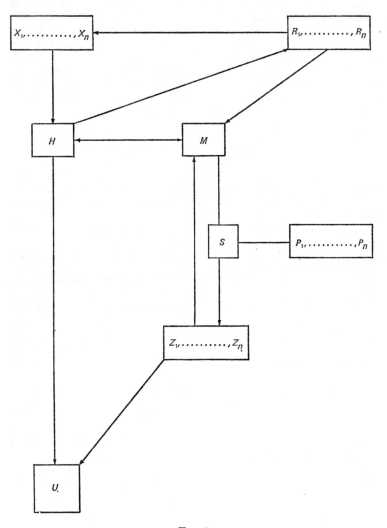

FIG. 1

able to bear the costs of illness. Mme Sandier closed by admitting that some of the resulting expenditures may not be well applied, and pointed to provision of frills and the duplication of facilities in hospital construction.

In reply, *M. Dupuy* feared that Mme Sandier had misunderstood the point of his paper to some extent, and illustrated his argument with a diagram designed with Professor Fuchs's help and reproduced as Fig. 1. In this flow diagram, let H be health, M medical care and U the economist's notion of utility. In addition, let $Z_1 \ldots, Z_n$ represent a group of services ancillary to medical care, including the quality of the patient's life, his feeling of security, and the quality of the doctor–patient relationship. M produces at the same time H and $Z_1 \ldots, Z_n$,so that no separation is possible. However, M can be partially substituted in producing $Z_1 \ldots, Z_n$ by $P_1, \ldots, P_n$, which are a collection of other goods and services (non-medical inputs). Furthermore, the $M{\to}H$ connection is what M. Dupuy has in mind while speaking of technical effects, while the $M{\to}Z$ connection (filtered through S, the social code) is what he means by non-technical effects.

Professor Fuchs added on this diagram $R_1, \ldots, R_n$, the resources in the whole economy, and $X_1, \ldots, X_n$ which are a set of non-medical inputs producing H (environmental variables, way of life . . .). He stressed the fact that most economists concentrate on $R{\to}M{\to}H{\to}R$ connections (human capital approach) and too often neglect the $X{\to}H$ connection (in which he is personally interested) and symmetrically the $M{\to}Z$ connection (in which M. Duputy is interesed).

Professor Lévy thought he sensed a certain contradiction between M. Dupuy's technical and non-technical effects, even if they are related. The non-technical effects may be carried out using the services of less highly trained personnel, such as social workers. Furthermore, where could one stop (beyond taking over a great part of all social work) once one began taking account of the non-technical effects of illness and medical officers? Certainly, it would be wasteful to entrust medical officers with social-worker functions, as well as vice versa. In conclusion, Professor Lévy felt that insofar as non-technical effects are complementary with the technical ones, they need no special consideration, while insofar as they are competitive, they should be obtained by non-medical expenditures.

M. Foulon opened his interpellation by recalling the Trumbo novel, *Johnny Got His Gun*. Should the quadriplegic anti-hero of that novel have been kept alive, when he wanted to die? This case exemplified M. Dupuy's conflict, as he himself saw it, and similar problems come up quite often in psychiatric practice, when the quality of a patient's life is so bad that euthanasia may be preferable. Professor Dupuy is probably right to distinguish two sorts of medical outputs, but the two are more closely related than he perhaps realizes. The non-technical effects are more variable and less well defined, especially because psychological factors and social integration issues are so intimately involved. His own suggestion (for Fig. 2, for example) would make the non-technical output of medical care dependent upon the technical, but add a third socio-psychological output unrelated to either of the others.

As an example of M. Dupuy's over-emphasis on the non-technical side, M. Foulon believes that pharmacological outputs of the health care system are treated here. This is not, in fact, the case, except for the psychedelics, depressants and other psychologically related drugs, whereas the conventional or 'regular' drugs are much more important.

Professor Evans, on the other hand, viewed the tie between the technical and non-technical aspects of medical care as highly intimate, and denied the feasibility of dividing them as sharply as M. Dupuy's critics were suggesting. On the other hand, he wondered whether the discussion was not simply reinventing old effects and giving them new names.

At this point, *M. Dupuy* himself re-entered the discussion. He felt that he had been better understood by Professor Evans than by any of his fellow-countrymen who had criticized his paper. The main point of his present interpolation, however, would be expository. In particular, he proposed to distinguish between the descriptive and normative aspects of his position.

The key point, he thought, was the rationality of considering the non-technical aspects of health care. Economists were using special assumptions stressing the technical side, striving for optimality on these limited bases, and criticizing the actual situation as non-optimal. Such criticisms, he thought, revealed a common habit among economists, which is to call 'non-optimal' or 'irrational' what in fact they have not succeeded in explaining.

In astronomy, continued M. Dupuy, we modify or even abandon our theorems when they do not fit the facts. We recognize that rationality does not exist in Nature, but only in the minds of observers. In medical economics, however, we compare the marginal utility obtained from equal health expenditures on different sectors. Their equality may, of course, be a criterion of rationality, but their inequality in practice may mean only that one is using the wrong indicators and too few dimensions. Health actions and expenditures are not, in fact, adequately explained by reference only to mortality, morbidity and the physical comfort of the ill. These dimensions alone cannot explain what goes on. If we allocate so far as to maximize or rationalize, for example on the basis of Professor William's proposal, this would involve treating human beings like industrial equipment, where we deliberately permit equipment to depreciate at optimal rates. This proposal suggests (to M. Dupuy) killing people who are too old or useless, and does not fit people, except, perhaps, in concentration camps. What he (M. Dupuy) would like to do is to explain the rationality of decisions actually made on the basis of non-technical as well as technical values. This is especially important in the case of terminal patients. Of course, agreed M. Dupuy, the expenditures made for their benefit are economically wasteful, but they are important from the viewpoint of the dying, of their families and of their physicians. (This is the sort of decision he is talking about.)

His critics, M. Dupuy went on, had tried to divide health actions into two sorts, a technical and a non-technical sort. The first involved medical people, the second not. This division is nonsense. Actually, all health actions have both sorts of effects, and ostensibly technical actions (in particular) have important non-technical effects. The great part of actual expenses is for the benefit of the really ill, and it is a great mistake to think of 'non-technical effects' as directed mainly at persons not really ill who need something other than medical care.

Mme Sandier felt that the important distinction between the technical and the non-technical aspects of health care was one of motivation rather than of oractical effect, while *M. Foulon* repeated his earlier view that the non-technical effects were imprecise and of relative unimportance. *Professor Williams* also entered this final discussion, claiming that he had been attacked personally. His own indicators, he felt, include psychological effects; his specialty is geriatrics; he does not favor, and never has favored, treating people like animals or industrial equipment. Nevertheless, people are, in fact, allowed to die when they might have been kept alive a little longer, and some form of analogy does hold between human and non-human capital.

B. *Mr Kaser's paper*

In introducing this paper, *Professor Imai* interpreted it as basically a survey of previous studies of a number of topics taken up at the present Conference. As such, it was difficult to criticize as a whole. He proposed to concentrate upon two points.

Though Mr Kaser's paper is entitled 'Choice of Technique', the problem of choice which he discusses is not the capacity of medical care supply, but only the allocation of variable inputs under given capacity. That is to say, his main theme is how the place and time for medical care are chosen when the supply capacity, as represented by hospitals, medical equipment, doctors, etc., is given – in other words, the problem of efficient use of the capacity of medical care supply. Professor Imai, however, feels that the problem of efficient use cannot be considered unless the determination of the supply capacity – including the choice between capital- or labor-intensive techniques – is clearly defined. Mr Kaser says that 'the aggregate resources of health are determined by a political process'. This may be true, but the political determination must be a reflection of the actual constraints on the availability of resources. For example, when the supply of funds for the construction of hospitals is sufficient, any increase in the supply of doctors is also difficult because of institutional constraints. The question, whether or not the use of the capacity determined under such a constraint is efficient, must be considered in the light of the shadow cost of the constraint itself. If the limited availability of hospital beds is the greatest bottleneck, for example, a method of medical care by which to minimize the stay of patients should be evaluated highly from the standpoint of efficiency.

Generally speaking, Professor Imai feels that the efficiency of medical care should be evaluated in the light of a set of existing constraints on the capacity to supply it. The problem covered by Mr Kaser should be considered with the basic factors determining the supply capacity clearly defined. It may be misleading to evaluate the efficiency of medical care by *ad hoc* criteria like the place of treatment and the optimum time.

Professor Imai was also concerned with incentive schemes for improving the efficiency of medical care. Evaluation of medical treatment from the viewpoint of efficiency aims to improve the medical supply system by means of some such policy measures.

But to make such an evaluation effective and meaningful, it is necessary, according to Professor Imai, to clarify how the efficiency of the supply of medical care would be affected if changes were made only on the basis of private incentives, without reference to possible policy changes.

An example of private incentives is a profit incentive for the doctor, such as operates in Japan. In England, medical care is publicly provided with almost no profit incentive given to the doctors, but public provision does not necessarily mean public production. Therefore, Professor Imai hopes for greater use of private incentive. For instance, it is quite natural that a general practitioner should try to make a reputation by increasing the number of the persons who register for his care. Moreover, when medical drugs are supplied by a profit system, it is natural that they should be used to an excessive degree, as has been pointed out by Professor Liefmann-Keil.

But as far as Mr Kaser's paper is concerned, Professor Imai felt that little consideration is given to the relationship of private incentives, especially under the condition of public provision, with the efficiency of medical care.

Mr Cooper opened the discussion from the floor by claiming that the paper had misunderstood certain aspects of his own earlier work. Specifically, he had been cited as having criticized the British National Health Service for allowing too much freedom of drug price movements. His argument had actually been for other controls (than drug prices) upon physicians' freedom to prescribe, i.e. that the N.H.S. had been too cautious in placing limitations upon this freedom.

Dr Kehrer believed that, under American conditions, a similar paper would have had to deal specifically with the problems raised by malpractice suits and malpractice insurance. An American physician may be faced with premiums of $10,000 per year, and also with the possibility of becoming uninsurable. The threats of rising premiums and of lawsuits prevent American physicians from experimenting both with new techniques and with the delegation of routine duties to paramedical personnel. Perhaps equally important, they force an overuse of routine testing, so that data can be readily available to support their decisions if they are ever called into question in court.

Professor Liefmann-Keil expressed the opinion that most commentators on the choice of techniques – Professor Imai being an exception here – underestimate both the importance of the individual physician's role and the constraints under which the individual physician operates. Doctors do have political constraints and special regulations upon their behavior. They have neither complete freedom nor perfect knowledge. Moreover, they are egoists as well as agents of the public in general or of their individual patients. Professor Liefmann-Keil felt that the medical care sector of the representative economy was less different from other sectors, producing other goods and services, than most speakers had been willing to admit. One must distinguish between the situation the doctors themselves desire, namely, special treatment of the health care sector, from the actual situation, in which health care is subject to the same resource limitations as any other economic sector.

Dr Christiansen commented upon the case that Mr Kaser had made for randomized control trials of such new techniques as special coronary-care units, attempted in certain British cities (Belfast, Oxford). He felt that the paper had underestimated the importance of statistical problems in testing the results of such trials, and in applying these results outside the countries in which the trials had been made. For example, he felt that British results might not be meaningful in Denmark, because the constraint on hospital beds is less severe there than in Britain. Another disturbing factor, for many conditions, is the length of time that patients can be kept under supervision. He suspected that in Britain, again because of the shortage of hospital beds, patients are sent home earlier than best practice would suggest in some other countries. In general, he thought that United Kingdom results were not applicable elsewhere without adjustment for the consequences of the British shortage of hospital beds.

Mr Culyer, like Mr Cooper, felt that his own views had been misinterpreted, or at least, presented too elliptically. He and his colleagues, he explained, favor direct quantitative measurement of health outputs. Furthermore, they favor state-of-health indicators to specific or arbitrary health targets. They accept such targets only where they imply, and are based upon, prior sets of state-of-health indicators.

Mr Kaser, in an interim reply to his critics, said that his paper was intended primarily to expose the need to link medical economics more closely with medical technology, and also the need for a health-outcome objective function to be maximized, despite the problems raised by the differences between self-perception and other-perception of the medical states of individual patients.

It was also important, Mr Kaser's view, to consider the process of technological innovation in medicine explicitly. He disagreed with Professor Fuchs's remarks at earlier sessions on the need to apply a 'technological imperative' to physicians to use new techniques; Professor Fuchs in his earlier paper, had ascribed to technical progress a substantial share of the aggregate improvement of levels of health. Professor Imai had interpreted his own paper correctly as taking the choice of techniques as in fact given at any particular time. In the case of the British N.H.S., he (Mr Kaser) saw the cumulative results of efficiency improvements as filtering to the 'monitors' of the system and governing the particular additions to capacity which these monitors would approve, but admitted that this point was not clear in the paper itself.

[1] V. R. Fuchs, 'The Contribution of Health Services to the American Economy', *Milbank Memorial Fund Quarterly*, part II (Oct 1966).

On the subject of the clinical freedom of physicians (regarding which Professor Atkinson and Mr Cooper had disagreed), his paper was concerned with the results of this freedom. By and large, the medical profession was extremely cautious on the techniques of economic analysis and the applicability of the results of such techniques to its own bailiwick. His paper represented, said Mr Kaser, an attempt to provide incentives to minimize costs acceptable to the profession and which would promote the behavior economists would regard as desirable.

Since his own work had been mentioned, *Professor Fuchs* asserted, he agreed that he had looked more favorably upon a technical change in medicine during what he called the 'antibiotic period' between 1930 and 1960, but that he did not now believe that the same could be said for it either earlier or later. Some innovations are decidedly deleterious to the level of health care. Bleeding was one such in the past; organ transplants may now be another.

Professor Williams rose to discuss measurability, with special reference to pain. Pain has been investigated in this regard, and its physiological and biochemical correlates are undoubtedly measurable. It is often judged and compared in practice; surgeons and dentists commonly compare different procedures on precisely this basis. Also, the doctors and the courts seem to have achieved a high degree of agreement among themselves.

Professor Liefmann-Keil suggested that the group consider what economists call induced, as well as autonomous, technical change. Both physicians and drug companies can influence the direction of change when it becomes obvious what they are looking for and/or what they are willing to finance economically.

Professor L. Lave entered the discussion with further evidence on the points raised by Professors Fuchs and Williams. With regard to the measurability of pain, psychiatrists at the University of Washington have been comparing, quantitatively, the degrees of pain associated with various conditions. They have achieved a good degree of replication of results from one experimenter to another and it is safe to say that pain is at least ordinally (if not cardinally) measurable.

Passing to Professor Fuchs's comparison between the 1930–60 generation of technological progress and the period since 1960, Professor L. Lave asserted that, generally, the new drugs (not merely the antibiotics) were able, in that period, to provide, simultaneously, higher life expectancy and symptomatic relief in a surprisingly large proportion of cases. Since 1960 the two desiderata seem to be in conflict more frequently, via the side-effect phenomenon. There seems to be a trade-off between life expectancy and symptomatic relief in an increasing proportion of cases. How this trade-off should be settled he could not, as an economist, venture to decide, but it seemed to him that the relevance of higher life expectancy was no longer quite so great as it had formerly been.

Mr Cooper wished to endorse Professor Liefmann-Keil's views, both on doctors being 'only human' and on the drug industry's ability to dominate the direction of technical progress by its own market orientation. He went on to discuss the problem of clinical freedom. He would grant, he said, that it operates only within the bounds of reason, but in the longer run it also can affect political decisions as well as the directions of medical innovation. His criticism of the N.H.S. has been, and remains, that it is too uncritical in accepting the notion that clinical freedom assists patients under any and all circumstances. After all, it includes the freedom to be (1) eccentric and (2) wrong.

Whereas the 'wicked' United States system encourages doctors, in Mr Cooper's opinion, to do entirely too much surgery, the N.H.S. encourages them to shift responsibility and so maximize leisure by using too many psychotropic drugs, and also by referring patients too frequently back and forth between specialists and general practitioners. The incentive system is important – just as important in a non-market as in a market economy – and should be studied, as per his own paper.

Mr Pole objected that two-thirds of N.H.S. expenditures is on hospital care, and that such expenditures are increasing only slowly. Also, as to the referral pattern, Mr Pole said that 95 per cent of all cases are treated by general practitioners, but *Mr Cooper* was concerned about the high degree of variability in this proportion. *Dr Phelps* added that 'treating patients as ping-pong balls' by numerous referrals is also a feature of United States prepaid practice plans, causing members to go outside the prepaid plans for difficult surgical procedures.

Professor Rosett, while unable really to argue with Professors Williams and L. Lave, expressed a certain skepticism about the measurability of pain. In any case, he did not want measures of pain used as part of mechanisms to limit clinical freedom. Along the same lines, *Professor Fuchs* wondered whether measurements of pain had allowed adequately for individual differences in the ability to endure it. *Mr Culyer* believed that the main use of the Williams measures of pain should be in connection with macro-decisions about the direction of innovation, not in the day-to-day practices (micro-decisions) of individual physicians.

An additional point relative to Mr Cooper's remarks on British doctors' 'leisure maximization' was then made by *Dr Christiansen* with special reference to older practitioners. These men know that hospital physicians are more nearly up to date than they themselves, and so put patients in hospitals rather than attempting to close the gap between their own knowledge and the best contemporary practice.

The discussion was closed by the author of each paper making a final statement of his position. *M. Dupuy* wished to elaborate on his insistence on the difference between the technical and non-technical aspects of health care. He believed that most conventional economists maintain that people are concerned only with the physical and physiological effects of their states of health, but he knew this is not true, particularly among the poor. To them, social integration and security are also important, both in general and with regard to health care. He also added (referring to his diagram, reproduced above as Fig. 2) that non-technical effects of a given sort of health care vary with the country, culture and social class, while the technical effects generally do not.

Mr Kaser feared that he had indeed misread Mr Cooper's paper. He also accepted Dr Christiansen's last interpellation, and found Mr Culyer's distinction (between macro- and micro-decisions and measures) useful. He would leave quantifying the sensation of pain to the experts among whom it was currently being debated, but would add that the statement in his paper had been based on opinion in the Medical Faculty at Oxford University.

Mr Kaser went on to say that the N.H.S. was scheduled for an important reorganization in 1974, and might then be more receptive to micro- rather than macro-indicators. The government's proposals laid particular stress on better evaluation procedures on the medical side and management methods on the support side. This was inevitably a compromise, but it was premature to expect an early application of macro-guidance.

Mr Cooper had described the N.H.S. as geared to (though not achieving) a 'medical ideal', and Mr Kaser was concerned lest, through misunderstanding, physicians might reject the criteria proposed by social scientists (economists and statisticians particularly). This situation was not, however, peculiar to the British health care system. Czechoslovakia, for example, set up its present health service at the same time as the N.H.S. (1948), but under a government dominated by the Communist Party, and had to determine whether its administrative echelons should be staffed by physicians, or by personnel from the pre-existing health insurance system, who were, presumptively, more cost-oriented. The choice was consciously made in favor of the physicians, perhaps to counteract the overly economic pressures that centralized planning might be held to impose.

Index

Entries in **bold type** under the names of participants in the conference indicate their papers or discussions of their papers. Entries in *italic* indicate contributions by participants in the dicussions.